D1526999

AMERICAN PSYCHIATRIC PRESS

REVIEW OF PSYCHIATRY

VOLUME
8

EDITED BY ALLAN TASMAN, MD,
ROBERT E. HALES, MD, and
ALLEN J. FRANCES, MD

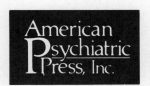
American Psychiatric Press, Inc.

1400 K Street, N.W.
Washington, DC
1989

Manufactured in the United States of America.

Typeset by VIP Systems, Alexandria, VA
Manufactured by Arcata Graphics, Fairfield, PA

Review of Psychiatry: Volume 8
ISSN 1041-5882
ISBN 0-88048-247-8

To Cathy, Joshua, David, and Sarah with love and thanks for your patience while I did my homework.

A.T.

To Dianne, who keeps me up-to-date and Julia, who wakes me up each day. With love,

R.E.H.

To Mel Sabshin, a man for all seasons and a great inspiration.

A.J.F.

PSYCHIATRY UPDATE: THE AMERICAN PSYCHIATRIC ASSOCIATION ANNUAL REVIEW, VOLUME 4 (1985)

Robert E. Hales, M.D., and Allen J. Frances, M.D., Editors

An Introduction to the World of Neurotransmitters and Neuroreceptors
Joseph T. Coyle, M.D., Section Editor

Neuropsychiatry
Stuart C. Yudofsky, M.D., Section Editor

Sleep Disorders
David J. Kupfer, M.D., Section Editor

Eating Disorders
Joel Yager, M.D., Section Editor

The Therapeutic Alliance and Treatment Outcome
John P. Docherty, M.D., Section Editor

PSYCHIATRY UPDATE: THE AMERICAN PSYCHIATRIC ASSOCIATION ANNUAL REVIEW, VOLUME 5 (1986)

Allen J. Frances, M.D., and Robert E. Hales, M.D., Editors

Schizophrenia
Nancy C. Andreasen, M.D., Ph.D., Section Editor

Drug Abuse and Drug Dependence
Robert B. Millman, M.D., Section Editor

Personality Disorders
Robert M.A. Hirschfeld, M.D., Section Editor

Adolescent Psychiatry
Carolyn B. Robinowitz, M.D., and Jeanne Spurlock, M.D., Section Editors

Psychiatric Contributions to Medical Care
David Spiegel, M.D., and W. Stewart Agras, M.D., Section Editors

Group Psychotherapy
Irvin D. Yalom, M.D., Section Editor

PSYCHIATRY UPDATE: THE AMERICAN PSYCHIATRIC ASSOCIATION ANNUAL REVIEW, VOLUME 6 (1987)

Robert E. Hales, M.D., and Allen J. Frances, M.D., Editors

Bipolar Disorders
Frederick K. Goodwin, M.D., and Kay Redfield Jamison, Ph.D., Section Editors

Neuroscience Techniques in Clinical Psychiatry
John M. Morihisa, M.D., and Solomon H. Snyder, M.D., Section Editors

Differential Therapeutics
John F. Clarkin, Ph.D., and Samuel W. Perry, M.D., Section Editors

Violence and the Violent Patient
Kenneth Tardiff, M.D., M.P.H., Section Editor

Psychiatric Epidemiology
Myrna M. Weissman, Ph.D., Section Editor

Psychopharmacology: Drug Side Effects and Interactions
Philip Berger, M.D., and Leo Hollister, M.D., Section Editors

AMERICAN PSYCHIATRIC PRESS REVIEW OF PSYCHIATRY, VOLUME 7 (1988)

Allen J. Frances, M.D., and Robert E. Hales, M.D., Editors

Panic Disorder
David H. Barlow, Ph.D., and M. Katherine Shear, M.D., Section Editors

Unipolar Depression
Martin B. Keller, M.D., Section Editor

Suicide
J. John Mann, M.D., and Michael Stanley, Ph.D., Section Editors

Electroconvulsive Therapy
Robert M. Rose, M.D., and Harold Alan Pincus, M.D., Section Editors

Cognitive Therapy
A. John Rush, M.D., and Aaron T. Beck, M.D., Section Editors

AMERICAN PSYCHIATRIC PRESS REVIEW OF PSYCHIATRY, VOLUME 9 (1990)

Allan Tasman, M.D., Stephen M. Goldfinger, M.D., and Charles A. Kaufmann, M.D., Editors

Treatment of Refractory Affective Disorders
Robert M. Post, M.D., Section Editor

AIDS
Stephen M. Goldfinger, M.D., and Carolyn B. Robinowitz, M.D., Section Editors

Geriatric Psychiatry
Charles A. Shamoian, M.D., Ph.D., Section Editor

Psychiatric Consultation to Special Populations
Robert E. Hales, M.D., and Troy L. Thompson II, M.D., Section Editors

Contributions of Self Psychology to Psychotherapy
Jerald Kay, M.D., Section Editor

Contents

Section

IV

Psychiatry and the Law

Foreword to Volume 8

by Allan Tasman, M.D., Robert E. Hales, M.D., and
Allen J. Frances, M.D.

Volume 8 of the *Review of Psychiatry* marks the third transition in the editorial leadership for this series as well as personal transitions for each of us. Allan Tasman has assumed the duties of Editor as well as the Chair of the Scientific Program Committee of the American Psychiatric Association. Robert Hales has concluded his very successful tenure as Chair of the Scientific Program Committee of the APA and as an Editor in this series, and he has begun work as a member of the APA Task Force on DSM-IV and as Deputy Editor of the new *Journal of Neuropsychiatry and Clinical Neurosciences*. Allen Frances also leaves his position as an Editor in this series to assume the Co-editorship this year, and he has taken on the important task of Chairing the APA's Task Force on DSM-IV. The volumes of this series edited by Allen and Bob have set a high standard, and they are owed a strong debt of thanks from those of us who have enjoyed and learned from them. Although this is a year of transition, we think you will find that the standards of excellence for the *Review of Psychiatry* are upheld in the present volume.

It is never easy choosing five topic areas for each volume of the *Review of Psychiatry*. As we discussed the various options for Volume 8, the overriding concern was to continue to make the *Review of Psychiatry* an outstanding reference for the practicing clinician. The success of previous volumes has demonstrated the important role that knowledge of the advances that have occurred in our field plays in providing the highest quality care to our patients. As you read through Volume 8, those of you who have been regular readers of each *Review* will see that certain topic areas have appeared in previous volumes. This is a testament to the success and longevity of the series, and the explosion of new knowledge which requires a more up-to-date review.

The Section on Borderline Personality Disorder, edited by John G. Gunderson, M.D., illustrates the major advances that have been made since the previous section was published in 1982 in the understanding of the heterogeneity of the disorder, the refinement of clinical diagnosis, and the variety of treatment approaches now available. Likewise, readers will find equally dramatic breakthroughs in our understanding of the epidemiology, pathogenesis, and treatment of alcoholism reviewed in the section edited by Roger E. Meyer, M.D. The section on Child Psychiatry, edited by Jerry M. Wiener, M.D., will provide the general practitioner with an up-to-date review of the diagnosis, course of illness, and treatment alternatives for a number of the most commonly encountered and important psychiatric disorders in children.

The interface between psychiatry and the legal system has changed dramatically since the last section on Psychiatry and the Law was published in 1982. This section, edited by Paul S. Appelbaum, M.D., not only provides a scholarly review of major legal issues relating to psychiatric practice, but also discusses the relevance of the law to daily clinical activities. We believe you will find the section on Difficult Situations in Clinical Practice, edited by William H. Sledge,

M.D., to be of special interest. This section provides an in-depth and practical discussion of various factors which complicate our clinical practice.

A book of this scope would not be possible without the help of many people. We would like to acknowledge the work of our Section Editors, Drs. Gunderson, Wiener, Meyer, Appelbaum, and Sledge. They have each brought a scholarly approach to their work and have provided valuable guidance and support to their chapter authors. Each of the chapter authors has shown a remarkable capacity to bring together information from a variety of research areas, and to present it in a clinically relevant way. The publication schedule for this volume is extremely tight, and it has been a pleasure to deal with such a conscientious group of Section Editors and authors who needed little extra motivation from us to complete their tasks.

The valuable editorial assistance provided by Sharon DellaVecchia and Mickey Hunt made the task possible, and brought a high level of organization to the correspondence and many details required to publish the book. We want to thank all of the individuals at the American Psychiatric Press involved with Volume 8, especially Ronald E. McMillen, Timothy R. Clancy, Richard E. Farkas, and Karen Loper. Particular thanks go to our Project Editor at APPI, Eve Shapiro, who has worked on the *Review* for the past five years. Professional growth has taken her to greater responsibilities in another organization, but we are especially grateful for the detailed editing she provided for this volume. Her contributions have been invaluable. The final coherence and readability of the volume are in great measure a reflection of her work. We would also like to thank our Department Chairmen for their guidance and support. Most importantly we are appreciative of our wives, Cathy Tasman, Dianne Hales, and Vera Frances, who endured with good humor and perseverance the time away from family activities that work on this volume entailed.

We hope that you find Volume 8 as rewarding to read as we have found it to prepare.

Contributors

Gerald Adler, M.D.
Director of Medical Student Education in Psychiatry, Massachusetts General Hospital, Boston, Massachusetts

Victor A. Altshul, M.D.
Associate Clinical Professor of Psychiatry, Yale University School of Medicine, New Haven, Connecticut

Paul S. Appelbaum, M.D.
A.F. Zeleznik Professor of Psychiatry; Director, Law and Psychiatry Program, University of Massachusetts Medical Center, Worcester, Massachusetts

Thomas F. Babor, Ph.D.
Professor of Psychiatry, University of Connecticut Health Center, Department of Psychiatry, Farmington, Connecticut

George W. Bailey, M.D.
Assistant Professor, Department of Psychiatry, George Washington University Medical School; Director of Inpatient Psychiatry, Children's Hospital National Medical Center, Washington, D.C.

Floyd E. Bloom, M.D.
Head, Division of Preclinical Neuroscience and Endocrinology, Department of Basic and Clinical Research, Research Institute of Scripps Clinic, La Jolla, California

Ian A. Canino, M.D.
Associate Clinical Professor, Columbia University College of Physicians and Surgeons, Division of Child Psychiatry, New York, New York

Dennis P. Cantwell, M.D.
Joseph Campbell Professor of Child Psychiatry; Director of Residency Training in Child Psychiatry, UCLA Neuropsychiatric Institute, Los Angeles, California

Sara C. Charles, M.D.
Professor of Clinical Psychiatry, University of Illinois College of Medicine at Chicago, Chicago, Illinois

C. Robert Cloninger, M.D.
Professor of Psychiatry and Genetics, Washington University Medical School, the Jewish Hospital of St. Louis, St. Louis, Missouri

Stephen H. Dinwiddie, M.D.
Instructor, Department of Psychiatry, Washington University, St. Louis, Missouri

James H. Egan, M.D.
Professor of Psychiatry, George Washington University Medical School; Professor and Chairman, Department of Psychiatry, Children's Hospital National Medical Center, Washington, D.C.

W. Lawrence Fitch, J.D.
Associate Professor and Director of Forensic Evaluation Training and Research, Institute of Law, Psychiatry and Public Policy, University of Virginia, Charlottesville, Virginia

Allen J. Frances, M.D.
Professor, Cornell University Medical College, Department of Psychiatry, New York, New York

Richard J. Frances, M.D.
Professor of Clinical Psychiatry; Vice-Chairman, Department of Psychiatry, University of Medicine and Dentistry of New Jersey, Newark, New Jersey

Marc Galanter, M.D.
Professor of Psychiatry, Director, Division of Alcoholism and Drug Abuse, New York University Medical School, New York, New York

Jeffrey L. Geller, M.D., M.P.H.
Associate Professor, University of Massachusetts Medical Center, Department of Psychiatry, Worcester, Massachusetts

John G. Gunderson, M.D.
Director of Psychotherapy and Psychosocial Research, McLean Hospital, Belmont, Massachusetts; Associate Professor of Psychiatry, Harvard Medical School, Boston, Massachusetts

Robert E. Hales, M.D.
Chief, Department of Clinical Investigation, Letterman Army
Medical Center, Presidio of San Francisco, California; and
Clinical Professor of Psychiatry, Georgetown University School
of Medicine, Washington, D.C.

Seymour L. Halleck, M.D.
Professor, Department of Psychiatry, University of North
Carolina School of Medicine, Chapel Hill, North Carolina

Gregory L. Hanna, M.D.
Assistant Professor in Residence, UCLA Neuropsychiatric
Institute, Los Angeles, California

Dianna E. Hartley, Ph.D.
Assistant Professor in Residence, Langley Porter Institute,
University of California-San Francisco, San Francisco, California

Steven K. Hoge, M.D.
Assistant Professor, University of Massachusetts Medical
Center, Department of Psychiatry, Worcester, Massachusetts

Javad H. Kashani, M.D., F.R.C.P.(C)
Professor of Psychiatry, Psychology, Pediatrics, and Medicine,
University of Missouri, Columbia, Missouri

Clarice J. Kestenbaum, M.D.
Columbia University College of Physicians and Surgeons,
Division of Child Psychiatry, New York, New York

Henry R. Kranzler, M.D.
Assistant Professor of Psychiatry, Department of Psychiatry;
Associate Director, Alcohol and Drug Abuse Treatment Center,
University of Connecticut School of Medicine, Farmington,
Connecticut

Henrietta L. Leonard, M.D.
Research Fellow, Child Psychiatry Branch, National Institute of
Mental Health, Bethesda, Maryland

Marsha M. Linehan, Ph.D.
Associate Professor of Psychology, University of Washington,
Seattle, Washington

Roger E. Meyer, M.D.
Professor and Chairman, University of Connecticut Health
Center, Department of Psychiatry, Farmington, Connecticut

Sheldon I. Miller, M.D.
Professor and Chairman, Department of Psychiatry, University
of Medicine and Dentistry of New Jersey, Newark, New Jersey

Richard L. Munich, M.D.
Associate Professor of Clinical Psychiatry, The New York
Hospital–Cornell Medical Center, Westchester Division, White
Plains, New York

Barbara Orrok, M.D.
Assistant Professor, University of Connecticut School of
Medicine; Co-Director, Alcohol Treatment Program, Veterans
Hospital, Newington, Connecticut

Richard R. Pleak, M.D.
Research Fellow in Child Psychiatry, Columbia University
College of Physicians and Surgeons, New York, New York

Judith L. Rapoport, M.D.
Chief, Child Psychiatry Branch, National Institute of Mental
Health, Bethesda, Maryland; Clinical Professor of Psychiatry,
George Washington University Medical School, Washington,
D.C.

Theodore Reich, M.D.
Professor of Psychiatry and Genetics, Washington University
Medical School, The Jewish Hospital of St. Louis, St. Louis,
Missouri

William H. Reid, M.D., M.P.H.
Clinical Professor of Psychiatry, University of Texas Health
Sciences Center, San Antonio, Texas

Loren H. Roth, M.D., M.P.H.
Professor of Psychiatry, Western Psychiatric Institute and
Clinic, Pittsburgh, Pennsylvania

Bruce J. Rounsaville, M.D.
Associate Professor of Psychiatry, Yale University School of
Medicine; Substance Abuse Treatment Unit, Connecticut
Mental Health Center, New Haven, Connecticut

I. Leslie Rubin, M.D.
Assistant Professor of Pediatrics, Harvard Medical School;
Director of Pediatrics, Developmental Evaluation Clinic,
Children's Hospital, Department of Psychiatry, Boston,
Massachusetts

Michael H. Sacks, M.D.
Associate Professor of Psychiatry, New York Hospital, Payne
Whitney Psychiatric Clinic, New York, New York

Diane H. Schetky, M.D.
Rockport, Maine

Harold I. Schwartz, M.D.
Chief, Program in Psychiatry and Law, Beth Israel Medical
Center, New York; Associate Professor of Clinical Psychiatry,
Mt. Sinai School of Medicine, New York, New York

Daniel D. Sherman, M.A.
Ph.D. Candidate in Clinical Psychology, Department of
Psychology, University of Missouri, Columbia, Missouri

C. Robert Showalter, M.D.
Clinical Associate Professor of Behavioral Medicine and
Psychiatry, Department of Psychiatry; Associate Medical
Director, Institute of Law, Psychiatry and Public Policy,
University of Virginia, Charlottesville, Virginia

William H. Sledge, M.D.
Associate Professor of Psychiatry, Yale University School of
Medicine, Connecticut Mental Health Center, New Haven,
Connecticut

Paul H. Soloff, M.D.
Associate Professor of Psychiatry, Western Psychiatric Institute
and Clinic, Pittsburgh, Pennsylvania

Michael H. Stone, M.D.
Professor of Psychiatry, Columbia College of Physicians and
Surgeons, New York, New York

Ludwik S. Szymanski, M.D.
Assistant Professor of Psychiatry, Harvard Medical School,
Developmental Evaluation Clinic, Children's Hospital, Boston,
Massachusetts

George Tarjan, M.D.
Professor of Psychiatry, University of California, Los Angeles, California

Allan Tasman, M.D.
Professor of Psychiatry, Director of Residency Training and Medical Student Education, Department of Psychiatry, University of Connecticut Medical School, Farmington, Connecticut

Robert M. Wettstein, M.D.
Co-Director, Law and Psychiatry Program, and Assistant Professor of Psychiatry, Western Psychiatric Institute and Clinic, Pittsburgh, Pennsylvania

Jerry M. Wiener, M.D.
Chairman, Department of Psychiatry, George Washington University Medical School, Washington, D.C.

Thomas A. Widiger, Ph.D.
Associate Professor, University of Kentucky, College of Arts and Sciences, Department of Psychology, Lexington, Kentucky

Mary C. Zanarini, Ed.D.
Assistant Psychologist, Psychosocial Research Program, McLean Hospital, Belmont, Massachusetts; Instructor in Psychology, Harvard Medical School, Boston, Massachusetts

I

Borderline Personality Disorder

Borderline Personality Disorder

Contents

Section I
Borderline Personality Disorder
Foreword
by John G. Gunderson, M.D., Section Editor

The first effort to provide an in-depth review of selected subjects in psychiatry occurred in 1982. At that time, Dr. Otto Kernberg accepted responsibility for organizing and editing a section of *Psychiatry Update* entitled "Borderline and Narcissistic Personality Disorders." The current editors of the series, now entitled *American Psychiatric Press Review of Psychiatry*, have requested a new review. That this updated review is needed is a testimonial to the fundamental clinical problems which borderline patients present, and it is a testimonial to the burgeoning knowledge about them.

The chapters that follow offer interesting contrasts with the chapters written in 1982 on similar subjects. In 1975, Margaret Singer and I published a review on the available literature related to borderline personality, and, by stretching the definition greatly, could come up with, at most, 100 references (Gunderson and Singer, 1975). By 1980 there were already 1,000 references which specifically related to borderline personality, and by 1983 this total had reached 3,000! Drs. Widiger and Frances point out that borderline personality disorder has become by far the most extensively studied personality disorder—constituting 40 percent of the literature on all personality disorders. So numerous have the studies on diagnosis alone become that Widiger and Frances offer a "meta-analysis" as an effort of statistically summarizing their findings. The exponential rise in research and the literature defies any one expert's ability to comprehend or master.

As a group, the chapters that follow dramatically expose the deeper knowledge and more diverse clinical approaches now available for diagnosing and treating borderline personality disorder. Chapter 1—the overview on diagnosis prepared by Drs. Widiger and Frances—contrasts with my earlier review on this subject in 1982 (Gunderson, 1982). The current review includes many more studies, uses positive and negative predictive power to judge criteria more than reliance upon discriminant function analysis, rests upon still flawed but better informed estimates of epidemiological distributions, and is organized by much more uniform reliance upon the *Diagnostic and Statistical Manual of Mental Disorders, Third Edition (DSM-III)* (American Psychiatric Association, 1980) criteria set. The reliance upon *DSM-III* has drawn attention to unexpected relationships between borderline personality disorder and many other categories which might otherwise be overlooked. The reliance has also led researchers to utilize the existing criteria set to assure replicable usage, but at the cost of doing research on better defining the disorder itself.

The initial studies of pathogenesis consisted of efforts to examine its possible genetic components. This was carefully described by Siever (1982), and, indeed, his empirical studies and careful thinking have been an important stimulus to the development of biogenetic research into borderline personality disorder.

There was no chapter on the broader issues related to pathogenesis in the 1982 Psychiatry Update. Indeed, most all of the research reviewed by Dr. Zanarini and me in Chapter 2 has been done in the 1980s. In 1982 there were only a few family prevalence studies and the biological marker studies were limited to one study on dexamethasone suppression, one study on rapid eye movement (REM) latency, and one study on electroencephalograms (EEGs). The profusion of studies in these areas is joined by a growing number of studies into the environmental, developmental, and familial interaction characteristics that are associated with the development of borderline personality disorder. In our review, Dr. Zanarini and I demonstrate how research occurs against the backdrop of a few broad theories derived from the clinical observations from such diverse sources as Kernberg, Andrulonis, and Klein.

The chapter on psychotherapy in borderline personality disorder was written by Kernberg in 1982. It emphasized the modifications of standard psychoanalytic technique required for such patients but maintained a psychoanalytic emphasis upon technical neutrality, transference, and transference interpretation. In his current review on the same subject, Dr. Adler now suggests, in Chapter 3, that the divisions used by Kernberg between supportive and exploratory methods are artifactual, and attempts to place transference and transference interpretations into a broader context of how therapeutic relationships work. As in Kernberg's earlier review, there remains a remarkable absence of any controlled research. Moreover, Adler cites a number of contributors to the literature whose work has appeared or gained popularity since Kernberg's seminal contributions.

Chapter 4, Dr. Soloff's review of psychopharmacology, contrasts with the review written by Cole and Sunderland in 1982. Cole and Sunderland's review largely consisted of efforts to apply findings from other clinical groups to the phenomenology associated with borderline personality disorder. They concluded by suggesting that "A reasonable drug is worth trying if it offers at least some hope of substantially improving the patient's disruptive dysphoric state and particularly if attempts at short-term psychotherapy have proved inadequate" . . . and by expressing the hope "that somewhere double-blind controlled studies of drug therapies are being done with patients who need explicit criteria for borderline stage" (p. 470). Soloff's review documents that such studies have now been done, prominent amongst them being his own. As a result of such studies, Soloff's review contains much better informed and more specific suggestions which psychiatrists can use and by which the modern borderline patient should benefit. Strikingly, the current review still points toward the heterogeneity of drug response among borderlines. It is clear the pharmacotherapy still relies upon very pragmatic trials but that this pragmatism is much better informed than it was in 1982.

Chapter 5, by Dr. Linehan on cognitive–behavioral therapy, is a new area with respect to borderline personality disorder. As such, her chapter had no precedent in 1982, but can be expected to have the same stimulating effect that the earlier chapters on biogenetics and psychopharmacology had for the development of research and clinical practices in those areas. Linehan's own work is, of course, central to her chapter, and it is time that the psychiatric field becomes informed by it. This chapter gives encouragement and precedent for psychiatrists to think in terms of more discrete, prescriptive, and focused forms of intervention which may be able to assist sectors of the borderline patient's problems.

Chapter 6, by Dr. Stone, documents the much greater knowledge we now have about what happens to borderline patients in the first few years and even decades following their identification as psychiatric patients. Stone, like the other chapter authors, speaks from the expertise gained by being a central contributor to the literature he reviews. The most broadly noted finding from these follow-up studies has been the significant number of borderline patients who function well and stop using psychiatric care in the second decade after their index diagnosis. Less often noted is the continued dysfunction for the first decade and for many thereafter. Stone's chapter goes further by showing more about what factors may predict or determine the nature of the borderline person's outcome—the highly varied pathways that defy easy prognostication.

The chapter subjects are by no means comprehensive. Certainly there are considerable bodies of literature that have also grown around other treatment modalities that are not covered here. Nevertheless, the reader is welcomed to a series of chapters that provide a broad and scholarly synthesis of much of the current knowledge about borderline personality disorder.

REFERENCES

American Psychiatric Association: Diagnostic and Statistical Manual of Mental Disorders, Third Edition (DSM-III). Washington, DC, American Psychiatric Association, 1980

Cole JO, Sunderland III P: The drug treatment of borderline patients, in Psychiatry 1982: The American Psychiatric Association Annual Review, vol. 1. Edited by Grinspoon L. Washington, DC, American Psychiatric Press, 1982

Gunderson JG: Empirical studies of the borderline diagnosis, in Psychiatry 1982: The American Psychiatric Association Annual Review, vol. 1. Edited by Grinspoon L. Washington, DC, American Psychiatric Press, 1982

Gunderson JG, Singer MT: Defining borderline patients: an overview. Am J Psychiatry 1974; 133:1–10

Kernberg OF: The psychotherapeutic treatment of borderline personalities, in Psychiatry 1982: The American Psychiatric Association Annual Review, vol. 1. Edited by Grinspoon L. Washington, DC, American Psychiatric Press, 1982

Kernberg OF (Ed): Borderline and Narcissistic Personality Disorders (Part V), in Psychiatry 1982: The American Psychiatric Association Annual Review, vol. 1. Edited by Grinspoon L. Washington, DC, American Psychiatric Press, 1982

Siever LJ: Genetic factors in borderline personalities, in Psychiatry 1982: The American Psychiatric Association Annual Review, vol. 1. Edited by Grinspoon L. Washington, DC, American Psychiatric Press, 1982

Chapter 1

Epidemiology, Diagnosis, and Comorbidity of Borderline Personality Disorder

by Thomas A. Widiger, Ph.D., and Allen J. Frances, M.D.

Borderline personality disorder (BPD) is currently by far the best researched of the personality disorders, accounting for 40 percent of the 262 articles published on personality disorders in 1985 (Blashfield and McElroy, 1987). This popularity reflects a variety of factors, including high prevalence, difficulties in diagnosis and treatment, frequency of comorbidity with other disorders, and numerous controversies that make this a fascinating but also ambiguous category. In this chapter we will review the epidemiology, diagnosis, and comorbidity of BPD. We will provide a summary of the research and in some cases aggregate the findings with the statistical technique of meta-analysis (Rosenthal, 1984). The literature on BPD is extensive, with 105 articles published in 1985 alone (Blashfield and McElroy, 1987). Simply providing the reference list on all of the articles concerned with the epidemiology, diagnosis, and/or comorbidity of BPD would consume the space allocated for this chapter. Therefore, our review will be necessarily restrictive and will emphasize studies that have appeared since the last review in this series by Gunderson (1982). We will also discuss the implications of this research for clinical practice.

EPIDEMIOLOGY

Prevalence

Borderline personality disorder is certainly one of the most common psychiatric diagnoses. Whether this reflects the actual prevalence of a widespread disorder, faddish popularity, or nonspecific diagnostic criteria, is unclear. Prevalence is difficult to estimate because of the variability in criteria, settings, and procedures used in psychodiagnostic studies. There have been no systematic studies of the prevalence of BPD in community settings. Estimates of the prevalance in the general population have been as high as 15 percent based on Kernberg's (1984) criteria (Gunderson, 1984), as low as .2 percent based on the *Diagnostic and Statistical Manual of Mental Disorders, Third Edition (DSM-III)* (American Psychiatric Association, 1980) criteria (Merikangas and Weissman, 1986), and between 2 and 4 percent based on the prevalence in the relatives of normal comparison groups (Gunderson and Zanarini, 1987).

Prevalence in clinical samples has ranged from 8 percent (Manos et al, 1987)

We would like to express our appreciation to Drs. Harris and Rosenthal for their consultation with respect to the meta-analyses and to Drs. Morey and Dubro for providing unpublished data.

to 63 percent (Zanarini et al, 1987). A substantial proportion of this variability can be accounted for by setting and selection criteria. For example, the proportion of patients with BPD is likely to be higher in inpatient than in outpatient settings and in samples that exclude patients with schizophrenia, than it is likely to be in samples with no exclusion criteria. Twenty-two studies (identified by a superscript a in the reference list) that most closely approximated systematic sampling were coded with respect to how the selection criteria and setting should affect the prevalence of BPD, and a correlation of .79 was obtained between the rating of each study and the prevalence estimate. That is, 62 percent of the variation in prevalence could be accounted for by variation in the setting and selection criteria. Based on these studies, an estimated prevalence of borderlines among all outpatients would be 11 percent (Kass et al, 1985); among all inpatients it would be 19 percent (Barrash et al, 1983; Koenigsberg et al, 1985; Manos et al, 1987; Piersma, 1987; Plakun et al, 1985; Stone et al, 1987; Trull and Widiger, 1988); among inpatients who are not schizophrenic, mentally retarded, or have an organic mental disorder it would be 23 percent (Dahl, 1986; Dubro et al, 1988; Kroll et al, 1981; McGlashan, 1983b; Mellsop et al, 1982; Modestin, 1987; Pfohl et al, 1986); among outpatients with a personality disorder it would be 33 percent (Frances et al, 1984; Morey, 1988); and among inpatients with a personality disorder it would be 63 percent (Widiger et al, 1986a; Zanarini et al, 1987). It should be emphasized, however, that the studies varied with respect to a number of other factors, and a more confident estimate of prevalence requires more systematic sampling across many settings.

Demographic Data

Although most BPD studies usually report sex prevalence data, some of these may be biased by the nature of the setting (for example, Veterans Administration hospital) or patient selection. The average proportion of females in 38 reasonably appropriate BPD studies was .74, with a 95 percent confidence interval of .70–.77 (space limitations prohibit a listing of all 38 studies; the complete list can be obtained on request and 15 of them are noted by the superscript b in the reference list). The significance of this proportion depends on the comparison group and the setting. Borderline personality disorder groups will have more females than schizophrenic or antisocial groups, but not necessarily more females than groups of depressed or histrionic and dependent patients (Reich, 1987b). Most borderline personality disorder patients seen in clinical settings are female, but the results might be different if more studies were conducted in military, Veterans Administration, or correctional settings.

The data on socioeconomic variables are insufficient and/or inconsistently reported across studies to allow meaningful interpretation. It does appear that BPD patients tend to be younger than nonborderline comparison groups (Akhtar et al, 1986). This may be consistent with the tendency of personality disorder symptomatology in general, and BPD in particular, to decrease in severity and prevalence into middle age (Paris et al, 1987). Akhtar and colleagues also reported a tendency across seven studies for there to be a significantly lower proportion of blacks in borderline groups. They suggested that this might be due to the assignment of black BPD patients to correctional rather than mental health settings. Castaneda and Franco (1985) also found a lower proportion of black borderline patients than black nonborderline patients, with no difference for whites or

Hispanics. They also found no differences between the sexes in the diagnosis of BPD for Hispanics, with a higher proportion of male Hispanic borderline patients (.47) than male white or male black borderline patients (.27 and .20, respectively). They suggested that this could be due to either greater instability in the identity of male immigrant Puerto Ricans, or to the exuberant mannerisms and dramatic behavior of Hispanic males being overdiagnosed by unfamiliar white clinicians. Castaneda and Franco also suggested that BPD might be under-diagnosed in Hispanic women as a result of clinicians dismissing the BPD symp-tomatology as being normative of Hispanic women. This is an interesting sex bias hypothesis that is opposite to the usual sex bias expectation of an overdi-agnosis in women.

In sum, it is possible that BPD varies in its prevalence or manifestation across cultural, sex, and ethnic groups, but it might also be overdiagnosed in some groups and underdiagnosed in others (Castaneda and Franco, 1985; Gunderson and Zanarini, 1987). It would be helpful in interpreting these demographic findings to determine whether the differential prevalence is confined largely to particular BPD items (e.g., identity disturbance versus affective instability) and assessment instruments (e.g., interviews versus self-report inventories). In any case, clinicians should exercise caution when diagnosing BPD in patients from different ethnic, sex, or cultural groups.

DIAGNOSIS

Reliability

The literature suggests that when using systematic assessment methods the diagnosis of BPD can be made quite reliably. This has been a gratifying and somewhat surprising finding, given the modest *DSM-III* field trial reliability (kappa = .54) for the presence of any personality disorder and the negligible reliability for the diagnosis of BPD in a clinical practice setting (kappa = .29) obtained by Mellsop and colleagues (1982) (kappa is an index of reliability that contrasts the percent of interrater agreement with the rate of agreement that would be expected by chance). However, when a systematic interviewing and/or scoring procedure has been used, kappa values have typically been above .70, both for clinical interviews (Cornell et al, 1983; Frances et al, 1984; Gunder-son, 1982; Pfohl et al, 1986; Widiger et al, 1986a; Zanarini et al, 1987) and for chart review (McGlashan, 1983a; Paris et al, 1987). It is not yet clear, however, how reliably BPD is diagnosed in general clinical practice. Researchers have indicated that their personality disorder diagnoses based on systematic assess-ment have not been consistent with clinical diagnoses (Morey and Ochoa, 1987; Pfohl et al, 1986). It should also be noted that surprisingly few BPD studies obtain interrater reliability data. Most refer the reader to prior studies.

Very few studies have reported kappa for individual items. The highest reli-ability is typically found for physically self-damaging acts and the lowest for identity disturbance (Frances et al, 1984; Pfohl et al, 1986; Widiger et al, 1986a). The *Diagnostic and Statistical Manual of Mental Disorders, Third Edition, Revised (DSM-III-R)* (American Psychiatric Association, 1987) criteria for identity disturb-ance are somewhat more specific than *DSM-III* (requiring uncertainty in at least two areas); but identity disturbance is likely to remain difficult to assess. Hampering reliability is the absence of specific criteria for the presence and for the threshold of clinical significance of each item. Researchers can obtain interrater reliability within their own site by developing their own implicit or explicit criteria, but it is likely that the threshold for some of the items varies across research settings.

One potential solution to low reliability is to make the criteria unambiguous and less inferential by using behavioral indicators to describe each item. It must be noted, however, that the listing of specific acts, even prototypic ones (Livesley and Jackson, 1986), might not adequately represent borderline psychopathology and might lose the construct in an effort to improve the reliability of its assessment (Frances and Widiger, 1986). For example, there will be many different behaviors that represent or suggest inappropriate, intense, or lack of control of anger, and the relevance of any particular behavior to this BPD item will depend on the situation, setting, and context in which it occurs. The particular acts or incidents that suggest BPD pathology will then vary across patients. A list of acts can offer illustrative examples but it is likely to be both incomplete and inadequate by itself.

Clinical assessments, however, should be based on the acts and incidents that have occurred across various situations and time periods (Widiger and Frances, 1985, 1987). It is tempting to assess anger by asking patients if they are frequently angry or often lose control of their temper, but patients will vary in how they interpret what is meant by "anger" and "loss of control." One should instead ask for descriptions of episodes of anger and assess their duration, chronicity, and interference with social and occupational functioning (e.g., resulted in failure to resolve disagreements, development of marital discord, or negative evaluation by employer).

Diagnostic Efficiency

There is no one way to describe the value of an item to the diagnosis of BPD. The most commonly reported statistics are sensitivity (proportion of patients with the disorder who have the symptom); specificity (proportion of patients without the disorder who do not have the symptom); and positive and negative predictive power (PPP and NPP, respectively). PPP is the probability of the diagnosis given the item and NPP is the probability of not meeting the criteria for the disorder given the absence of the item. PPP indicates which items are optimal for identifying the presence of the disorder, NPP indicates which are optimal for ruling out the presence of the disorder, and sensitivity indicates what proportion of the patients with the disorder will be identified by the symptom (Widiger et al, 1984).

We calculated the average of these statistics across 14 studies (identified by a superscript c in the reference list). Physically self-damaging acts, unstable–intense relationships, and impulsivity were the most useful items for diagnosing BPD across the 14 studies (as indicated by the overall hit rate and PPP values). Impulsivity and affective instability were the most characteristic of the BPD patients (as indicated by the sensitivity rate) and their absence was a very strong indication that the patient would not be diagnosed with BPD (as indicated by the NPP values). McGlashan (1987b) also concluded on the basis of his review of the empirical research that the core BPD criteria were unstable relationships, impulsivity, and self-damaging acts, and the least characteristic were inappropriate anger and intolerance of being alone. Modestin (1987), as well, suggested that unstable–intense relationships is the most consistently diagnostic feature of BPD across studies. Nurnberg and colleagues (1987), using their own criteria set for BPD, also found impulsivity and unstable–intense relationships to be the two items with the highest positive and negative predictive power. "Acting-out behaviors" and chronic depressive emptiness, boredom, and loneliness were also useful, but only when used in combination with impulsivity and/or unstable relationships, consistent with the findings of Clarkin and colleagues (1983).

These findings might be inconsistent to some extent with clinical expectations. Gunderson and Zanarini (1987) suggested that the three most important clinical features of BPD were intense, unstable relationships, repetitively self-destructive behavior, and chronic abandonment fears. Impulsivity was rated next to last in a list of seven items. Livesley and colleagues (1987) reported in a survey of 45 psychiatrists that the items considered to be the most prototypical were unstable relationships, identity disturbance, and inappropriate, intense anger. Hilbrand and Hirt (1987), in a survey of 30 clinicians, found that the three most frequently cited features of BPD were impulsivity, anger, and identity disturbance. However, it is not unusual to find that the features judged to be the most characteristic of classical cases are not the most useful in routine clinical practice (Widiger and Frances, 1985).

The *DSM-III* item, intolerance of being alone, obtained the lowest hit rate across the 14 studies and the lowest prototypicality ratings in studies by Livesley and colleagues (1987) and Hilbrand and Hirt (1987). This item was replaced in *DSM-III-R* by "frantic efforts to avoid real or imagined abandonment" (American Psychiatric Association, 1987) which, it is hoped, represents more accurately the intense dependency and separation anxiety that have often been described in BPD patients (Goldstein, 1987; Gunderson and Zanarini, 1987; Kernberg, 1984; Livesley et al, 1987).

Any summary across studies, however, must be qualified by the fact that the importance of each item to the diagnosis of BPD is dependent upon the setting and time in which the diagnosis occurs and the differential diagnosis that is at issue. Intolerance of being alone obtained the lowest average hit rate across the 14 studies, but it is the BPD criterion which best discriminates borderlines from patients with narcissistic or schizotypal personality disorders. For these comparisons, the criterion had a PPP rate of 1.00 in the studies by Plakun (1987) and McGlashan (1987b). Narcissistic and schizotypal patients tend to display many BPD characteristics, but not an intolerance of being alone. Impulsivity obtained a high average PPP across the 14 studies, but it had the lowest PPP (.33) in the study by Malow and Donnelly (1987) that was conducted at a Veterans Administration Medical Center drug dependence treatment unit. Impulsivity was so prevalent in this population that it was not specific to patients with borderline personality disorder.

When the diagnosis is confined largely to outpatients with personality disorders (as in Clarkin et al, 1983; Jacobsberg et al, 1986; Morey, 1988), physically self-damaging acts might be the best item for identifying the presence of BPD. It obtained an average PPP of .69 in this situation, in comparison to PPP rates of .51 to .58 for all of the other items. If the diagnosis is confined largely to inpatients with personality disorders (as in Dahl, 1986; Dubro et al, 1988; Modestin, 1987; Pfohl et al, 1986; Widiger et al, 1986a), then unstable–intense relationships may be the best item for identifying the presence of BPD. It obtained an average PPP of .82 in this situation, in comparison to PPP rates of .57 to .68 for all of the other items. Physically self-damaging acts are less prevalent in outpatient settings and are then more specific to BPD patients. Unstable–intense relationships might be a more common phenomenon of outpatients than inpatients, and more specific to BPD patients in samples of inpatients with personality disorders. These results illustrate that the relative importance of an item to the diagnosis of BPD is affected by the setting and the differential diagnosis that is at issue. The systematic nature of this effect will become more apparent when a sufficient number of settings, populations, and differential diagnoses have been sampled.

Cutoff Points

The *DSM-III-R* diagnosis of BPD is categorical, determining whether a person has or does not have a borderline personality disorder. The cutoff point for this decision is the presence of five of the eight items (American Psychiatric Association, 1987). This cutoff point is to some extent arbitrary. Patients with only four borderline symptoms may be more similar to patients with five than with those who have fewer, and patients with five may be more similar to those with four than with those who have all eight (Widiger et al, 1986b). Patients can be diagnosed with BPD without having unstable–intense relationships, affective instability, or impulsivity (Clarkin et al, 1983). Substantial information might be lost by lumping together persons with 0 to 4 items and 5 to 8 items (Frances, 1982; Frances and Widiger, 1986).

Clinicians may then find it useful to record the number of BPD items each patient possesses. This would provide a measure of the degree to which the patient displays borderline psychopathology. However, it should also be recognized that the number of BPD items is not itself an infallible measure of the severity of borderline psychopathology. The items are not equivalent with respect to severity of dysfunction, and the severity of dysfunction represented by each item varies across patients. For example, patients will differ considerably with respect to the severity of their affective instability. There is currently no simple way to include all of the information necessary for a comprehensive assessment. The number of BPD items and the Axis V global assessment of functioning rating (American Psychiatric Association, 1987) together provide some indication of the severity of borderline psychopathology.

Other Items

At least for research purposes and during this time of rapid progress and evolution in psychiatric diagnosis, one should not be committed to a specific set of BPD criteria. Historically, there has been a variety of formulations for borderline personality (Gunderson, 1982, 1984; Kernberg, 1984). A limitation of most psychodiagnostic studies is that the *DSM-III-R* criteria tend to receive the exclusive attention, and viable alternative formulations and criteria sets do not receive adequate consideration. For example, brief psychotic experiences were not included in the *DSM-III-R* criteria for BPD because they may have a low frequency in outpatients and may be more characteristic of schizotypal patients (Frances et al, 1984; Jacobsberg et al, 1986; McGlashan, 1987b; Torgersen, 1984; Widiger et al, 1986a). Psychotic symptoms that do occur are often secondary to an Axis I syndrome, such as substance abuse or a major affective disorder, and the psychotic symptomatology that is specific to BPD may reflect manipulative, exaggerated, and/or factitious tendencies (Pope et al, 1985). However, brief psychotic experiences and psychotic-like symptoms have been associated with BPD (Goldstein, 1987; Gunderson and Zanarini, 1987; Kernberg, 1984; Livesley et al, 1987) and research that has used alternative formulations for BPD suggests more support for including these features (Gunderson, 1982; Nurnberg et al, 1987). Future research should include alternative criteria to allow for comparative results. Other features that might receive further consideration are the tendency to be unusually demanding in interpersonal relationships (Hurt et al, 1986; Livesley et al, 1987) and somatization and hypochondriasis (Nurnberg et al, 1987).

Assessment Instruments

There are now five semistructured interviews used to assess *DSM-III-R* personality disorders. These include the Structured Interview for *DSM-III* Personality Disorders (SIDP; Pfohl et al, 1986); Personality Disorder Examination (PDE); Structured Clinical Interview for *DSM-III-R* (SCID-II); Personality Interview Questions-II (PIQ-II; Widiger et al, 1986a); and Diagnostic Interview for Personality Disorders (DIPD; Zanarini et al, 1987). Overviews of these instruments are presented elsewhere (Reich, 1987a; Widiger and Frances, 1987).

The Diagnostic Interview for Borderlines (DIB; Gunderson, 1982, 1984) warrants particular attention because it offers an alternative diagnostic system for BPD. The DIB includes 29 items to assess five areas of functioning, two of which are not included in the *DSM-III-R* formulation (that is, affectivity, interpersonal relations, and impulsivity/action, plus psychotic symptoms and social adaptation). It has obtained supportive validity and interrater and test–retest reliability (Cornell et al, 1983; Gunderson, 1982, 1984; Reich, 1987a; Widiger and Frances, 1987). Barrash and colleagues (1983) and Kroll and colleagues (1981) reported the DIB to be more inclusive than the *DSM-III*; Nelson and associates (1985) found the *DSM-III* criteria to be somewhat more inclusive; and Frances and colleagues (1984), Loranger and co-workers (1984), and McGlashan (1983a) reported no substantial difference. The concordance of DIB and *DSM-III* BPD diagnoses has been moderate to good (Barrash et al, 1983; Frances et al, 1984; Hurt et al, 1986; Kroll et al, 1981; Loranger et al, 1984; Nelson et al, 1985), but disagreement can be advantageous because it indicates the DIB might offer an alternative approach to BPD diagnosis (McGlashan, 1983a). The DIB has recently been revised and is now somewhat less inclusive in diagnosis (Gunderson and Zanarini, 1987; Pope et al, 1987).

Another alternative formulation is Kernberg's (1984) concept of borderline personality organization. "Borderline" in Kernberg's formulation refers to a level of personality organization (distinguished from the "neurotic" and "psychotic") shared by all of the severely dysfunctional *DSM-III-R* personality disorders. Kernberg has also been critical of relying on overt symptomatology for diagnosis, indicating, for example, that some nonborderlines display *DSM-III* BPD impulsivity (e.g., patients with high level hysterical character disorders) and some patients at a borderline level of personality organization do not present anger or depression (e.g., schizoid patients). He also suggests that a reliance on overt behaviors or acts diminishes the clinical utility of the diagnosis. "The nature of the primitive transferences that these patients develop . . . and the techniques for dealing with them stem directly from the structural characteristics of their internalized object relations" (Kernberg, 1984, p. 4). The difficulty in testing this hypothesis is the absence of a reliable, replicable method for assessing these internalized object relations. Only very preliminary and/or pilot data for the assessment of borderline personality organization (Kernberg et al, 1981; Selzer et al, 1987) has been provided. Moderate kappa values of .49 (Kernberg et al, 1981) and .45 (Koenigsberg et al, 1983) in assessing the concordance of the DIB and structural diagnoses have been reported, but it is not clear if this is good news or bad news since the amount of convergence that should occur is unclear. It is conceivable that an assessment of internalized object relations and primitive defenses are important in the diagnosis of BPD (Goldstein, 1987; Kernberg, 1984), but it is necessary to demonstrate that an interview or inventory can measure them reliably, distinguish them from the overt behaviors or acts, and provide incremental validity to a DIB or *DSM-III-R* diagnosis.

There are also many self-report measures of BPD, such as the MMPI Personality Disorder Scales (PDS), Millon Clinical Multiaxial Inventory-II (MCMI-II), and the Personality Diagnostic Questionnaire-Revised (PDQ-R). Overviews of these instruments are presented elsewhere (Reich, 1987a; Widiger and Frances, 1987). The MMPI PDS offers a useful alternative to profile interpretations of the MMPI clinical scales because the latter may not provide the optimal dimensions with which to identify and differentiate among the *DSM-III-R* personality disorders (Morey et al, 1985; Widiger and Frances, 1987). For example, the MMPI profile characterized by elevations on the Schizophrenia, Depression, and Psychopathic Deviate scales has been associated most often with BPD, but it lacks specificity and typically occurs in less than one-third of the samples of BPD patients (Widiger et al, 1986b).

Borderline patients obtain significantly higher elevations than patients with other personality disorders on the borderline scales from the PDS, MCMI(-II), and PDQ(-R) (Hurt et al, 1984; Morey et al, 1988; Reich, 1987a). The BPD scales have also obtained significant correlations with the total number of BPD symptoms as assessed by various semistructured interviews. The PDQ correlated .64 with the SIDP (Reich et al, 1987) and the MCMI correlated .51 with the PIQ (Widiger et al, 1986b), although Reich and colleagues (1987) also reported a correlation of only .32 between the MCMI and the SIDP. Agreement with interview-based BPD diagnoses tends to be moderate at best, with kappa agreement rates of .05 to .32 for the MCMI (Piersma, 1987; Reich et al, 1987) and .43 for the PDQ (Reich et al, 1987). All of the self-report inventories tend to be most useful in ruling out persons who are unlikely to be diagnosed with BPD, with NPP rates of .83 for the PDS, .91 for the MCMI, and .82 to .97 for the PDQ (Hurt et al, 1984; Dubro et al, 1988). They may not be as useful in identifying persons with BPD, with PPP rates ranging from .15 to .58 (Hurt et al, 1984; Dubro et al, 1988), unless they are used as inclusive screening instruments. All of the self-report inventories tend to diagnose more patients with BPD than are diagnosed by interviews (Dubro et al, 1988; Hurt et al, 1984; Reich et al, 1987). This may reflect, in part, the arbitrariness of the cutoff point for BPD, but this explanation would then suggest that the substantial prevalence of BPD already provided by semistructured interviews is an underestimate. It is more likely that self-report inventories are more susceptible to state factors and exaggeration tendencies than semistructured interviews (Reich, 1987a; Widiger and Frances, 1987). Although the PDQ BPD scale obtained a test–retest kappa of .63 in the study by Hurt and colleagues (1984), the test–retest kappa for a semistructured interview was substantially higher (.89). Piersma (1987) found that the MCMI diagnosed 25 percent of 151 patients with BPD at admission (N = 38) but only 11 percent at discharge (N = 11), obtaining a test–retest kappa of only .11. Borderline patients are themselves characterized by exaggeration tendencies and affective symptomatology (Hurt et al, 1984; Widiger et al, 1986b), but this exaggeration and affectivity may be especially problematic for the self-report inventory measurement of BPD.

COMORBIDITY

Comorbidity is most simply interpreted as the co-occurrence of independent disorders, but it may also reflect a common underlying cause shared by both disorders, a causal relationship between the disorders, or a definitional artifact resulting from shared diagnostic criteria. Interpreting comorbidity data is complicated by a variety of methodological problems. Comorbidity may be exagerated in settings populated by persons with the most severe forms of the disorders. A diagnostic system can increase comorbidity by delineating numerous new diagnoses, emphasizing multiple diagnoses rather than differential diagnosis, demarcating different categories along a spectrum of disorders, lowering the threshold for diagnosis, and including overlapping criteria.

A broad array of Axis I syndromes often coexist with BPD, including panic disorder, substance use disorders, affective disorders, gender identity disorder and homosexuality, attention deficit disorder, and eating disorders (Gunderson, 1984). The earlier borderline research focused on the association with schizophrenia (Gunderson, 1982), but this has become largely a moot issue with the *DSM-III* extraction of the schizotypal personality disorder. The attention is focused now on the association with other personality, eating, substance use, and affective disorders.

Other Personality Disorders

Borderline personality disorder typically obtains the most overlap with the other personality disorders, and a BPD patient will usually meet the criteria for at least one other personality disorder (Dahl, 1986; Pfohl et al, 1986; Widiger et al, 1986a). Clinicians should not stop in their personality disorder assessment once a BPD diagnosis has been made. Borderline personality disorder overlaps in particular with the histrionic, antisocial, schizotypal, narcissistic, and dependent personality disorders, and to a lesser but still substantial degree with the passive–aggressive, avoidant, and paranoid personality disorders (Clarkin et al, 1983; Dahl, 1986; Kass et al, 1985; Livesley and Jackson, 1986; Morey, 1988; Pfohl et al, 1986; Widiger et al, 1986a; Siever and Klar, 1986; Zanarini et al, 1987).

Patients with BPD have been differentiated from patients with other personality disorders on a number of variables, consistent with the hypothesis that the criteria set is identifying a qualitatively distinct disorder (Gunderson and Zanarini, 1987). However, these distinctions are strongest when overlapping cases are deleted (Baron et al, 1985). Even as one distinguishes BPD from one personality disorder (e.g., schizotypal) one is left with cases that are difficult to distinguish from other personality disorders (e.g., antisocial and histrionic; Pope et al, 1983; Torgersen, 1984). Because of the considerable overlap, many studies now report data for overlapping and nonoverlapping groups (e.g., Perry, 1985). For example, the overlapping BPD and schizotypal patients tend to be closer to nonoverlapping BPD cases than to nonoverlapping schizotypal cases on treatment, biological marker, and follow-up data (Plakun et al, 1985; McGlashan, 1986a; Siever, 1985); but the prevalence of these overlapping cases, their tendency to fall somewhere between the nonoverlapping cases, and to be closer at times to the nonoverlapping schizotypal patients on some variables (e.g., heterosexual contact) and closer to the nonoverlapping borderline group on others (e.g., frequency and closeness of social activities; McGlashan, 1986a), suggest that the degree of overlap of BPD and schizotypal personality disorder might be as compelling as the degree of differentiation. There does not appear to be a sharp boundary between BPD and the schizotypal, antisocial, histrionic, narcissistic, or perhaps any other personality disorder, at least as they are presently defined.

Direct tests of a categorical distinction between the personality disorders, however, have not been done. It is not yet clear if BPD refers to a discrete diagnostic entity (Gunderson and Zanarini, 1987) or a dimension of instability or impulsivity that cuts across many diagnostic categories (Kernberg, 1984; Millon, 1981). The research to date is consistent with both models (Frances, 1982; Fyer et al, 1988).

Clinically, one may possibly differentiate between BPD and other personality disorders (Gunderson, 1984; Gunderson and Zanarini, 1987). The borderline's exploitative use of others is often an angry response to disappointment and frustration and is usually accompanied by feelings of guilt or shame, whereas the antisocial's exploitative use of others tends to be a guiltless effort for personal gain. Manipulation by the borderline is also typically impulsive and even self-destructive, whereas the antisocial tends to be more calculating, cunning, and successful. Self-destructive tendencies are also less common in antisocial persons, unless they are being confined or restrained from acting-out. Both the narcissistic and antisocial patients tend to be more disaffiliated, detached, and/or self-absorbed than the borderline. Narcissistic persons are primarily interested in using others to bolster their fragile self-esteem, whereas borderlines are intensely dependent and desperate to avoid being alone. Narcissistic persons also tend to be somewhat more stable and successful in social and occupational functioning. Both the borderline and histrionic patients tend to be clinging, manipulative, dependent, and needy of attention. Histrionic patients, however, tend to be somewhat less self-destructive and hostile, experience periods of sustained well-being, and obtain more stability in their relationships. Sexuality may also play a more central role in the interpersonal relations, self-esteem, and pathology of histrionic patients, evident in their erotization of relationships and communications, rivalry with members of the same sex, and seductiveness. The schizotypal patient lacks the intense emotionality and interpersonal involvements, is more socially isolated, and is more peculiar and odd in mannerisms, thinking, and behavior.

Many (if not most) patients with BPD, however, will present with mixed features. The above suggestions for differential diagnosis should not imply that a differential diagnosis must be made, as if these diagnoses are mutually exclusive and a patient has either a borderline or a narcissistic personality disorder. If a patient presents with both features of BPD and another personality disorder, then the most accurate description might be to provide both diagnoses rather than attempt to determine a potentially illusory distinction of which is the "correct" diagnosis.

Eating and Substance Use Disorders

The impulsivity and self-destructiveness of borderline patients can be expressed in a variety of behaviors, including promiscuity, fighting, self-mutilation, suicide attempts, shoplifting, reckless driving and spending, and running away, and can result in a variety of related Axis I syndromes—bulimia and substance use disorders, in particular. Substantial rates of BPD have been reported in persons with bulimia (Levin and Hyler, 1986). Pope and colleagues (1987), however, have cautioned that the comorbidity might at times be an artifact of overlapping diagnostic criteria. Levin and Hyler (1986), for example, acknowledged that "bulimic behavior invariably satisfies the poor impulse control and affective instability criteria (two of the five criteria needed for the disorder)" (p. 51). Pope and colleagues administered the revised DIB in a blind format to bulimic, depressed, and nonpsychiatric controls with the item pertaining to eating disorders omitted. The bulimic group obtained a significantly higher DIB score than the nonpsychiatric controls, but only 1.9 percent met the DIB criteria for BPD, and the elevation that did occur was associated with a comorbid major affective disorder.

Substance use disorders also occur with BPD (Gunderson, 1984). Loranger and Tulis (1985) reported no change in the diagnosis of BPD when substance abuse was excluded as a criterion for impulsivity. They also found that the family history of alcoholism in BPD patients could be accounted for by comorbid alcoholism in the BPD patients, indicating that the comorbidity may not be the result of a common underlying disorder.

In sum, clinicians should consider the presence of BPD in patients with Axis I disorders that involve impulsive and/or self-destructive behavior. The presence of a comorbid BPD would suggest a more difficult treatment and poorer prognosis. Similarly, clinicians treating BPD patients should be cognizant of the possible presence of additional syndromes, such as bulimia and substance abuse, that may warrant separate attention. However, one must also be careful not to overdiagnose BPD in patients with impulse dyscontrol or affective disorders.

Mood Disorders

The comorbidity that has received the most attention and is the most important with respect to the validity and interpretation of the BPD diagnosis concerns the affective disorders. The comorbidity of BPD with affective disorders, particularly dysthymia and major depression, is extensive (Davis and Akiskal, 1986; Gunderson and Elliott, 1985; McGlashan, 1987a). The three traditional explanations are that BPD predisposes a person to the development of depression (Gunderson, 1984; Kernberg, 1984); BPD is a subaffective disorder (Akiskal et al, 1985); and BPD and affective disorders are independent disorders that often coexist in severely dysfunctional populations (McGlashan, 1983b). The findings, however, suggest a more complicated relationship (Fyer et al, 1988; Gunderson and Elliott, 1985; McGlashan, 1987a). Some (but not all) borderlines have a comorbid affective disorder (McGlashan, 1987a; Pope et al, 1983) at a rate that is at times no greater than for other personality disorders (Barasch et al, 1985 Perry, 1985; Shea et al, 1987) It will suggest in some cases a relatively good prognosis in the first four to seven years (Pope et al, 1983) but a relatively poorer prognosis thereafter (McGlashan, 1986b; Plakun et al, 1985). The association of BPD with affective disorders may even be reversed in its effect by the presence of third (often) comorbid antisocial personality disorder (Perry, 1985). Comorbidity may at times involve the co-occurrence of independent disorders (Barasch et al, 1985) and at other times a confusion of a major affective disorder with BPD (Pope et al, 1983). Early studies suggested that a substantial proportion of BPD patients eventually developed a primary affective disorder diagnosis, but it now appears that a substantial proportion do not (Barasch et al, 1985; Pope et al, 1983). Follow-up diagnosis is in any case equivocal, because affective disorder diagnoses can be more unstable (McGlashan, 1987a) and unreliable (Perry, 1985) than the BPD diagnosis. The *DSM-III-R* affective disorder diagnoses themselves may be identifying a broad, heterogeneous array of psychopathology (McGlashan, 1987a). In sum, the BPD diagnosis identifies a heterogeneous group of persons with affective dyscontrol, many of whom never develop a specific affective disorder (Barasch et al, 1985; McGlashan, 1986b; Perry, 1985; Plakun et al, 1985; Pope et al, 1983), but some of whom have instead a major affective disorder (Pope et al, 1983), a "double depression" (Perry, 1985), hysteroid dysphoria, or some other form of atypical depression.

Complicating the interpretation of the research is the inherent overlap of the diagnostic criteria for BPD and affective disorders. Most of the criteria for BPD directly or indirectly tap affective dyscontrol (e.g., affective instability, inappropriate or intense anger, suicidal behavior, and chronic feelings of emptiness or boredom). An association of BPD and affective disorders may be tautological. One could delete from studies those borderlines whose diagnoses were influenced by affective symptomatology, but are borderlines who are without affective instability, suicidal behavior, and intense anger, really borderlines? Including these patients, however, renders research results uninterpretable. Consider, for example, a study by Akiskal and colleagues (1985). They replicated rapid eye movement (REM) latency data in 24 BPD patients and suggested that these data (along with prior findings) "supports the proposal that conditions considered borderline by contemporary operational criteria belong to a broadly conceived affective spectrum" (p. 197). However, 71 percent of their borderlines carried lifetime affective diagnoses and it was primarily these BPD patients who obtained the affective REM latencies. It may be better for future comorbidity research to focus on particular BPD characteristics, such as identity disturbance or splitting, rather than the disorder itself (Akiskal et al, 1985), or use a dimensional model of a classification that allows for varying degrees of BPD and affective disorder pathology and an overlap between them (McGlashan, 1987a).

Some of the difficulty with this controversy is also the result of unnecessary assumptions with respect to the distinction between Axis I and Axis II disorders (Gunderson and Pollack, 1985). There tends to be an assumption that personality disorders should be psychosocial in origin and treated with psychosocial therapies, and affective disorders imply a biogenetic etiology and are treated pharmacologically. Few practicing clinicians might hold these assumptions but they are implied in the interpretation of comorbidity research. Determining that patients have disturbances in biogenic amine functioning, a family history of affective disorder, or are responsive to pharmacologic interventions does not necessarily imply the absence of a personality disorder. Personality disorders can have an

innate, inherited biogenetic substrate and be responsive to pharmacologic interventions.

Gunderson and Zanarini (1987) suggested that BPD and chronic depression
can be differentiated clinically, with the depressive experiences of BPD patients
being characterized by sustained feelings of emptiness, inner badness, and
impulsive destructiveness and, in contrast, an affective depression involving
guilt themes, actual losses, and unconflicted dependency. These distinctions
may be useful, but inferences regarding the quality of a depression are difficult
to make reliably and the effort implies a necessity in making a differential diagnosis. Borderline personality disorder and affective disorders probably possess
overlapping and interactive etiologies and pathogeneses (Davis and Akiskal,
1986; Gunderson and Elliott, 1985). There will be some borderlines without a
strong association with affective disorders, but many will lie along the interface.
In some cases, BPD may represent a characterological variant along an affective
spectrum, identifying persons with a personality style that often involves affective dysregulation and is a predisposition to affective dyscontrol. Borderline
personality disorder would often, but not always, share biogenetic covariates
with other disorders along the affective spectrum. Some patients with BPD
would at times be responsive to treatments for relatively pure affective disorders,
and most would have a relatively low threshold for affective dyscontrol. The
distinction between personality and affective disorders would then be more fluid
and at times somewhat moot.

CONCLUSIONS

The inclusion of BPD in *DSM-III* was controversial (Frances, 1980) but clearly
appropriate, evidenced in part by the fact that it is currently the most heavily
researched and one of the most prevalent of the personality disorder diagnoses.
Borderline personality disorder should be considered in any clinical assessment,
and particularly in populations of subjects with impulse dyscontrol (e.g., bulimia
and substance abuse) or affective disorders. Borderline personality disorder can
be diagnosed reliably if clinicians perform a systematic assessment of each item.
It may at times be overdiagnosed, particularly by self-report inventories, in
subjects with affective disorders, and when the term is used in a nonspecific
way without attention to the criteria set. One difficulty is the confusion of state
and trait factors. Borderline personality disorder is a personality disorder that
involves a long-term problem with affective dyscontrol, and acute affective
dyscontrol is therefore at times confused with BPD.

The diagnostic criteria for BPD were not changed markedly in *DSM-III-R*, in
part because the original criteria performed well and there was a lack of convincing data warranting any substantial revisions, and also because of the need for
continuity in ongoing research. Possible additional or alternative criteria should
be included in future BPD studies in order to identify the optimal set of items
for *DSM-IV*. The construction of alternative instruments for the assessment of
BPD is useful in this respect, but their relative advantages and disadvantages,
and their association with etiological, course, and treatment variables, need to
be studied further. An additional consideration for *DSM-IV* is to weight the
diagnostic criteria with respect to their relative efficiency within and across
particular settings, populations, and differential diagnoses. In order to do this,

the performance characteristics of the items need to be assessed in diverse samples and settings.

Another consideration for *DSM-IV* is the use of a dimensional rather than a categorical classification. One could classify patients with respect to the extent to which they manifest borderline personality disorder, rather than simply categorize BPD as present or absent. A dimensional model would be more accurate in representing the variation in the extent to which patients display borderline psychopathology. There is also considerable overlap of BPD with other personality and with depressive disorders, with no clear point of demarcation between them. However, a variety of dimensional models have been proposed (Frances, 1982; Frances and Widiger, 1986), and the optimal set of dimensions that would provide a comprehensive yet manageable system is unclear.

REFERENCES

Akhtar, S, Byrne J, Doghramji K: The demographic profile of borderline personality disorder. J Clin Psychiatry 1986; 47:196–198

Akiskal H, Yerevanian B, Davis G, et al: The nosologic status of borderline personality: clinical and polysomnographic study. Am J Psychiatry 1985; 142:192–198

American Psychiatric Association: Diagnostic and Statistical Manual of Mental Disorders, Third Edition (DSM-III). Washington, DC, American Psychiatric Association, 1980

American Psychiatric Association: Diagnostic and Statistical Manual of Mental Disorders, Third Edition, Revised (DSM-III-R). Washington, DC, American Psychiatric Association, 1987

Barasch A, Frances A, Hurt S, et al: Stability and distinctness of borderline personality disorder. Am J Psychiatry 1985; 142:1484–1486

Baron M, Gruen R, Asnis L, et al: Familial transmission of schizotypal and borderline personality disorders. Am J Psychiatry 1985; 142:927–934

Barrash J, Kroll J, Carey K: Discriminating borderline disorder from other personality disorders. Arch Gen Psychiatry 1983; 40:1297–1302[a,b]

Blashfield R, McElroy R: The 1985 journal literature on the personality disorders. Compr Psychiatry 1987; 28:536–546

Castaneda R, Franco H: Sex and ethnic distribution of borderline personality disorder in an inpatient sample. Am J Psychiatry 1985; 142:1202–1203[b]

Clarkin J, Widiger T, Frances A, et al: Prototypic typology and the borderline personality disorder. J Abnorm Psychol 1983; 92:263–275[c]

Cornell D, Silk K, Ludolph P, et al: Test–retest reliability of the Diagnostic Interview for Borderlines. Arch Gen Psychiatry 1983; 40:1307–1310

Dahl A: Some aspects of the DSM-III personality disorders illustrated by a consecutive sample of hospitalized patients. Acta Psychiatr Scand 1986; 73 (Suppl 328):61–66[a,b,c]

Davis G, Akiskal H: Descriptive, biology, and theoretical aspects of borderline personality disorder. Hosp Community Psychiatry 1986; 37:685–692

Dubro A, Wetzler S, Kahn M: A comparison of three self-report questionnaires for the diagnosis of DSM-III personality disorders. Journal of Personality Disorders (1988)[a,c]

Frances A: The DSM-III personality disorders section: a commentary. Am J Psychiatry 1980; 137:1050–1054

Frances A: Categorical and dimensional systems of personality diagnosis: a comparison. Compr Psychiatry 1982; 23:516–527

Frances A, Widiger T: The classification of personality disorders: an overview of problems and solutions, in Psychiatry Update: American Psychiatric Association Annual Review, vol. 5. Edited by Frances A, Hales R. Washington, DC, American Psychiatric Press, 1986

Frances A, Clarkin J, Gilmore M, et al: Reliability of criteria for borderline personality disorder: a comparison of DSM-III and the Diagnostic Interview for Borderline Patients. Am J Psychiatry 1984; 141:1080–1084[a,b]

Fyer M, Frances A, Sullivan T, et al: Comorbidity of borderline personality disorder. Arch Gen Psychiatry 1988; 45:348–352

George A, Soloff P: Schizotypal symptoms in patients with borderline personality disorders. Am J Psychiatry 1986; 143:212–215[b]

Goldstein W: Current dynamic thinking regarding the diagnosis of the borderline patient. Am J Psychother 1987; 41:4–22

Gunderson J: Empirical studies of the borderline diagnosis, in Psychiatry 1982: The American Psychiatric Association Annual Review, vol. 1. Edited by Grinspoon L. Washington, DC, American Psychiatric Press, 1982

Gunderson J: Borderline Personality Disorder. Washington, DC, American Psychiatric Press, 1984

Gunderson J, Elliott G: The interface between borderline personality disorder and affective disorder. Am J Psychiatry 1985; 142:277–288

Gunderson J, Pollack W: Conceptual risks of the Axis I-II division, in Biologic Response Styles: Clinical Implications. Edited by Klar H, Siever L. Washington, DC, American Psychiatric Press, 1985

Gunderson J, Zanarini M: Current overview of the borderline diagnosis. J Clin Psychiatry 1987; 48 (Suppl):5–11

Hilbrand M, Hirt M: The borderline syndrome: an empirically developed prototype. Journal of Personality Disorders 1987; 1:299–306

Hurt S, Hyler S, Frances A, et al: Assessing borderline personality disorder with self-report, clinical interview, or semistructured interview. Am J Psychiatry 1984; 141:1228–1231

Hurt S, Clarkin J, Koenigsberg H, et al: Diagnostic interview for borderlines: psychometric properties and validity. J Consult Clin Psychol 1986; 54:256–260

Jacobsberg L, Hymowitz P, Barasch A, et al: Symptoms of schizotypal personality disorder. Am J Psychiatry 1986; 143:1222–1227[a,b,c]

Kass F, Skodol A, Charles E, et al: Scaled ratings of DSM-III personality disorders. Am J Psychiatry 1985; 142:627–630[a]

Kernberg O: Severe Personality Disorders. New Haven, CT, Yale University Press, 1984

Kernberg O, Goldstein E, Carr A, et al: Diagnosing borderline personality. J Nerv Ment Dis 1981; 169:225–231

Koenigsberg H, Kernberg O, Schomer J: Diagnosing borderline conditions in an outpatient setting. Arch Gen Psychiatry 1983; 40:49–53

Koenigsberg H, Kaplan R, Gilmore M, et al: The relationship between syndrome and personality disorder in DSM-III: experience with 2,462 patients. Am J Psychiatry 1985; 142:207–212[a,b]

Kroll J, Sines L, Martin K, et al: Borderline personality disorder: construct validity of the concept. Arch Gen Psychiatry 1981; 38:1021–1026[a,b]

Levin A, Hyler S: DSM-III personality diagnosis in bulimia. Compr Psychiatry 1986; 27:47–53

Livesley WJ, Jackson D: The internal consistency and factorial structure of behaviors judged to be associated with DSM-III personality disorders. Am J Psychiatry 1986; 143:1473–1474

Livesley WJ, Reiffer L, Sheldon A, et al: Prototypicality ratings of DSM-III criteria for personality disorders. J Nerv Ment Dis 1987; 175:395–401

Loranger A, Tulis E: Family history of alcoholism in borderline personality disorder. Arch Gen Psychiatry 1985; 42:153–157

Loranger A, Oldham J, Russakoff LM, et al: Structured interviews and borderline personality disorder. Arch Gen Psychiatry 1984; 41:565–568

Malow R, Donnelly J: Psychometric evaluation of borderline and antisocial personality disorder criteria. Unpublished manuscript, Veterans Administration Medical Center, New Orleans, Louisiana, 1987[a,c]

Manos N, Vasilopoulou E, Sotiriou M: DSM-III diagnosed borderline personality disorder and depression. Journal of Disorders 1987; 1:263–268[a]

McGlashan T: The borderline syndrome, I: testing three diagnostic systems. Arch Gen Psychiatry 1983a; 40:1311–1318[a]

McGlashan T: The borderline syndrome, II: is it a variant of schizophrenia or affective disorder? Arch Gen Psychiatry 1983b; 40:1319–1323

McGlashan T: Schizotypal personality disorder: Chestnut Lodge follow-up study, VI: long-term follow-up perspectives. Arch Gen Psychiatry 1986a; 43:329-334

McGlashan T: The Chestnut Lodge follow-up study, III: long-term outcome of borderline personalities. Arch Gen Psychiatry 1986b; 43:20–30

McGlashan T: Borderline personality disorder and unipolar affective disorder: long-term effects of comorbidity. J Nerv Ment Dis 1987a; 175:467–473

McGlashan T: Testing DSM-III symptom criteria for schizotypal and borderline personality disorders. Arch Gen Psychiatry 1987b; 44:143–148[c]

Mellsop G, Varghese F, Joshua S, et al: The reliability of Axis II of DSM-III. Am J Psychiatry 1982; 139:1360–1361[a]

Merikangas K, Weissman M: Epidemiology of DSM-III Axis II personality disorders, in Psychiatry Update: American Psychiatric Association Annual Review, vol 5. Edited by Frances A, Hales R. Washington, DC, American Psychiatric Press, 1986

Millon T: Disorders of Personality: DSM-III Axis II. New York, Wiley, 1981

Modestin J: Quality of interpersonal relationships: the most characteristic BPD criterion. Compr Psychiatry 1987; 28:397–402[a,c]

Morey L: A psychometric analysis of five DSM-III categories. Personality and Individual Differences 1985; 6:323–329[c]

Morey L: Personality disorders under DSM-III and DSM-III-R: an examination of convergence, coverage, and internal consistency. Am J Psychiatry 1988; 145:573–577[a,c]

Morey L. Ochoa E: An investigation of influences upon misdiagnosis: borderline and antisocial personality. Paper presented at the 95th Annual Meeting of the American Psychological Association, New York, NY, August 31, 1987

Morey L, Waugh M, Blashfield R: MMPI scales for DSM-III personality disorders: their derivation and correlates. J Pers Assess 1985; 49:245–251

Morey L, Blashfield R, Webb W, et al: MMPI scales for DSM-III personality disorders: a preliminary validation study. J Clin Psychol 1988; 44:47–50

Nelson H, Tennen H, Tasman A, et al: Comparison of three systems for diagnosing borderline personality disorder. Am J Psychiatry 1985; 142:855–858

Nurnberg H, Hurt S, Feldman A, et al: Efficient diagnosis of borderline personality disorder. Journal of Personality Disorders 1987; 1:307–315

Paris J, Brown R, Nowlis D: Long-term follow-up of borderline patients in a general hospital. Compr Psychiatry 1987; 28:530–535[b]

Perry J: Depression in borderline personality disorder: lifetime prevalence at interview and longitudinal course of symptoms. Am J Psychiatry 1985; 142:15–21[b]

Pfohl B, Coryell W, Zimmerman M, et al: DSM-III personality disorders: diagnostic overlap and internal consistency of individual DSM-III criteria. Compr Psychiatry 1986; 27:21–34[a,c]

Piersma H: The MCMI as a measure of DSM-III Axis II diagnoses: an empirical comparison. J Clin Psychol 1987; 43:478–483[a]

Plakun E: Distinguishing narcissistic and borderline personality disorders using DSM-III criteria. Compr Psychiatry 1987; 28:437–443[c]

Plakun E, Burkhardt P, Muller J: Fourteen-year follow-up of borderline and schizotypal personality disorders. Compr Psychiatry 26:448–455, 1985[a]

Pope H, Jonas J, Hudson J, et al: The validity of DSM-III borderline personality disorder:

a phenomenologic, family history, treatment response, and long-term follow-up study. Arch Gen Psychiatry 1983; 40:23–30

Pope H, Jonas J, Hudson J, et al: An empirical study of psychosis in borderline personality disorder. Am J Psychiatry 1985; 142:1285–1290[b]

Pope H, Frankenburg F, Hudson J, et al: Is bulimia associated with borderline personality disorder? A controlled study. J Clin Psychiatry 1987; 48:448–455

Reich J: Instruments measuring DSM-III and DSM-III-R personality disorders. Journal of Personality Disorders 1987a; 1:220–240

Reich J: Sex distribution of DSM-III personality disorders in psychiatric outpatients. Am J Psychiatry 1987b; 144:485–488[a,b]

Reich J, Noyes R, Troughton E: Lack of agreement between instruments assessing DSM-III personality disorders, in Conference on the Millon Inventories. Edited by Green C. Minnetonka, MN, National Computer Systems, 1987

Rosenthal R: Meta-Analytic Procedures for Social Research. Beverly Hills, CA, Sage Publications, 1984

Selzer M, Kernberg P, Fibel B, et al: The Personality Assessment Interview: preliminary report. Psychiatry 1987; 50:142–153

Shea T, Glass D, Pilkonis P, et al: Frequency and implications of personality disorders in a sample of depressed outpatients. Journal of Personality Disorders 1987; 1:27–42

Siever L: Biological marker studies in schizotypal personality disorder. Schizophrenia Bull 11:564–575, 1985

Siever L, Klar H: A review of DSM-III criteria for the personality disorders, in Psychiatry Update: American Psychiatric Association Annual Review, vol 5. Edited by Frances A, Hales R. Washington, DC, American Psychiatric Press, 1986

Spitzer R, Endicott J, Gibbon M: Crossing the border into borderline personality and borderline schizophrenia. Arch Gen Psychiatry 1979; 36:17–24[c]

Stone M, Hurt S, Stone D: The PI 500: long-term follow-up of borderline inpatients meeting DSM-III criteria, I: global outcome. Journal of Personality Disorders 1987; 1:291–298[a,b]

Torgersen S: Genetic and nosological aspects of schizotypal and borderline personality disorders. Arch Gen Psychiatry 1984; 41:546–554[b]

Trull T, Widiger T: The categorical versus dimensional status of borderline personality disorder. Paper presented at the 96th Annual Meeting of the American Psychological Association, August 14, 1988, Atlanta, GA[a,c]

Widiger T, Frances A: The DSM-III personality disorders. Perspectives from psychology. Arch Gen Psychiatry 1985; 42:615–623

Widiger T, Frances A: Interviews and inventories for the measurement of personality disorders. Clin Psychol Rev 1987; 7:49–75

Widiger T, Hurt S, Frances A, et al: Diagnostic efficiency and DSM-III. Arch Gen Psychiatry 1984; 41:1005–1012

Widiger T, Frances A, Warner L, et al: Diagnostic criteria for the borderline and schizotypal personality disorders. J Abnorm Psychol 1986a; 95:43–51[a,b,c]

Widiger T, Sanderson C, Warner L: The MMPI, prototypal typology, and borderline personality disorder. J Pers Assess 1986b; 50:540–553

Zanarini M, Frankenburg F, Chauncey D, et al: The Diagnostic Interview for Personality Disorders: interrater and test–retest reliability. Compr Psychiatry 1987; 28:467–480[a]

Chapter 2

Pathogenesis of Borderline Personality

by John G. Gunderson, M.D., and Mary C. Zanarini, Ed.D.

This chapter will begin with a review of the clinical theories about the etiology of borderline personality disorder (BPD). These theories are divided into those which are psychodynamic and those which are biogenetic. The second part of this chapter concerns empirical examinations into possible etiological factors. The studies here are divided into three parts: 1) family characteristics; 2) family pedigree and possible genetic contributions; and 3) possible neurobiological substrates. This chapter concludes by looking at the connections between the empirical findings and the etiological theories. From this synthesis of the state of present knowledge, implications for a next generation of investigation will be identified.

ETIOLOGICAL THEORIES

Psychodynamic Theories

Three major theories about the origins of borderline personality disorder can be distinguished from the many psychoanalytic papers which have been written about such patients. More detailed examinations of alternative views and refinements on these theories are available elsewhere (Grotstein et al, 1987; Rinsley, 1982).

EXCESSIVE AGGRESSION. The most widely recognized theory for borderline patients is that of Kernberg (1975, 1976), who suggested that the basic pathology involves too much aggression. This excessive aggression can be derived from either a constitutional excess in the aggressive drive which then leads to disproportionate reactions to usual parental frustrations, or from an excessive amount of early frustration from which the excessive aggression is secondary and reactive. The effect in either case is that the small child vacillates between the views that he is dangerous and potentially murderous person, and that he lives in a very hostile and dangerous world. In effect, either he sees himself as "all bad" or he sees his object world as "all bad."

Kernberg states that this splitting of internal perceptions occurs in the context of being able to differentiate self from object. Such differentiation coincides with Mahler's developmental phase of separation–individuation (16 to 26 months old), which she had suggested was particularly critical in the development of borderline personality (Mahler, 1971). When the child believes that the badness exists externally, this reinforces the use of projection and the search for an idealized other; whereas the alternative belief, that the badness resides internally, leads to dissociative splits and masochism. These processes and defenses in turn prevent the development of a stable identity and compromise the development of affect tolerance and other ego strengths.

MATERNAL WITHDRAWAL. A second theory derives more directly from Mahler's identification of the developmental importance of the rapprochement subphase of separation-individuation. In this theory, Masterson and Rinsley (1975) highlight the withdrawal of libidinal (that is, loving) availability by a child's mother in response to the child's efforts toward separation and developing autonomy. This theory places responsibility squarely on the shoulders of mothers. Masterson originally suggested that the mothers of borderlines are themselves borderline (due to the severity of their abandonment fears). The theory has subsequently been expanded by both Rinsley (1982) and Masterson (1987) by noting that the mothers may have a variety of disorders (e.g., psychosis, depression) and by noting the possible presence of a pre-existing constitutional and genetically determined vulnerability in the child. Recurrence of this dilemma in adolescence revives and repeats the pathogenic interactions postulated to occur in the rapprochement subphase. Notably, Shapiro and colleagues (1975) ascribed unresolved conflicts concerning their offspring's emerging autonomy to both parents, and they emphasized the role of both parents' overinvolved separation-resistant dependency upon their children.

Because of the loss of such mothers' affection, attention, and availability in response to the child's efforts toward separation-individuation, the child does not complete a clear differentiation of self from object. According to Masterson and Rinsley, the child then splits the image of the mother into two parts; one is rewarding and gratifying in response to dependency and the other is punitive and withdrawing in response to autonomy. Due to this split, the child sacrifices attention and investment in reality (because it is unpleasurable) in favor of maintaining a positive relationship with the mother.

INTROJECTIVE FAILURE. A third theory on the etiology of borderline personality remains tied to Mahler's object relations developmental paradigm but also utilizes concepts from Kohut's self-psychology (1971). Adler and Buie (1979; Buie and Adler, 1982; Adler, 1985) identify a failure to develop evocative memory as a core element in the psychopathology of borderline patients. This refers to the inability to remember an outer object (person) without tangible external cues. This defect is attributed to parental and especially maternal failures to provide sufficient holding and soothing for the child to develop positive introjects—hence the borderline's inner emptiness and reliance upon transitional objects or upon the presence of significant relationships.

The pathogenic maternal failure is specifically related to the misapprehension of and inappropriate responsiveness to the child's internal psychological attitudes and feelings. The consequence of this is the child's failure to internalize (that is, introject) a coherent, stable, and lovable sense of self. The angry, manipulative, and impulsive actions of borderline patients are secondary features by which such patients then attempt to evoke involvement and reassuring holding responses. Adler (1985) anchors this developmental failure to the period up to and around 18 months of age.

Biogenetic Theories

Paralleling the more general shifts within psychiatry away from a dynamic paradigm, has been a growing interest in theories by which the origins of borderline personality disorder are traced to biogenetic problems.

AFFECTIVE DYSREGULATION. Klein (1975, 1977) first suggested that a subgroup of borderline patients whom he called "hysteroid dysphorics" have a basic underlying problem in affective regulation. This theory derived from his observation that such patients were responsive to antidepressants, most notably to the monoamine oxidase (MAO) inhibitors. He noted that such drugs could modify their pathologically heightened emotional sensitivity to admiration or rejection and this had secondary effects in diminishing their involvement in self-destructive, provocative, and manipulative relationships. More generally, Klein reasoned that "the maladaptive interpersonal tactics and object relations may be viewed as secondary reverberations and miscarried repairs related to the basic affective difficulty" (Klein, 1977, p 374). Noting the similarities between the borderline's emotional reactions to rejection or disapproval and the reactions observed upon withdrawal of amphetamines, Klein hypothesized that the affective dysregulation may be due to the poorly regulated release of an endogenous amphetamine-like substance such as phenylethylamine. This regulatory problem could be either an inherited or acquired defect (Klein, 1975; Liebowitz and Klein, 1981).

In a subsequent refinement of this theory, Akiskal and colleagues (1985a, 1985b) noted that many patients who met criteria for borderline personality disorder have shortened rapid eye movement (REM) latency—a characteristic associated with primary depressive illnesses. This suggested a neurophysiological disturbance which may underlie and explain much of the dysthymic, irritable, somatization-prone symptoms of BPD. Since shortened REM latency is predictive of response to tricyclic antidepressants, Akiskal argued that this could signal an underlying disturbance in cortical indolamine metabolism.

Even more recently, Cowdry and Gardner (1988), like Klein, suggested that the favorable responses observed to an MAO inhibitor reflects defects in the brain's catecholamine-releasing properties that might mimic the effects of stimulants. In addition, because responsiveness to an MAO inhibitor was often associated with a history of attention deficit disorder, he proposed that the biological difficulty might involve insufficient catecholamine release as much as it did an excess of monoamine oxidase.

NEUROLOGICAL DYSFUNCTION. In a study of adolescents with BPD, Andrulonis (1981) found such high rates of neurological dysfunction (38 percent), episodic dyscontrol (65 percent), histories of head trauma, encephalitis, epilepsy (11 percent), or minimal brain dysfunction and/or learning disabilities (27 percent) that he proposed a theory that many patients with early onset BPD have underlying brain dysfunctions. Such dysfunctions were postulated to cause an underlying depletion of monoamines, which might be located in the subcortical temporal lobe–limbic system. Andrulonis suggested that this neurophysiological dysfunction might have either a genetic basis or be due to an "early organic insult."

Cowdry and Gardner (1988) subsequently noted the positive benefits he observed from an anticonvulsant (carbamazepine) whose neurophysiological effects are known to be anatomically located in the limbic area (as opposed to other anticonvulsants which act in cortical brain areas). Because the limbic sites are thought to be involved in control of a variety of aggressive behaviors, Cowdry speculated that an inherited or acquired low threshold for activation of the limbic structures may be a neurological predisposition in those borderline patients who have considerable behavioral and aggressive dyscontrol.

EMPIRICAL EXAMINATIONS

Family Environment Studies

Despite the widespread belief that the etiology of borderline personality disorder can be traced to a pathogenic family environment, the families of these patients have received modest attention in both the psychoanalytic (explanatory) and empirical (descriptive) literature. Many empirical efforts have addressed issues identified by the prior clinical literature (Gunderson and Englund, 1981, for review); that is, the issue of separation and loss of parents, the issue of disturbed parental involvement, and the issue of conflicted family relationships. Another issue overlooked in prior accounts has emerged from empirical studies; that is, physical and sexual abuse. Table 1 provides a background for the review of the empirical studies that follow.

PARENTAL SEPARATION/LOSS.   In a small study Walsh (in Grinker and Werble, 1977) found that a majority of families of borderline patients (57 percent) had histories of parental loss through divorce or death; a significantly higher percentage than was found in a group of matched schizophrenic controls. In addition, one-half of the borderline patients had experienced a serious chronic parental illness which often required extensive hospitalization. Only 21 percent of the patients with BPD came from families that had not experienced the loss of a parent through death, divorce, or serious illness. In another small study, Bradley (1979) found that most (64 percent) children or adolescents with BPD had separations in the first five years of life and that they were significantly more likely to have had such separations than either psychotic or personality-disorder controls. Soloff and Millward (1983a) compared separation experiences in the background of 45 patients with BPD to those of depressive and schizophrenic comparison groups. They found that patients with BPD were significantly more likely to come from broken families than either control group. They also found that patients with BPD had a significantly higher incidence of loss of their fathers by death or divorce (47 percent).

These three initial studies had methodological problems by virtue of either small or clinically diagnosed samples and/or by use of nonblind assessments. Two more recent studies with stronger methodology have also examined the issues of parental separation and loss. Zanarini and colleagues (in press, a) compared the separation experiences of 50 outpatients with borderline personality disorder to those of patients with other forms of personality disorder. Nearly one-half (46 percent) of the patients with BPD reported experiencing a significant (> 1 month) separation before the age of six and 74 percent reported such a separation before the age of 18. The frequency of the early separations was not significantly higher compared to early separations found in patients with antisocial personality disorder, but was significantly higher than that found in patients with other personality disorders. Links and associates (1988) found that a significantly greater number of inpatients with BPD (25 percent) reported having been separated (> 3 months) from their primary caretaker during early childhood than did controls who exhibited borderline traits.

DISTURBED PARENTAL INVOLVEMENT. The original empirical study to characterize the families of borderline personality disorder patients (Grinker et al, 1968) found that a minority (12.8 percent) were characterized by relationships in which the parents were overinvolved and overprotective. Another nine families were characterized by a pervasive denial of problems, which was evidenced by the absence of marital discord and the lack of strong parental affect of either a positive or negative nature. Subsequently, Walsh (Grinker and Werble, 1977) found that a greater percentage (57 percent) of patients with BPD felt that they were overinvolved with one parent with whom they had a special relationship. In accordance with Masterson's theory, these relationships were judged as supportive of the parent's "need to be needed" but destructive to the patient's need to have a life of his or her own. Walsh also found that most (87 percent) of the patients with BPD characterized their relationships with one or both parents as lacking in feelings of attachment. These patients described their parents variously as "aloof," "detached," "remote," and "preoccupied."

Gunderson and colleagues (1980) studied three groups of patients who had intact families: those with borderline personality, paranoid schizophrenia, and neurosis/other Axis II disorders. The group with BPD had parents who were found to be more likely than the parents of schizophrenics, and less likely than the parents of neurotics, to invest in their children at the expense of their marriage. The families of probands with BPD also exhibited more paternal psychopathology and maternal ineffectiveness than found in the parents of either comparison group. More generally, results failed to show a high level of overinvolved families for the patients with BPD, but rather a "rigid tightness of the marital bond to the exclusion of the attention, support, or protection of the children."

Frank and Paris (1981) compared the accounts of parental attitudes of three female samples: those with BPD, those with neuroses/other personality disorders, and normal controls. All three groups reported disturbed attitudes in their mothers. The groups with BPD remembered their fathers as significantly less interested in and less approving of them in general than did the other two groups. Their fathers, more specifically, were reported to be less interested in and less approving of dependent behaviors than controls with neuroses/other personality disorders. The investigators speculated that BPD in females may be due, in part, to the failure of such fathers to protect their daughters from the disturbed dependency concerns of their mothers. In a subsequent small study of parental attitudes, Frank and Hoffman (1986) found that females with BPD remembered both their mothers and fathers as significantly less nurturant and less affectionate than did neurotic controls.

Soloff and Millward (1983a) found that inpatients with BPD, as well as controls with depression and schizophrenia, saw their mothers as being overinvolved with them. The patients with BPD were, however, significantly more likely to see their fathers as being underinvolved than patients from either control group.

Goldberg and colleagues (1985) retrospectively assessed the parental attitudes of 24 patients with BPD, 22 general psychiatric controls, and 10 normal controls using a self-report questionnaire. They found that patients with BPD remem-

Table 1. Childhood Environment Studies

Study	BPD+ (N)	Controls	Separation From or Disturbed Behavior of Parents/Other Caretakers					
			Loss/ Separation	Over-involvement	Under-involvement	High Conflict	Physical Abuse	Sexual Abuse
Grinker et al (1968)	47							
Walsh (1977)	16	schizophrenic	57 %[a]	12.7%	19.2%	34%		
Bradley (1979)	14	psychotic nonpsychotic delinquent	64 %[b]	57 %	86 %	64%		
Gunderson et al (1980)	12	schizophrenic neurosis/other Axis II disorder			[c]			
Frank and Paris (1981)	?	neurosis/other Axis II disorder normal			[d]			
Soloff and Millward (1983a)	45	schizophrenic major depressive	8.9%(m) 46.7%(f)[e]	48 %(m) 14 %(f)[e]	29 %(m) 72 %(f)[f]			
Goldberg et al (1985)	24	general psychiatric normal				69%(m)[e] 60%(f)[e]		

Table 1. Childhood Environment Studies (Continued)

Study	BPD† (N)	Controls	Separation From or Disturbed Behavior of Parents/Other Caretakers					
			Loss/ Separation	Over- involvement	Under- involvement	High Conflict	Physical Abuse	Sexual Abuse
Zanarini et al (in press, a)	50	antisocial other Axis II (+ dysthymia)	46 %[g]				46.0%[g]	26.0%[g]
Links et al (1988)	88	borderline traits	25 %[h]				29.4%[h]	25.9%[h]

†All studies pertain to DIB or *DSM-III* BPD, except Grinker et al (1968) and **Walsh** (1977), which pertain to a clinical diagnosis of BPD.

[a-g]Pertain to significant differences between borderlines and controls.

[a]Higher rate of loss of parents through divorce or death than schizophrenic controls.

[b]Higher rate of early childhood separation from primary caretaker than any of control groups.

[c]Results suggest parents involved with one another to exclusion of children.

[d]Results suggest that fathers of borderlines are less approving and more disinterested than fathers of both types of controls.

[e]Higher rate of loss of father through divorce or death than either control group; lower rate of overinvolvement and higher rate of underinvolvement of fathers than either control group; higher rate of conflict with both mothers and fathers than either control group.

[f]Results suggest that parents of borderlines are less caring than parents of both types of controls.

[g]Higher rate of early separation and sexual abuse than dysthymic or other personality disorder controls.

[h]Higher rate of early separation, physical, and sexual abuse than borderline trait controls.

bered both their parents as significantly less caring than did those in either control group. They also found that patients with BPD remembered their parents as significantly more overprotective than did the normal controls.

FAMILY CONFLICT. The most common (approximately one-third) pattern that Grinker and colleagues (1968) observed in their families with BPD was a high degree of discord between the mother and her children and between the two parents. Walsh (1977) found that 64 percent of her cohort with BPD reported strongly negative, highly conflictual relationships with their parents, which were characterized by parental hostility, devaluation, or frank abuse. Patients with BPD also commonly (79 percent) reported that their parents had a highly conflicted relationship, marked by the presence of demeaning attitudes and outright rejection.

Soloff and Millward (1983a) reported that their patients with BPD saw their relationships with their mothers and fathers as being significantly more negative and conflictual than did the two control samples. Moreover, patients with BPD were less likely than control patients to characterize their parental relationships as positive. In addition, 80 percent of patients with BPD saw their parents' marriages as being conflictual in nature. However, 75 percent of the depressed patients and 43 percent of the patients with schizophrenia also characterized their parents' marriages in this manner.

PHYSICAL AND SEXUAL ABUSE. Since Walsh's (1977) original comment about parental abuse in the history of patients with BPD, two studies have directly addressed this issue. In the first of these studies, Zanarini and colleagues (in press, a) found that nearly one-half of a group of borderline outpatients with BPD reported a childhood history of physical abuse and 26 percent reported a childhood history of sexual abuse. The frequency of sexual abuse, but not of physical abuse, differentiated the patients with BPD from two groups of controls with other personality disorders. Links and colleagues (1988) found that 29.4 percent of inpatients with BPD reported a childhood history of physical abuse and 25.9 percent reported a childhood history of sexual abuse. Both forms of abuse were significantly more common in patients with BPD than in their inpatient control group.

OVERVIEW OF FAMILY ENVIRONMENT STUDIES. The validity of studies based on retrospective reports of the involvement between patients with BPD and their families is difficult to judge. In particular, the studies that depend upon the patient's reconstruction of his or her past are invariably contaminated by conscious and unconscious distortions. Reports from the parents are similarly contaminated by possible biases.

A few conclusions that are sufficiently repetitious to be assigned good credibility, however, are the following: 1) mothers are sometimes but not always overinvolved and/or resistant to separations; 2) patients with BPD usually see their relationships to their mothers as highly conflictual, distant, or uninvolved; 3) the father's failures to be present and involved is an even more discriminating aspect of these families than the mother's problems; 4) childhood sexual and physical abuse are common antecedents whose effects may predispose to borderline psychopathology; and 5) disturbed relationships with both parents may be more pathogenic and specific than that with either one alone.

Family History Studies

Family history studies usually refer to studies of the familial prevalence of psychiatric disorders in biological relatives. If a diagnostic group such as patients with borderline personality disorder is found to have an excess occurrence of any type of disorder in its relatives, this is believed to reflect an etiological linkage. Although this type of study cannot distinguish between genetic and environmental effects, if a disorder has an excess of its own type of disorder in its relatives then it is thought to "breed true." This is considered strong evidence of the validity of that disorder (Robins and Guze, 1970). More definitive separation of genetic and environmental effects on the origins of borderline personality disorder depend upon twin and adoption studies.

FAMILIAL PREVALENCE STUDIES. In the past 10 years there have been about 10 studies on the family prevalence of psychiatric disorders in the relatives of patients with BPD. Aspects of these studies are summarized in Table 2. The comparison of the results of these studies is handicapped by the variable diagnostic standards used for the proband group, the variable methods of assessment used for the relatives (often combining direct interviews, chart information, and patient reports), and the variable ways in which results are reported (that is, some studies report the percentage of the probands with an affected relative, whereas most report the percentage of affected relatives; some studies report prevalence rates, while others report the morbid risk of developing such a disorder). Moreover, reports vary about whether to limit or subdivide the relatives into those which are first degree, second degree, or third degree. Finally, the reports are highly variable as to which diagnostic categories in the relatives are studied. Despite these handicaps, this review reveals some areas of consensus.

Stone (1977, 1979, 1981) pioneered studies on the families of patients with BPD. His first two efforts (1977, 1979) involved samples diagnosed as having a borderline personality organization (Kernberg, 1975) and contrasted them with proband groups having neuroses or psychoses. Relatives were categorized according to the degree to which they fit into a schizophrenia spectrum or into a manic-depressive spectrum. His results suggested a high frequency of affectively ill relatives for the patients with BPD and a low frequency of schizophrenia-spectrum disorders. These results were important, despite methodological problems, because they reoriented psychiatrists away from linking borderline personality to schizophrenia and toward the idea of a possible linkage to affective illness. A third study (Stone et al, 1981) compared another sample of borderline probands to psychotic patients as well as nonpsychiatric controls. This study confirmed his earlier finding that patients with BPD appeared to have a higher than expected frequency of affective disorder in their relatives but no increase in schizophrenia-spectrum disorders. Stone's familial history studies led him to conclude that borderline personality was linked to the affective disorders, and even to suggest that the nature of this linkage was genetic.

In a similar vein, Akiskal conducted several studies on the family prevalence of psychiatric disorders in relatives of patients with BPD (Akiskal, 1981; Akiskal et al, 1985a, 1985b). Akiskal and colleagues (1985a) found that the borderline probands had a significantly higher rate of familial affective disorder (bipolar disorder or major depression) than either the schizophrenic group (35 percent versus 9 percent, respectively) or than a group with other forms of personality

Table 2. Family History Studies†

Study	BPD†† (N)	Controls	Schizophrenia	Affective Disorder	Substance†† Abuse	BPD	APD	SPD
Stone (1977)	28	neurotic	8.9	12.5	1.8			
Stone (1979)	23	psychotic	0.0[a]	18.7[a]	5.5			
Stone et al (1981)	39	psychotic normal	0.7[b]	14.1[b]	7.4			
Akiskal et al (1985a)††††	97	schizophrenic bipolar major depressive other Axis II	3.0[c]	35.0[c]				
Akiskal et al (1985b)††††	24	major depressive other Axis II		33.3				
Andrulonis and Vogel (1984)††††	106	schizophrenic affective	4.0[d]	32.0	35.0			
Loranger et al (1982)††††	83	schizophrenic bipolar	0.0	6.9[e]		11.7[e]		
Loranger and Tulis (1985)††††	83	schizophrenic bipolar			18.4[f]			
Soloff and Millward (1983b)	48	schizophrenic major depressive	2.6	8.7[g]	11.8		7.0	
Pope et al (1983)	33	schizophrenic bipolar	0.0	6.2[h]	11.5	7.7[h]		
Schulz et al (1986)	26	schizophrenic antisocial	4.9	16.8[i]	12.9[i]		7.6[i]	
Zanarini et al (in press, b)	50	other Axis II (+ dysthymia)	0.0	28.4[j]	28.4	22.3[j]	12.2	

Percent Diagnosable First Degree Relatives††

Table 2. Family History Studies† (Continued)

Study	BPD†† (N)	Controls	Percent Diagnosable First Degree Relatives					
			Schizophrenia	Affective Disorder	Substance††† Abuse	BPD	APD	SPD
Links et al (1988)†††††			0.0	31.1	21.0	15.3	9.6	
Baron et al (1985)†††††	17	schizotypal normal		13.3	13.6	17.9[k]		3.1[k]

†BPD indicates Borderline Personality Disorder; APD indicates Antisocial Personality Disorder; SPD indicates Schizotypal Personality Disorder.

††All studies pertain to DIB or DSM-III BPD, except Stone (1979) and Stone et al (1981), which pertain to the broader concept of borderline personality organization.

†††All studies, except Andrulonis and Vogel (1984) and Zanarini et al (in press, b) pertain to alcohol abuse, as opposed to alcohol + drug abuse.

††††These studies pertain to percent of patients who had at least one first degree relative with the disorder, as opposed to percent of first degree relatives with the disorder.

†††††These studies pertain to lifetime expectancy (morbid risk) rates, as opposed to unadjusted prevalence rates.

[a-k]Pertain to significant differences between rates of borderlines and controls (see below for details).

[a]Lower rate of schizophrenia and higher rate of affective disorder than psychotic controls.

[b]Lower rate of schizophrenia than psychotic controls; higher rate of affective disorder than normal controls.

[c]Lower rate of schizophrenia than schizophrenic controls; higher rate of affective disorder than schizophrenic or Axis II controls.

[d]Lower rate of schizophrenia than schizophrenic controls.

[e]Higher rate of depression than schizophrenic controls; higher rate of BPD than either control group.

[f]Higher rate of alcohol abuse than either control group.

[g]Lower rate of depression than depressed controls.

[h]Higher rate of affective disorder than schizophrenic controls; higher rate of "dramatic" cluster personality disorders than either control group.

[i]Higher rate of depression, alcohol abuse, and APD than schizophrenic controls.

[j]Higher rate of affective disorder than antisocial controls; higher rate of BPD than either control group.

[k]Higher rate of BPD than either control group; lower rate of SPD than schizotypal controls.

disorder (35 percent versus 12 percent, respectively). Similar to Stone's studies, no increase in the frequency of schizophrenia was found among the relatives. In a second study, Akiskal and colleagues (1985b) again found that one-third of the borderline probands had a first degree relative with an affective disorder and that this rate was about the same as the rate seen in probands with affective disorder, but was greater than that found in probands with other personality disorders. Like Stone, Akiskal concluded that these results supported the idea of a genetic linkage between affective disorders and borderline personality. The results, however, have been criticized because many of the borderline patients had concurrent major affective disorders that were not identified or controlled for and which might account for the frequency of affective disorder in the relatives.

Andrulonis (Andrulonis et al, 1982; Andrulonis and Vogel, 1984) found a higher than expected prevalence of affective disorder in the relatives of both the borderline (32 percent) and the schizophrenic comparison group (33 percent), but these prevalence rates were somewhat less than that observed in the relatives of patients with affective disorders (46 percent). Because they tried explicitly to exclude patients with BPD who had a concurrent affective disorder from their sample, this offers an explanation for the disparity of the results from the earlier studies by Stone and Akiskal. Like the latter authors, they confirm that patients with BPD were significantly less likely than patients with schizophrenia to have a family history of schizophrenia. Moreover, they found that a sufficiently high rate of substance abuse (35 percent) in the first degree relatives of the patients with BPD suggests a possible linkage to substance use disorders.

Loranger and colleagues (1982) compared the family history of female inpatients with BPD with those of patients with bipolar disorder and schizophrenia. Raters reviewed the chart information on the relatives and assigned them diagnoses of borderline, bipolar, schizophrenic, or depressive disorders. Modifications on the prevalence rates were made to yield an estimate of the lifetime expectancy of each disorder. The rate of major depression (6.4 percent) was similar to that seen in the relatives of the bipolar patients, whereas there was no increase in bipolar disorder. Like Akiskal's study, it was unclear to what extent the affective disorder in the relatives was linked to the presence of a concurrent affective disorder in the borderline probands. Like all previous studies, the frequency of schizophrenia in the relatives (.54 percent) was quite low. Of particular note was Loranger's observation that the patients with BPD were 10 times more likely than relatives of either comparison group to have been treated for a "borderline-link" disorder. Despite the fact that the borderline disorder could not be well documented among the relatives, this finding is the first evaluation of the possibility and the first evidence that showed borderline personality "breeds true." Loranger and Tulis (1983) also found a prevalence of alcoholism/alcohol abuse (18.4 percent) in the relatives of the patients with BPD, which was significantly higher than either of the comparison groups—even when the comparison was between the probands who had never themselves abused alcohol. The possible linkage with substance abuse is similar to that noted by Andrulonis and Vogel (1984).

Soloff and Millward (1983b) studied the family history of borderline patients compared to patients with schizophrenia and unipolar depression. They found a higher prevalence of affective disorder in the families of the patients with BPD compared to those with schizophrenia, but significantly less than in the families of the depressed probands. Borderline personality disorder patients were also significantly less likely than the relatives of the depressed probands to have neurological disorders. Coupled with the observation that the relatives of the schizophrenic patients were not only more apt to have schizophrenia but also epilepsy, the results weigh against a theory which would link borderline personality to neurological dysfunction.

Although they unfortunately did not look for the prevalence of borderline personality in the relatives, Soloff and Millward found that the frequency of antisocial personality was almost twice that in the families of the patients with BPD than in either comparison group. This observation, which partially offsets the failure to find an increase in substance abuse, encourages theories that link borderline personality to disorders of impulse and action. More specifically, it suggests there may be some underlying linkage in genetics and/or environmental origins for borderline and antisocial personality disorders.

Pope and colleagues (1983), like Loranger before them, compared the prevalence of psychiatric disorder in the families of a borderline sample to groups of bipolar and schizophrenic controls. Borderline patients had an increased prevalence of affective disorder in their relatives—but only if the index borderline had an affective disorder. Without this distinction the rate of affective disorder in the first degree relatives of patients with BPD resembled those observed in the studies of Loranger and of Soloff and Millward. Concurrent presence of an affective disorder in the patients with BPD increased the prevalence of affective disorder fivefold in the family. Although being borderline did not increase the likelihood of either substance abuse or schizophrenia in the relatives, it did significantly enhance the likelihood of having a "dramatic cluster" (histrionic, borderline, antisocial) type of personality disorder. This finding, like Loranger's, raises the specter that patients with BPD "breed true" and, like Soloff and Millward, suggests a possible linkage to antisocial personality.

Three subsequent studies explored the familial relationship between BPD, unipolar affective disorder, substance abuse, and antisocial personality disorder. Schulz and colleagues (unpublished manuscript, 1986) looked at a sample of inpatients with BPD and found that the prevalence rate of major depression was significantly higher in the families of borderline probands (15.3 percent) than in the families of schizophrenic controls. They also noted that the rate of alcoholism (13 percent) and antisocial personality disorder (7.6 percent) was significantly greater than in the relatives of schizophrenics.

Zanarini and colleagues (in press, b) studied the family histories of 48 outpatients with BPD and two groups of personality disordered controls. High prevalence rates were found for unipolar affective disorders, substance use disorders, and personality disorders of either a borderline or antisocial nature. No first degree relative of a borderline proband, however, met *Diagnostic and Statistical Manual of Mental Disorders, Third Edition (DSM-III)* (American Psychiatric Association, 1980) criteria for schizophrenia. Borderlines were significantly more likely than either antisocial or dysthymic/other personality disorder controls to have a family history of BPD. They were also significantly more likely than antisocial controls to have a first degree relative who met *DSM-III* criteria for dysthymic disorder. However, they were significantly less likely than antisocial controls to have an impaired relative who met *DSM-III* criteria for antisocial personality disorder. Taken together, these results suggest that BPD breeds true. They also suggest a nonspecific link to affective disorder as well as a link to both Axis I and Axis II impulse disorders.

Links and colleagues (1988) studied the family histories of 69 borderline inpatients. Although control groups were not used, the results of this study indicate a high prevalence of depression, alcoholism, drug abuse, borderline personality disorder, and antisocial personality disorder as well as an absence of schizophrenia among the first degree relatives of borderline probands.

Baron and associates (1985) were the first to undertake a family history study specifically directed at examining the relationship between borderline and schizotypal personality disorders. Both the schizotypal and borderline probands were recruited from nonclinical populations and most (15 to 17) of the borderline sample was made up of people who met only three or four of the *DSM-III* criteria. Schizotypal probands had a significantly greater risk of schizotypal personality disorder in their relatives than did either the borderline probands or normal controls. The relatives of the borderlines had a significantly greater risk of borderline personality than did the relatives of the schizotypal or normal controls. The latter finding again supports the idea of borderline personality breeding true but this conclusion must be viewed with suspicion due to the idiosyncracies in the sampling in this study. The relatives of the borderline probands were at greater risk for major depression than the relatives of the schizotypals. More generally, the differences in the familial patterns of psychiatric illnesses led Baron and colleagues to conclude that schizotypal and borderline disorders are separate diagnostic entities—at least regarding their familial transmission—whether genetic or environmental.

TWIN AND ADOPTIVE STUDIES. Baron's conclusion that borderline and schizotypal disorders are genetically separate echoes the conclusion from an adoptive sample (Gunderson et al, 1983). Gunderson and colleagues reexamined the 27 interview records of biological relatives of schizophrenic adoptees who had been called "borderline schizophrenics" in the original Danish extended family study (Kety et al, 1968). A syndrome was identified in these relatives that was clearly distinct from borderline personality disorder. This syndrome overlapped with—but in some ways clearly differed from—the *DSM-III* definition of schizotypal personality disorder. The results helped distinguish between borderline and schizotypal personality and pointed toward the value of redefining the latter. The results failed to show any linkage in the genetic transmission of borderline and schizophrenic disorders.

Torgersen (1984) has conducted the only twin study of patients with BPD. When he looked at co-twins of the probands with borderline personality, he found that none of three monozygotic co-twins, and two of seven dizygotic co-twins, were concordant. In contrast, he found that 7 of 21 monozygotic co-twins of schizotypal probands were schizotypal, while only 1 of the 23 dizygotic co-twins was—a difference significant at $p<.02$. From these results, Torgersen concluded that genetic factors seemed to influence the development of schizotypal personality but not borderline personality disorder. Because he also found that no schizotypal proband had a borderline co-twin, and no borderline proband had a schizotypal co-twin, he also concluded the disorders were genetically independent of one another. However, the 29 percent concordance of borderline personality disorder in the dizygotic twins can be seen as supporting the familial nature of this disorder, even though the lack of concordance for borderline personality disorder in the three monozygotic twin pairs speaks against this genetic influence being very powerful. Clearly, further studies using larger twin samples are needed.

OVERVIEW OF FAMILY HISTORY STUDIES.   As noted above, the methodological limitations and variations among these studies make generalizations or firm conclusions difficult. To a large extent these studies were initially prompted by an interest in identifying a linkage between borderline personality and schizophrenia. No studies support such a linkage. The early failure to find confirmation of this by Stone and Akiskal was accompanied by results which pointed toward a link with affective disorders. Subsequent studies have shown quite uniformly an elevated prevalence of affective disorder in the relatives of borderline probands, but also have shown clearly that the linkage between these disorders is neither uniform nor strong. The studies have shown a failure for borderline personality to be associated with bipolar disorder, and have shown that even depressive disorders in the relatives is usually related to concurrent depressions in the borderline probands. Moreover, the studies have rarely employed a comparison group with a different type of personality disorder to determine whether the observed rates of affective disorder in the relatives implies any specificity for the borderline type of personality disorder.

After pursuing the linkage to schizophrenia and affective disorder, a third major direction in which the family prevalence studies has moved is toward the prevalence of personality disorders or traits. Here some of the studies have suggested that borderline personality breeds true (Loranger et al, 1982; Pope et al, 1983; Links et al, 1988; Zanarini et al, in press; Baron et al, 1985), an observation that lends credibility to the validity of this disorder. A number of these studies have also suggested that the borderline personality is linked to types of impulse or action disorder such as antisocial personality (Soloff et al, 1982; Schulz et al, 1986; Links et al, 1988; Zanarini et al, in press, b). These results are particularly interesting. Whereas the original putative linkage to schizophrenia might have suggested an underlying disorder in cognition, and the subsequent theory of a linkage to affective disorder suggested that the problem might be in relation to affect, this third set of studies suggests that the core problem for patients with BPD may be in the arena of impulse and action. Such a linkage would join borderline personality to antisocial and perhaps other forms of personality disorder in a way that harkens back to Kernberg's conceptualization of a similar underlying personality organization for many Axis II disorders.

Neurobiological Studies

BIOLOGICAL MARKER STUDIES.   *Dexamethasone Suppression Test (DST)*: Nine studies have attempted to assess the response of borderline patients to the DST (Carroll et al, 1981; Soloff et al, 1982; Sternbach et al, 1983; Val et al, 1983; Beeber et al, 1984; Krishnan et al, 1984; Steiner et al, 1984; Silk et al, 1985). This work is set against the backdrop of prior studies which have suggested that failure to suppress dexamethasone reflects an abnormal limbic system–neuroendocrine regulation problem that is seen frequently in seriously depressed patients. Hence, much of this work was done with borderline samples to evaluate a relationship to affective disorders.

Table 3 summarizes the series of studies done on DST response in borderline samples. In general, these studies have shown a broad range of nonsuppressive responses from a low of 16 percent (Soloff et al, 1982) to a high of 73 percent (Baxter et al, 1984). When the samples of borderline patients were divided into those with or without concurrent major affective disorder, it was found that the presence of a concurrent major affective disorder could account for most or all of the positive DSTs (Carroll et al, 1981; Soloff et al, 1982; Sternbach et al, 1983; Val et al, 1983; Beeber et al, 1984; Steiner et al, 1984; Silk et al, 1985). The only exception in this regard was in the study by Krishnan and colleagues (1984), which found that 33 percent (8 of 24) of his borderlines had a positive DST response, but only three of the seven with a concurrent major depression had a positive response.

Four of these DST studies used nonborderline comparison samples. When these samples were composed of patients with major affective disorder, no difference in the frequency of positive DSTs from the borderline samples was found (Beeber et al, 1984; Silk et al, 1985). However, in two other studies that used either normal (Sternbach et al, 1983) or general psychiatric controls (Baxter et al, 1984), a significantly higher percentage of borderlines were nonsuppressors.

In general, these studies suggest that many borderline patients have a problem with limbic system–neuroendocrine regulation similar to that found in many patients with major affective disorder. However, frquently those patients with BPD who evidence this also have major affective disorder; and because there are ongoing questions about the specificity of the DST to affective disordered patients, these results do little to inform the nosologic questions about the interface between borderline and affective disorders.

Thyrotropin-Releasing Hormone Test (TRH): Like the DST, this test too has been

Table 3. Dexamethasone Response Studies

Study	BPD† (N)	Controls	Percent of Borderlines		
			Depressed	Positive DST	Both
Carroll et al (1981)	21		62%	62%	62%
Soloff et al (1982)	19		74%	16%	21%
Sternbach et al (1983)	24	normal	71%	54%[a]	65%
Val et al (1983)	10		100%	50%	50%
Baxter et al (1984)	26	general psychiatric	54%	73%[a]	?
Beeber et al (1984)	13	depressive	100%	62%	62%
Krishnan et al (1984)	24		29%	33%	43%
Steiner et al (1984)	21		100%	29%	29%
Silk et al (1985)	22	depressive	100%	50%	50%

†All studies pertain to DIB or *DSM-III* borderline personality disorder.
[a]Significantly higher rate of positive response than controls.
? = unknown.

used on borderline samples to test whether they share some biological predisposition with affectively disordered patients.

Garbutt and colleagues (1983) found that a significantly greater number of patients with BPD (47 percent) than normal controls (0 percent) had a blunted thyroid-stimulating hormone (TSH) response to TRH. However, 57 percent (4 of 7) of those with the abnormal response had concurrent affective disorders. In a later study, Garbutt and colleagues (1987) found that 3 of 12 patients (25 percent) with borderline personality disorder had a blunted response. Sternbach and associates (1983) found that 38 percent of their borderline sample had a blunted TSH response to TRH compared to 1 of 11 normal controls. The borderline patients who had concurrent depressions were more likely to have a blunted response than those without depressions.

Like the DST studies, these studies show a high frequency of abnormal tests, but the abnormal tests frequently reflected concurrent affective disorders.

Rapid Eye Movement (REM) Sleep Studies: Depressed patients have been found to have shortened REM latencies on electroencephalographic (EEG) studies. Hence, the performance of borderline patients on this measure has also assumed interest.

Six sleep studies of criteria-defined borderline personality disorder patients have been conducted to date. Five of these studies have found that the REM latencies of patients with BPD and depressed controls are very similar (Akiskal, 1981; Akiskal et al, 1985b; Bell et al, 1983; McNamara et al, 1984; Reynolds et al, 1985), while one (King et al, 1987) found that the mean REM latency of a depressed control group was significantly shorter than that of borderline probands. One-half of these six studies have also found that the mean REM latency of the patients with BPD was significantly shorter than that of normal controls (Akiskal et al, 1985b; McNamara et al, 1984; Reynolds et al, 1985). In addition, two studies have found that the mean REM latency of personality-disordered controls was significantly longer than that of borderline probands (Akiskal, 1981; Akiskal et al, 1985b).

These studies of REM latency point toward similarities with depressive patients and show that both groups are distinct from the sleep records found in normals. Most of the studies have not controlled carefully for depressions within the borderline cohorts nor used comparison groups with other psychiatric disorders. These methodological problems limit the degree to which a linkage with affective disorders can be inferred.

Neurological Studies: Kutcher and colleagues (1987) compared the event-related auditory EEG potentials of patients with BPD to groups with nonborderline Axis II disorders, schizophrenics, depressives, and normals. Patients with BPD and schizophrenia were found to have similar event-related potentials, but they differed significantly from those in the two other groups by having a longer P3 latency and a smaller P3 amplitude.

Snyder and associates (1983) found that the CT scans of male patients with BPD were normal (that is, there was no evidence of cerebral ventricular enlargements). Subsequently, Snyder and Pitts (1984) compared the EEG records of male inpatients with BPD to those with dysthymic disorder. Both samples had similar rates of marginally abnormal EEGs, but those with BPD had significantly more (19 percent) definitely abnormal EEGs. In addition, both slow wave activity and wave fusing were significantly more common in the borderline than in the dysthymic controls.

Cowdry and colleagues (1985) also found significantly more definitely abnormal EEG records ($p = .003$) in a borderline sample than in depressed controls. In addition, significantly more patients with BPD (41 percent) than depressed controls (5 percent) exhibited some form of definite posterior sharp abnormality.

Although the difference was not statistically significant, Cornelius and associates (1986) found more temporal lobe dysrhythmias in their borderline sample (18.8 percent) than in patients with other Axis II disorders (9 percent). However, the dysrhythmias found in the borderline cohort did not correlate with the clinical symptoms usually associated with temporal lobe difficulties.

Gardner and co-workers (1987) compared soft signs of neurological disorder (e.g., dysarthric speech, right–left confusion, mixed lateral dominance) in female patients with BPD to normal controls. Over one-half (65 percent) of the borderline subjects had two or more of these neurological soft signs, which was significantly higher than the 32 percent found in the normal control group.

OTHER NEUROBIOLOGICAL STUDIES. Schulz and colleagues (1985) compared the responses of patients with BPD and normal controls to administration of amphetamine, a substance that increases dopamine transmission. Fifty percent of the patients with BPD, but no controls, were rated as psychotic after amphetamine administration; a difference significant at the $p<.02$ level. In addition, global ratings of well-being were significantly elevated in the borderline group compared to the normal group.

Work by Lucas and associates (1987) has also stimulated interest in abnormal central dopaminergic activity for borderline patients. They studied the response to methylphenidate infusion of three subjects with BPD, four with major depression, and five with schizophrenia. Two borderline but no control subjects developed episodes of intense dysphoria that closely resembled their spontaneously occurring dysphorias. As methylphenidate enhances dopaminergic activity, Lucas and colleagues reasoned that the dysphoric experiences of BPD patients may derive from excess dopamine. As noted earlier, Garbutt and colleagues (1987) studied the TSH response to TRH of 12 BPD patients. They subsequently administered haloperidol for seven days, and a second TRH test was given. This revealed that haloperidol did not increase the TSH response of the borderlines as a group or, more particularly, the three subjects who had shown a blunted response to the first TSH test. Garbutt and associates concluded that reductions in TSH response in patients with BPD are not secondary to excess dopamine.

Chapin and co-workers (1987) administered a reaction time test to 5 groups of 12 subjects: borderline, schizophrenic, depressed, schizotypal, and normal control subjects. Borderlines had a significantly longer crossover time than schizotypal and schizophrenic patients, and a significantly longer reaction latency than schizotypal (but not schizophrenic) patients, findings which support the distinctness of the two Axis II disorders and suggest that schizotypal (but not borderline) personality disorder is a schizophrenia spectrum disorder.

OVERVIEW OF NEUROBIOLOGICAL STUDIES. In general, the studies on biological markers are rapidly proliferating. Most involve tests (DST, TRH, REM latency) that have been useful in looking at other psychiatric disorders—notably affective types. Though the fact that many patients with BPD have abnormalities (especially in REM latency) keeps Klein's theory of affective dysregulation alive, the fact that the apparent similarities to affective disorders lessens when a concurrent affective disorder is absent weakens the evidence for that theory.

The exploration of neurological dysfunction has been mainly through EEG studies, which show increased abnormalities but have defied any consensus on localization. They do, however, validate Andrulonis's theory about the possible etiological role of such dysfunction. Some of the more exciting work has concerned infusion studies with amphetamines (Schulz et al, 1985; Lucas et al, 1987). This work implicates possible metabolic vulnerability in the central nervous system similar to that earlier put forth in the "dopamine hypothesis" for schizophrenia; that is, an excess of dopamine (or norepinephrine) at the synapses. As explicated by Cloninger (1987) this, in turn, might help explain "novelty seeking" aspects of borderline personality such as being impulsive, excitable, and quick-tempered.

SUMMARY

The broadest question that can be raised about the pathogenesis of borderline personality disorder concerns the relative contribution of genetic and environmental factors. Most theorists have included the likelihood that both are possible and are consistent with the core vulnerabilities which they identify. It seems highly unlikely that any serious type of psychopathology would not have some type of genetic predisposition. Indeed, even personality variants of healthier types appear to have unexpectedly powerful genetic determinants. It is equally transparent that the developmental histories and familial environments of patients with BPD are very disturbed. Their backgrounds are marked by highly conflicted and distorted parental involvement, a high frequency of separations from the parents during early childhood, and a high frequency of sexual and physical abuse. Despite the dangers of retrospective distortions, the variety of means by which these histories were obtained and their consistency across studies leaves little doubt about their general validity.

What is less certain than the likelihood of both genetic and environmental contributions is the question of whether either the genetic or the environmental factors have specificity for this type of personality development. It seems more likely that the genetic contribution is a broad predisposition which is insufficient in itself. Likewise, the broad range of developmental problems, such as parental loss, abuse, and emotional neglect, suggests that these two are nonspecific predisposing antecedents which are not sufficient to explain the origins of borderline personality.

These studies raise considerable doubts about the psychodynamic formulations on the origins of borderline personality, which suggest that the maldevelopment is determined by a specific development phase. Despite the frequent stipulation that a phase-specific parent–child interactional failure occurs between roughly 1 and 2½ years of age, there is little reason to expect that this is a necessary or sufficient antecedent for patients with BPD. Mahler herself (Mahler and Kaplan, 1977) noted that a child with severe problems during this "rapprochement" subphase could grow up without borderline psychopathology, and that another child with no problems during this period could grow up to be quite typically borderline. Moreover, such phase-specific theories fail to take into consideration the pathogenic influence of severe traumas that occur in later life, such as sexual and physical abuse, and more generally, the degree to which personality is shaped by ongoing, stable patterns of familial interactions, beliefs, communication, and social "fit" (Thomas and Chess, 1984).

There is a strong need for prospective studies on samples who are at "high risk" for the later development of borderline psychopathology. Such samples could now be identified by the presence of borderline psychopathology in the parents, identifiable separation problems in early childhood, and, in the future, perhaps by a biological marker. Such studies would allow a more definitive identification of the developmental factors that mitigate both for and against development of borderline psychopathology. It is timely that studies be done on patients with BPD through detailed pedigree analyses over multiple generations. This would help isolate the putative modes of genetic transmission and allow the identification of ameliorating or provoking environmental conditions. The many studies on family prevalence which have been done implicate familial factors in transmission but they do little to sort out to what extent this is genetic. Though future familial prevalence studies can add methodological advantages, they seem unlikely to add much to our understanding of links to psychiatric disorders. The major remaining frontier in this area is for more definitive studies on prevalence of personality types in relatives. Those which have been done largely concur in showing a linkage to impulse–action disorders (such as antisocial personality and substance abuse) and to depressive disorders and, most importantly, to borderline personality itself. The relative strengths of these linkages and their separation into environmental and genetic components depend upon more definitive twin and adoption strategies.

A variety of conceptualizations for the core sector of psychopathology for patients with BPD are apparent. Perhaps the one which has generated the most empirical research is the possibility of a basic failure of affective regulation. Two alternatives have presented themselves: that this, basic affective problems may relate to aggression as suggested by Kernberg, or to depression as suggested by Klein. The inquiries into the possible core affective dysfunction have been most extensive and were reviewed previously (Gunderson and Elliott, 1985). These studies have suggested that depressive disorders are neither necessary nor sufficient for the development of borderline personality, but that there are many overlaps in both biological features and developmental factors. Much less research has been done concerning the hypothesis of a basic problem of the regulation of aggresion. This is largely due to the lack of methodology for studying heightened aggressiveness. Nevertheless, this remains a viable and important theory insofar as it appears to be more specific than that which is offered by the emphasis upon depression. It may offer a way of understanding some of the most discriminating aspects of borderline phenomenology such as the hostility, manipulativeness, devaluation, and the self-concept of being evil.

A second sector that has been identified as a possible basis for borderline psychopathology involves cognition. Efforts to study cognitive failure via possible linkage to schizophrenia or even schizotypal personality have quite uniformly indicated that this is not a means of understanding the origins of borderline personality. Still, the failures to develop evocative memory, which were suggested by Adler and Buie, are tightly linked to neurophysiological maturational processes that may yet yield an important insight into the origins of this disorder which has not yet been studied. Moreover, the revival of a "dopamine hypothesis" for borderline personality keeps alive theories of a basic cognitive fault.

Andrulonis's suggestion that there may be a neurological dysfunction has been confirmed by the studies that have looked at EEG abnormalities—at least for a significant subset of people diagnosed as borderline. However, these studies have offered little evidence to localize or specify the nature of the neurological problem; and it is highly unlikely that these neurological problems, when present, alone are sufficient to explain the development of a borderline personality, or are sufficiently common in borderline subjects even to contribute to the origins of this disorder in many.

A final sector in which the core deficits have been suggested involves the management of impulses. Here, too, there is both dynamic theory and familial evidence in support of such a theory. It is a pattern of behavior to which patients with BPD are often extensively exposed in their families. Those reports that have linked borderline personality to substance abuse and antisocial personality suggest there may be some broader underlying mechanisms that join borderline personality to other types of impulse disorder. Although impulsivity has been noted in most dynamic formulations about borderline personality, usually it has been considered secondary.

While these sectors of basic or core psychopathology appear quite variable and often appear to be competing, it is wise to consider them as coinciding components for most patients with BPD. This kind of formulation lends itself to an understanding of pathogenesis that is in line with a systems theory and which includes such diverse pathogenic influences as neurophysiological limitations, traumatic childhoods, and ongoing environmental stresses.

The studies reviewed here show an era of great activity. These studies also indicate that continued development of our understanding of pathogenesis will require greater sophistication in research design to concurrently explore the biological, social, and psychological domains.

REFERENCES

Adler G: Borderline Psychopathology and Its Treatment. New York, Jason Aronson, 1985

Adler G, Buie D: Aloneness and borderline psychopathology: the possible relevance of child development issues. Int J Psychoanal 1979; 60:83–96

Akiskal HS: Subaffective disorders: dysthymic, cyclothymic and bipolar II disorders in the "borderline" realm. Psychiatr Clin North Am 1981; 4:25–46

Akiskal HS, Chen SE, Davis GC, et al: Borderline: an adjective in search of a noun. J Clin Psychiatry 1985a; 46:41–48

Akiskal HS, Yerevanian BI, Davis GC, et al: The nosologic status of borderline personality: clinical and polysomnography study. Am J Psychiatry 1985b; 142:192–198

American Psychiatric Association: Diagnostic and Statistical Manual of Mental Disorders, Third Edition. Washington, DC, Amerian Psychiatric Association, 1980

Andrulonis PA, Vogel NG: Comparison of borderline personality subcategories to schizophrenic and affective disorders. Br J Psychiatry 1984; 144:358–363

Andrulonis P, Glueck B, Stroebel C, et al: Organic brain dysfunction and the borderline syndrome. Psychiatr Clin North Am 1981; 4:61–66

Andrulonis P, Glueck B, Stroebel C, et al: Borderline personality subcategories. J Nerv Ment Dis 1982; 170:670–679

Baron M, Gruen R, Asnis L, et al: Familial transmission of schizotypal and borderline personality disorders. Am J Psychiatry 1985; 142:8

Baxter L, Edell W, Gerner R, et al: Dexamethasone suppression test and Axis I diagnosis of inpatients with DSM-III borderline disorder. J Clin Psychiatry 1984; 45:150–153

Beeber AR, Kline MD, Pies RW, et al: Dexamethasone suppression test in hospitalized depressed patients with borderline personality disorder. J Nerv Ment Dis 1984; 172: 301–303

Bell J, Lycaki H, Jones D, et al: Effect of preexisting borderline personality disorder on clinical and EEG sleep correlates of depression. Psychiatry Res 1983; 9:115–123

Bradley SJ: The relationship of early maternal separation to borderline personality in children and adolescents: a pilot study. Am J Psychiatry 1979; 136:424–426

Buie DH, Adler G: Definitive treatment of the borderline personality. Int J Psychoanal Psychother 1982; 9:51–87

Carroll BJ, Greden JT, Feinberg M, et al: Neuroendocrine evaluation of depression in borderline patients. Psychiatr Clin North Am 1981; 4:89–99

Chapin K, Wightman L, Lycaki H, et al: Difference in reaction time between subjects with schizotypal and borderline personality disorders. Am J Psychiatry 1987; 144:948–950

Chess TA: Genesis and evolution of behavioral disorders: from infancy to early adult life. Am J Psychiatry 1984; 141:1–9

Cloninger CR: A systematic method for clinical description and classification of personality variants. Arch Gen Psychiatry 1987; 44:579–588

Cornelius JR, Brenner RP, Soloff PH, et al: EEG abnormalities in borderline personality disorder: specific or nonspecific. Biol Psychiatry 1986; 21:974–977

Cowdry RW, Gardner DL: Pharmacotherapy of borderline personality disorder. Arch Gen Psychiatry 1988; 45:111–119

Cowdry RW, Pickar D, Davies R: Symptoms and EEG findings in the borderline syndrome. Int J Psychiatry Med 1985; 15:201–211

Frank H, Hoffman N: Borderline empathy: an empirical investigation. Compr Psychiatry 1986; 27:387–395

Frank H, Paris J: Recollections of family experience in borderline patients. Arch Gen Psychiatry 1981; 38:1031–1034

Garbutt JC, Loosen PT, Tipermas A, et al: The TRH test in patients with borderline personality disorder. Psychiatry Res 1983; 9:107–113

Garbutt JC, Loosen PT, Glenn M: Lack of effect of dopamine receptor blockade on the TSH response to TRH in borderline personality disorder. Psychiatry Res 1987; 21: 307–311

Gardner D, Lucas PB, Cowdry RW: Soft sign neurological abnormalities in borderline personality disorder and normal control subjects. J Nerv Ment Dis 1987; 175:177–180

Goldberg RL, Mann LS, Wise TN, et al: Parental qualities as perceived by borderline personality disorders. Hillside Journal of Clinical Psychiatry 1985; 7:134–140

Greenman DA, Gunderson JG, Cane M, et al: An examination of the borderline diagnosis in children. Am J Psychiatry 1986; 143:998–1003

Grinker RR Sr, Werble B, Drye RC: The Borderline Syndrome: A Behavioral Study of Ego-Functions. New York, Basic Books, 1968

Grotstein JS, Solomon MF, Lang J (Eds): The Borderline Patient: Emerging Concepts in Diagnosis, Psychodynamics and Treatment. Hillsdale, NJ, The Analytic Press, 1987

Gunderson JG: Borderline Personality Disorder. Washington, DC, American Psychiatric Press, Inc., 1984

Gunderson JG, Elliott GR: The interface between borderline personality and affective disorders. Am J Psychiatry 1985; 142:277–288

Gunderson JG, Englund DW: Characterizing the families of borderlines. Psychiatr Clin North Am 1981; 4:159–168

Gunderson J, Kerr J, Englund D: The families of borderlines: a comparative study. Arch Gen Psychiatry 1980; 37:27–33

Gunderson J, Siever L, Spaulding E: The search for a schizotype. Arch Gen Psychiatry 1983; 40:15–22

Kernberg O: Borderline Conditions and Pathological Narcissism. New York, Jason Aronson, 1975

Kernberg O: Object Relations Theory and Clinical Psychoanalysis. New York, Jason Aronson, 1976

Kety SS, Rosenthal D, Wender PH, et al: The types and prevalence of mental illness in the biological and adoptive families of adopted schizophrenics, in The Transmission of Schizophrenia. Edited by Rosenthal D, Kety SS. Oxford, Pergamon Press Ltd, 1968

King R, Benson KL, Zarcone BP Jr: REM latency in borderlines and depressed. Sleep Research 1987; 16:280

Klein DF: Psychopharmacology and the borderline patient in borderline states, in Psychiatry. Edited by Mack JD. New York, Grune & Stratton, 1975

Klein DF: Psychopharmacological treatment and delineation of borderline disorders, in Borderline Personality Disorders: The Concept, the Syndrome, the Patients. Edited by Hartocollis P. New York, International Universities Press, 1977

Kohut H: The Analysis of the Self. New York, International Universities Press, 1971

Krishnan KR, Davidson JRT, Rayasam K, et al: The Dexamethasone Suppression Test in borderline personality disorder. Biol Psychiatry 1984; 19:1149–1153

Kutcher SP, Blackwood DHR, St. Clair D, et al: Auditory P300 in borderline personality disorder and schizophrenia. Arch Gen Psychiatry 1987; 44:645–650

Liebowitz MR, Klein DG: Interrelationship of hysteroid dysphoria and borderline personality disorder. Psychiatr Clin North Am 1981; 4:67–87

Links PS, Steiner M, Huxley G: The occurrence of borderline personality disorder in the families of borderline patients. Journal of Personality Disorders 1988; 2:14–20

Links PS, Steiner M, Offord D, et al: Characteristics of borderline personality disorder: a Canadian study. Can J Psychiatry 1988; 33:336–340

Loosen PT, Prange AJ Jr: Serum thyrotropin response to thyrotropin-releasing hormone in psychiatric patients: a review. Am J Psychiatry 1982; 139:405–414

Loranger AW, Tulis EH: Family history of alcoholism in borderline personality disorder. Arch Gen Psychiatry 1983; 42:153–157

Loranger AW, Oldham JM, Tulis EH: Familial transmission of DSM-III borderline personality disorder. Arch Gen Psychiatry 1982; 39:795–799

Lucas PB, Gardner DL, Wolkowitz OM, et al: Dysphoria associated with methylphenidate infusion in borderline personality disorder. Am J Psychiatry 1987; 144:1577–1579

Mahler M: A study of the separation-individuation process and its possible application to borderline phenomena in the psychoanalytic situation. Psychoanal Study Child 1971; 26:403–424

Mahler M, Kaplan L: Developmental aspects in the assessment of narcissistic and so-called borderline personalities, in Borderline Personality Disorders: The Concept, the Syndrome, the Patients. Edited by Hartocollis P. New York, International Universities Press, 1977

Masterson JF: Borderline and narcissistic disorders: an integrated development object-relations approach, in Diagnosis, Psychodynamics and Treatment. Hillsdale, NJ, The Analytic Press, 1987

Masterson JF, Rinsley D: The borderline syndrome: the role of the mother in the genesis and psychic structure of the borderline personality. Int J Psychoanal 1975; 56:163–177

McNamara E, Reynolds CF III, Soloff PH, et al: EEG sleep evaluation of depression borderline patients. Am J Psychiatry 1984; 141:182–186

Pope HG, Jonas JM, Hudson JI, et al: The validity of DSM-III borderline personality disorder. Arch Gen Psychiatry 1983; 40:23-30

Reynolds CF III, Soloff PH, Kupfer DJ, et al: Depression in borderline patients: a prospective EEG sleep study. Psychiatry Res 1985; 14:1–15

Rinsley D: Borderline and Other Disorders. New York, Jason Aronson, 1982

Robins E, Guze SB: Establishment of diagnostic validity in psychiatric illness: its application to schizophrenia. Am J Psychiatry 1970; 126:983–987

Schulz PM, Kelly T, Di Franco R, et al: Borderline Personality Disorder: Family Histories. Paper presented at the 139th Annual Meeting of the American Psychiatric Association, Washington, DC, May 1986

Schulz SC, Schulz PM, Dommisse C, et al: Amphetamine response in borderline patients. Psychiatry Res 1985; 15:97–108

Schulz SC, Cornelius J, Brenner R, et al: Can amphetamine solve borderline heterogeneity? Proceedings of the IVth World Congress of Biological Psychiatry (in press)

Shapiro E, Zinner J, Shapiro R, et al: The influence of family experience on borderline personality development. International Review of Psychoanalysis 1975; 2:399–411

Siever L, Gunderson JG: Genetic determinants of borderline conditions. Schizophrenia Bull 1979; 5:59–86

Silk KR, Lohr NE, Cornell DG, et al: The Dexamethasone Suppression Test in borderline and nonborderline affective patients, in The Borderline: Current Empirical Research. Edited by McGlashan TH. Washington, DC, American Psychiatric Press, Inc., 1985

Snyder S, Pitts WM Jr, Gustin Q: CT scans of patients with borderline personality disorder (letter). Am J Psychiatry 1983; 140:272

Snyder S, Pitts WM Jr: Electroencephalography of DSM-III borderline personality disorder. Acta Psychiatr Scand 1984; 69:129–134

Snyder S, Sajadi C, Pitts WM Jr, et al: Identifying the depressive border of the borderline personality disorder. Am J Psychiatry 1982; 139:814–817

Soloff PH, Millward JW: Developmental histories of borderline patients. Compr Psychiatry 1983a; 24:574–588

Soloff PH, Millward JW: Psychiatric disorders in the families of borderline patients. Arch Gen Psychiatry 1983b; 40:37–44

Soloff PH, George A, Nathan RS: The Dexamethasone Suppression Test in patients with borderline personality disorder. Am J Psychiatry 1982: 139:1621–1623

Steiner M, Martin S, Wallace JE, et al: Distinguishing subtypes within the borderline domain: a combined psychoneuroendocrine approach. Biol Psychiatry 1984; 19:907–911

Sternbach HA, Fleming J, Extein I, et al: The dexamethasone suppression and thyrotropin-releasing hormone tests in depressed borderline patients. Psychoneuroendocrinology 1983; 8:459–462

Stone MH: The borderline syndrome: evolution of the term, genetic aspects, and prognosis. Am J Psychother 1977; 31:345–365

Stone MH: Contemporary shift of the borderline concept from a subschizophrenic disorder to a subaffective disorder. Psychiatr Clin North Am 1979; 2:577–594

Stone MH, Kahn E, Flye B: Psychiatrically ill relatives of borderline patients: a family study. Psychiatry Q 1981; 53:71–84

Thomas A, Chess S: Genesis and evolution of behavioral disorders. Am J Psychiatry 1984; 141:1–9

Torgersen S: Genetic and nosological aspects of schizotypal and borderline personality disorders: a twin study. Arch Gen Psychiatry 1984; 41:546–554

Val E, Nasr SJ, Gaviria FM, et al: Depression, borderline personality disorder and the DST. Am J Psychiatry 1983; 140–819

Walsh F: The family of the borderline patient, in The Borderline Patient. Edited by Grinker RR Sr, Werble B. New York, Jason Aronson, 1977

Zanarini MC, Gunderson JG, Marino MF, et al: Childhood experiences of borderline patients. Compr Psychiatry (in press, a)

Zanarini MC, Gunderson JG, Marino MF, et al: DSM-III disorders in the families of borderline outpatients. Journal of Personality Disorders (in press, b)

Chapter 3

Psychodynamic Therapies in Borderline Personality Disorder

by Gerald Adler, M.D.

OVERVIEW

The contributions of different theorists and clinicians who have written about the psychodynamic psychotherapeutic treatment of the borderline personality disorder must be examined in the context of several factors. First, it is not clear whether the patients they describe would meet the *Diagnostic and Statistical Manual of Mental Disorders, Third Edition, Revised* (*DSM-III-R*) (American Psychiatric Association, 1987) criteria for borderline personality disorder. For example, Kernberg's (1975) discussion of borderline personality organization is a broad category that includes a whole spectrum of patients with personality disorders, a portion of whom would have borderline personality disorder. In addition, many writers describe their work with "primitive" or "difficult" patients, some of whom clearly have borderline personality disorder. Thus, patients with borderline personality disorder are often lumped together with a heterogeneous group of patients. In spite of these difficulties, it is possible to get a sense from the literature of a spectrum of difficult patients, many of whom probably fulfill *DSM-III-R* criteria for borderline personality disorder.

Another factor that complicates this discussion relates to disagreements in the literature about the degree of "support" or "holding" such patients require in treatment, and how much the essence of the treatment involves confrontation and interpretation. Related are the issues of: 1) how much is deficit and how much is conflict in the etiology of these patients' difficulties, and 2) how to determine whether they need a "supportive" psychotherapeutic approach or one which is defined as "expressive" or "modified analytic" (Kernberg, 1975, 1976, 1982) or "exploratory" (Gunderson, 1984). Although there is a literature that debates these distinctions with valuable heuristic results, clinical and research experience reveal their complexity. Wallerstein (1986) demonstrates that these boundaries are not only blurred in clinical practice, but "supportive" approaches may lead to permanent changes as profound as those seen in the expressive or exploratory models.

The personalities of the clinicians who describe their work with their patients, including patients with borderline personality disorder, play an important role in their views of these patients (Adler, 1986; Gunderson, 1984). The fit between patient and therapist, the theoretical models the therapists bring to their work, and their basic personality characteristics interdigitate with these patients to determine an important aspect of the data obtained, and therefore result in both theoretical and clinical precepts about the understanding and treatment of patients with borderline personality disorder. Such factors must be considered in discussions which involve recommendations to clinicians.

Finally, it is not possible to discuss the psychodynamic treatment of patients with borderline personality disorder without emphasizing the importance of countertransference in the work with them. These are the patients who have the reputation of eliciting intense responses from their therapists, which often determine whether the therapy will survive and lead to constructive results or be a repetition of these patients' failed interpersonal experiences involving abandonment, rage, and self-punishment.

The literature about the psychotherapeutic treatment of patients with borderline personality disorder is vast and includes both theoretical and clinical as well as empirical studies. In a brief review, it is not possible to detail the work of many significant contributors. Among those who deserve careful study are Abend and colleagues (1983), Chessick (1977), Giovacchini (1979, 1984) Meissner (1984), Modell (1984), and Volkan (1987). There are also several recent excellent summaries available detailing current views in the understanding and treatment of the borderline patient that are useful: Goldstein (1985), Gunderson (1984), and Waldinger and Gunderson (1987).

MAJOR MODELS COMPARED

Attempts to categorize the different contributors to the understanding and treatment of the borderline personality disorder within certain dimensions present the dangers of oversimplification. While keeping this caveat in mind, the models of psychodynamic psychotherapy of five major contributors will be examined.

Waldinger and Gunderson (1987) have emphasized that intensive treatment of patients with borderline personality disorder must address a series of issues which include:

1. a stable framework that defines the boundaries of the treatment setting
2. demonstrating greater therapist activity than is usual with neurotic patients because of the borderline's reality testing problems, tendency to project and distort, and his or her tenuous sense of the therapist's presence
3. tolerating the negative transference
4. helping the patient with connections between actions and feelings
5. making self-destructive behaviors ungratifying, by clarification and confrontation
6. blocking the patient's acting-out behaviors by setting limits on actions that endanger either the person or the therapy
7. clarifying and interpreting the transference in the "here and now" in the early phases of treatment when genetic interpretations (i.e., those defining early environmental factors) can be disruptive
8. emphasizing the importance of countertransference feelings in work with these patients.

In this section and in those that follow, these considerations will be explored.

Kernberg

Kernberg's contributions (1975, 1976, 1980, 1982, 1984) have been in the forefront of advancing our understanding of patients with borderline personality disorder and their treatment. Although the borderline concept has been used since 1938 (Stern), and was gradually being defined in the growing literature as well as in everyday clinical discussions, Kernberg's 1967 paper (in Kernberg, 1975) was an exciting moment in advancing work with these patients. He brought together a descriptive, genetic, and dynamic understanding, and spelled out the clinical ramifications of these formulations. His descriptions of the treatment of borderline patients, by the relatively clear positions he takes on many of the basic theoretical and clinical issues, allows us to compare and contrast his work with other formulations.

By emphasizing the concept of splitting, Kernberg defines his understanding of these patients as one in which this conflictual basis of their psychopathology is central. Their conflicts are reflected in the primitive defenses they use to ward off their intense anger and longings. Kernberg sees the major difficulty of patients with a borderline personality organization as their inability to bring together positive self and object representations with those that have negative affects associated with them. This defensive constellation is a manifestation of their inability to tolerate ambivalence toward a person, and is a result either of an excessive amount of inborn aggression, or an environment that has not helped them integrate libidinal and aggressive self and object representations.

The result of this splitting process has profound clinical implications. These relatively unrepressed and dissociated parts readily and prematurely become activated in the transference, leading to the well-known intense transference and countertransference manifestations that are part of the experience in the treatment of the borderline patient. Since they are split-off parts, they are not an aspect of a more coherent reliving of actual childhood experiences that make up the transferences of healthier patients. The overriding insistence of the aggressive components elicits the intensification of the splitting process, with projective identification as a related major defense, and the increasing tendency to act out these primitive conflicts. Controlling this transference acting-out becomes a major task, since the analysis of the transference, to whatever extent it is possible, is at the core of Kernberg's work.

In his treatment of these patients Kernberg emphasizes three factors: interpretation, the maintenance of technical neutrality, and transference analysis. Kernberg clarifies that technical neutrality does not mean an absence of empathy. He emphasizes the therapist's capacity to maintain this neutrality in the face of the patient's regressive angry verbal assaults. In addition, the patient's potential for acting out threatens this technical neutrality. Although the therapist may be required to deviate from a neutral stance at such times, the goal is to return to it as soon as possible. The sharing with the patient of the therapist's dilemma when structure must be provided, the attempt to analyze the meanings of the patient's actions and the therapist's responses to them, and a position that expects the patient to assume responsibility for his or her actions help in this goal.

Kernberg carefully differentiates "supportive" from "expressive" psychotherapy. Supportive psychotherapy is reserved for those patients who have severe antisocial features, seriously disorganized life circumstances, a paucity of real people in their lives, or evidence of significant ego weakness; that is, lack of a capacity to tolerate anxiety or control impulses. In contrast to other writers (Knight, 1954; Zetzel, 1971), Kernberg's description of supportive psychotherapy emphasizes the importance of the transference. Although the therapist is aware of the transference, only the negative transference is explored in supportive psychotherapy. In addition, the therapist does not connect the transference interpretively to the patient's unconscious relationship to the therapist or to the past. The emphasis is the connection of the transference distortions within the treatment setting to distortions in the patient's other interpersonal experiences. In contrast, in expressive psychotherapy, which is a modification of psychoanalysis, the therapist will explore the full meaning of the transference to whatever extent it is possible. However, the usual interpretation of the transference with neurotic patients must be modified because the borderline patient has difficulties with reality testing in the transference situation and also cannot use genetic interpretations early in treatment. The therapist is required to be vigilant to the patient's distortions of the therapist's statements. These distortions must first be interpreted by the therapist before basic interpretations can be utilized by the patient.

Kernberg addresses the "holding environment" aspects (Winnicott, 1965) of treatment in his discussions of the therapist tolerating the patient's rage. Yet, the reader of his work may be left with the impression that his treatment is carried out in a cold, abstinent environment. In addition, his clinical examples may at times appear to illustrate a series of interpretations to patients that contain so much material that they cannot conceivably be integrated by that patient. Kernberg (1986) has clarified that such vignettes condense many sessions and cannot be taken literally. However, opportunities to see videotapes of Kernberg's actual treatment of patients and to hear his discussions of them reveal that there are many elements of his everyday work in his expressive psychotherapy that would be considered to be "supportive" by others who write about the treatment of patients with borderline personality disorder. Although he probably is more "abstinent" and "neutral" than some other workers in the field, his basic caring and concern for his patients, which is obviously present, is an area that he rarely addresses in his writing, and may give a one-sided impression of his treatment.

Masterson and Rinsley

Masterson (1976, 1981) and Rinsley (1982), separately and together (Masterson and Rinsley, 1975), have defined a therapeutic approach that has its roots, in part, in an extension of Kernberg's concept of splitting, and in part in Mahler's stages of separation–individuation (Mahler et al, 1975), especially the rapprochement subphase. Masterson and Rinsley originally described (1975) that borderline patients had mothers who rewarded their child's continued attachment and punished or withdrew from their child when he or she began to separate. The result of this interaction was a splitting process in which the rewarding, but pathological, relationship with the mother was dissociated from the punishing or withdrawing one. Psychotherapy with the borderline patient addresses this split, which is accompanied by an abandonment depression, the use of primitive defenses, and problems with separation–individuation.

The borderline patient in psychotherapy tends to repeat the experience with his or her pathological mother in the transference. Thus, the patient will form a relationship with the therapist that maintains the attachment at the expense of emotional growth and separation–individuation. Confrontation is required by the therapist in order to help the patient examine and work through this pathological splitting process. It is evident that Masterson and Rinsley view the transference experience as the reliving of actual early experiences with the patient's mother. This contrasts with Kernberg, who describes the reactivation early in treatment of primitive part-objects; that is, an affect associated with a specific self and object representation that does not necessarily correspond to real experiences with a parent.

Masterson describes the therapist, in work with these patients, as functioning in many ways that can be considered "supportive" or "real." The therapist, as a new and nonpathological object, appreciates and approves of the patient's healthy attempts to become a separate individual. This approach is related to the "communicative matching" that Mahler describes as central to the resolution of the rapprochement subphase of separation–individuation.

Adler and Buie

Adler and Buie (Adler, 1981, 1985; Adler and Buie, 1979; Buie and Adler, 1982) emphasize the aloneness issues in their treatment of patients with borderline personality disorder. They describe the core difficulty with these patients as occurring prior to the splitting that Kernberg defines. In their view, patients with borderline personality disorder have an inability to count upon their internal resources to tolerate separations. Under the stress of their mounting anger, they lose their capacity to maintain an evocative memory for the important people in their lives, including their therapist. Adler and Buie emphasize that these patients long for the holding and soothing qualities of these important people, and also conceptualize their difficulties as a failure to maintain holding and soothing introjects of them when under the stress of separation. Added to these problems are their tenuous capacity to maintain a relationship with the other person, based upon the "need–fear dilemma" (Burnham et al, 1969). Their longings for closeness, accompanied by fears of merger when they begin to obtain it, in part accounts for their attempts to flee from therapy as it intensifies, and to act out in different ways. Finally, their primitive guilt is responsible for their potentially dangerous self-punishment, the ease with which they project their feelings of badness, and the negative therapeutic reaction that frequently tends to occur in therapy with them.

In working with the aloneness issues that occupy the first phase of treatment, Adler and Buie stress the experience of the therapist and the patient surviving the patient's rage and emphasize the therapist's countertransference response to it. Adler (in press) also describes the creative experience with projective identification during this phase. Depending upon the therapist's capacity to "contain" the projections, the patient's use of projective identification can be constructive, leading to the internalization of new structures rather than a destructive repetition of childhood experiences. The outcome, which can require months or years, is the development of dependable holding and soothing introjects.

At this point the patient is no longer seen by Adler and Buie as borderline (Adler, 1981). The patient has entered the part of the continuum from borderline to narcissistic personality disorder that deals with the issues of worthlessness and incompleteness, rather than the borderline personality disordered patient's problems with aloneness and annihilation. In the second phase of treatment,

Adler and Buie utilize Kohut's (1971, 1977) framework, which examines the selfobject transferences that occur with narcissistic personality disorders. They define the patient in the second phase as someone who tends to idealize the holding and soothing qualities of the relatively stably experienced therapist. The process of disillusionment that occurs with the everyday imperfections of the therapist ultimately addresses these issues through the analysis of these experiences and their relationship to past disappointments. At the end of this phase the patient has a relatively solid sense of worth and completeness. Kohut defines the process of taking in the needed functions from the therapist—through the experience of optimal frustration—as transmuting internalization.

In the final phase of treatment, structures are consolidated. The patient ultimately develops a love and respect for him- or her-self, trusts and values his or her capacities, and has values and ideals that are consonant with the sense of self, and which are experienced as part of the self. An important experience during this final phase is the process of validation; that is, the therapist's acknowledgement of and appreciation for the genuine achievements of the patient. Adler and Buie describe the need for validation in order for a person, from childhood on, to consolidate gains and make them a permanent part of the individual.

Although Adler and Buie's formulations have been described as emphasizing the borderline patients' deficits (Waldinger and Gunderson, 1987), they also define important conflictual issues in these patients; that is, their conflicts about the need–fear dilemma and their anger, with anxiety and guilt as a response to it. Adler and Buie also describe an approach that has more supportive aspects early in treatment than Kernberg's. However, they also do stress the expressive or exploratory aspects of the treatment.

Gunderson

Gunderson (1984) has presented a framework for understanding and treating the patient with borderline personality disorder that defines three levels of the patient's functioning, as well as a formulation of the four phases of treatment in work with them.

Level I occurs with the borderline patient's experience of feeling supported in treatment. Although the patient may long for closeness, there is a stability in the relationship and a capacity to be reflective to some extent. At the same time, the patient has a sense of tentativeness about the therapist's solidity, and fears becoming dependent on or being controlled by the therapist. These concerns are part of the patient's feelings of dysphoria and depression; present are aspects of emptiness, which may be expressed as passivity, accompanied by masochistic fantasies. In Level II, the intensity of the borderline transference has emerged. At this time, the patient experiences the therapist as a major object who is frustrating; the angry, devaluing, manipulative behavior so well described as part of borderline psychopathology is most manifest. Interpretation as well as confrontation and limit-setting become major activities of the therapist. At Level III, the patient with borderline personality disorder may experience periods of aloneness or objectlessness, as well as a sense of badness, which can be accompanied by panic states, impulsive action to avoid the panic, or brief psychotic episodes. This level of psychopathology is akin to the aloneness experiences described by Adler and Buie (1979). Gunderson also emphasizes the primitive superego aspects involving intense feelings of badness, and the projection of these feelings, that can accompany the aloneness experiences.

Gunderson's four stages of treatment in the exploratory psychotherapy of patients with borderline personality disorder utilize these three levels. In Stage I, the issue revolves around the establishment of the boundaries that make the therapy possible. The patient will test the therapist's commitment to him or her and the established boundaries. During this stage the therapist struggles with concerns about being either too frustrating or seductive. When successfully negotiated, the patient tends to settle down in treatment, accompanied by a diminution in self-destructive acting-out. Stage II is characterized as focusing on negativity and control. Many of the issues of Gunderson's Level II are present at this time, as the patient experiences the therapist as a major frustrating figure. When confrontation and interpretation are successful, the patient may begin to recover early memories and work effectively by being able to weave past experiences into the here-and-now of the transference. Thus, the intense experience of the emerging anger is worked through to a point where the patient becomes more stable. The process occurs through the internalization of needed aspects of the therapist; as part of it, the patient is able to explore the disillusionment that occurs in the treatment. Stage III, which deals with separation and identity, is one in which gains in role functioning and social relationships are consolidated. The separation anxiety that emerges is within tolerable and analyzable bounds. Identity issues are addressed by exploration as well as by the therapist's support for the importance of the patient's gains. In Stage IV, termination assumes center stage; the issues that were largely worked through in the earlier stages reemerge in a way that can be reexamined usefully and further integrated.

There are parallels between Gunderson's four stages of treatment and the stages described by Masterson (1976) and Adler and Buie (Adler, 1985; Buie and Adler, 1982). Masterson's first "testing" phase parallels Gunderson's Stage I. His Stage II relates to Masterson's second phase of "working through." Stage III has elements of Masterson's second as well as third phase; in the latter, the patient demonstrates a diminution of anger and better social functioning as splits are beginning to be resolved, leading to the capacity for ambivalence. Gunderson's Stages I and II are similar to Adler and Buie's first phase of treatment. The more stable part of his Stage II parallels Adler and Buie's second phase. Stage III has similarities to the issues of consolidation and validation that Adler and Buie discuss in their last phase.

Searles

Searles (1986), in his work with borderline patients, has built upon his significant intensive inpatient psychotherapeutic experiences with chronic schizophrenics (1960, 1979). His sensitivity to the impact of subtle verbal and nonverbal interchanges in the treatment of these chronic patients has enabled him to make useful contributions to the understanding and treatment of patients with borderline personality disorder. He defines the patient with borderline personality disorder as having serious difficulties in differentiating unconsciously between fantasy and reality, as well as between words and actions. The patient does not have a reliable, stable image of him- or herself, or of the therapist. Therefore, any interaction between patient and therapist is bound to have an unpredictable and perhaps profound impact on the patient.

Searles emphasizes that the therapist's nonverbal participation with the patient is far more significant than any interpretation; that is, the emotional environment of the therapy is more important than any verbal interchange between the two participants. The therapist may experience the countertransference burden in the early phases of treatment of not having the freedom to make interpretations. As part of these constraints, the therapist must become aware of the wish to impose his or her own reality upon the patient, and the ease with which the patient will comply, stalemating the treatment. The danger in treatment is a repeat of the pathological experience with parents, resulting in a "pseudo-reality and pseudo-identity" for the patient. However, there is also the opportunity for a new experience with the therapist. The therapist's capacity to be aware of the impact of the transference, which is experienced from the patient's perspective as a "reality," allows the patient to develop ego-nuclei and, ultimately, a stable identity. In addition, the therapist who can acknowledge aspects of him- or herself that are similar to those of the patient is in a most useful position to help the patient with identifications; otherwise, the patient may experience each participant struggling with projected and disavowed parts of the other. Clinically, the therapist working with such issues may be tempted to make premature interpretations of the patient's identifications with others.

Searles's sensitive observations help enrich the contributions of the other workers who have been described. Some of his formulations are also similar to those involving the therapeutic use of projective identification (Adler, in press; Kernberg, 1975; Ogden, 1979).

Countertransference

The importance of countertransference issues has been emphasized by all the contributors to the understanding of patients with borderline personality disorder. In this literature, countertransference is viewed in its broader context, involving conscious as well as unconscious feelings aroused by the patient in the therapist, not only in response to the patient's transference, but also as a result of projective identification and real aspects of the relationship between the participants. In addition, the differing personalities of the therapists and their interaction with their patients' personalities can lead to idiosyncratic responses in the therapists. These responses can at times be difficult to label as pathological, for they may be unique and creative within that specific therapeutic dyad (Gunderson, 1984).

Many countertransference issues relate to the two poles of the borderline patient's dilemma; the patient's feelings of neediness and longings to be held and nurtured on one hand, and the rage when these wishes and needs are not responded to consonant with the patient's hopes on the other. The therapist often can experience a wish to rescue, hold, or contain, which can be part of a useful countertransference awareness of the patient's wishes or needs. However, it can also become part of a pathological countertransference rescue of the patient, perhaps a manifestation of the therapist's own unresolved wishes to be rescued, or a part of the therapist's discomfort with the patient's anger and a wish to avoid it (Adler, 1985). Gunderson (1984) refers to these countertransference issues as the "good mother," "strong father" paradigms, and relates them to

Kernberg's (1975) "withdrawal from reality" type of countertransference, in which the patient and therapist collude to deny the patient's anger and project the source of difficulty to the outside.

Countertransference issues in response to the patient's anger can include the therapist's tendency to withdraw, or retaliate, sometimes in the guise of carrying out a useful confrontation, as well as feelings of helplessness, hopelessness, and despair (Adler, 1985). Countertransference to the borderline's aloneness issues can include these responses as well as panic, and a need to take some action in the face of the therapist's unbearable countertransference aloneness.

All contributors emphasize the importance of the therapist's work in being aware of countertransference as much as possible with such patients. Many stress the therapist's capacity to acknowledge to him- or herself that many of the patient's feelings are also present in the therapist. To the degree that the therapist can do this, the likelihood of pathological countertransference acting-out is diminished.

MANAGING COMMON PROBLEMS: ENGAGEMENT IN THE TREATMENT

The Relationship Between the Therapist's Technique and the Patient's Symptoms

The technical approach to the treatment of the borderline personality disordered patient's symptoms is paradoxical: In theory, we can argue that a therapeutic approach that more actively defines the boundaries of the treatment and its limits is most likely to contain and minimize the symptoms of the patient with borderline personality disorder. However, as most of the contributors have described, such patients are exquisitely sensitive to feeling misunderstood, invaded, or abandoned. Thus, an approach that relatively quickly defines boundaries and attempts to limit acting-out is in danger of being experienced by the patient as intrusive, requiring either compliance or flight. Therapists who are active in this regard therefore must be sensitive to the patient's tenuous sense of self, and the ease with which the therapist can be experienced as invasive and unempathic. On the other hand, therapists who are slow to define the therapeutic boundaries may be experienced by these patients as abandoning them, or allowing frightening closeness; both can endanger the patient's tenuous sense of impulse control. Thus, these need–fear dilemma issues of patients with borderline personality disorder require the therapist's sensitivity to the impact of the uniqueness of the therapist's personality, or to his or her specific way of working with these patients. If appropriately utilized, any of the theoretical frameworks presented can contain the borderline patient, thereby minimizing symptoms early in treatment.

The Processes and Problems in Building an Alliance

All the contributors recognize, either explicitly or implicitly, that patients with borderline personality disorder establish therapeutic alliances only with diffi- culty, and that the alliance is stable only toward the end of the treatment. Masterson (1981) describes the pathological alliances that accompany the acti- vation of the pathological splitting process. Through confrontation, the patient learns about the destructive price paid for maintaining these pathological configurations. The end result of this process is the patient's capacity to have a reality-based alliance with the therapist, who represents a new object helping with healthy separation–individuation. Adler (1979) believes that a therapeutic alliance with borderline patients is only solidly present at the end of treatment. He believes that selfobject transferences (that is, transferences in which the patient experiences the self-esteem regulating functions that the therapist performs as part of himself) are often confused with the therapeutic alliance; he ascribes the therapist's need to believe that a therapeutic alliance exists to countertransference problems, in which the therapist feels so painfully alone during the treatment of the borderline patient.

The issues described in the preceding section and earlier are relevant to issues of therapeutic alliance formation. Any intervention that is experienced by the patient with borderline personality disorder as intrusive or abandoning will temporarily destroy anything resembling such an alliance. The therapist's work of monitoring this delicate balance and the accompanying countertransference responses is an important part of the therapeutic experience, which leads to the patient's ultimate capacity to form a relatively stable therapeutic alliance. It requires that the therapist be open to his or her feelings in working with the patient, and learn to utilize them as clues to the patient's experience in the treatment. Rather than the therapist knowing with certainty that his or her feelings and fantasies are similar or identical to the patient's, the therapist has the task of learning to tolerate the ambiguity and uncertainty that accompanies a questioning stance (Adler, in press). Under such circumstances, the therapist is less likely to disrupt the tenuous therapeutic alliance these patients have. In addition, using countertransference feelings in this way also allows the therapist to be sensitive to experiences of projective identification, in which the patient may attempt to provoke intrusive or abandoning responses, as split-off or dissociated aspects of the patient become mobilized and projected.

Compliance With the Treatment Schedule and Boundaries

Compliance, in addition to describing the process of patients collaborating in the treatment, can relate to patients who conform on the surface and, at the same time, have a false self; for survival, they have to hide who they really are (Winnicott, 1965). Since patients with borderline personality disorder are sensitive to the needs of their therapists and others—and since they have problems that frequently can be defined as relating to a false self—in discussing compliance in the treatment of these patients we must be careful to distinguish between interactions between patient and therapist that reenforce their serious psychopathology, and those that foster their mature participation in the treatment. The discussions about the therapeutic alliance and the transferences that attach the patient to the therapist have addressed aspects of this issue. In addition, the need–fear dilemma that is apparent in working with these patients always poses difficulties: Longings for closeness that are part of the positive transference and bond with the therapist may yield to fears of merger and disruption of the treatment. At the same time, therapist activity that is experienced as intrusive will lead to the same fears.

These formulations relate to the common problems in working with borderline patients, since they often tax the therapist's skills and equanimity by missing appointments, coming late, demanding extratherapeutic contacts, or threatening some destructive or self-destructive action. The above considerations define the dilemma in working with these patients: The therapist who sets no limits will have a patient who feels out of control, which can lead to a disruption or ending of the treatment; limits that are too firm can be experienced as sadistic and lead to compliance or to an identification with the aggressor (that is, the patient becomes like the sadistically experienced therapist). At the same time, it is important that the therapist have a formulation, even if it is a tentative one, that explains the meaning of the patient's current behavior in the context of the patient's life story and experience in the therapy. Thus, demands for telephone contact may be a manifestation of the patient's transient loss of holding and soothing introjects (Adler, 1985) as the patient's rage has become manifest in therapy. Under these circumstances, brief phone contacts can be indicated to help the patient evoke the affective memory of the therapist. However, the patient's demands still can escalate into a neediness and insistence on long telephone calls that tax the therapist's capacity beyond the therapist's limits.

Patients with borderline personality disorder force their therapists to consider their own limits if they are to work successfully with their patients. The neediness of these patients, coupled with their potentially destructive anger, can exhaust therapists who have not resolved the limits of their capacity to give while at the same time maintain a private life apart from their work. Therapists who have not resolved this issue are most likely to "burn out," withdraw from, or sadistically attack their patients in potentially destructive ways. Therapists who are comfortable with their personal limits are more able to suggest alternatives to their patients when their demands are beyond their therapists' capacities; for example, use of an emergency room, partial or full hospitalization, or even termination. Of course, therapists must monitor their countertransference feelings so that their decisions are made on the basis of their personal limitations and not because of countertransference hate. When based on the former, patients are often grateful for their therapists' stance, and can ultimately identify with their therapists' capacities to care about themselves.

Although Gunderson and Kernberg are more often described as therapists who have firmer personal limits that Adler and Buie, no therapist can work successfully with borderline patients unless these issues have been resolved adequately by the therapist. In addition, the therapist's constant vigilance about these issues, and the countertransference involved in them, can allow for the possibility of clarification, confrontation, interpretation, and limit-setting, and the minimization of therapeutic disruption.

The Use of Psychotherapy as a "Trial"

Since patient and therapist do not know each other well, there are advantages in defining the early sessions as an opportunity for two people to find out whether the form of psychotherapy chosen is appropriate and the therapist–patient fit is good. Such a position allows the therapist time to learn more about the strengths and regressive potential of the patient, and his or her capacity to utilize a form of individual psychotherapy. At the same time, it is important for the therapist to be aware that patients with borderline personality disorder have the issues of separation and abandonment in the forefront. Hearing about a "trial" of therapy can be experienced by them as an actual or potential abandonment. However, the therapist's sensitivity to the abandonment theme allows for the opportunity to offer clarifications and interpretations that also help define the patient's capacity to work in a supportive or exploratory psychotherapeutic framework. Of course, the therapist's need to monitor countertransference is crucial. If the therapist is using the therapeutic trial because of possible dislike for or uncertainty in working with the patient, or for other countertransference reasons, these sensitive patients are very likely to grasp such therapist feelings, leading to a potentially disastrous trial period.

It is important that both patients and therapists be aware that they have choices throughout the therapy. If the patient does not wish to accept the form of therapy offered by the therapist at this beginning point of treatment, he or she may explore treatment possibilities with other therapists, or work with the current therapist to understand the concerns. Similarly, if a therapist concludes that a patient is unsuitable for an exploratory form of therapy, but does not wish to supply the supportive treatment, he or she should have the option of referring the patient to another therapist. As a result of this evaluation or trial period, either patient or therapist may modify his or her understanding or position based on further data obtained as part of this discussion. Of course, the therapist who is aware of the borderline patient's concerns about abandonment or invasion will be sensitive to these issues in treatment negotiations with the patient.

Choices for the therapist also include a decision about his or her wish to work with the patient based upon feelings of liking or disliking the patient in the early sessions. Since it is inevitable that the therapist will feel countertransference hate for the patient once the transference has intensified, it is crucial that the therapist experience the patient in positive ways at the beginning of treatment in spite of the serious pathology also present. If such feelings are not present in the therapist, serious questions should be raised about continuing treatment with the patient after an evaluation or trial period. It is also important for the therapist to be aware that feelings of dislike, hatred, and a wish to terminate with the patient once the transference has intensified are most likely related to countertransference feelings, and should be examined carefully by the therapist without acting on them impulsively.

SELF-DESTRUCTIVE ACTIONS

Self-destructive behavior occurs most often at times when the patient experiences the therapist as frustrating or not present at all (Gunderson, 1984). At those times, self-destructive acts may be a manifestation of anger and/or desperation expressed in an interpersonal context, or an attempt to numb feelings or to feel alive at times of panicky aloneness. Intrapsychically, such behavior may be a wish to punish a hated introject, rid the self of badness associated with it, or punish oneself for hateful thoughts. In work with the borderline patient, it is important for the therapist to formulate which of the above mechanisms is related to the current self-destructive acts, and their connection to the current state of the transference.

All the contributors to the literature on the treatment of the patient with borderline personality disorder have addressed issues in working with self-destructiveness. Although there are differences in the rapidity and style in which different workers would confront or interpret this behavior, and the extent to which they would tolerate self-destructive acts, all of them are aware that such acts threaten the viability of the treatment and may endanger the patient's life. They all point to countertransference feelings as playing an important role in determining whether self-destructive acts will either escalate or be contained. Labeling the patient's behavior as only manipulative, or being involved in regressive rescuing of the patient, can be manifestations of such countertransference difficulties. A careful formulation and constant scrutiny of countertransference feelings, as described in earlier sections, are essential ingredients in working with self-destructive behavior, regardless of the specific details described by the various contributors. Protection and containment of the patient sometimes requires hospitalization, or use of some other extratherapeutic holding and containing measures.

INADEQUATE SOCIAL/FAMILY SUPPORT

Among the criteria for accepting a borderline patient for expressive or exploratory psychotherapy are that social and family supports are available to the patient. The patient's capacity for relatively mature friendships is an important measure of ego strength. These friendships, as well as available family, can be turned to for support during the inevitable crises in treatment. However, many patients with borderline personality disorder have pathological relationships with family members who themselves may have severe psychopathology (Gunderson and Englund, 1981). These family interactions become particularly important with adolescent borderlines, or with borderline patients who require hospitalization. Thus, most of the literature on family treatment involves patients who have been hospitalized. Indeed, borderline patients who lack solid social and family supports are most apt to need hospital settings. The problems in working with such patients usually require hospitalization and conjoint family therapy, or some other form of milieu treatment, in addition to the individual psychotherapy.

Rinsley (1971), in his work with hospitalized borderline adolescents, developed a therapeutic approach that kept the family from contact with the patient. In order for the staff to assume a surrogate parent role and help the patient with separation–individuation, he felt that involving parents directly would continue the pathological family interaction. Instead, a caseworker met with the family members apart from the patient in order to help them in their difficulties with separation, while supporting them to understand the role of the hospital staff with the patient.

Gunderson (1984) feels that such an approach may be appropriate only for those borderline patients who have very disturbed relationships with their parents. He also points out the disruptive dangers of not involving families when borderline patients are hospitalized. Parents who have supported the patient's admission may quickly shift to a position of agreeing with the patient's complaints about the hospital. The patient may feel that the hospital is trying to force separation from the parents, or that the hospital is trying to save him or her from such difficult parents. Family sessions with the patient and family together, as well as work with the family apart from the patient, allows these issues to be aired, interpreted, and to be worked through as much as possible during the hospitalization.

Kernberg (1984) believes that the families of hospitalized patients should work largely with their social workers, since the patient is already involved in so many therapeutic activities within the hospital. It is only when specific issues involving the entire family need to be addressed that sessions with patient and family are held.

INDICATIONS/CONTRAINDICATIONS, LIMITATIONS

The literature describing the psychotherapy with borderline personality disordered patients does convey a sense of agreement about those patients who can most likely be treated successfully. Patients with previous positive therapeutic experiences, who have relatively good object relationships (e.g., stable friendships and a capacity for intimacy) and solid abilities to work productively, would certainly be in the group with the best prognosis. On the other hand, patients who are socially isolated, who have antisocial or serious acting-out histories (including previous therapies with competent therapists in which there has been serious acting-out of aggressive and/or self-destructive impulses), and evidence of significant incapacities to tolerate impulses, affects, and anxiety, would clearly be in the group with a poor prognosis. In addition, this group would most likely require hospitalization, psychopharmacology, or other supportive or containing modalities added to the psychotherapy.

Apart from Kernberg's (1982) relatively clear distinctions between supportive and expressive psychotherapy, most of the literature defines a mixture of supportive and expressive/exploratory techniques. The therapist who is capable of being active to the degree the patient requires, in touch with inevitable countertransference feelings that can be used to formulate the meaning of current material, able to define boundaries, interpret, and contain when necessary, is described as someone who can work most usefully with these patients.

The research literature on the psychotherapy of patients with borderline personality disorder is in its early stages, and leaves many questions unanswered. However, it suggests (Gunderson, 1984) that a combined supportive–expressive/exploratory approach can be successful with some of these patients. The studies point to the high dropout rates, the problems in separating the results of psychotherapy from the natural course of the disorder, and the fact that psychoanalysis is generally contraindicated. All of the studies have serious methodological problems and report results that can be only suggestive. The need for more controlled, systematic, prospective studies is obvious.

The clinical, theoretical, and research literature, in spite of all its limitations, conveys an optimism that borderline personality disorder patients are amenable to a flexible, psychodynamic psychotherapeutic approach. Not all of these patients are recommended for individual psychotherapy, particularly those who have the qualities described above in the poor prognosis group. Ancillary forms of treatment and hospitalization may be required. But a thoughtful, flexible approach seems to be effective with those patients who are willing to remain in treatment for a sufficiently long period of time. Even those who drop out often return to treatment with the same or another therapist; some of them ultimately become patients who are successfully treated.

SUMMARY

Some of the major models for understanding patients with borderline personality disorder have been described, with an emphasis on an understanding of the psychotherapeutic implications of these formulations. Although these models use different frameworks and terminology, they do define a group of patients with significant psychopathology who develop intense transference relationships, and tax the skill and fortitude of their therapists, as they elicit intense countertransference reactions in them.

Although the research findings are methodologically flawed, and the theoretical and clinical literature can only be suggestive, there is a sense that many of these difficult patients are treatable ultimately by a flexible psychotherapeutic approach that at times uses ancillary modalities of treatment. The models presented have many areas of overlap, and seem to stress the need, in working with these patients, to understand, contain, confront, interpret, and support when necessary. In the hands of their authors and those who adapt them, the various models address many of the core issues in the treatment of these patients.

Further systematic, prospective research can help to clarify whether certain formulations are more useful than others in understanding and treating patients with borderline personality disorder. Such work would also define which approaches are most efficacious at which points in the treatment. At the same time, contributors to the theoretical and clinical literature are continuing to add to our understanding with further observations and formulations about this patient population.

REFERENCES

Abend S, Porder M, Willick M: Borderline Patients, Psychoanalytic Perspectives. New York, International Universities Press, 1983

Adler G: The myth of the alliance with borderline patients. Am J Psychiatry 1979; 136:642–645

Adler G: The borderline–narcissistic personality disorder continuum. Am J Psychiatry 1981; 138:46–50

Adler G: Borderline Psychopathology and Its Treatment. New York, Jason Aronson, 1985

Adler G: Psychotherapy of the narcissistic personality disorder patient: two contrasting approaches. Am J Psychiatry 1986; 143:430–436

Adler G: Transitional phenomena, projective identification, and the essential ambiguity of the psychoanalytic situation. Psychoanal (in press)

Adler G, Buie DH: Aloneness and borderline psychopathology: the possible relevance of child development issues. Int J Psychoanal 1979; 60:83–96

American Psychiatric Association: Diagnostic and Statistical Manual of Mental Disorders, Third Edition, Revised (DSM-III-R). Washington, DC, American Psychiatric Association, 1987

Buie DH, Adler G: The definitive treatment of the borderline personality. Int J Psychoanal Psychother 1982; 9:51–87

Burnham DG, Gladstone AI, Gibson RW: Schizophrenia and the Need–Fear Dilemma. New York, International Universities Press, 1969

Chessick R: Intensive Psychotherapy of the Borderline Patient. New York, Jason Aronson, 1977

Giovacchini P: Treatment of Primitive Mental States. New York, Jason Aronson, 1979

Giovacchini P: Character Disorders and Adaptive Mechanisms. New York, Jason Aronson, 1984

Goldstein W: An Introduction to the Borderline Conditions. New York, Jason Aronson, 1985

Gunderson JG: Borderline Personality Disorder. Washington, DC, American Psychiatric Press, 1984

Gunderson JG, Englund DW: Characterizing the families of borderlines. Psychiatr Clin North Am 1981; 4:159–168

Kernberg OF: Borderline Conditions and Pathological Narcissism. New York, Jason Aronson, 1975

Kernberg OF: Object-Relations Theory and Clinical Psychoanalysis. New York, Jason Aronson, 1976

Kernberg OF: Internal World and External Reality. New York, Jason Aronson, 1980

Kernberg OF: The psychotherapeutic treatment of borderline personalities, in Psychiatry 1982: American Psychiatric Association Annual Review, vol. 1. Edited by Grinspoon L. Washington, DC, American Psychiatric Press, 1982

Kernberg OF: Severe Personality Disorders. New Haven, Yale University Press, 1984

Kernberg OF: Panel Discussion: Treatment of Personality Disorders. Boston, MA, Massachusetts General Hospital Department of Psychiatry, April 6, 1986

Knight RP: Management and psychotherapy of the borderline schizophrenic patient, in Psychoanalytic Psychiatry and Psychology. Edited by Knight RP, Friedman CR. New York, International Universities Press, 1954

Kohut H: The Analysis of the Self. New York, International Universities Press, 1971

Kohut H: The Restoration of the Self. New York, International Universities Press, 1977

Mahler MS, Pine F, Bergman A: The Psychological Birth of the Human Infant. New York, Basic Books, 1975

Masterson J: Psychotherapy of the Borderline Adult. New York, Brunner/Mazel, 1976

Masterson J: The Narcissistic and Borderline Disorders. New York, Brunner/Mazel, 1981

Masterson J, Rinsley D: The borderline syndrome: the role of the mother in the genesis and psychic structure of the borderline personality. Int J Psychoanal 1975; 56:163–177

Meissner W: The Borderline Spectrum. New York, Jason Aronson, 1984

Modell AH: Psychoanalysis in a New Context. New York, International Universities Press, 1984

Ogden TH: On projective identification. Int J Psychoanal 1979; 60:357–373

Rinsley D: Theory and practice of intensive residential treatment of adolescents. Adolesc Psychiatry 1971; 1:479–509

Rinsley D: Borderline and Other Self Disorders. New York, Jason Aronson, 1982

Searles HF: The Nonhuman Environment in Norman Development and in Schizophrenia. New York, International Universities Press, 1960

Searles HF: Countertransference and Related Subjects. New York, International Universities Press, 1979

Searles HF: My Work with Borderline Patients. Northvale, NJ, Jason Aronson, 1986

Stern A: Psychoanalytic investigation and therapy in the borderline group of neuroses. Psychoanal Q 1938; 7:467–489

Volkan VD: Six Steps in the Treatment of Borderline Personality Organization. Northvale, NJ, Jason Aronson, 1987

Waldinger RJ, Gunderson JG: Effective Psychotherapy with Borderline Patients. New York, MacMillan, 1987

Wallerstein RS: Forty-Two Lives in Treatment. New York, Guilford, 1986

Winnicott DW: The Maturational Processes and the Facilitating Environment. New York, International Universities Press, 1965

Zetzel E: A developmental approach to the borderline patient. Am J Psychiatry 1971; 127:867–871

Chapter 4

Psychopharmacologic Therapies in Borderline Personality Disorder

by Paul H. Soloff, M.D.

OVERVIEW: PROBLEMS IN PHARMACOTHERAPY OF BORDERLINE DISORDER

The "borderline" concept is the inevitable result of efforts to define clean boundaries between neurotic and psychotic functioning. In its many representations, as a state, syndrome, or personality disorder, the term has come to describe a spectrum of symptoms bounded by mild thought disorder at one extreme and affective instability at the other. The schizotypal borderline, the patient "at the psychotic border," defines a group of odd, eccentric individuals who demonstrate mild peculiarities of thinking, especially under stress. Historically, these patients were termed latent, ambulatory, or pseudoneurotic schizophrenics and defined the borderline as a "sub-schizophrenic disorder" (Bleuler, 1911; Zilboorg, 1941; Hoch, 1949; Knight, 1954). Many of these patients now fall within the *Diagnostic and Statistical Manual of Mental Disorders, Third Edition, Revised (DSM-III-R)* (American Psychiatric Association, 1987) definition of schizotypal personality disorder (SPD).

At the "neurotic border" are affectively unstable, rejection-sensitive individuals with wide mood swings, impulsive, and often self-destructive behavior. Recent efforts to redefine the borderline as a "subaffective disorder" arise from observations of patients who had been called primitive oral hysterics, those with emotionally unstable character disorders, and hysteroid dysphorics (Marmor, 1953; Easser and Lesser, 1965; Klein and Davis, 1969; Rifkin et al, 1972a). Comprehensive constructs such as psychotic character and borderline personality organization acknowledge the vulnerability to psychotic thinking in these unstable patients, bridging the conceptual gap between the affective and cognitively unstable patients (Frosch, 1964; Kernberg, 1967). Empirical study shows that the overlap between the schizotypal and unstable borderline diagnoses is extensive, more than one-half of *DSM-III* borderline patients meeting *DSM-III* criteria for SPD. (Spitzer et al, 1979) When schizotypal symptoms are systematically sought among unstable borderline patients, at least one (and an average of six) such symptoms are found in each patient (George and Soloff, 1986). Efforts to resolve this heterogeneity and define the relationship of unstable and schizotypal borderlines to affective and schizophrenic spectrum disorders have included family history studies, neuroendocrine and sleep studies, pharmacologic challenge, and drug treatment studies. This review updates recent efforts to study this heterogeneous syndrome through the methods of psychopharmacology.

This work is supported by NIMH grants #MH35392, #MH00658, and CRC #MH30915

A pharmacologic approach to the study of patients with borderline personality disorder (BPD) has an immediate and practical appeal to the clinician. Treatment indications may be defined through the main effects of drugs on individual symptoms, while patterns of response to medication may lead to definition of meaningful clinical subtypes (e.g., pharmacologic behavioral dissection). Surveys of clinical practice indicate that more than one-half of patients with BPD admitted to hospital receive some form of pharmacotherapy, generally neuroleptics directed at schizotypal symptoms or antidepressants directed toward affective symptoms, alone or in combination (Soloff, 1981). No "treatment of choice" has emerged.

Methodologic problems in the pharmacologic study or treatment of borderline personality disorder are formidable and include:

1. delineation of borderline from related Axis I "next neighbor" disorders, especially in the "soft affective spectrum" (e.g., dysthymic, cyclothymic, and bipolar II disorders)
2. delineation from other Axis II "dramatic disorders": histrionic, antisocial, and narcissistic personality disorders
3. true comorbidity between borderline and discrete Axis I disorders (especially major depression)
4. the marked heterogeneity of affective, schizotypal, and impulsive behavioral symptoms found in this disorder
5. confusion surrounding the "state versus trait" definition of many borderline symptoms, especially during stress-related decompensations
6. lack of a coherent etiology for borderline disorders

Given the heterogeneity of symptom presentation, an empirical, atheoretical approach is preferred for both study and treatment of the patient with BPD. Target symptoms include: all of the patient's affective symptoms (e.g., lability, reactive depression, inappropriate anger); schizotypal symptoms (e.g., referential thinking, illusions, dissociation, paranoid ideation); and impulsive behaviors, regardless of whether they are deemed state or trait in origin.

REVIEW OF LITERATURE

When first presented in *Psychiatry 1982* (Grinspoon, 1982), the drug treatment of patients with BPD was a controversial approach to a poorly defined clinical problem. Cole and Sunderland (1982) reported that there were "no controlled studies using clear criteria for borderline diagnosis." They reviewed "the vestigial literature" on drug therapy with borderline patients (which consisted of two papers presenting seven patients), and chose instead to discuss "the effectiveness of drugs in other clinical conditions which fall in the same no-man's land between schizophrenia, depression and neurosis." These disorders included pseudoneurotic schizophrenia, adult attention deficit disorder, emotionally unstable character disorder, rejection-sensitive dysphoria, impulsive anger, panic agoraphobia, and nonendogenous depression. In the intervening years, reliable diagnostic criteria for borderline personality disorder have been proposed and field tested (Spitzer, 1979). Structured interview methods have been developed to allow definition of patient samples for research. In particular, Gunderson's

Diagnostic Interview for Borderlines (DIB) has achieved widespread acceptance among research workers and has been shown to discriminate patients with BPD from those with depression and schizophrenia, as well as other personality disorders, in a wide variety of inpatient and outpatient settings (Kolb and Gunderson, 1980; Gunderson et al, 1981; Soloff, 1981; Barrash et al, 1983). Gunderson's concept of the borderline includes vulnerability to transient psychotic episodes and is closer to the historical origin of the construct than the *DSM-III*. Using the DIB, or similar reliable criteria for the diagnosis of BPD, a small but expanding literature of controlled clinical trials has appeared in the past five years. This update will focus primarily on recent clinical reports or controlled trials of *criteria-defined* borderline patients, reporting on older literature or "next neighbor" diagnoses only when the overlap with BPD is widely accepted or the contribution is significant. The literature review is organized by medication class, focusing on main effects to allow some definition of indications for treatment. This will be followed by a discussion of medication efficacy against empirically derived symptom patterns in patients with BPD in an effort to relate medication response to clinically meaningful subtypes.

Neuroleptics

Given the origin of the borderline construct as a "pre-psychotic" or "sub-schizo-phrenic" disorder, and the prominence given schizotypal symptoms in early definitions, the use of neuroleptics in patients with BPD would seem to be a rational choice. Case reports of low dose neuroleptic therapy in criteria-defined borderline patients were described by Brinkley and colleagues in 1979. Using low dose neuroleptic strategies, these investigators reported improvements in mood, anxiety, and cognitive disturbances in borderline patients clinically defined by Gunderson and Singer (1975) criteria. Brinkley (1980) called particular attention to the mild thought disorders found in these patients. These "soft signs" included tangentiality, circumstantiality, off-target and nonsequitur responses to questions, eccentricities of expression, and magical thinking. Improvement in these symptoms was achieved rapidly, often after only one or two weeks of low dose neuroleptic treatment. The widespread acceptance of diagnostic criteria for borderline personality disorder soon led to systematic drug trials of low dose neuroleptic agents.

Initial studies by Leone (1982), and by Serban and Siegel (1984), were parallel comparison trials of two neuroleptic agents in criteria-defined borderline outpatients (e.g., chlorpromazine versus loxapine, thiothixene versus haloperidol). Patients experienced improvement in affective symptoms such as depressed mood, sleep disturbance, anger, hostility, anxiety, somatic concerns, and tension, but also in cognitive symptoms such as paranoid ideation, suspiciousness, derealization, and confusion. These studies were not placebo controlled and left unanswered the question of the effects of time alone.

Goldberg and associates (1986), at the Medical College of Virginia, addressed this issue in a double blind, placebo-controlled study using thiothixene (mean = 8.67 mg/day) for 12 weeks in a highly functional outpatient population. Borderline personality disorder was diagnosed by *DSM-III* criteria with the additional requirement of "at least one psychotic symptom." Statistically significant drug effects were found against cognitive symptoms such as illusions, ideas of reference, and self-reported measures of psychoticism. Derealization and depersonalization also showed some improvement. Among the affective-spectrum symptoms that responded to thiothixene were obsessive-compulsive and phobic-anxiety symptoms, with some drug effects against anger, hostility, and somatization. The more severely ill patients showed the greatest response to the low dose neuroleptic treatment.

The sample of Goldberg and colleagues was skewed toward the schizotypal symptom spectrum by the inclusion requirement of one psychotic symptom. Cowdry and Gardner (1988) conducted a study skewed toward the affective spectrum with 16 female outpatients diagnosed as borderline by DIB and *DSM-III* criteria, who also met the additional inclusion requirement of a hysteroid dysphoric presentation. In a complex placebo-controlled, random-assignment, crossover design, patients received one of four active medications (trifluoperazine, alprazolam, tranylcypromine, or carbamazepine) for six-week periods. All patients were simultaneously treated in psychotherapy outside of the drug study. Patients assigned to neuroleptics received trifluoperazine in 2 mg capsules in a dose averaging 7.8 mg/day. Trifluoperazine trials were hampered by a low rate of completion, with only 5 of 10 trifluoperazine-treated patients finishing the trial. For patients able to tolerate the medication for a three-week period, the investigators noted that the ratings were "among the best observed with any medication, with statistically significant improvement in depression, anxiety, and sensitivity to rejection, despite the small number of subjects ($n = 7$)" (Cowdry and Gardner, 1988, p. 114). Trifluoperazine also showed a trend toward lessened behavioral dyscontrol compared with placebo.

Severity of illness was an important factor in a series of reports by Soloff and associates (1986b, 1987a) at the University of Pittsburgh. These investigators reported results of a double blind, placebo-controlled study conducted primarily in an inpatient setting. Two active medications were compared: haloperidol and amitriptyline. Patients were defined as borderline by the DIB and subtyped by the *DSM-III* into BPD, SPD, or mixed (BPD/SPD) variants. They received haloperidol in an average daily dose of 4.8 mg and were followed for 5 weeks. As in the previous studies, the low dose neuroleptic was associated with improvement in both affective and cognitive symptoms. Among 90 inpatients, haloperidol was markedly superior to placebo on measures of global functioning, depression, hostility, schizotypal symptoms, and impulsive behavior. The neuroleptic effect was not related to borderline subtype (e.g., BPD versus BPD/SPD) and appeared to diminish symptom severity independent of the specific content of symptoms.

These five studies reflect neuroleptic efficacy in the *acute* treatment of symptomatic borderline patients. A role for continuation therapy following acute treatment is suggested by Montgomery and colleagues (1982), who studied 37 hospitalized patients with personality disorders, selected for histories of "multiple-episode parasuicide attempts." Patients were randomly assigned to flupenthixol 20 mg injection every 4 weeks and compared to placebo injections in a double blind 6-month trial. Among 30 patients completing the 6-month study, 14 were receiving the neuroleptic drug and 16 the placebo. Episodes of repeat "parasuicide" in the 6-month period were found in 75 percent of placebo patients compared to only 21 percent of the neuroleptic group, a significant difference.

Antidepressant Medications

The comorbidity of borderline personality disorder with Axis I affective syndroms has been the topic of several recent reviews (Gunderson and Elliott, 1985; Perry, 1985; Soloff et al, 1987b). In some series, up to 62 percent of hospitalized patients with BPD meet criteria for Axis I major depression (Carroll et al, 1981). Although the diagnostic significance of depressive symptoms in patients with BPD is a topic of controversy, the prevalence of mood disturbances in general, and depression in particular in this population, strongly suggests a role for antidepressant medication. Drug surveys and open clinical trials confirm the usefulness of antidepressants in some borderline patients, generally related to Axis I disorders rather than BPD itself (Soloff, 1981; Cole and Sunderland, 1982; Sternberg, 1987). Sternberg (1987) found that 90 percent of patients with BPD and concurrent Axis I major depression improved with tricyclic antidepressant medication, while only 25 percent of dual diagnosis patients improved without medication. In general, one would expect higher response rates among borderline patients with valid Axis I diagnoses of endogenomorphic depressive disorder, and lower rates among borderline patients with atypical depressive diagnoses or diagnoses not validated by longitudinal observations of behavior.

The study by Soloff and colleagues (1987a) represents the only placebo-controlled trial of a tricyclic antidepressant in criteria-defined borderline patients. Amitriptyline was given in a daily treatment range of 100 to 175 mg (average, 149.1 mg/day), corresponding to an average plasma level of 240.4 ± 99.4 ng/ml (mean $\pm$ SD) of combined metabolites amitriptyline and nortriptyline by the fourth week on medication. Significant antidepressant effects favoring amitriptyline over placebo were found; however, antidepressant effects attributed to amitriptyline were *not* superior to the antidepressant effects of haloperidol on the same outcome measures. Many patients who failed to respond to amitriptyline did significantly *worse* than patients on placebo. These patients developed increased referential thinking, behavioral impulsiveness, suicidal threats, and assaultive behavior (Soloff et al, 1986a). *The presence of a concurrent diagnosis of major depression (by RDC criteria) did not predict response to the amitriptyline.*

The prevalence of atypical depression in borderline personality disorder has led other investigators to systematic trials of monoamine oxidase inhibitor (MAOI) antidepressants. Liebowitz and Klein (1981) studied phenelzine in patients with "hysteroid dysphoria," the majority of whom met *DSM-III* criteria for borderline personality disorder. In an open treatment phase of 3 months' duration, patients received phenelzine in doses ranging from 15 to 75 mg per day, along with intensive psychotherapy. Open treatment produced significant improvement in typical borderline diagnostic criteria such as "problems being alone," "complaints of chronic emptiness and boredom," and "behavioral impulsivity." At the end of three months, responding patients entered a double blind, randomized, cross-over study and were assigned to continue either phenelzine or placebo. Patients receiving active drug continued to show reduction in borderline diagnostic criteria, while patients switched to placebo appeared to worsen.

Cowdry and Gardner (1988) reported their experience with tranylcypromine in patients meeting DIB and *DSM-III* criteria for borderline personality disorder as well as criteria for hysteroid dysphoria. For the tranylcypromine trials, patients received 20 to 60 mg daily (average, 40 mg) for a 6-week period. Patients improved in their mood, suicidality, and impulsivity. Their capacity for pleasure was increased while rejection sensitivity and angry affect were decreased. As in the Soloff study, *Cowdry and Gardner found no correlation between medication response and a concurrent diagnosis of major depression in borderline patients.* This suggests that either the research diagnosis of major depression in patients with BPD lacks validity, or the affective state of patients with BPD reflects a different ("atypical") mood disorder. One can also speculate that the medications compared in these studies are equally effective (or ineffective) against the mood disorder of patients with BPD.

While these three studies address acute treatment of symptomatic borderline patients, Montgomery and colleagues (1982, 1983) studied the prophylatic use of antidepressant medication against recurrent impulsive "parasuicidal" acts in patients with personality disorders. The efficacy of the antidepressant mianserin was studied in a sample of 58 patients with a past history of 2 or more acts of deliberate self-harm. These patients were not clinically depressed at the onset of the drug trial and received diagnoses of *DSM-III* borderline personality disorder (65 percent) and *DSM-III* histrionic personality disorder (35 percent). This double blind placebo-controlled trial utilized 30 mg of mianserin daily for 6 months. Among the 38 patients completing the study, there were no significant differences in recurrence rates of "parasuicidal" acts between groups at 3-month or 6-month follow-up.

Hirsch and associates (1983) compared mianserin 60 mg/day to nomifensine 150 mg/day and placebo in high risk patients with histories of multiple episodes of "parasuicide." At 6 weeks, the recurrence rate for parasuicidal acts was not significantly different among groups: 21 percent for patients on mianserin; 13 percent for patients on nomifensine; and 13 percent for those on placebo. The diagnostic composition of the study sample was not given in detail, perhaps in deference to the authors' view that "parasuicide" is "not a single disorder but a state defined by its outcome." They note that since drug therapy (alone) or psychotherapy (alone) addresses only one part of the etiology, recurrence of parasuicidal acts is not surprising with selective treatment modalities.

Minor Tranquilizers

There are few systematic treatment trials involving the use of minor tranquilizers in criteria-defined borderline patients. In an oral presentation, Reus and Markrow (1984) reported favorable responses in 9 of 18 borderline inpatients treated with alprazolam (up to 5 mg daily) in a double blind, placebo-controlled, crossover design. Although there was no significant group difference between drug and placebo periods, a few individuals did exceptionally well. The best predictors of favorable response included baseline measures of cognitive and sleep disturbance, hostility, and suspiciousness, and pathologic interpersonal relationships on the DIB. These variables predicted 93.8 percent of the cases correctly (Reus, personal communication, 2/16/88). Faltus (1984) reported favorable case experience using alprazolam against anxiety, paranoia, suspiciousness, anger, and irritability in patients with BPD. His report suggested that borderline patients are better able to withstand stress on the minor tranquilizer medication without developing further schizotypal symptoms. A less optimistic report was given by Gardner and Cowdry (1986a), who used alprazolam as one of the four active drug conditions in their multidrug, crossover design (described above). Among female outpatients with BPD receiving a daily dose of 1 to 6 mg of alprazolam (average 4.7 mg), there was a significant increase in episodes of behavioral dyscontrol compared to the placebo condition. Indeed, 7 of 12 (58 percent) patients assigned to alprazolam were overtly self-destructive or assaultive during the medication trial, compared to only 1 of 13 patients on placebo. A history of disinhibition of impulsive and aggressive behavior and a concern for abuse and habituation are relative contraindications to the use of the benzodiazepine family in patients with borderline personality disorder. Nonetheless, the brief, reactive nature of many symptoms in patients with BPD make minor tranquilizers an attractive group for further systematic study.

Anticonvulsant Medication

The possibility that some manifestations of borderline pathology are secondary to central nervous system (CNS) dysfunction has important implications for pharmacotherapy. A neurobehavioral etiology for borderline personality disorder suggests that borderline personality traits may represent both direct and indirect (e.g., conditioned) effects of seizure disorders, minimal brain dysfunction/attention deficit disorder, or other early CNS insult. Symptoms often related to these origins include impulsivity, aggressive outbursts, mood swings, suicide attempts, episodes of depersonalization, feelings of rage, emptiness, or loneliness, identity confusion, antisocial behavior, drug and alcohol abuse, and eating problems. Anticonvulsants and psychostimulants would seem worth investigating in this small group of patients with borderline-like presentations, abnormal EEG and/or histories of attention deficit disorder, learning disability, or other markers of neurodevelopmental pathology.

Cowdry and Gardner (1988) included carbamazepine in their outpatient multidrug, placebo-controlled, crossover study (described above). Patients received carbamazepine 200 to 1200 mg per day for the 6-week trial period. Plasma levels were adjusted to 8 to 12 mcg/ml. Carbamazepine treatment was associated with significantly less behavioral dyscontrol compared to the placebo trial. The basis for this effect is unclear. The authors noted that carbamazepine is effective in treating mood disorders (especially mania) as well as epileptic disorders. The presence of therapeutic effects in impulsive borderline patients *in the absence of EEG evidence of abnormal temporal or limbic discharges* suggests the possibility of a purely "affective" effect of the medication. These authors have also reported the development of melancholia in three patients with BPD during carbamazepine treatment (Gardner and Cowdry, 1986b). All had prior episodes of melancholia or major depression but were free of these disorders when starting carbamazepine.

Lithium Carbonate

For the sake of completeness, one must include lithium carbonate in the armamentarium of medications that play a possible role in treating borderline personality disorder. Although there are no recent systematic studies using lithium in patients defined by modern criteria for borderline personality disorder, an earlier study of patients with emotionally unstable character disorder (EUCD) remains relevant. Rifkin and colleagues (1972b) found that lithium carbonate demonstrated significant efficacy compared to placebo against mood lability in hospitalized adolescent girls with EUCD. Lithium also produces a "reflective delay" and a decrease in overt aggressive behavior in impulsive criminal subjects in several placebo-controlled studies (Tupin et al, 1973; Sheard, 1975). Case experience suggests that the antiaggressive effects of lithium have clinical application with borderline patients (Shader et al, 1974).

MAJOR MODELS

The Primacy of Axis I

How does one determine priorities for pharmacotherapy in the borderline patient when the definition of the disorder falls somewhere between "sub-affective", "sub-schizophrenic" and personality disorder? The separation of Axis I and Axis II becomes problematic in such patients. Descriptive psychiatrists often use multiaxial diagnoses to label the acute symptom presentations of the patient with BPD. Analytic writers prefer to view the patients' affective, cognitive, and impulsive state symptoms within the context of the personality disorder. Each perspective is probably accurate in some patients. Comorbidity undoubtedly exists between borderline and some Axis I disorders, especially major depression, justifying a careful differential diagnosis for all patients presenting in distress. However, the reactive and transient nature of many state symptoms in the borderline patient confounds simple descriptive formulations. Many borderline symptoms fail to meet criteria for duration or intensity sufficient to warrant an Axis I diagnosis. For example, symptoms of depression, agitation, anxiety, panic, or mild thought disorder may appear transiently in the context of a stress response and fail to meet duration or severity criteria for a separate Axis I designation. Authors reviewing this dilemma generally agree that any clearly differentiable Axis I disorder for which specific therapy exists warrants primary consideration for pharmacotherapy (Cowdry, 1987; Schulz, 1986). Diagnoses of melancholic (endogenous) depression, bipolar disorder, panic disorder, paranoid, or schizophreniform disorder warrant primary attention in any decision hierarchy. The position of Axis I "next neighbors" is less clear. Disorders of temperament such as dysthymic or cyclothymic disorders are often difficult to separate from borderline character pathology and have only recently been "elevated" to Axis I status from their previous (DSM-II) personality classification. In these cases, Axis II may be the proper focus for pharmacotherapy. Disorders of impulse, such as substance abuse or bulimia, may reflect symptomatic expression of the underlying borderline character rather than independent and discrete diagnostic entities. Depressive diagnoses such as "chronic and intermittent depression," hysteroid dysphoria, and atypical depression are made according to fashion and can not reliably be discriminated from the affective dysphoric states of borderline patients. Multiple complaints of mild somatization, anxiety, and dissociative disorder may well represent the "pan-neurosis" of the borderline patient. Where such symptoms appear to arise with stress in the context of a borderline syndrome, a philosopy of parsimony should prevail and pharmacotherapy be directed toward Axis II.

The duration of treatment depends on target symptoms and medication class. Low dose neuroleptics suppress hostility and schizotypal symptoms within days, while antidepressants may require weeks for proof of efficacy. The length of therapy has not been empirically studied. Research protocols from six weeks to three months offer rough guidelines. At present, There are no good studies of maintenance treatment in criteria-defined borderline patients.

Where the stress is specific and transient and the patients' response known to be intense but short-lived (days to weeks), the "as needed" use of neuroleptics or minor tranquilizers may prove useful (within the limits described for each drug). This strategy applies more to the functional patient engaged in psychotherapy than to the more severely impaired or vulnerable patient who requires a "course" of medication (e.g., weeks to months).

Specific versus Nonspecific Approaches to Treatment

Choice of medication for borderline patients follows a target-symptom approach, yet some effective treatments are surprisingly nonspecific. For example, neuroleptic therapy affects both affective and cognitive symptoms, diminishing symptom severity regardless of content. Response to neuroleptic treatment does not selectively separate schizotypal from unstable borderline patients. In general, empirical trials tend to broaden indications for a given drug, suggesting relationships between groups of symptoms by similar medication responses or nonspecific effects on overall symptom severity. There is no single drug treatment specifically for the borderline disorder. Some may view this as further evidence that the borderline does not exist as a discrete psychiatric disorder. Others suggest that the multiplicity of state symptoms presented by the patient are merely epiphenomena of an underlying disease process which medication trials are not addressing (that is, the patient's vulnerability to dyscontrol). At this time, there is no scientific resolution to this debate. In *Psychiatry 1982*, Sunderland and Cole chose to compare the acute symptoms of the patient with BPD to other constructs for which pharmacotherapy trials had been described. The implication was that treatments specifically for these next neighbors might also apply to similar presentations in patients with BPD (that is, perhaps "borderline" is a term describing this diverse group of disorders). The lack of specificity in pharmacologic response tends to challenge this approach. An atheoretical empirical approach would be to identify responsive symptom patterns in the patient with BPD. While not clear enough to distinguish borderline subtypes at the present time, symptom patterns offer practical clinical guidelines for treatment.

Pharmacotherapy by Symptom Pattern

All pharmacotherapy with the borderline patient should be viewed as single case research with clearly defined target symptoms, systematic assessments of change, single drug trials of adequate dose, and duration. The recent empirical literature enables us to suggest symptom patterns that may be responsive to specific classes of medication. In our own research sample, a factor analysis of 90 DIB-defined hospitalized patients produced the following patterns of acute symptom presentations: 1) a hysteroid depressive pattern (representing 42.6 percent of the variance); 2) an observed affective pattern (20 percent of the variance); 3) a schizotypal symptom pattern (15 percent of the variance); and 4) an impulsive trait pattern (9 percent of the variance). Studying medication response among empirically defined symptom patterns is a first step in developing meaningful subtypes of the borderline personality disorder.

THE HYSTEROID DEPRESSIVE PATTERN. Two independent clusters of

Table 1. A Review of Medication Response in Criteria Defined Borderline Patients

Medication(s) (Average Daily Dose)	Authors	Summary of Main Effects
Neuroleptics		
loxepine (14.5 mg) *vs* chlorpromazine (110 mg)	Leone (1982)	Improvement in: anger, hostility, suspiciousness
thiothixene (9.4 mg) *vs* haloperidol (3 mg)	Serban and Siegel (1984)	psychoticism: illusions, ideas of reference, paranoia, derealization
thiothixene (8.67 mg) haloperidol (4.8 mg)	Goldberg et al (1986) Soloff et al (1987)	anxiety, phobic anxiety, somatization, obsessive-compulsive symptoms
trifluoperazine (4.8 mg)	Cowdry and Gardner (1988)	subjective depressed mood, suicidality, sensitivity to rejection
flupenthixol (20 mg inj. q 4 wks)	Montgomery and Montgomery (1982)	global symptom severity
Antidepressants		
tricyclic antidepressants amitriptyline (149.1 mg)	Soloff et al (1987)	Improvement in: subjective depression Untoward Effects: increased suicidality, assaultiveness and referential thinking in some nonresponders
Monoamine Oxidase Inhibitors 1. tranylcypromine (40 mg)	Cowdry and Gardner (1988)	Improvement in: depressed mood, suicidality, capacity for pleasure, impulsivity, euphoria, anger, rejection sensitivity, global functioning
2. phenelzine (15–75 mg)	Liebowitz and Klein (1981)	Improvement in: behavioral impulsivity, problems being alone, complaints of chronic emptiness and boredom; hysteroid dysphoric patterns: mood reactivity, hypersomnia, hyperphagia, leaden paralysis, rejection sensitivity

Table 1. A Review of Medication Response in Criteria Defined Borderline Patients (Continued)

Medication(s) (Average Daily Dose)	Authors	Summary of Main Effects
other antidepressants mianserin (30 mg)	Montgomery et al (1983)	No prophylactic effects on recurrent suicidal acts for mianserin or nomifensine
mianserin (60 mg) vs nomifensine (150 mg)	Hirsch et al (1983)	
Minor Tranquilizers alprazolam (5 mg)	Reus and Markrow (1984)	Improvement in: hostility, suspiciousness, cognitive disturbance, sleep disturbance
alprazolam (4.7 mg)	Gardner and Cowdry (1986a) Cowdry and Gardner (1988)	Untoward effects: increased suicidality, serious behavioral dyscontrol, "disinhibition" in some nonresponders
Anticonvulsants carbamazepine (820 mg)	Gardner and Cowdry (1986b) Cowdry and Gardner (1988)	Improvement in: impulsivity, behavioral dyscontrol, anger, suicidality, anxiety, euphoria, global functioning
	Gardner and Cowdry (1986c)	Untoward effects: precipitation of melancholic depression
Related Trials lithium carbonate (0.6–1.5 mEq/Li)	Rifkin et al (1972a, 1972b) Tupin et al (1973) Sheard (1975)	Improvement in: mood lability (in emotionally unstable character disorder) aggressiveness in antisocial personality disorder

acute depressive symptoms are found in borderline patients recently admitted to hospital. One is defined by dramatic subjective complaints (the hysteroid depressive pattern); the other, by more objective measures of depressive symptom severity (the observed affective pattern). Clinicians will recognize the subjective complainer as the angry, demanding, and entitled borderline patient. These patients demonstrate hostility and resentment of others, and are provocative and manipulative. They describe a chronic history of dysphoric moods though demonstrate little distress in the company of other patients on the ward. Their affective complaints are generally of "atypical" depression, with mood reactivity, hypersomnia, hyperphagia, "leaden paralysis," and marked rejection sensitivity. They readily endorse the hysteroid dysphoric pattern defined by Liebowitz and Klein (1981). They report mood "crashes" when alone and brighten with attention. Multiple somatic complaints and anxiety symptoms are common.

Phenelzine appears useful in borderline patients with the hysteroid depressive pattern. In a dose range of 45–90 mg daily (averaging 1 mg/kg), phenelzine has been shown effective against the depressive mood, lability, and "mood crashes" of the hysteroid patient. Liebowitz and Klein (1981) reported improvement in symptoms considered diagnostic traits of borderline disorder: complaints of chronic emptiness, problems being alone, and behavioral impulsivity. These changes suggest that some of the "core features" of the borderline diagnosis may be mood-dependent.

Tranylcypromine in doses of 30-60 mg daily has been shown effective against depressed mood, suicidality, impulsivity, anger, and rejection sensitivity in borderline outpatients with similar affective presentations. Low dose neuroleptics are useful in containing the anger and hostility of these patients. This strategy may provide relief sufficient that antidepressant medication is not required.

THE OBSERVED AFFECTIVE PATTERN. The second affective presentation (the observed affective pattern) is more objectively described and defines a quiet, withdrawn depressive patient with a mix of atypical and "classical" depressive symptoms, including (but not limited to): pervasive low mood; guilt; suicidal ideation; sleep disturbance; appetite disturbance; and loss of interest. These patients often project a needy, helpless, dependent picture which immediately solicits attention and involvement of staff. The apparently pervasive low mood and mild neurovegetative symptoms make differential diagnosis especially important to identify any concurrent Axis I effective diagnosis. If tricyclic antidepressants have any role in treating the depressed borderline patient, it would be in this group. However, given our experience with behavioral toxicity in depressed borderline patients treated with amitriptyline, we prefer to begin treatment of these patients with an MAOI.

THE SCHIZOTYPAL PATTERN. Referential thinking, paranoid ideation, and derealization/depersonalization in the borderline patient generally present as transient, stress-related state symptoms rather than fixed character traits. Patients with the mixed BPD/SPD pattern may demonstrate sensory distortions, illusions, magical thinking, thought blocking, intrusive thoughts, unusually violent or perverse fantasies, a preference to be alone, hypersensitivity to criticism, marked ambivalence, anhedonia, and pan-anxiety (George and Soloff, 1986). Much of the severity of these symptoms resolves spontaneously with hospitalization and supportive care (Soloff, 1987a).

Low dose neuroleptics appear especially useful for persistent or frequent cognitive and dissociative symptoms in the mixed BPD/SPD patient. Ideas of reference, paranoid ideation, derealization/depersonalization, and illusions are very responsive to this approach. Despite the presence of depressive symptoms, schizotypal features in a borderline patient predict poor outcome with tricyclic antidepressants (Soloff et al, in press). In general, the schizotypal symptoms should be addressed before any remaining depression.

THE IMPULSIVE PATTERN. While accounting for only a small percentage of symptom patterns, impulsive behavior is most difficult to manage in its many destructive presentations. Impulsive behavior can include overdose, self-mutilation, suicidal threat, food or alcohol binges, dystonic promiscuity, and assaultive or antisocial acts. The etiology of impulsiveness in the patient with BPD may reflect: 1) functional disinhibition of ego controls; 2) impulsive temperament; 3) a residual of early life CNS insult (as in minimal brain dysfunction/attention deficit disorder or episodic dyscontrol syndromes); or 4) current cerebral dysrhythmia or epileptiform disorders. (Although one may challenge the placement of syndromes with possible organic etiologies within the borderline spectrum, their resemblance to "functional" borderline disorders requires careful assessment in the impulsive patient.)

Medication strategies against behavioral impulsiveness in borderline patients may include low dose neuroleptics, carbamazepine, tranylcypromine, or lithium carbonate. The neuroleptic appears the least specific agent but has been shown to decrease actual impulsive ward behavior in an inpatient borderline sample (Soloff et al, 1987a). An abnormal electroencephalogram (EEG) (grade II or greater dysrhythmia), and perceptual disturbances, associated with a history of impulsive behavior, suggests a role for carbamazepine (Cowdry, 1985). This drug is also effective against impulsiveness in patients without a dysrhythmic EEG, possibly reflecting its mood stabilizing potential (Cowdry and Gardner, 1988). Tranylcypromine is useful against behavioral impulsiveness occurring in the context of atypical depression. The antiaggressive effects of lithium have been demonstrated in patients with character disorder (Tupin et al, 1973; Shader et al, 1974; Sheard, 1975)

MANAGING COMMON PROBLEMS

Engagement in Treatment

Pharmacotherapy facilitates "accessibility." Patients are unable to establish a therapeutic alliance and proceed with psychotherapy until affect, perception, and cognition are under sufficient control to allow for new learning. Pronounced depression, hostility, anxiety, or mild thought disorder disrupts the basic functions of attention, concentration, and reflection necessary to engage in psychotherapy. Decompensations in affective, cognitive, or behavioral controls during the process of psychotherapy may require instituting medications to preserve engagement and facilitate the process under controlled conditions.

Concerns about possible deleterious effects of medication upon psychotherapy were reviewed in depth by the Group for the Advancement of Psychiatry (1975). At that time, therapists' fears included: a) harmful effects upon the psychotherapeutic relationship, and upon the attitudes of patient and therapist; b) loss of patient motivation for psychotherapy through effective relief of anxiety or other symptoms; c) development of new symptoms when anxiety, depression, or tension are reduced; and d) the "academic" question of state dependence of psychotherapeutic learning under medication. Clinical experience has shown these early concerns to be without merit. The principle barrier to adding medication to psychotherapy *when indicated* is clinician prejudice rather than chemical interference with the psychodynamic process. In skilled hands, the two approaches are entirely complementary.

Engagement in treatment and development of a working relationship with the borderline patient is always difficult. Under the best of circumstances, only one-third of borderline patients treated by "experienced expert therapists" in private practice actually complete treatment. Forty-six percent break treatment within the first six months (Waldinger and Gunderson, 1984). Attrition is similar in some outpatient pharmacotherapy studies (Goldberg et al, 1986). Data reported from research studies, especially pharmacotherapy studies, represent the experience of a few cooperative patients. These individuals are sufficiently motivated to participate in structured interviews, weeks of research ratings, and the uncertainties of random assignment of treatment. Generalizing conclusions from this cooperative sample to more or less impaired patients must consider this bias.

The working agreement between doctor and patient needs to be explicit in any pharmacotherapy of the borderline personality disorder. Since pharmacotherapy is, at best, an empirical trial, the risks and benefits must be presented to the patient much as an informed consent is obtained from the research participant. There is no certainty of outcome. The patient is engaged as a research partner for what is, essentially, a single case study. Target symptoms, probable effects and side effects, dose, and duration are explained in this consent process without any unwarranted promises made by the clinician. An authoritarian posture is avoided since 1) the medication may not work, and 2) a power struggle would surely ensue over the efficacy of the medication or compliance with doctor's orders.

Engagement of the patient as a research partner requires the patient to take periodic observations of his or her behavior and to report accurately relevant experiences. This is a difficult task for any person, let alone one prone to distortion and exaggeration. Borderline patients, along with other "dramatic cluster" personalities, manipulate the clinician by their manner of presentation. Exaggeration and distortion serve an interpersonal process at the expense of reliability of content. Perspectives provided by family, friends, or hospital staff are needed to corroborate the picture presented by the patient with BPD.

Compliance

As in all pharmacotherapies, patients may develop dissatisfaction with treatment for a wide variety of reasons, some related to side effects of the medication or lack of progress, others to the doctor–patient relationship. Patients with BPD complain frequently of multiple side effects which may be described with an exaggerated intensity, suggesting a manipulation of the therapeutic relationship. Dissatisfaction with treatment may be based on realistic failure of response or the patient's disappointment with unrealized expectations. The patient's (and doctor's) expectations for pharmacotherapy may far exceed relief of symptom distress and blur the distinction between state symptoms and character traits. State symptoms of distress are legitimate targets for pharmacotherapy, while character traits, based on intrapsychic dynamics, generally require an interpersonal approach. Medication will never "cure character" or protect the patient from the vicissitudes of life.

The introduction of medication may be viewed by the patient (or the doctor) as an indication of the failure of psychotherapy. In some settings, pharmacotherapy may be viewed as "second class" treatment for patients too impaired for traditional interpersonal approaches, or worse, as "clinic treatment" for patients unable to afford psychotherapy. In other settings, the reverse prejudice applies, as all behavior is "biologized" and medication trials are directed against interpersonal dynamics.

Noncompliance is the most frequent problem in any effort at pharmacotherapy of the borderline patient. Failure to comply with recommendations or actual abuse of dose or duration can represent acting out of interpersonal conflicts between doctor and patient. In the specific case of MAOI pharmacotherapy, cooperation must extend to dietary restrictions. It is not uncommon for patients to test the therapeutic relationship by willful indiscretion of the tyramine-free diet. Fortunately, the physician's fantasy of patients "overdosing" on cheese or chocolate rarely materializes. More often, the compliance struggle focuses on side effects and failure of expected results. Faced with the complaint that "promised" results have not occurred, the physician increases dosage, only to be met by the complaint of intolerable side effects. A change in medication usually occurs and the process repeats itself until both are aware of the underlying therapeutic struggle. In the extreme case, suicidal threat or overdose may act out patient anger.

Overdose is the complication most feared by clinicians treating borderline patients. It is interesting to note how rarely this actually occurs among patients followed in our own research clinic. Among the first 46 patients participating in a current double blind placebo-controlled trial (haloperidol versus phenelzine), only one trial was terminated by virtue of overdose. (After 11 weeks of outpatient follow-up, this patient took all of her study medication in a successful effort to reenter the hospital. She had been randomly assigned to placebo and complained of lack of progress.) Overdose is most commonly an interpersonal event, a nonverbal message directed toward the therapist or other dynamically significant people in the patient's life. In our experience, patients with BPD generally provide sufficient opportunity for "rescue" to diminish the risk of the event and to deliver the nonverbal message to the intended object. Unfortunately, impulsive behavior and poor judgment occasionally result in serious or even lethal outcomes. This is especially likely when alcohol is mixed with medication or multiple drugs are taken. Patients who have been thoroughly and explicitly forewarned about the danger of abusing certain medications (e.g., MAOIs and diet) may overdose with over-the-counter agents rather than the more hazardous medication. As in all pharmacotherapy, the clinician weighs risks and benefits, carefully assessing the patient's impulsiveness, affective state, and past history of self-destructiveness before prescribing. In situations of high risk, especially those in which social or family support is lacking, a period of hospitalization is indicated to begin pharmacotherapy and obtain symptom relief in a controlled setting. This would seem preferable to withholding medication from a symptomatic patient out of fear of suicide (in other words, if the risk is that great, the patient belongs in the hospital).

While noncompliance usually refers to failure to take medication, some patients take excessive doses to produce sedation, arousal, or a chemical "high." Some patients cause more problems trying to enhance the drug effect: that is, "If some is good, more is better."

Many patients with BPD admit to abusing street drugs or alcohol regularly. Mixing medication with street drugs or alcohol can have serious physical consequences. The abuse of stimulants (e.g., amphetamines) by borderline patients on MAOI medication is especially hazardous. Whether such patients can be medicated reasonably as outpatients is a matter of fine clinical judgment.

Pharmacotherapy in a Social Context

In our culture, taking medication is an affirmation of illness. The act carries both stigma and status. For families looking to explain the disturbing behavior of borderline members, pharmacotherapy suggests the "chemical imbalance" that reduces feelings of guilt and personal responsibility. Other families view the patient as willfully deviant and oppose medication as unwarranted. To the extent that the treatment reduces symptom intensity, the patient will better be able to relate to family and friends. The quality of these relationships, however, depends more on long-standing patterns of behavior than on transient symptoms. In our own experience, patients successfully relieved of symptoms return to their baseline life styles, which may involve antisocial behavior in the "street culture." Pharmacotherapy enhances sociability; however, social outcome depends more on character than on chemical.

By the time they seek help, borderline patients have often alienated family and friends. They quickly wear out their welcome at the mental health clinics through demands, manipulation, and coercion of care and attention. These patients create emergencies (e.g., suicidal threat, overdose) which force social supports (including the clinic) to reengage. After the emergency, family, friends and clinic may distance once again, setting the stage for the next round. Successful pharmacotherapy—directed at anxiety, hostility, and impulsiveness—coupled with family and social support and consistent limits, breaks this common pattern. The family plays a pivotal role in supporting the clinician's efforts to engage the patient in the initial stages of therapy. Relieving the intensity of anxiety, anger, and depression through pharmacotherapy enables the patient to cooperate with family, tolerate frustrating but therapeutic limits, and utilize therapeutic efforts.

Social structure is critical to patients' stability. School or work settings provide clear role expectations—with accountability, sanctions, and rewards. A highly structured job or school setting facilitates ego controls, provides an opportunity for achievement, and supports self-esteem. It is the one therapeutic area most neglected in the overall care of patients with BPD.

INDICATIONS/CONTRAINDICATIONS FOR PHARMACOTHERAPY

Pharmacotherapy is indicated for severe or persistent affective, schizotypal, or impulsive-behavioral symptoms in patients with BPD. Generally, a medication-free period of careful observation is required to define target symptoms. This may involve inpatient care, in cases where impulsiveness or self-destructiveness are primary concerns. Unreliability, social instability, or active self-abuse are other factors favoring inpatient treatment. Outpatient study is feasible for less severely impaired patients, although support and cooperation of family or friends is necessary.

SUMMARY

Our review of literature suggests the use of low dose neuroleptics when anger, hostility, impulsiveness, and schizotypal symptoms are present (though depression will also improve). For atypical depression, MAOIs may be added, reserving the tricylic antidepressants for clear diagnoses of comorbid endogenous depression. Carbamazepine and lithium have less empirical support and greater medical risk. They are "second-line" drugs for labile mood and impulsiveness. The role of minor tranquilizers is poorly defined, though disinhibition of impulse and dependence with long-term use diminish the appeal of these drugs. While the empirical study of medication in borderline patients is in its infancy, some broad principles of use have been established to date. These include the following:

1. Medication effects are modest. Patients improve from severely to moderately impaired.
2. Pharmacotherapy works best in a treatment plan which includes family support, social structure, and psychotherapy. Such a combined effort enhances compliance and reliability, and minimizes self-destructive behavior.
3. There are no adequate studies on long-term continuation or maintenance therapies to test for prophylactic effects. Given the risks (e.g., tardive dyskinesia), maintenance treatment must be justified carefully by persistence of symptoms or extreme vulnerability.
4. Borderline personality disorder remains a heterogeneous syndrome with no single "treatment of choice."

Further research is needed to define pharmacologically responsive subtypes and symptom patterns.

REFERENCES

American Psychiatric Association: Diagnostic and Statistical Manual of Mental Disorders, Third Edition (DSM-III). Washington, DC, American Psychiatric Association, 1980

American Psychiatric Association: Diagnostic and Statistical Manual of Mental Disorders, Third Edition, Revised (DSM-III-R). Washington, DC, American Psychiatric Association, 1987

Barrash J, Kroll S, Carey K, et al: Discriminating borderline disorders from other personality disorders. Arch Gen Psychiatry 1983; 40:1297–1302

Bleuler E: Dementia Praecox, or the Group of Schizophrenias (1911). Translated by Zinkin J, New York, International Universities Press, 1950

Brinkley JR: Haloperidol and other neuroleptics in the treatment of borderline patients, in Haloperidol Update 1958–1980. Edited by Ayd FJ. Baltimore, MD, Ayd Medical Communications, 1980

Brinkley JR, Beitman BD, Friedel RO: Low dose neuroleptic regimes in the treatment of borderline patients. Arch Gen Psychiatry 1979; 36:319–326

Carroll BJ, Greden JF, Feinberg M, et al: Neuroendocrine evaluation of depression in borderline patients. Psychiatr Clin North Am 1981; 4:89–99

Cole JO, Sunderland P III: The drug treatment of borderline patients, in Psychiatry 1982: American Psychiatric Association Annual Review, vol. 1. Edited by Grinspoon L. Washington, DC, American Psychiatric Press, 1982

Cowdry RW, Gardner DL: Pharmacotherapy of borderline personality disorder: alprazolam, carbamazepine, trifluoperazine and tranylcypromine. Arch Gen Psychiatry 1988; 45:111–119

Cowdry RW, Pickar D, Davies R: Symptoms and EEG findings in the borderline syndrome. Int J Psychiatry Med 1985–1986; 15:201–211

Cowdry RW: Psychopharmacology of borderline personality disorder: a review. J Clin Psychiatry 1987; 48:(Suppl) 15–25

Cowdry RW, Pickar D: Symptoms and EEG findings in the borderline syndrone. Int J Psychiatry Med 1985–1986; 15:201–211

Easser BR, Lesser SR: Hysterical personality: a re-evaluation. Psychoanal Q 1965; 34:390–405

Faltus F: The positive effect of alprazolam in the treatment of three patients with borderline personality disorder. Am J Psychiatry 1984; 141:802–803

Frosch J: The psychotic character: clinical psychiatric considerations. Psychiatr Q 1964; 38:81–96

Gardner DL, Cowdry RW: Alprazolam-induced dyscontrol in borderline personality disorder. Am J Psychiatry 1986a; 143:519–522

Gardner DL, Cowdry RW: Positive effects of carbamazepine on behavioral dyscontrol in borderline personality disorder. Am J Psychiatry 1986b; 143:519–522

Gardner DS, Cowdry RW: Development of melancholia during carbamazepine treatment in borderline personality disorder. J Clin Psychopharmacol 1986c; 6:236–239

George A, Soloff PH: Schizotypal symptoms in patients with borderline personality disorders. Am J Psychiatry 1986; 143:212–215

Goldberg SC, Schulz SC, Schulz PM, et al: Borderline and schizotypal personality disorders treated with low-dose thiothixene vs placebo. Arch Gen Psychiatry 1986; 43:680–686

Grinspoon L: Psychiatry 1982: American Psychiatric Association Annual Review, vol. 1. Washington, DC, American Psychiatric Press, Inc., 1982

Group for the Advancement of Psychiatry: Pharmacotherapy and Psychotherapy: Paradoxes, Problems and Progress. New York, Brunner/Mazel, 1975

Gunderson JG, Elliott GR: The interface between borderline personality disorder and affective disorder. Am J Psychiatry 1985; 142:277–288

Gunderson JG, Kolb JE: Discriminating features of borderline patients. Am J Psychiatry 1978; 135:792–796

Gunderson JG, Singer MT: Defining borderline patients: an overview. Am J Psychiatry 1975; 132:1–10

Gunderson JG, Kolb JE, Austin V: The Diagnostic Interview for Borderline Patients. Am J Psychiatry 1981; 138:896–903

Hirsh SR, Walsh C, Draper R: The concept and efficacy of the treatment of parasuicide. Br J Clin Pharmacol 1983; 15:1895–1945

Hoch P, Polatin P: Pseudoneurotic forms of schizophrenia. Psychiatric Q 1949; 23:248–276

Kernberg O: Borderline Personality Organization. Am J Psychoanal 1967; 15:641–685

Klein DF, Davis JM: Diagnosis and Drug Treatment of Psychiatric Disorders. Baltimore, Williams & Wilkins, 1969

Knight RP: Management and psychotherapy of the borderline schizophrenic patient, in Psychoanalytic Psychiatry and Psychology. Edited by Knight RP, Friedman DR. New York, International Universities Press, 1954

Kolb JE, Gunderson JG: Diagnosing borderline patients with a semi-structured interview. Arch Gen Psychiatry 1980; 37:37–41

Leone NF: Response of borderline patients to loxapine and chlorpromazine. J Clin Psychiatry 1982; 43:148–150

Liebowitz MR, Klein DF: Inter-relationship of hysteroid dysphoria and borderline personality disorder. Psychiatr Clin North Am 1981; 4:67–89

Marmor J: Orality in the hysterical personality. Am J Psychoanal 1953; 656–671

Montgomery SA, Montgomery D: Pharmacological prevention of suicidal behavior. J Affective Disord 1982; 4:291–298

Montgomery SA, Roy D, Montgomery DB: The prevention of recurrent suicidal acts. Br J Clin Pharmacol 1983; 15:1835–1885

Perry JC: Depression in borderline personality disorder: lifetime prevalence at interview and longitudinal course of symptoms. Am J Psychiatry 1985; 145:15–21

Reus MD, Markrow S: Alprazolam in the treatment of borderline personality disorder. Paper presented at the Society of Biological Psychiatry, Los Angeles, CA, May 1984

Rifkin A, Levitan SJ, Galewski J, et al: Emotionally unstable character disorder—a follow-up study. Biol Psychiatry 1972a; 4:65–79

Rifkin A, Quitkin F, Carrillo, et al: Lithium carbonate in emotionally unstable character disorders. Arch Gen Psychiatry 1972b; 27:519–523

Schulz SC: Response to medication in borderline patients. Paper presented at the 139th Annual Meeting of the American Psychiatric Association. Washington, DC, May 14, 1986

Serban G, Siegel S: Response of borderline and schizotypal patients to small doses of thiothixene and haloperidol. Am J Psychiatry 1984; 141:1455–1458

Shader RI, Jackson AH, Dodes LM: The anti-aggressive effects of lithium in man. Psychopharmacologia (Berl) 1974; 40:17–24

Sheard MH: Lithium in the treatment of aggression. J Nerv Ment Dis 1975; 160:108–118

Soloff PH: Pharmacotherapy of borderline disorders. Compr Psychiatry 1981; 22:535–543

Soloff PH, Ulrich RF: The Diagnostic Interview for Borderlines: a replication study. Arch Gen Psychiatry 1981, 38:686–692

Soloff PH, George A, Nathan RS, et al: Paradoxical effects of amitriptyline in borderline patients. Am J Psychiatry 1986a; 143:1603–1605

Soloff PH, George A, Nathan RS, et al: Progress in pharmacotherapy of borderline disorders. Arch Gen Psychiatry 1986b; 43:691–697

Soloff PH, George A, Nathan RS, et al: Amitriptyline vs haloperidol in borderlines. Paper presented at the 140th Annual Meeting of the American Psychiatric Association, Chicago, IL, May 12, 1987a

Soloff PH, George A, Nathan RS, et al: Characterizing Depression in Borderline Patients. J Clin Psychiatry 1987b; 48:155–157

Soloff PH, George A, Nathan RS, et al: Patterns of response among borderline patients with amitriptyline and haloperidol. Psychopharmacol Bull (in press)

Spitzer RL, Endicott J, Gibbon M: Crossing the border into borderline personality and borderline schizophrenia: the development of criteria. Arch Gen Psychiatry 1979; 36:17–24

Sternberg DE: Pharmacotherapy and affective syndromes in borderline personality disorder. Paper presented at 140th Annual Meeting of the American Psychiatric Association, Chicago, IL, May 12, 1987

Tupin JP, Smith DB, Classon TL, et al: Long-term use of lithium in aggressive disorders. Compr Psychiatry 1973; 14:311–317

Waldinger RJ, Gunderson JG: Completed psychotherapies with borderline patients. Am J Psychotherapy 1984; 38:190–202

Zilboorg G: Ambulatory schizophrenia. Psychiatry 1941; 4:149–155

Chapter 5

Cognitive and Behavior Therapy for Borderline Personality Disorder

by Marsha M. Linehan, Ph.D.

REVIEW OF LITERATURE

Behavior therapists have written very little on the topic of borderline personality disorder and, when mentioned, attention is often brief (Turkat and Maisto, 1985). (There are many schools of therapy within the general behavior therapy fold. Although there are important theoretical differences, in the context of this chapter their similarities are more important than their differences. Thus, unless otherwise stated, the term "behavior therapy" includes "behavior modification," "applied behavioral analysis," "cognitive–behavior therapy" and "cognitive therapy.") Before 1988, the only authors who had published behavioral treatments for borderline personality disorder were Turner (1983) and Linehan (1987b, 1987c, 1987d). Interestingly, none of the first publications have appeared in behavior therapy journals! Factors inhibiting attention to borderline personality disorders among behavior therapists are discussed by Linehan and Wasson (in press) and include general problems with both the construct of personality itself and with categorical classification systems, as well as more specific problems having to do with the validity of the borderline personality disorder construct. To date, only two experimental studies have been conducted evaluating empirically the efficacy of behavior therapy (or *any* psychological therapy for that matter) with borderline patients (Linehan, 1987a; Turner, 1987). Turner conducted a single case, multiple baseline, across-subjects evaluation of cognitive–behavioral treatment combined with pharmacotherapy. Of the seven patients who began treatment, three dropped out prior to completion of the program. Thus, the study tracked progress for only four patients. Treatment reduced self-reported frequency of worst symptoms as well as mood disturbance for three of the four patients. In a randomized, treatment control design, Linehan (1987a) compared her treatment, dialectical behavior therapy (DBT), with treatment-as-usual in the community. Dialectical behavior therapy is described more fully in a later section. Linehan's patients were severely dysfunctional women who were actively parasuicidal, had high suicidal ideation, and met criteria for borderline personality disorder. In comparison to the control group, DBT reduced the frequency and medical severity of parasuicide and tended to improve the employment rate. In addition, no patients (out of the 11 who began DBT treatment) dropped out of the one-year treatment program. This is in contrast to the control group in which only 50 percent of the patients were still with the same therapist at the end of one year, indicating that DBT is effective in enhancing treatment

Preparation of this chapter was funded by National Institute of Mental Health Grant MH34486.

alliance and reducing premature therapy termination. Although DBT patients clearly were behaving more functionally, there were no between-group differences on reported symptoms, depression, hopelessness, or suicidal ideation at any point. A slight but significant improvement could be detected overall on self-reported symptoms.

In contrast to the paucity of data on treatment efficacy with patients diagnosed as borderline, the empirical literature on treatment of specific behavioral patterns comprising borderline personality disorder is extensive. Certainly, the efficacy of these treatments may be seriously compromised when the patient has the multitude of problems associated with borderline personality disorder in combination with the specific behavioral syndrome under study. Individuals meeting criteria for various affective disorders, impulse control disorders, or interpersonal behavior disorders who do not also meet criteria for personality disorder at the same time may respond to standard behavior therapies quite differently from those who meet such criteria. However, it must be acknowledged that since personality disorder assessments are not, as a rule, carried out in behavior therapy research, these multiple diagnoses individuals were also not excluded from the research studies.

The evidence for the efficacy of behavioral and cognitive therapies in treating at least some affect regulation difficulties (*Diagnostic and Statistical Manual of Mental Disorders, Third Edition, Revised, [DSM-III-R]* criteria 3, 4) (American Psychiatric Association, 1987), including problems with excessive anger, anxiety, and depression is strong (Masters et al, 1987; O'Leary and Wilson, 1987). There is also an extensive empirical literature on the effectiveness of cognitive and behavior therapies for problems of impulse control in specific areas (*DSM-III-R* criteria 2), including eating disorders and substance abuse disorders (Masters et al, 1987; O'Leary and Wilson, 1987). Especially relevant to the borderline personality disorder, two studies (Bartman, 1976; Liberman and Eckman, 1981) found behavior therapy to be superior to insight therapy in reducing parasuicidal behavior (*DSM-III-R* criteria 5). Finally, there is extensive literature on behavioral treatments of both specific and generalized interpersonal problems (*DSM-III-R* criteria 1, 8; Turner and Hersen, 1981; Linehan, 1979; Curran, 1985). It is beyond the scope of this chapter to review the extensive outcome data on behavior therapy for specific behavior problems here. The interested reader is referred to general reviews of behavior therapy such as Barlow (1985), O'Leary and Wilson (1987) and Masters and colleagues (1987).

Missing in the behavioral literature is attention to problems of identity disturbance, as well as chronic feelings of emptiness or boredom (*DSM-III-R* criteria 6, 7). Perhaps a partial explanation for this is an attitude toward treatment among behavior therapists exemplified by Kanfer and Saslow (1969), who stated:

> When a behavioral analysis reveals that a patient's problems lie mainly in his dissatisfactions with or uncertainties about his self-attitudes, or a loss of meaning or purpose, there is further a serious question . . . whether such patients should be treated by the traditional professional groups, the psychiatry, psychology, and social work members of the "mental healing" professions. (p. 429)

MAJOR MODELS

Cognitive Models

THEORY.   The cognitive model of borderline personality disorder is based on the proposition that emotional and behavioral patterns associated with the disorder are mediated by maladaptive cognitive processes. Generally, standard cognitive theory and associated therapy (Beck, 1976; Beck et al, 1979) focus on three levels of cognitive phenomena: automatic thoughts, cognitive distortions, and underlying assumptions. Padesky (1986) and Young (1983) suggest that in contrast to Axis I disorders, where the primary dysfunction is in automatic thoughts and underlying assumptions, in Axis II disorders the core problem involves dysfunctional cognitive schemas developed during early childhood. Although Pretzer (in press) does not refer to schemas, he does identify underlying cognitive assumptions common in borderline patients which seem quite similar to the schemas proposed by Young. Padesky further suggests that a critical difference between Axis I and Axis II patients is that the former have adaptive schemas available, even though not activated, whereas Axis II patients have never developed adaptive schemas. Thus, Axis I patients can switch to adaptive schemas when the maladaptive ones are invalidated. Axis II patients, however, have no easy alternative and, in fact, cannot even conceive of alternatives.

Young identifies nine specific maladaptive schemas as central to borderline personality disorder. With two exceptions, these fall into the categories of schemas about autonomy (the sense that one can function independently in the world without continual support) and connectedness (the sense that one is connected to others in a stable, enduring, and trusting manner). In contrast, Pretzer proposes that three basic assumptions characterize borderlines: "The world is a dangerous and malevolent place"; "I am powerless and vulnerable"; and "I am inherently unacceptable."

Pretzer also stresses the role of cognitive distortions—in particular, dichotomous thinking—in the etiology of borderline personality disorder. Extreme and abrupt shifts in emotional responses and action are a natural result of dichotomous thinking, since such thinking forces extreme interpretations on relatively neutral events, and, thus, when a perception of a situation changes, it necessarily changes from one extreme to another. Although it does not seem to grow out of the usual theory underpinning cognitive therapy, Pretzer further suggests that a core component in the borderline personality is a weak or unstable sense of identity. Consistent with cognitive theory, however, "identity" in Pretzer's work refers to goals, priorities, self-efficacy, and self-concept. While acknowledging that biology and temperament play some role, cognitive theorists generally assume that there are no exceptional biological traits that significantly influence the development of maladaptive schemas, cognitive distortions, and identity issues. Instead, the emphasis is on the role of early social learning experiences.

TREATMENT.   Cognitive therapy (CT) focuses on identifying and changing automatic thoughts, processes of cognitive distortions, and underlying assumptions. Both Young (1983) and Pretzer (in press) suggest that CT as usually practiced is unlikely to be particularly effective with borderline patients. Issues that Pretzer highlights include problems in developing and maintaining a collaborative patient–therapist relationship; problems maintaining a consistent, focused strategic approach; power struggles, especially around agenda setting and homework assignments; noncompliance on homework assignments; and patients' fears of change and of termination. Generally, Pretzer's approach to these problems is to refocus on identifying and critically examining the thoughts, assumptions, and cognitive distortions surrounding the therapy problem (i.e., the focus of CT becomes the cognitive processes interfering with therapy). Pretzer's main contention is that, flexibly applied, CT strategies should be effective with the borderline patient.

The cornerstone of Young's (1983) therapy is his emphasis on targeting early maladaptive schemas. The treatment consists of steps for identifying schemas and techniques for changing schemas. The first stage of treatment requires the patient and therapist to identify schemas relevant to the patient's problems, schema avoidance strategies and coping behaviors, and schema trigger events. This is done by discussing the patient's presenting problems, current events, past memories, the therapeutic relationship, dreams, and by assigning relevant books and films, group therapy, and written homework assignments such as diary keeping. More so than in usual CT, the therapist focuses on triggering the patient's maladaptive schemas within the therapy session and on identifying and confronting schema avoidance strategies of the patient.

Schema change techniques include all of the usual hypothesis testing strategies used in CT. However, Young suggests that these techniques alone are insufficient in changing early maladaptive schemas. Instead, it is essential to challenge the schemas when they are actually triggered and accompanied by their usual intense affect. Many of the proposed techniques are drawn from gestalt therapy. They include creating imaginary dialogues with patients, encouraging patients to express or "ventilate" emotions in sessions, reading counterschema flashcards outside of sessions when schemas are triggered, and actively countering schemas when activated during the therapy session. In addition, Young recommends a directive focus on changing the patient's environment, the adjunctive use of medication, pushing the patient to change schema coping behaviors, using the therapeutic relationship to "re-parent" the patient, providing experiences that counteract early maladaptive schemas. Unfortunately, these latter techniques are touched on only briefly by Young, and guidelines for implementing them are not provided.

Classic Behavior Therapy

Turner (1983, 1984, 1987) and Linehan (1987a, 1987b, 1987e, unpublished treatment manual) have applied and expanded more mainstream behavioral therapies to borderline personality disorder. Neither Turner nor Linehan ignore cognitive processes in the etiology and maintenance of borderline phenomena, but both emphasize a wider range of treatment strategies than do their cognitively oriented colleagues.

TURNER'S COGNITIVE—BEHAVIORAL TREATMENT MODEL. Turner (1984) proposes a cognitive–analytic model of borderline personality disorder that in many respects is indistinguishable from the cognitive theory presented above. Like cognitive theorists, Turner proposes that maladaptive schema learned early in life profoundly effect and limit later learning and strongly influence behavior and affect. With respect to borderline personality disorder, specifically, maladaptive schema are responsible for rapid dysjunctive shifts in mental and emotional sets, leading to a disturbance in the sense of temporal continuity, and a sense of cognitive confusion, disorientation, and derealization whenever a feared stressor occurs. Several behavioral sequelae of these difficulties are paramount from Turner's perspective: interpersonal difficulties, social anxiety, cognitive dysfunction problems, depression, and impulsive behavior.

LINEHAN'S BIOSOCIAL (BEHAVIORAL) MODEL. Although Linehan's model of borderline personality also recognizes the role of cognitive processes in the disorder (1987a; Linehan and Wagner, in press), she differs from the cognitive and cognitive–behavioral theorists in that she proposes a diathesis/environment model which holds that the primary dysfunction is one of inadequate affect regulation. Given an initial affective vulnerability, together with an invalidating social-developmental environment, Linehan's theory specifies both how borderline personality disorder develops and which behavioral patterns are central to it, once developed. The behavioral patterns are organized along three dialectical poles: 1) emotional vulnerability versus invalidation; 2) active–passivity versus the apparently competent person; and 3) unremitting crises versus inhibited grieving. The first behavioral patterns in each pair are originally most heavily influenced by biological factors associated with emotion regulation. The second patterns in each pair are most heavily influenced by past and current social responses to emotional behaviors. From Linehan's point of view, these behavioral syndromes, when not recognized by the therapist, can account for much of the trouble encountered when conducting therapy with this population.

The *emotional vulnerability* syndrome refers to high sensitivity to emotional stimuli, intense responses to even low-level stimuli, and slow return to emotional baseline. The mechanisms of this emotion dysregulation are unclear, although limbic system reactivity and difficulties in attention control are suggested. The *invalidating* syndrome refers to the tendency of the social environments and, subsequently, the borderline individual, to invalidate affective experiences and to oversimplify the ease of solving life's problems. The invalidating family is similar to the high expressed emotion families described in research on schizophrenia (Leff and Vaughn, 1985). Developmentally, without validating environments, borderline individuals do not learn how to label or control emotional reactions adequately, how to tolerate emotional distress, or when to trust their own emotional responses as reflections of valid interpretations of events. Thus, affective intolerance and lability continue, together with impulsive behaviors, which terminate or completely avoid the recurrent, painful emotional states. This emphasis on avoidance of negative affect is similar to Young's emphasis on maladaptive schema avoidance. The difference is that Linehan does not assume cognitive mediation. Since emotional consistency and predictability, across time and similar situations, are prerequisites for the development of a sense of self, a stable sense of identity fails to develop. Within an invalidating environment, extreme emotional displays and/or extreme problems are necessary to provoke a helpful environmental response. Thus, the social contingencies favor the development of extreme reactions on the part of the borderline individual. A stable sense of self as well as emotion control skills are necessary ingredients in stable interpersonal relationships. Their absence, therefore, is an important factor in the chaotic relationships so typical of borderline individuals.

The other two behavioral poles are derivatives of the emotion vulnerability/invalidating syndrome. *Active–passivity* refers to the tendency to approach problems passively and helplessly, as well as a corresponding tendency under extreme distress to actively demand solutions from the environment. This passive, self-regulation style is a result of both a disposition to high autonomic reactivity as well as to the individual's history of failing in attempts to control both negative affects and associated, maladaptive avoidance and/or escape behaviors (i.e., learned helplessness). The *apparently competent person* syndrome refers to the tendency of borderline patients to appear deceptively competent, both interpersonally and in other ways. The deception is that the real competencies these individual have are not generalized across all relevant situations. The failure in generalization is due to a number of factors, including an inability to avoid extreme affect unconditionally. This discrepancy between appearance and actual competence perpetuates the invalidating environment and is at the cost of almost total inhibition of negative affective experiences and expression in certain situations.

The *unrelenting crisis* syndrome refers to the seemingly never-ending personal crises that borderline individuals are faced with and their inability to return to the baseline of neutral emotional functioning. Biological factors exacerbate initial emotional responses and rate of return to baseline after each stressor. The magnitude and number of subsequent stressors are then increased by both the individual's responses to the initial stressor as well as by equally inadequate social support networks (the invalidating environment). The cycle is self-perpetuating. The *inhibited grieving* syndrome refers to the pattern of repetitive, significant trauma and loss together with an inability to experience and personally integrate these events. The accumulation of such losses leads to bereavement overload, and necessary grieving is inhibited.

Behavior Therapy

The critical first step in behavior therapy with any individual, including those with personality disorders, is a behavioral assessment to identify behavioral referents for the patient's presenting complaints, as well as to formulate hypotheses about current mechanisms (i.e., controlling variables) maintaining those complaints and their etiology. The theories presented by Linehan and Turner, respectively, offer hypotheses about possible treatment targets and controlling variables. Although both caution clinicians to assess, not assume, the formulation in the individual case, they each, nonetheless, have developed comprehensive treatment packages based on their respective formulations. Interestingly, although they identify different etiological mechanisms (maladaptive schemas versus affect dysregulation), their treatments share many similar components.

Both treatments assume that borderline individuals have several important behavioral deficits. Turner focuses on interpersonal skill and anxiety management deficits. Linehan also targets interpersonal skills, but expands anxiety management to general emotional regulation and adds a focus on developing distress tolerance skills. Both treatments consist of simultaneous group and individual therapy. Group treatment in both is psychoeducational, consisting of didactic training in the appropriate skills, behavior rehearsal, in vivo practice and exposure in the problematic situations, and discussion of the in vivo practice assignments. Turner, in his research treatment protocol, offers a 15-week interpersonal skill training group. Linehan offers four sequential group treatments over the course of one year: 1) core skills (training in observing, describing, spontaneous participation, mindfulness, nonjudgmentalness, and focusing on effectiveness); 2) interpersonal skills; 3) emotion regulation skills; and 4) distress tolerance skills.

Although there is substantial overlap, the individual treatments recommended by Linehan and Turner differ considerably. Turner's treatment is defined by four cognitive–behavior therapy components offered sequentially to the patient as follows: 1) cognitive therapy, very similar to standard cognitive therapy described above, but with an added emphasis on teaching problem-solving skills; 2) self-control desensitization to stress-producing situations, a procedure similar to the treatment developed by Goldfried (1971); 3) supportive psychotherapy; and 4) "states of mind modification." This latter technique was developed by Turner and is based on the theorizing and clinical insights of Horowitz and colleagues (1984). Briefly, it involves analyzing the patient's usual problematic states of mind, a concept similar to that of schema in cognitive theory, then imaginally exposing the patient to those "states of mind" and affective experiences that normally lead to dysjunctive or decompensation episodes. The goal is to expose the patient to troublesome affects so that their cue saliency is reduced. It is not clear from Turner's writings whether the method of exposure is always flooding, as in the research study described above, or is sometimes graded much like desensitization.

Linehan's therapy has three overriding characteristics; a problem-solving focus, an emphasis on dialectical processes, and observation and management of the contingencies operating in the patient–therapist relationship. The problem-solving focus requires that the therapist address all problematic patient behaviors (in and out of sessions) and therapy situations in a systematic manner, including conducting collaborative behavioral analyses, formulating hypotheses about possible variables influencing the problem, generating possible changes (behavioral solutions), and trying out and evaluating the solutions. The term dialectical has two meanings in the context of Linehan's therapy. First, it provides a philosophical underpinning, similar to a systems approach, which addresses the multiple tensions that coexist and must be balanced and synthesized in conducting therapy with this population. Second, it suggests the necessity of both dialectical thinking on the part of the therapist as well as targeting non-dialectical, rigid, and dichotomous thinking on the part of the patient. (For the interested reader, Bassecus, 1984, provides an excellent description of dialectical thinking and adult development.)

Dialectics, as used by Linehan, refers to a world view that emphasizes the wholeness, interconnectedness, and nonreducibility of all things, a unity of opposites (i.e., all things are inherently heterogeneous, composed of opposing forces), identity as fundamentally tied to relationships, and change as the nature of reality. All of nature, therefore, is seen as continual process rather than as static. Change from this perspective is the result of continual resolution or synthesis of tensions (thesis and antithesis) occurring within each whole. This viewpoint influences conceptualization on all levels. For example, a dialectical view favors a systems approach, a developmental viewpoint, dimensional rather than categorical analyses, and is incompatible with assignment of blame or truth in a dichotomous manner.

Dialectical behavior therapy (DBT) is defined by its philosophical underpinnings, described above, its treatment targets, and the treatment strategies guiding the conduct of the therapist. Treatment targets (goals) in individual DBT are hierarchically arranged as follows: 1) suicidal behaviors; 2) behaviors interfering with the conduct of therapy (similar to Pretzer's emphasis on problems implementing CT); 3) avoidance and escape behaviors interfering with a reasonable quality life (similar to Young's emphasis on reducing avoidance); 4) behavioral skill acquisition (emotion regulation, interpersonal effectiveness, distress tolerance, self-management; similar to Turner's emphasis on skill training); and 5) other goals suggested by the individual case formulation. Attention is shifted to a target earlier on the list when problems in that area surface. Thus, therapy is somewhat circular in that target focal points revolve over time.

There are eight basic treatment strategy groups in DBT. Four strategies common to other behavior therapies are:

1. *problem-solving strategies*: an active attempt to "reframe" suicidal and other dysfunctional behaviors as part of the patient's learned problem-solving repertoire with emphasis on active problem-solving (includes behavioral analysis, insight, solution generation, analyses and implementation, and environmental intervention strategies)
2. *contingency management strategies*: the use of interpersonal reinforcement to shape adaptive behaviors and extinguish those that are maladaptive (includes contingency clarification and application, instructions about "how the world operates," therapists observing their own limits in contrast to setting arbitrary limits, and shaping strategies)
3. *irreverent communication strategies*: matter-of-fact, somewhat literal-minded attitude about current and previous parasuicidal and other dysfunctional patient behaviors (but not matter-of-fact about patient suffering)
4. *capability enhancement strategies*: active teaching of the skills necessary to cope with one's self and with a sometimes invalidating environment (includes response acquisition, response strengthening, response generalization, and response inhibition reduction strategies)

The *dialectical* strategies include many techniques used by cognitive therapists but also add a focus on dialectical thinking, metaphor, paradox, comfort with ambiguity and inconsistency, and attention to the dialectical tensions in the therapeutic relationship. The *consultant* strategy is a simple rule in DBT theory (though hard to carry out) which states that the role of the DBT therapist and treatment team is to consult with the patient about how to interact with others, not to consult with others about how to interact with the patient. The *validation* strategies contrast somewhat with usual cognitive and behavior therapies in that they require the therapist to search for the inherent validity and wisdom of the patient's response patterns, even when these patterns are apparently maladaptive. Finally, a number of *relationship* strategies are suggested to both enhance the patient–therapist alliance and to use the relationship as a vehicle for interpersonal change. Linehan has further polarized DBT strategies into those representing primarily *acceptance* of the patient in the moment, and those focusing on enhancing *change*. Dialectical behavior therapy, done correctly, balances the two strategic poles.

APPROACHES TO COMMON PROBLEMS

As noted above, very little has been written about conducting cognitive or behavior therapy with borderline patients. I have, however, been conducting behavior therapy treatment outcome research with this population for the past 10 years. Dialectical behavior therapy is the outcome of this research. In what follows, I will draw mostly on my work with these patients to discuss how one might approach various common treatment problems behaviorally.

Engagement in Treatment

Patients with borderline personality disorder are notoriously difficult to engage in an *active* collaborative relationship. However, with the exception of contingency management, all cognitive and behavior therapies require just such a relationship. A first step in getting patients engaged is "getting their attention," as Frances once put it (1988). This can be done in a variety of ways. Most important, the therapists must show an initial, genuine interest in and understanding of the hell in which these patients are currently living. In fact, it is sometimes useful if therapists describe patients' suffering even more dramatically than they themselves describe it (dialectical and validating strategies). Ameliorating this state of affairs is the first target of therapy. Then, one must persuade the patient (using contingency strategies) of the ways in which suicidal (especially chronic parasuicide) behaviors, therapy-interfering behaviors, and avoidance behaviors are contributing to this never-ending suffering. The reciprocal role of skill deficits in interpersonal problem-solving, emotional control, distress tolerance, and self-management as both precipitants and consequences of the overall problem is discussed extensively. Generally, we present our entire theoretical notions (described above) and in the process of active discussion, refine the theory to fit the particular patient. Once the goals of treatment and a theoretical approach are agreed upon, we elicit a commitment from the patient to work on reducing problematic behaviors and not drop out of treatment for one year (suicide, of course, would constitute dropping out of treatment). It is essential, here, that the therapist be very explicit about how hard this joint task will be, while all the time offering hope that the task can be negotiated if the two work together. Difficulties are predicted, relapses are to be expected, but eventual success is likely. The metaphor here is that of building a house in the middle of a raging hail storm. It is understandable that patients would want to run into their old and trusty tents from time to time.

Next, the therapist must get the patient to agree on the form of therapy; that is, how the two (or group) are going to actually bring about all of these changes. We are very clear: First we have to get behavior under control, then we will deal with other problems. It often comes as quite a surprise when we clearly state that we expect the patient to learn to *be* miserable but not *act* miserable. Although we are very clear about our belief in a biological factor in their misery, we point out that to date there is no biological treatment that will cure their misery. Thus, learning to act, feel, and think differently is the only way out for the moment. It is essential at each point here that therapists weave patient validation strategies (especially validating patients' emotional suffering, their analyses of what the important maintaining factors might be, and their wisdom about what types of therapy might be effective) with a similar emphasis on relationship enhancement strategies, such as communicating a sense of the therapist's own expertise, credibility, and efficacy as a therapist.

Relationship of Technique to the Borderline Patient's Presenting Symptoms

In cognitive therapy, automatic thoughts, cognitive distortions, underlying assumptions, and early maladaptive schemas are presumed to underlie all symptoms. Once those relevant to the patient's symptoms are identified, cognitive treatment is implemented, aimed at changing those maladaptive processes. Thus, in cognitive therapy, both the general focus of treatment (cognitive processes) and treatment techniques employed usually do not change. The specific target (i.e., specific cognitive distortion, underlying assumption, early maladaptive schema), of course, varies according to the individual patient.

To date, both DBT and Turner's treatment have been offered in very standard manners. This is primarily due to the research focus of our respective treatment programs. Also, at least in our DBT research, the program varies little due to the extremely dysfunctional nature of the patients referred to the program. Generally, the first year is spent getting parasuicide and therapy-interfering behaviors under control and teaching basic self-management skills. We have yet to have many patients for whom these were not significant initial issues. Dialectical behavior therapy however, is a very flexible treatment, and the ebb and flow of the use of various strategies as well as emphasis on various targets (symptoms) changes as the patient changes.

Treatment changes in DBT are usually related to stages of therapy, the state of the treatment relationship, and patient progress. For example, validation strategies are used from the very beginning of treatment, whereas relationship contingencies cannot be used until there is a significant, strong bond between the patient and therapist. Shaping might dictate much more environmental intervention at early stages, before the patient has acquired sufficient skills, and little or no intervention at later points. Likewise, before patients learn to label and communicate their current emotional state we might be quite likely to engage in "mind reading." At a later point in therapy, we would likely refrain from such activities. Focused skill training groups are usually "graduated from" after a year or so. With court referred or nonvoluntary patients, skill training groups may be delayed until we modify motivation for treatment. The point I am making here is that strategies and targets depend very much on the capabilities the patient has at each point in time. Unfortunately, however, how to make the appropriate judgment about which strategies to use, and when to use them, is still very much an art rather than a science.

The Processes and Problems in Building an Alliance

In cognitive therapy, difficulties in the alliance are resolved by attempting to identify and critically examine the patient's schemas relevant to the relationship problem. In DBT, validation and relationship strategies are essential in developing and maintaining a working relationship. Validation strategies require the therapist to observe and describe the patient's behavior accurately (emotions, beliefs, overt behavioral patterns); to empathize or understand the responses in question; and to communicate the essential understandability or sensibility of the patient's responses. In essence, the therapist searches for the inherent validity and functionality of the patient's reponses. This is in contrast to usual cognitive and behavior therapy, in which a primary focus of treatment is to search for and replace dysfunctional behavioral processes.

There are six specific DBT relationship strategies: relationship acceptance, reciprocal vulnerability, relationship enhancement, relationship problem-solving, relationship contingencies, and relationship generalization. Acceptance and reciprocal vulnerability strategies dictate therapist behaviors that enhance acceptance of both the patient as he or she is right at the moment (i.e., patience), as well as acceptance and communication to the patient of where the therapist is (including a certain amount of self-disclosure and using oneself as a model). The reciprocal vulnerability strategy in DBT is similar to Pretzer's admonitions to the cognitive therapist to exercise care in communicating clearly and honestly, and to maintain congruence between verbal statements and nonverbal cues. Relationship problem-solving recommends use of ordinary problem-solving techniques in the treatment relationship situation. This is similar to the notion, prominent in some forms of psychodynamic therapy, that relationship repair is an essential vehicle for the efficacy of therapy. From a DBT point of view, I would suggest that avoiding mistakes is far less important than repairing mistakes well. Contingency strategies focus on the use of therapist-administered reinforcing contingencies for responses on the part of the patient, which are in the direction of a positive treatment alliance. The use of natural reinforcers (e.g., therapist warmth, keeping agreements) instead of arbitrary reinforcers (e.g., saying "good") is emphasized.

An additional important factor in maintaining a good alliance in DBT is the supervision and theory offered the therapists. Stone and colleagues (1987), and Woollcott (1985), have suggested that likability of the patient is an important factor in patient improvement. The theoretical underpinnings of DBT were developed partially to offer an explanatory system for borderline patient behaviors, which would enhance therapist compassion no matter what the patient does. Thus, in DBT supervision, the emphasis is on helping the therapist replace pejorative conceptualizations (e.g., "She is manipulating me") with less judgmental theoretical positions (e.g., "Social responses are maintaining her behavior; I feel manipulated"). Dialectical strategies (e.g., "How could both points of view here be correct?") are practiced within therapists' supervisory sessions to prevent staff splitting. A major task of DBT supervision is to help therapists both observe their own limits and continue to reach out to patients, even when such responses are extremely difficult.

Compliance With the Treatment Schedule and Boundaries

Two types of noncompliance are important in cognitive and behavior therapy: 1) the patient will not engage in a focused, strategic approach to achieving goals and treatment priorities, and 2) the patient will not engage in recommended homework practice assignments or will not follow through with other treatment requirements. In cognitive therapy, a consistent focus is maintained by discussing the pros and cons of such a steady focus, by agreeing to set aside part of each session for current issues and then shifting to ongoing goals, and, if necessary to maintain continuity, by each week addressing the issues underlying the immediate crisis (Pretzer, in press). In DBT, I have addressed this problem by dividing DBT into two sections: group skills training and individual therapy.

Essentially, I gave up trying to keep the patient focused on a consistent, goal-oriented topic in individual therapy. Focused skills training can be done individually or in pairs, but is easier in groups. Group norms explicitly discourage discussion of individual crises or nonskill related events. During individual therapy, there are only two topics that the patient must focus on like it or not—reducing parasuicide and "solving" therapy-interfering problems. If either of these surface between (or during) sessions, the therapist insists on devoting some therapy session time to them. Patients, of course, often get very angry about this: The therapist uses contingency and relationship strategies (e.g., "I can't work with you effectively if these problems are not addressed"). With these two exceptions, however, the direction of individual therapy is usually left up to the patient. The therapist keeps sessions focused by judicious use of questioning and comments.

Other noncompliant behaviors are addressed as problems to be collaboratively solved. Pretzer suggests that cognitive therapists be alert to maintaining flexibility, adhering to the collaborative model, and examining patients' thoughts and assumptions about treatment recommendations as well as those surrounding fears of change. In DBT, noncompliance could require use of any or all of the DBT strategies and, in particular, the validation, problem-solving, and contingency strategies. With respect to homework practice (usually only given in the group treatment component), DBT stresses the importance of shaping (a contingency management strategy).

Patient behaviors which transgress the therapist's comfortable "boundaries," such as excessive phone calls, not leaving after sessions, inappropriate suicide threats, expecting the therapist to figure out and solve problems, overdemanding behaviors, and so on, are addressed in a number of ways in DBT. First, such behaviors are therapy-interfering behaviors (primarily because they cause undue wear and tear on the therapist) and, thus, are second only to suicidal behaviors as a treatment target. This means they are discussed directly with the patient. Problem-solving, relationship, and contingency strategies are likely to be employed. A most important contingency strategy is the "observing limits" strategy. In DBT, arbitrary limits on patient behavior are not set. Instead, each therapist is required to monitor his or her own limits closely, with each particular patient at each point in time. The supposition of DBT is that when therapists allow patients to push them past their own limits, burn-out will occur and the patient will be harmed. Either the therapist will reject the patient or will not reach out when the patient pulls away. This rationale for observing limits is explained clearly to patients. Generally, we try not to deny the role of our own welfare in determining the treatment strategies and limits (an example of reciprocal vulnerability). As with parasuicidal behavior, when limit-pushing (boundary-crossing) behaviors occur, the therapist insists on addressing them in each session until they are under control. In very extreme and recalcitrant cases, the therapist might implement an arbitrary contingency schedule. The key element here is that the required behavior for reinforcement or to avoid losing reinforcement is clearly specified, and the contingencies, once set, are implemented surely and consistently.

The Use of Treatment as a Trial

The notion of treatment as a trial is integral to behavior therapy. Generally, one is admonished to switch treatments if the current one is not working. A number of questions, however, arise when treating borderline patients. How soon should one expect progress? That is, at what points should assessments be conducted? How much progress should be expected? That is, how little is too little suggesting a treatment change? Are there alternative treatments appropriate to the specified goal? There is very little empirical data to answer these questions. Stone and colleagues' data (1987) suggests that appreciable improvement among discharged borderline inpatients should not be expected for 5–10 years, at least when type of follow-up treatment is not controlled. Some pharmacotherapy studies with inpatients suggest that measurable improvement in affect can be expected by five weeks (Soloff et al, 1985). In Turner's work (1987), and in our first outcome study of DBT (Linehan, 1987d), reduction in worst symptoms (always parasuicide in my work) occurred within 16 weeks.

The emphasis on shaping in DBT suggests that it is particularly important for the therapist to be very precise both in specifying the treatment goals and in operationally defining progress at each step. Breaking down the targeted goal into its component parts is essential. For example, affect control may require the component skills of observing and labeling negative affect; analytic skills for identifying precipitating stimuli; interpersonal skills for changing various problem situations; cognitive skills for testing and changing automatic thoughts, assumptions, schemas, and cognitive styles; relaxation or other self-management skills for directly modifying biological states; and motivational skills for identifying and overcoming impediments to change.

Management of Self-Destructive Behavior

Dialectical Behavior Therapy was developed specifically for the chronically suicidal, actively parasuicidal patient. In general, suicidal behaviors are treated as maladaptive problem-solving behaviors (Linehan, 1981). Thus, the treatment plan is designed to: 1) teach other, more adaptive strategies such as interpersonal skills for coping with problematic situations, affect regulation skills for coping with negative affect, and distress tolerance skills for impulse control (capability enhancement strategies); 2) use the validation strategies to defuse crises situations and overwhelming affect; and 3) use contingency strategies to highlight (and effect) negative outcomes for suicidal behaviors and positive outcomes for nonsuicidal coping. In this respect, from a DBT point of view, it is essential that the treatment be arranged so that suicidal behaviors are not followed by positive consequences, and nonsuicidal coping is. Attention to the power of intermittent reinforcement schedules is very important here.

In our research, a large number of patients receive their individual treatment from non-DBT therapists. One of the most important differences between DBT and other treatments is the in-session attention paid to suicidal behaviors. Many therapists seem to believe that attention to suicidal behavior will reinforce it. This belief is based, I suspect, on the assumption of many that the preferred outcome of suicidal behavior among borderline patients is attention. Not only is such an assumption unwarranted in the absence of assessment data, but it is often not the case. Even when attention is the preferred outcome, attention to every nitty gritty detail (every emotion, thought, act, event) that led up to and followed the suicidal behavior (threat, parasuicide), as well a similar analysis of how the chain of events could have been altered prior to the suicidal response, is generally not the kind of attention a patient has in mind. Thus, rather than attending to why the patient was distressed (the attention sometimes desired), we attend to how it was that that distress led to suicidal behavior.

In the absence of any empirical data that outpatient pharmacotherapy or that hospitalizing suicidal, borderline patients actually reduces suicide risk, DBT rarely recommends medication or hospitalization as a response to suicide risk. Suicide risk is further reduced by attention to the types of medications allowed the suicidal outpatient. The general protocol is to eliminate lethal drugs, including antidepressants and oral neuroleptics, from the treatment regime of patients with overdose histories. The notion here is that all pharmocotherapy is ineffective with a dead patient. If medication is required (e.g., lithium in a patient also meeting criteria for bipolar disorder), the medication must be controlled by a third party and blood levels are required every two days to prevent medication hoarding. Once the suicide risk is very low, these precautions can, of course, be relaxed.

INADEQUATE SUPPORT SYSTEMS. Inadequate support systems are usually dealt with in two ways: providing support until changes can be made, and addressing the inadequate support system as a treatment target. Therapist availability is crucial. This need for greater contact with the therapist is met in DBT by including between-session phone calls as an expected part of the treatment. Although extra sessions may be needed at times during great crises, day-to-day needs for between-session support are usually handled via the telephone. (Proper use of the phone is often one of the early targets in DBT). Young suggests that therapists often need to "re-parent" borderline patients, providing direction and experiences crucial for development but nevertheless missed. I would suggest, further, that the therapist often must function much like an extended family member, ready to assist the patient when needed and refrain from overassisting when not needed.

Several DBT strategies are relevant in dealing with inadequate support systems. Validating strategies involve the therapist providing a supportive, validating emotional atmosphere in the therapeutic relationship, which is often missing in patients' external environments. Although DBT requires a therapist with reasonably flexible and compassionate limits, the observing limits strategy requires therapists to avoid overextending themselves in the long run. Demands for impossible amounts of support are dealt with as problems-to-be-solved in therapy, using relationship strategies. Problem-solving strategies are used to help patients analyze their current support systems, determine the types of changes needed and wanted, and generate possible solutions. Capability enhancement strategies are implemented to teach the patient the interpersonal skills necessary to implement the solutions. Such skill training might focus on one-to-one interpersonal skills, family interactions, or more general skills for obtaining institutional support. Relationship generalization strategies might be implemented to help generalize the gains accrued via the patient–therapist relationship to other intimate relationships. Once the patient has entered into some supportive relationships, whether with other professionals, the state, mental health organizations, friends, or family, the therapist uses the consultant strategies to help the patient interact in a skillful way to maintain the support.

A note here should be made about enhancing patient dependence versus independence. A dialectical framework stresses the fundamental interrelatedness and wholeness of reality. From this perspective, independence without dependence is a myth. Often, the problem for borderline patients is not too much dependence, but too much fear of dependence (with good reason, of course). Teaching independence is not a fundamental goal of DBT. Indeed, the world would perhaps be better off if we stressed interdependence more and independence less. This is not to suggest that the ability to function effectively in spite of inadequate support systems is not a goal of DBT. Self-management, affect regulation, distress tolerance, and interpersonal skills, all targeted in DBT, stress individual self-care and self-soothing in the face of an inadequate and often invalidating social environment.

INDICATIONS/CONTRAINDICATIONS.   There simply are no reliable, empirical data to suggest when or with which type of borderline patient cognitive and behavior therapy (or any other therapy) is more or less effective. Dialectical behavior therapy was developed for chronically parasuicidal, borderline patients. The research on DBT has been with severely dysfunctional women, most of whom have not been able to work effectively with other therapists. But the treatment is also intended to be useful with individuals once they substantially improve but before they achieve all of their treatment goals. As in any treatment, modifications in the application of techniques is needed as the patient progresses.

Cognitive and behavior therapies require active participation on the part of the patient. Neither is likely to be effective with a patient who does not want to be in the treatment and is there only under duress. Although individual DBT can be applied in this instance, its success would depend on the effectiveness of the treatment in changing the patient's motivation to change. With borderline patients who are also actively psychotic or meet criteria for bipolar disorder, adjunctive pharmocotherapy is required. When current severe substance abuse is indicated, treatment targeting the borderline syndrome is more useful after the substance abuse is under control.

Finally, cognitive and behavior therapies require a therapist who is willing to participate actively in treatment, who is not uncomfortable being directive, and who has the requisite skills to pass along to the patient. In addition, abilities to remain compassionate under adverse conditions, to be hopeful in the midst of very slow progress, to take phone calls at home, to withstand the stress of a patient who might commit suicide at any minute, to refrain from blaming the victim, and to be flexible, vulnerable, and centered within one's self are prerequisites to working with this population. If these characteristics are not present, at least most of the time, cognitive and behavior therapy and probably any psychotherapy with this population is contraindicated for that particular therapist.

SUMMARY

While both cognitive and behavior therapy are promising interventions with borderline patients, very little empirical work has been done to validate this claim. Only Linehan and Turner have subjected their treatments to experimental tests. Their data, while encouraging, also make clear that much more work needs to be done. No treatment approach, including cognitive and behavior therapy, has so far demonstrated a "cure" for borderline personality disorder. At best, behavior therapy can demonstrate significant improvement in reducing dysfunctional behaviors. Behavior therapy, at least as implemented by Linehan, does not seem very efficient at reducing self-reported negative affect. Faster results were obtained by Turner, who combined behavior therapy with alprazolam. However, he does not report follow-up data for mood stability once the alprazolam is removed. Sustained improvement is not particularly likely.

As usual, much more research is needed. Particularly important are empirical tests of the effectiveness of cognitive therapy, and studies testing the relative effectiveness of behavior therapies with and without the addition of pharmacotherapy. Careful attention to documenting the relative cost, effectiveness, and rate of gain in treatment-as-usual in the community (as controls for the experimental treatments) would be particularly advantageous. An important research area, so far neglected, is the role of therapists' characteristics, training, and supervision/support on treatment outcome. Due to the length of treatment and the stress that these patients put on research staff, studies are extremely expensive. They need to be carefully designed, adequately funded, and provide for sufficient treatment documentation to allow simultaneous analyses of both process and outcome. Outcome and process measures need to be of sufficient breadth that researchers across theoretical orientations—psychodynamic, biological, cognitive, and behavioral—can have confidence that the data from any particular study are relevant to their clinical concerns.

Problems with the validity of the borderline personality construct need to be addressed. Overlaps with Axis I and other Axis II diagnoses are considerable in borderline clinical populations, and the effect of lumping all such patients together in treatment trials is questionable. For example, Linehan's treatment is designed specifically for the severely dysfunctional and suicidal patient. It has only been empirically tested with women. Will it work as effectively with men? Would it work as well with more functional patients? Would a two-year treatment be better than one? Are five years needed? When do costs outweigh benefits? These are empirical questions. It is essential that we leave aside polemical and theoretical arguments, clinical hunches, and unsupported clinical observations and begin the arduous task of conducting the clinical trials needed.

REFERENCES

American Psychiatric Association: Diagnostic and Statistical Manual of Mental Disorders, Third Edition, Revised (DSM-III-R). Washington, DC, American Psychiatric Association, 1987

Barley WD: Paper presented at the panel, New Developments in Understanding and Treating Borderline Personality Organization, Southological Association, Atlanta, GA, 1981

Barlow DH (ed): Clinical Handbook of Psychological Disorders. New York, Guilford, 1985

Bartman ER: Assertive Training with Hospitalized Suicide Attemptors. Unpublished doctoral dissertation. Washington, DC, Catholic University of America, 1976

Basseches M: Dialectical Thinking and Adult Development. Norwood, NJ, Ablex Publishing Corp., 1984

Beck AT: Cognitive Therapy and the Emotional Disorders. New York, Penguin, 1976

Beck AT, Rush AJ, Shaw BF, et al: Cognitive Therapy of Depression. New York, Guilford, 1979

Bowers K: Situationism in psychology: an analysis and a critique. Psychol Rev 1973; 80:307–336

Cantor N, Kihlstrom JF: Cognitive and social processes in personality, in Contemporary Behavior Therapy: Conceptual and Empirical Foundations. Edited by Wilson GT, Franks CM. New York, Guilford, 1982

Chatham PM: Treatment of the Borderline Personality. Northvale, NJ, Jason Aronson, 1985

Curran JP: Social skills therapy: a model and a treatment, in Evaluating Behavior Therapy Outcome. Edited by Turner RM, Ascher LM. New York, Springer, 1985

Endler NS, Magnusson D (Eds): Interactional Psychology and Personality. Washington, DC, Hemisphere Publishing Corp., 1976

Eysenck HJ: Neobehavioristic (S–R) theory, in Contemporary Behavior Therapy: Conceptual and Empirical Foundations. Edited by Wilson GT, Franks CM. New York, Guilford, 1982

Foa EB, Emmelkamp PMG (Eds): Failures in Behavior Therapy. New York, John Wiley & Sons, Inc., 1983

Francis A: Paper presented in symposium, Alternative Models and Treatments of Patients with Borderline Personality Disorder, in meeting of the Society for the Exploration for Psychotherapy Integration, Boston, MA, April 1988

Garfield SL, Bergin AE (Eds): Handbook of Psychotherapy and Behavior Change. New York, John Wiley & Sons, Inc., 1986

Glantz K: The use of a relaxation exercise in the treatment of borderline personality organization. Psychotherapy: Theory, Research & Practice 1981; 18:379–385

Goldfried M: Systematic desensitization as training in self-control. J Consult Clin Psychol 1971; 37:228–234

Gunderson JG, Kolb JE, Austin V: The diagnostic interview for borderline patients. Am J Psychiatry 1981; 138:896–903

Hollandsworth JG Jr: Physiology and Behavior Therapy: Conceptual Guidelines for the Clinician. New York, Plenum, 1986

Horowitz M, Marmar C, Krupenick J, et al: Personality Styles and Brief Psychotherapy. New York, Basic Books, 1984

Kanfer FH, Saslow G: Behavioral diagnosis, in Behavior Therapy: Appraisal and Status. Edited by Franks CM. New York, McGraw-Hill, 1969

Kazdin AE: History of Behavior Modification: Experimental Foundations of Contemporary Research. Baltimore, University Park Press, 1978

Leff JP, Vaughn C: Expressed Emotion in Families: Its Significance for Mental Illness. New York, Guilford, 1985

Liberman RP, Eckman T: Behavior therapy vs. insight oriented therapy for repeated suicide attempters. Arch Gen Psychiatry 1981; 38:1126–1130

Linehan MM: A structured cognitive behavioral treatment of assertion problems, in Cognitive Behavioral Interventions: Theory, Research and Procedures. Edited by Kendall PC, Hollon SD. New York, Academic, 1979

Linehan MM: A social-behavioral analysis of suicide and parasuicide: implications for clinical assessment and treatment, in Depression: Behavioral and Directive Intervention Strategies. Edited by Glaezer H, Clarkin J, New York, Brunner/Mazel, 1981

Linehan MM: Dialectical behavior therapy: a cognitive–behavioral approach to treating borderline personality and chronic suicidal behavior. Workshop presented at the Association for Advancement of Behavior Therapy Annual Convention, Houston, TX, 1985

Linehan MM: Dialectical behavior therapy: Treating borderline personality disorder and suicidal behaviors. Workshop presented at the Association for Advancement of Behavior Therapy Annual Convention, Chicago, IL, 1986

Linehan MM: Behavioral treatment of suicidal clients meeting criteria for borderline personality disorder, in Cognitive and Behavioral Approaches to Suicide. Symposium conducted at the Association for the Advancement of Behavior Therapy, Annual Convention, Boston, MA, November 1987a

Linehan MM: Dialectical behavior therapy: a cognitive behavioral approach to parasuicide. Journal of Personality Disorders 1987b; 1:328–333

Linehan MM: Dialectical behavior therapy for borderline personality disorder: theory and method. Bull Menninger Clin 1987c; 51:261–276

Linehan MM: Dialectical behavior therapy in groups: treating borderline personality disorders and suicidal behavior, in Women's Therapy Groups: Paradigms of Feminist Treatment. Edited by Brody CM. New York, Springer, 1987d

Linehan MM: Dialectical behavior therapy: treating borderline personality disorder. Workshop presented at the Association for the Advancement of Behavior Therapy Annual Convention, Boston, MA, 1987e

Linehan MM, Wagner A: Behavioral treatment of borderline personality disorder: a dialectical–feminist perspective. The Behavior Therapist (in press)

Linehan MM, Wasson E: Behavior therapy for borderline personality disorder, in Handbook of Comparative Treatments. Edited by Bellack AS, Hersen M. New York, John Wiley & Sons (in press)

Masters JC, Burish TG, Hollon SD, et al: Behavior Therapy: Techniques and Empirical Findings, 3rd edition. New York, Harcourt, Brace, Jovanovich, Inc., 1987

Millon T: Modern Psychopathology: A Biosocial Approach to Maladaptive Learning and Functioning. Prospect Heights, IL, Waveland Press, 1983

Mischel W: Personality and Assessment. New York, John Wiley and Sons, 1968

Mischel W: Toward a cognitive social learning reconceptualization of personality. Psychol Rev 1973; 80:252–283

O'Leary KD, Wilson GT: Behavior Therapy: Application and Outcome. Englewood Cliffs, NJ, Prentice-Hall, 1987

Padesky CA: Personality disorders: cognitive therapy into the 90's. Paper presented at the 2nd International Conference on Cognitive Psychotherapy, Umea, Sweden, September, 1986

Pervin LA: Current Controversies and Issues in Personality, 2nd edition. New York, John Wiley & Sons, Inc., 1984

Pretzer J: Borderline personality disorder, in Clinical Applications of Cognitive Therapy. New York, Plenum Press (in press)

Schwartz GE: Integrating psychobiology and behavior therapy: a systems perspective, in Contemporary Behavior Therapy: Conceptual and Empirical Foundations. Edited by Wilson GT, Franks CM. New York, Guilford, 1982

Soloff PH, George A, Nathan S, et al: Progress in pharmacotherapy of borderline disorders. Arch Gen Psychiatry 1985; 43:691–697

Staats AW: Social behaviorism. Homewood, IL, The Dorsey Press, 1975

Staub E: Social and prosocial behavior: personal and situational influences and their interactions, in Personality: Basic Aspects and Current Research. Edited by Staub E. Englewood Cliffs, NJ, Prentice-Hall, 1980

Stone MH, Stone DK, Hurt SW: Natural history of borderline patients treated by intensive hospitalization. Psychiatr Clin North Am 1987; 10:185–206

Turkat ID, Maisto SA: Personality disorders: application of the experimental method to the formulation and modification of personality disorders, in Clinical Handbook of Psychological Disorders. Edited by Barlow DH. New York, Guilford Press, 1985

Turner RM: Behavioral therapy with borderline patients. Carrier Foundation Letter, #88. Published by The Carrier Foundation, Belle Mead, NJ, April, 1983

Turner RM: Assessment and treatment of borderline personality disorder. Paper presented at the 18th Meeting of the Association for the Advancement of Behavior Therapy, Philadelphia, PA, November, 1984

Turner RM: A bio-social learning approach to borderline personality disorder. Paper presented at the Association for the Advancement of Behavior Therapy. Boston, MA, November 1987

Turner SM, Hersen M: Disorders of social behavior: a behavioral approach to personality disorders, in Handbook of Clinical Behavior Therapy. Edited by Turner SM, Calhoun KS, Adams HE. New York, John Wiley & Sons, Inc., 1981

Woolcott P Jr: Prognostic indicators in the psychotherapy of borderline patients. Am J Psychother 1985; 39:17–29

Young J: Borderline personality: cognitive theory and treatment. Paper presented at the American Psychological Assocation Annual Convention, Philadelphia, PA, August, 1983

Chapter 6

The Course of Borderline Personality Disorder

by Michael H. Stone, M.D.

Despite concentrated efforts that began half a century ago (Stern, 1938), we have advanced only a short way toward the development of effective treatment and good prediction in borderline conditions. In part this relates to their nature and complexity, but in part, to the relative paucity of studies bearing on their course (taking treatment into account) or their natural history (leaving treatment to one side). Lack of diagnostic uniformity (Pope et al, 1983; Akiskal et al, 1985; Dahl, unpublished manuscript, 1987) has contributed to the problem. In this area some progress has been made.

The recent definitions of borderline personality disorder (Gunderson and Singer, 1975; DSM-III, 1980) rely upon diagnostic features that are more amenable to consensual validation (i.e., more objectifiable) than the criteria upon which previous definitions (Kernberg, 1967; Grinker et al, 1968) rested.

The newer definitions represent improvements in both specificity and reliability, though one must be aware that certain patients diagnosed as borderline in the older literature would not be so labeled by current standards (Stone, 1987). The tendency during this decade to differentiate between borderline personality disorder (BPD) and schizotypal personality disorder (SPD) (Spitzer et al, 1979) has brought about a shift in the meaning of "borderline," in favor of cases exemplifying the items included in the Gunderson or DSM definitions. I have referred to this tendency as "biometric drift" (Stone, 1987b).

Both the Gunderson and the *Diagnostic and Statistical Manual of Mental Disorders, Third Edition* (*DSM-III*) (American Psychiatric Association, 1980) schemata are polythetic and allow for various combinations of traits and symptoms. The Gunderson definition is narrower and more cohesive, and has helped to outline a *prototypical* borderline case, in which impulsivity, self-damaging acts, and inordinate anger are all present. This cluster was the most common in Hurt's analysis (1988) of 465 patients with borderline personality disorder (BPD) by DSM-III criteria. Borderline personality disorder patients exhibiting only the other five DSM-III items might have a different outcome from those shown by the prototypical patients.

The long-term course of borderline conditions is the ultimate goal of follow-up study and can only be delineated by inquiry about outcome—at many fixed points in time after initial contact. Particularly because of the unpredictability and impulsivity of typical borderline patients, outcome study at only one chosen interval cannot serve as a good predictor of life course.

The most meaningful study of life-course would involve the near-100 percent follow-up of a patient cohort, ample in number for statistical purposes, whose status was examined at intervals frequent enough (approximately every two to three years) to minimize retrospective falsification of data. At least one such study is under way, with a prospective design, of the adolescent patients (mainly with borderline personality disorder and schizophrenia) at Chestnut Lodge (McGlashan, 1988).

All follow-up studies represent compromises. They fall short of an ideal design, partly because of practical considerations but, more important, because of currently unsuspected factors the next generation of clinicians will consider important.

In the sections that follow I will examine briefly the older reports and then, in greater detail, the results of short-, intermediate-, and long-term outcome studies for the contemporary literature.

EARLY FOLLOW-UP STUDIES OF PATIENTS IN THE BORDERLINE DOMAIN

Before the era of operationalized diagnostic criteria, follow-up studies of borderline patients were few in number, small in sample size, variable in interval, and unsystematic in design. Comparison with contemporary studies is difficult, particularly because of overlap in the former uses of the borderline concept with that of schizophrenia.

Hoch and colleagues (1962) reported on 109 patients 5–20 years after initial contact. Diagnoses as "pseudoneurotic schizophrenic" originally (Hoch and Polatin, 1949), a proportion would be borderline by current standards. Approximately one-half had been private outpatients; the others had been hospitalized. The only clear result concerns the greater likelihood of rehospitalization if one had been an inpatient. The ambulatory group seemed less likely to have a "poor" outcome. One patient in 10 had a course compatible with "chronic schizophrenia," as the latter was understood by the broad Bleulerian criteria then in vogue.

The study of Gidro-Frank and colleagues (1967), based on 24 male inpatients followed 5–10 years, provided only a few vignettes complete enough to permit rediagnosis. Their value is only anecdotal: An affectively ill and borderline patient eventually recovered; a schizophrenic man was still dysfunctional six years later.

Short-Term Studies

The follow-up study of Gunderson and colleagues (1975) used operational criteria for diagnosis. Twenty-four hospitalized patients selected according to the criteria for BPD outlined earlier that year by Gunderson and Singer (1975) were matched with 29 inpatients diagnosed as schizophrenic according to clinical, Schneiderian, and I.P.S.S. (Carpenter et al, 1973) criteria. Though the borderlines of this sample were, like Grinker's Type I patients, close to the psychotic border, they could be adequately differentiated from schizophrenics symptomatically. The patients with BPD did not, for example, show prolonged psychotic episodes and had relatively greater dissociative experiences, more anger, and less anxiety than their schizophrenic counterparts. Depression was a commonly encountered affective symptom in the borderline group. The two patient groups were closely matched at the outset with respect to prognostic variables (work history, previous hospitalizations, social and heterosexual relations). At two-year follow-up evaluation their function in four major areas (hospitalization, social contacts, employment, and symptoms) was remarkably similar, both achieving near-identical scores (all in the range of moderate impairment) on the four subscales. In contrast to the schizophrenics, all but four of whom still were diagnosed schizophrenic at follow-up, diagnostic changes were proposed by their evaluators for 60 percent of the borderlines. In a subsequent paper, follow-up of these patients at a five-year interval was reported (see below).

Akiskal et al (1981) carried out a short-term follow-up of 100 patients who met Gunderson criteria for borderline personality (though structured interviews were not done). The 100 patients could be further subtyped into a large fraction with concomitant affective disorder, along with smaller proportions with a) severe "neuroses," b) sociopathy/somatization disorder, c) schizotypal personality disorder, d) organic (grand mal epilepsy, temporal lobe epilepsy, attention deficit disorder), and e) a residual group of patients with chronic identity disorder. In Akiskal's series both family history and short-term follow-up suggested a close connection between BPD and primary affective disorder in many of the patients, 37 of whom had already experienced 52 episodes of the latter, in one form or another, two or three years later: depression/melancholia, hypomanic episodes, manic psychoses, or mixed states. Four had already committed suicide. In contrast, only one patient evolved in an unmistakably schizophrenic direction. Akiskal understands the high frequency of an affective disorder evolution as a consequence of the high concentration of affective traits already apparent in his borderline population—a coincidence that is not surprising in view of the DSM-III definition of BPD, which contains many affectively colored items (p. 37). Even a trait such as identity disturbance, central to the psychoanalytic definitions of borderline, but not customarily associated with affective illness, can arise as a function of wide mood swings that bring about an unstable and ever-shifting sense of self (p. 44).

Tucker and colleagues (1987) reported preliminary results of their follow-up study of borderline patients diagnosed by *DSM-III* criteria. They located 40 of 62 patients who had been hospitalized for up to 23 months (with an average of eight months) on a long-term unit. The typical patient was a single, Caucasian female with depressive symptoms besides the BPD traits. Alcohol abuse and affective illness were common among the close relatives. At short-term follow-up (one to two years after discharge), the patients tended to show less suicidal and substance abusing behavior and to socialize better. Overall outcome improved on average from "marginal" (GAS = 40) levels at discharge to "fair" (GAS = 50 at 1 year; 56 at 2 years) levels at follow-up.

Perry (1985) reported the results of several mood rating scales in 82 outpatients with borderline and other conditions. Since the subjects were asked to respond to the questionnaires at three-month intervals for one year, some longitudinal data became available for approximately three-fourths of the patients, though the study was not one of follow-up per se. Patients with BPD alone (N = 23) tended to show high levels of hostility, anxiety, and depressive symptoms throughout that year, whereas patients with BPD × ASP (N = 12) reported fewer symptoms of depression over time (especially those with the most prominent borderline pathology).

Subsequently, Perry and Cooper (1985) provided the outcome results, as measured by the GAS, of their original patient groups at a two- to three-year interval. Data were available for two-thirds of the original patients, yielding small numbers: 16 with BPD; 8 with BPD × ASP; 10 with ASP alone. The authors found no significant differences in global function: Average scores in all groups were in the "fair" range (GAS = 55 ± 3.5). Viewed from the perspective of the authors' symptom scales for BPD and ASP, it appeared, however, that ". . . borderline psychopathology was a more negative predictor of global functioning than ASP psychopathology" (Perry and Cooper, 1985, p. 35). This impression, not borne out by long-term follow-up, must be assessed in the light of a) possible sample artifact, and b) the self-destructive behavior of the borderlines, often still active at the three-year interval and capable of pulling the GAS score below that of the less blatantly self-injurious ASP group. These findings underscore the importance of evaluating outcome by specific (symptom, work, and social) as well as by global measures. By virtue of their better social attributes, as we shall see, borderlines without serious ASP traits usually outperform ASP patients eventually, provided the patients with BPD do not succumb to their self-destructive tendencies.

Intermediate Term Studies

THE I.P.S.S. STUDY: FIVE YEAR INTERVAL.   Approximately two-thirds of the patients with BPD and schizophrenia selected from the International Pilot Study of Schizophrenia and followed at a two-year interval (Gunderson et al, 1975) were also evaluated at five years (Carpenter and Gunderson, 1977). For most measures, significant differences did not emerge at the longer interval either (namely, useful employment, duration of nonhospitalization, ability to meet own needs). The one exception was quality of social contacts, which was superior in the borderline groups at the five-year follow-up. These findings are summarized and highlighted with a useful diagram in another report (Carpenter et al, 1977). The similarity of the pattern of presenting symptomatology in the borderlines to that of severe neurotic depression is also illustrated in this report.
THE GRINKER STUDY.   The reports on follow-up of patients diagnosed "borderline" by Grinker and his colleagues (1968, 1977) center chiefly on intermediate-range intervals, though some data reflect short- and long-term outcome. Their studies were based on 51 hospitalized patients in Chicago during the 1960s. As mentioned by Carpenter and associates (1977), "borderline" was used, in the Chicago study, as a dimensional term, signifying between psychotic and neurotic; their four subgroups can also be arranged sequentially from the border with psychosis (Group I) to the border with neurosis (Group IV). Some information concerning the course of illness emerges from their work, since material was obtained on 41 patients at 1½ to 3 years postdischarge; on 28 patients at 5 years (Werble, 1970) and on 7 patients at 10 years (Grinker and Werble, 1977). A schizophrenic evolution was most unusual (only 2 of the former borderlines from Group I). Outcome was analyzed according to several parameters, including work, social life, marital status, and family adjustment by means of standardized rating scales. In general, work went better for the borderlines, throughout their course, than did socialization. One-half of the patients of either sex were regularly employed; one-quarter, either minimally (12 percent) or never (12 percent). Only 7 of 41 achieved the 2 highest ratings (on a 5-point scale) for social participation. At the first follow-up, two-thirds of the males had never married; 5 of 18 females were also single/never married. Nearly one-half of the patients experienced significant difficulties in their relations with central family figures or were isolated from their families (Grinker and Werble, 1977, p. 201). Grinker and Werble mention the possibility that their recent respondents were

more stable and psychologically better off than those whom they could no longer contact. They speculated that the latter may have left the Chicago area for environments they could handle more easily (p. 215). Some of the anaclitically depressed (Group IV) patients, mostly women, married "motherly husbands" who helped create a stabilizing environment for their still fragile spouses. The borderline patients continued to show major difficulties in interpersonal relations; particularly, an ". . . inability to attain and maintain positive object relations" (p. 215). This the authors took as an indication that, for the most part, patients with BPD require direction, control, and education rather than insight.

THE STUDY OF POPE AND COLLEAGUES. Pope and colleagues at the McLean Hospital (1983) reported on the 4–7 year follow-up of 33 patients who fulfilled *DSM-III* criteria for BPD as well as less stringent criteria for Gunderson-BPD (cut off score of 6 instead of 7 on the DIB). These patients, all over 18 on admission, had been hospitalized between 1974 and 1977. The sample was preponderantly female (27:6). Outcome was analyzed via 5-point scales relating to social, occupational, residual symptom, and global status. The original group could be subdivided into those with concomitant major affective disorder (MAD) (N = 17) and those without (N = 16). The authors were able to trace 27 (82 percent) of their sample. None of these 27 had gone on to develop DSM-III schizophrenia. The BPD × MAD patients showed a greater tendency to exhibit affective symptoms (i.e., persistence of MAD) at follow-up (10/14 or 71 percent) than did the "pure" BPD group, as well as a schizophrenic comparison group, on the outcome scales pertaining to social function and residual symptoms. Nearly one-half the BPD × MAD patients no longer fulfilled BPD diagnostic criteria at follow-up, though most of them, along with the pure BPD group, did show signs of other personality disorders (chiefly, histrionic, narcissistic, and antisocial). A bipolar–manic comparison group did significantly better even than the BPD × MAD patients, demonstrating, as the authors mention, ". . . the serious morbidity of the BPD diagnosis with or without concurrent MAD" (p. 29). The patients comorbid for affective disorder seemed to respond more favorably to antidepressants or lithium than did the patients with pure BPD, raising the question as to whether this drug responsivity contributed to the more favorable course. Two patients (one with MAD)—that is, six percent of the traced sample—had completed suicide during the follow-up interval.

MASTERSON'S STUDY OF BORDERLINE ADOLESCENTS. The follow-up study conducted by Masterson and Costello (1980) concerned borderline adolescents hospitalized on a specialized unit at Payne Whitney Psychiatric Clinic. The diagnosis rested on clinical criteria, stressing acting-out behavior (namely, drug abuse, promiscuity, running away) and a history of "narcissistic oral fixation" (p. 44). These criteria are not easily brought into line with operational definitions; it remains unclear how many of these adolescents (average age at admission: 15.7) would be borderline by DSM-III or DIB criteria. Of 37 patients hospitalized between 1968 and 1975 and who remained a year or more on the unit, 31 were located from 1 to 7¼ years later (average interval = 3.9 years). Using a 4-point scale of impairment (minimal to severe), the authors noted that 16 percent of the traced patients showed only minimal impairment at follow-up; 42 percent showed mild impairment. The remaining 42 percent were categorized as moderately (23 percent) or severely (19 percent) impaired. A number of factors were associated with better outcomes: a history of good peer relations, acute onset of symptoms, ego alien symptoms, least impairment on admission, a supportive family, and a hospital stay greater than six months. Several factors augured poorly, including lower than average IQ, signs or organicity, and a history of academic underachievement.

THE NORWEGIAN STUDY OF HOLM AND HUNDEVADT. Holm and Hundevadt (1976, 1981) reexamined, after a five-year interval, a series of hospitalized patients diagnosed as borderline by Grinker criteria. Approximately one-half (30/64) did not require rehospitalization. In this group women outnumbered the men 3:1. In the rehospitalized group the gender ratio was near parity. These authors were of the impression that patients who could not be fit conveniently into one of the four Grinker subtypes had a worse prognosis than did those who were easily classified within that framework. The authors provided a number of brief vignettes, but did not report the percentages of good or bad outcomes within their total sample. Among the examples cited were Grinker type III or IV patients with excellent social recoveries (though they tended to be hyper-conventional); several type I or II patients were still symptomatic and socially awkward.

THE SWEDISH STUDY OF NYMAN. Nyman (1978) followed up 100 probands hospitalized in Lund, Sweden at intervals of 6–9 years. Hers was a study of "borderline schizophrenia" (one-half of her sample carried this diagnosis; one-half were "process" schizophrenics) and bears little relation to BPD as currently defined. No marked differences were discernible at follow-up; there was a slightly higher suicide rate (12 percent) in the process, as compared with the borderline, schizophrenics (8 percent). A special feature of her monograph is the appendix of clinical sketches on all 110 patients, facilitating sample comparison between investigators and across cultures.

THE MENNINGER STUDY. The monograph of Wallerstein (1986), which reports the results of the Menninger study of psychotherapy and psychoanalysis, describes 42 ambulatory and hospitalized patients treated by the Menninger Clinic staff beginning in the mid-1950s. The study, having been conceived in the 1950s, did not use operational diagnostic criteria. According to my somewhat arbitrary division, 24 of the patients were "neurotic"; 18, "borderline" by the clinical measures of the time. The borderlines were more likely to have been hospitalized at the Menninger Clinic (12/18) than the neurotic patients (3/24). Wallerstein used a 4-point scale for outcome (very good, moderate, equivocal, failed); this can be collapsed to good versus bad for statistical purposes, forming a 2×2 table as follows: outcomes in the neurotic patients, 19 good versus 5 bad (including one suicide); in the borderlines, 6 good versus 12 bad (including 5 suicides). Anecdotal material was available on many of the patients 10 to 20 or more years later. The results are not easy to compare with studies using standardized outcome measures (see below: McGlashan and colleagues). The relatively poor outcomes in the patients with BPD may be partly a reflection of the brief follow-up intervals in some cases and of the high proportion of alcoholics in the series as a whole (12/42). In other respects the demographic characteristics (Caucasian, average IQ = 124, middle or upper class) resemble those of McGlashan's Chestnut Lodge series. The high suicide rate in the borderlines (5/18 = 28 percent) is not unlike that of the BPD alcoholics in Stone's series (see below); 4 of the 5 Menninger borderline suicides abused substances (alcohol in 3 of them).

Long-Term Studies

THE CHESTNUT LODGE STUDY. The most elegant of the long-term BPD follow-up studies to date is that of McGlashan (1986a, 1986b). The BPD patients, rediagnosed by DIB–DSM-III criteria, had been treated 2–32 years earlier, in an average hospital stay of 2 years, at Chestnut Lodge in Rockville, Maryland. Eighty-six percent of the pure-BPD group (81/94) were traced. Chief comparison groups were unipolar depressives and schizophrenics. The *typical* BPD patient was female, had become symptomatic at age 20, had been hospitalized elsewhere at 25, and had been transferred to Chestnut Lodge at 27. A fair proportion eventually signed out against advice. In contrast to the patients with schizophrenia, rehospitalization *after* Chestnut Lodge was less frequent (1 or 2 times) and briefer. Seventy were still alive at follow-up. Two of the 11 who died were suicides. Intensive (three to four sessions per week) psychotherapy had been the mainstay of treatment for these borderline patients; only one-fourth had received psychotropic medications. At *follow-up*, one-half were still in some form of therapy. Two-thirds were working full time, a record similar to that of the patients with unipolar depression, and much better than that of the patients with schizophrenia. The BPD patients had either married or found a steady sexual partner, or lived alone in "studious avoidance of relationships" (p. 29). Whereas the schizophrenic and unipolar patients tended to function at follow-up about the same as they did at discharge from Chestnut Lodge years earlier, the BPD patients followed a more complex course. If they became symptomatic again, the symptoms were usually those reminiscent of BPD in general: substance abuse or other manifestations of impulsivity. Suicidal thoughts were still common; one in five had continued on occasion to perform suicidal acts. The average Health Sickness Rating Scale (HSRS) score at follow-up was 64 for the BPD group, as opposed to 37 for the schizophrenics (but 60 for the unipolars). The typical BPD life *trajectory* consisted of continuing poor adaptation through the 20s and into the early 30s, followed by good function during the 40s. Some patients, especially after the dissolution (through death, divorce, or rejection) of a close relationship, suffered another downturn during their late 40s–early 50s. McGlashan noted that the patients who most closely resembled Pope's BPD × MAD group, namely, the BPD × unipolar patients, usually exhibited lower scores on the key outcome variables than did Pope's group (whose BPD × MADs outperformed the pure BPDs).

In a separate paper, McGlashan (1987) noted that the rate of completed suicide was highest in the comorbid UNI × BPD group (16 percent), intermediate in the pure unipolars (8 percent), and lowest in the BPD-only group (2 percent). Though all three types of patients had been about equally prone to suicidal gestures at index admission, they pursued divergent courses over time with respect to suicide risk. As McGlashan observed, "it appears that mixing affective dysregulation with action-oriented personality style constitutes a particularly lethal combination" (p. 471). Alcohol abuse was quite common in the comorbid patients. Since long-term follow-up demonstrated changes in both directions in a proportion of patients—BPD to UNI but also UNI to BPD—McGlashan cautions that ". . . we are dealing with highly fluid and heterogeneous entities, among which we must also include the more 'classical' affective disorders" (p. 473).

The life-course of patients with BPD appears to depend upon the varying degrees of admixture of affective and impulsive tendencies.

McGlashan (1986a) also studied the long-term outcome in the Chestnut Lodge patients with schizotypal personality (STP). Global outcome measures could be aligned within a "spectrum." At one end were either schizophrenic (SZ) patients or schizophrenics who also manifested the STP profile: Both usually functioned only marginally (HSRS values in the mid-30s). Patients with STP alone or those with SZ × STP × BPD were less impaired (values in the mid-40s). At the opposite end, patients with STP × BPD did as well (average HSRS = 68) or slightly better than the pure-BPD group (average HSRS = 64). The schizotypal patients generally were loners, were less flamboyant, and were less self-destructive (and less often hospitalized) than the BPD patients. The latter, however, were "object-seeking" (p. 333) and more successful at establishing love relationships as well as friendships, whereas the schizotypal patients tended to have friends but not lovers. As in most American (in contrast to Scandinavian) studies, STP is uncommon in hospital settings and the numbers comparatively small (for the Chestnut Lodge–STP group, N = 10; STP × BPD, N = 18). While the pure STP patients seemed symptomatically, as well as genetically, closer to SZ, the STP × BPD group appeared closer to the affective pole symptomatically and often had both major depressive disorder and a family history of affective illness.

THE NEW YORK STATE PSYCHIATRIC INSTITUTE-500. The long-term follow-up of patients hospitalized at the New York State Psychiatric Institute was similar in scope and time-interval to the Chestnut Lodge study: 550 patients of the cohorts 1963–1976 (Stone et al, 1987). The Psychiatric Institute series contained more BPD patients (205) and fewer schizophrenics than the Chestnut Lodge study. Average follow-up interval was 16 years (range: 10–23 years). A quarter of the Psychiatric Institute patients were adolescents (under 18 at admission). The typical patient was 22 when hospitalized and came from a middle to upper class home (average SES = 2.7; Hollingshead and Redlich, 1958). Eighty percent of the borderlines were first admissions; those hospitalized earlier became severely symptomatic about 2–2½ years befor the index admission. Average IQ was 118. In the Psychiatric Institute series, affective comorbidity was especially common in the traced females: 100 showed BPD × MAD; only 37 were "pure" BPD cases. Among the traced males this tendency was less striking (BPD only = 24; BPD × MAD = 27). Altogether, 92 percent of the borderline patients were traced, as were 96 percent of the schizophrenic comparison group. The high trace-rate lent authenticity to the observed suicide rates—which were similar for the schizophrenics (10.3 percent) and the combined borderlines (9 percent). But within the BPD group, the suicide rate was lowest for the pure BPD females (5.4 percent), highest for the BPD × MAD males (18.5 percent), and 8 percent in the other groups. Mean GAS scores at follow-up were 65.6 for the combined borderlines, 39.4 for the schizophrenics. Within-subgroup averages were not different from the whole-group means, except in the pure-BPD males, who remained significantly more impaired (average = 55). This stood out even more clearly if one looked at the percentages of patients whose current function exceeded GAS-60. This level was achieved by two-thirds or more of all the borderline subgroups *except* the pure BPD males (37.5 percent) (and only by 8 percent of the schizophrenics). The authors felt the poor function of the BPD males was a reflection of the high proportion of antisocial traits in this subgroup. The suicides among the borderlines showed the same gender ratio (7F:3M) as in the BPD group as a whole, and occurred with few exceptions within four years after discharge. The ages at suicide varied between 15 and 32, clustering in the third decade (Stone et al, 1987). Alcohol abuse was common in the 17 suicides; the most lethal combination of circumstances in the Psychiatric Institute-500 was alcohol abuse in conjunction with BPD × MAD (5 of 11, or 45 percent).

The respondents (the former patients and their relatives) in the Psychiatric Institute-500 study were asked to reconstruct, as best as their memory would permit, the life trajectory postdischarge. A number of patterns could be discerned, similar to those categorized by Ciompi (1976) and Bleuler (1972). Some patients exhibited a slow progression upwards toward recovery or downwards toward rehospitalization or suicide. A large number showed rapid movement (steep slope) in one direction or the other. A number of borderlines who went on to develop unipolar or bipolar-II (or less often, -I) affective disorders had wavy trajectories with many ups and downs in function over the years. A few show flat trajectories, representing chronic impairment and little fluctuation in function. The latter pattern was common among the schizophrenic patients. Finally, a sizeable group showed an "atypical" course; particularly, the pattern alluded to by McGlashan (1986): 5–10 years of poor function, followed by rapid recovery and long-time maintenance of good clinical status (doing well socially and at work; few symptoms). Table 1 shows the number of borderline patients in each category of outcome pattern, subdivided according to whether their most recent status was good (GAS>60), fair (51–60), or poor (<60, including suicides). Information was available on 167 of the traced patients; no gender differences were noted, so both sexes are combined in the resulting figures.

As in the Chestnut Lodge series, only a few of the Psychiatric Institute-500 met the criteria either for schizotypal personality (STP) or combined STP × BPD. Of the 9 pure STP patients, 8 were traced: One had completed suicide; average GAS in the other was 67 (range: 50–84). Four were clinically "well" (GAS>60). The comorbid group contained 7 patients of whom 6 were traced: Their average GAS = 58 (range 40–76); two had scores >60.

In contrast to the *DSM-III* criteria for patients with schizophrenia of the Psychiatric Institute-500, most of whom led similar and constricted lives postdischarge, the borderlines exhibited greater *variability* in both course and outcome. In the

Table 1. Outcome Patterns in 167 Patients with BPD

Postdischarge Life Trajectory Pattern:	Functional Level at Follow-Up		
	Good (GAS > 60)	Fair (GAS 51–60)	Poor (Suicide or GAS <60)
Slow progression	20	4	7
Rapid progression	37	4	10
Wavy	7	7	11
Linear (flat)	15	7	4
Atypical	22	6	6

area of work, three had become professors; five, physicians; nine, psychologists; three, high corporate executives; three, ministers. But there were also three prostitutes (two male, one female), four murderers (all male) and several still hiding from the law. This variability cannot all be accounted for by comorbidity with one or another Axis I or Axis II condition. Much of the variance seemed related to attributes outside the realm of conventional nosography. Certain attributes, such as likeableness, though important as determinants (Woolcott, 1985), are elusive, especially in a retrospective study. A number of other factors were evaluated for the Psychiatric Institute borderlines as to whether their presence correlated with better than average or with worse than average outcome. These are shown in Table 2.

Given the large S.D. in outcome GAS (± 14.5), one might select as significant only those factors associated with group means greater than 1½ S.D. (i.e., 21.75 points) from the average for all BPDs (66), especially if one is to reduce Type II errors stemming from small numbers. By this standard, artistic talent and attractiveness in females were associated with distinctly better outcomes (and a more favorable life course); antisociality, parental brutality, male elopees, female rape victims, and those ever jailed predicted a worse than average outcome. Several

Table 2. Psychiatric Institute-500: Percentage of BPD Patients With Follow-Up GAS > 60

Variable	N	% with GAS>60
Artistic talent	9	88
Female patients with attractiveness		
1 S.D. above average	25	87
At least one "natural advantage"	36	85
I.Q. 2 S.D. above average (>138)	18	85
Alcoholics in Alcoholics Anonymous	15	80
Females without major affective disorder	37	75
Anorexia/bulimia	30	72
Females with major affective disorder	100	67
All traced BPD patients	188	64
Males with major affective disorder	27	63
Females who eloped	33	61
Alcoholics not in Alcoholics Anonymous	28	57
Female incest victims	26	52
Homosexual/bisexual (males and females)	22	50
Fire-setting history	8	50
Antisocial personality comorbidity	29	42
Schizotypal personality comorbidity	14	42
Males without major affective disorder	24	38
Victims of parental brutality	18	33
Males who eloped	9	22
Female rape victims	7	14
Patients of either sex jailed one day or more	10	10

other factors shown tend in one or the other direction. Incest, which appeared to lower global outcome only to a modest degree, probably had a more profound effect, in the sense that the victim, though doing fairly well compared with other BPD patients, might not have developed BPD in the first place in the absence of this traumatization (Stone, in press a, b).

THE AUSTIN RIGGS STUDY. The Study of Plakun and colleagues (1985) derived from their follow-up of 878 patients hospitalized for at least two months at Austin Riggs Center between 1950 and 1976. The authors used a mailed questionnaire/informed consent method and elicited 237 (27 percent) positive responses. Of the remainder, 94 had died; others either refused to answer or could not be contacted. Retrospective *DSM-III* diagnoses were made by two raters blind to the chart diagnoses. The authors felt the nonresponders did not differ appreciably from the responders with respect to the demographic variables examined. The main diagnostic groups within the traced patients consisted of schizophrenics (SZ, = 19), major affective disorder (MAD, = 24), schizotypal personality disorder (STP, = 13), borderline personality disorder (BPD = 63) and schizoid personality (SD, = 19). The borderlines were further subdivided into those with concomitant MAD (=9), BPD alone (=43), BPD × STP (=6) and BPD × SD (=5). Outcome was reported via the Global Assessment Score (GAS). The mean GAS levels in the Plakun study are all actually quite similar, ranging from the SZ group (=59.3) to the small BPD × STP group (=72). Their results differ from the Pope study (1983) in that their BPD × MAD group did worse than their pure BPDs (mean GAS = 67), and did not differ significantly in outcome from the SZs. Clinical vignettes and data concerning the sex-ratio within subgroups, socioeconomic status, and suicide rate were not provided. The authors make no claim to assess treatment effects, but felt ". . . there is no reason to assume that treatment has no effect and that we are dealing with the natural history of BPD . . ." (p. 453).

THE MINNEAPOLIS STUDY. In an effort to learn whether BPD represents a nonspecific collection of syndromes involving emotional lability and impulsivity, or whether BPD is a separate entity unified by a common etiology, Kroll and colleagues (1985), undertook a pilot study of borderlines hospitalized approximately 20 years earlier. Narrowing their focus to female inpatients with an "8–4–2" pattern on the Minnesota Multiphasic Personality Inventory (MMPI), they found 31 cases, out of which 15 were rated as having Gunderson-DIB scores of 7 or higher. Thirteen of these 15 borderlines were traced (87 percent). Four had already died: two by suicide (one, at six months postdischarge; the other, three years postdischarge); an amphetamine addict who died of breast cancer; and a diabetic "semisuicide" who helped death along via noncompliance with her medical regimen. Of the nine still alive, three were working at responsible jobs and doing well in general (two were married). Four had made only fair to marginal adjustments: They were unemployed and on public assistance. Two, including the only one to require rehospitalization, were doing poorly. One of the marginal patients was now schizophrenic by DSM-III critiera, though she also met criteria for major depressive disorder (MDD) and might therefore be considered schizoaffective. One other patient also showed MDD at follow-up. The authors felt their study did not support the notion of a close relationship between BPD and affective disorder.

THE MONTREAL STUDY. The most recent of the large-scale reports is that of Paris and colleagues (1987), who were able to trace and interview 100 of 322 patients (256 female; 66 male) admitted to the Jewish General Hospital, Montreal, between 1958 and 1978, and whose initial clinical characteristics justified rediagnosis as borderline by Gunderson DIB criteria. Outcome was measured via the Menninger Health/Sickness Rating Scale (Luborsky, 1963) and several 5-point scales of work, social and family adjustment, and of subsequent treatment. At follow-up, only one-fourth of the patients still had DIB scores of 7 or greater; the remainder would no longer be judged "borderline." Global function, by the HSRS, was 63.2, S.D. = 11. The suicide rate thus far was 8.5 percent. Of special interest about the Montreal study is the wider range of educational and socioeconomic status of the patients, one-half of whom had never completed high school and many of whom were from lower middle class origins. This suggests, given the similarity in outcome measures, at long-term, a wider applicability of the impressions of McGlashan and of Stone, both of whose studies centered around patients from presumably more favorable educational/S.E.S. backgrounds. The mean follow-up interval in the Montreal study was 15 years; the average age, when located, 41. Paris and his colleagues felt the interviewed patients constituted a representative sample of their borderline population as a whole.

PROGNOSTIC VARIABLES

The recent follow-up studies of BPD, especially those oriented toward the long term, have established that a reassuring proportion (more than one-half) of hospitalized patients with borderline personality disorder eventually make substantial improvement. But life-course and outcome at 10–20 years vary over a wide range, from suicide to full recovery, suggesting that diagnosis alone cannot account for all the variance. This observation has prompted the search for other variables, combinations of personality traits coexisting with those of BPD, preexisting demographic and family factors, and so on, that might exert an impact upon the life trajectory whether for good or for ill. As is customary when grappling with such a multiplicity of possible influences, investigators begin with the obvious and move gradually toward the elusive and the subtle.

Substance abuse, for example, a frequent concomitant of BPD (in all cohorts since 1965, in the United States), exerts a worsening effect upon the course. Persistent alcohol abuse more than doubles the suicide rate; abuse of cocaine or opiates appears to reduce the proportion of recovered cases to approximately one-half the expected level (Stone, 1988a). Many borderlines, if able at some point to conquer their drug habits, pulled out of their nose-dive and began to lead a reasonably productive and relatively symptom-free life. Some of the best outcomes have been noted among BPD patients who abused alcohol but finally became "dry" with the help of Alcoholics Anonymous (A.A.). The life-course in such patients appears to be a function of the intensity of personality aberrations and of antecedent traumatic factors in the families of origin. Those from the most traumatic environment and those with the most impulsive and help-repudiating personalities fail at A.A. and at all other forms of treatment and have the worst life-trajectories.

Major affective disorder (MAD) comorbidity did not exert uniform effects across the studies. This combination was associated with better than average outcome (compared with BPD alone) in Pope's series, with lower outcome scores and a higher suicide rate in the Chestnut Lodge and Austin Riggs studies, and with mixed results in the Psychiatric Institute-500 (better outcome than for males with BPD only, a higher suicide rate than in males with BPD only, and not much difference among female patients). Pope offered the possibility that a positive medication response rendered the comorbid group more amenable to treatment. It may be, however, that BPD × MAD only *appears* to do better, because BPD-"alone," especially in males, may be found in conjunction with antisocial traits that augur poorly for the life course—such that antidepressants did not so much help the BPD × MAD group as did ASP-comorbidity hurt those without MAD. Outcome in any given follow-up study would, in other words, be complicated by any one of a host of intervening variables and would also appear to be different depending upon the original proportion of males, upon the relative severity of the affective and antisocial components, and so on. The male borderlines in McGlashan's series, for example, had low ASP comorbidity and as a group outperformed the females (1985, p. 83), whereas in the Psychiatric Institute-500 males with BPD had more antisocial traits and a poorer outcome. The heightened suicide risks associated with MAD when combined with BPD is a more uniform finding and one that makes sense clinically (high risk for depression × high proclivity for impulsive and violent action). In several series, approximately 10 percent of cases originally diagnosed as BPD × MAD went on to develop one of the classic forms of manic depression. The life course was then compatible with the latter diagnosis.

Admixture with schizotypal elements, in what is sometimes called a "mixed" borderline personality, also does not by itself affect prognosis in a uniform direction. Depending, probably, upon the particular schizotypal trait that is most prominent, one may witness a borderline patient fail repeatedly to connect closely with other people, thus leading a marginal existence (worse than certain BPD cases), or leading a calm and measured, if somewhat colorless, existence—free of the affect storms and upheavals of certain other BPD cases. "Mixed" borderlines with strong paranoid trends are often particularly resistant to therapy because of their propensity to lose faith even with the most trustworthy of therapists. They are prone to pathological jealousy if they permit themselves any intimacy at all, and thus ultimately alienate and drive away their partners.

Similarly, McGlashan noted an adverse effect upon outcome if magical thinking (a "schizotypal" trait) were present in BPD or if either hostility or anhedonia were prominent (1985, p. 84).

Antisocial personality is usually associated with a dismal prognosis. Of the many combinations of antisocial traits, some are genuinely predictive of bad outcome; others, however, are associated with counterintuitive results. Some fundamentally decent adolescents in the studies cited above found themselves plunged, through death or divorce of a parent, into a hostile environment—from which they sought to escape via attachment to opportunistic peers, "street life," truancy, or petty thievery. Apprehended for a minor offense, they might, in lieu of jail, be remanded to a psychiatric hospital, where they would be diagnosed as cases of BPD × ASP. They usually responded poorly to conventional therapy and left the hospital unimproved (and often with confirmed drug habits). Their prospects for recovery were considered poor. Yet at long-term follow-up, about one-half are now leading conventional and productive lives, working steadily, and supporting families. A few "reformed" after near-death experiences with drug overdoses; others dropped their dyssocial traits for less dramatic reasons. Conversely, antisocial borderlines with a history of felonious assault or of chronic lying and "conning" (after the manner of the "psychopaths" described by Cleckley in 1976) have shown no improvement over time. Many committed suicide when cornered by the authorities. Thus, even the customary expectations about antisocial comorbidity need to be reexamined with greater attention to the subtle gradations along the spectrum between rebelliousness and true malice.

In the Psychiatric Institute-500, approximately one-sixth of the BPD patients showed concomitantly the features of narcissistic personality disorder (NPD). These patients had approximately the same long-term outcome, suicide rate, and life course patterns as did the BPD group as a whole (Stone, in press).

Eating disorders (ED) are common in BPD, especially among female patients. In the generation of the long-term studies cited above (1950s to 1970s), anorexia was the most typical disorder. Currently, anorexia with bulimia or episodic bulimia alone appear to be on the increase. From the standpoint of the life-course, eating disorder comorbidity did not adversely affect earlier cohorts of BPD patients: Course and outcome were similar to those of BPD in general; the suicide rate was also similar (2/22 = 9 percent), in BPD × ED cases in the Psychiatric Institute-500), as were the marriage (40–50 percent by an average age of 36) and fertility rate (1 in 4 has had a child).

Life trajectory appears to depend not only upon the admixture of borderline traits and of the traits of other personality disorders, but also upon the density of symptomatic expression. Patients exhibiting all 8 *DSM-III* borderline criteria when first hospitalized, for example, were more likely to complete suicide than were BPDs with 5–7 items (5/14 = 36 percent, as opposed to 12/174 or 7 percent, in the Psychiatric Institute-500). These highly volatile patients were apt to lead chaotic lives with extremely disruptive relationships and were less likely to "mellow out" with the years. Only one of the 14 has become asymptomatic.

In the Psychiatric Institute-500, impulsive, self-damaging patients constituted just over one-half the BPD cohort; their suicide rate was double that of BPD patients who did *not* show those features. Life course and outcome appears to be a function of *which* of the main trait-clusters (as outlined by Hurt, above) predominates in any particular borderline patient. Manipulativeness and devaluation were associated with lower outcome in McGlashan's series (1985). Elopement from hospital is often an index of impulsivity and was common among the borderlines both of the Chestnut Lodge (McGlashan, 1985) and Psychiatric Institute-500 studies, especially in the adolescents. This did not always correlate with persistence of impulse-ridden behavior and an unfavorable course, though *male* elopees seemed prone to both.

Analogous to those with all eight BPD criteria are the "pansymptomatic" inpatients studied at the Menninger Clinic (Colson et al, 1986). These patients, many of whom were borderline, showed all four attributes that the investigators had isolated as peculiar to the "most difficult" subgroup: withdrawn psychoticism, severe character pathology, suicidal–depressed behavior, and violence–agitation. Although the point needs to be examined in the light of follow-up study, presumably pansymptomatic BPD patients have a more irregular life-course and a worse outcome than those with pathology along only one or two of these dimensions. Subtle organic defects were detectable in many of the pansymptomatic patients (Colson and Allen, 1986).

Prognostic variables unrelated to conventional diagnostic or demographic categories have a way of being overlooked. Elsewhere I have attempted to examine some of these in detail (Stone, 1988a). Some, such as cruelty to animals, firesetting during childhood, and violence toward family members invite assumptions about a bad prognosis. A fair number of borderline patients give evidence of these acts, singly or in combination, in the initial histories. As a group the firesetters did perform, in their posthospital years, well below the norms for BPD. However, a number of sexually molested girls, future "border-lines," took out their vengeful feelings on their pets but never on another person, while one of the BPD murderers, the victim of bilateral parental violence, hated mankind and loved only his dog. Not all victims of parental cruelty became cruel in their turn, though the annals of criminology are replete with such examples (Leyton, 1986). The borderline patients who formed the cadres of the Chestnut Lodge and Psychiatric Institute studies, though very ill in many ways (these were hospitals of "last resort"), had had to appeal to the staff at these referral hospitals as being "good candidates" for intensive psychotherapy. Rarely had they been exposed to the harshest or most dehumanizing parental mistreatment. Borderline patients who have been subjected to these extremes do appear more prone to violence—against others or themselves—and become severely maladjusted, often leading wasted lives on the fringes of society. This phenomenon has not yet been studied systematically within the context of BPD research. In these situations the clinician is often confronting an example of posttraumatic stress disorder (Kolb, 1987), in which repeated early traumata have set in motion a self-perpetuating neuroregulatory dysfunction whose outward signs overlap with, and elicit the diagnosis of, BPD. The case of the serial killer, John Wayne Gacy, considered an example of BPD by his examiners, is illustrative (Cahill, 1986).

The suicide risk in BPD is appreciable, approximating the levels noted for schizophrenia and manic-depression. Kullgren and colleagues (1986) regard this as in line with expectation, given the impulsivity and interpersonal difficulties characteristic of borderlines. Though only a fraction of BPD patients who make suicidal acts eventually die of suicide, making repeated attempts is associated with a higher rate of completed suicide (Kotila and Lonnquist, 1987). Female patients are more prone to make suicidal acts that do not end in suicide than are male BPD patients, although their ultimate suicide rates are similar (owing to the higher lethality of the acts carried out by the males). The time of maximum risk appears to be the mid-twenties. Factors such as this may account for the higher suicide rate noted in the Psychiatric Institute-500 than in the Chestnut Lodge study. As McGlashan mentioned (personal communication, 1988), the borderlines were about 5 years older than those of the Psychiatric Institute-500, and may represent a patient sample less vulnerable to suicide (as they approached their 30s) than the younger patients at certain other treatment centers.

A number of factors had equivocal effects upon the life course. Adoptees and patients with homosexuality or bisexuality showed a tendency toward poorer outcomes and more difficult life course. But their numbers were not overrepresented among the BPDs as a group. These factors may, when present in someone with BPD, aggravate already existing problems, but do not appear to be associated with higher rates of mental illness than would be found in the general population.

Of the "natural advantages"—talent, attractiveness, high IQ, social position, fame, wealth—only the first three are associated (in descending order) with a better than average life course for patients with BPD. High I.Q. did not begin to show significant differences in the Psychiatric Institute-500 study until the level 2 S.D. above the group mean was reached. High I.Q. was a strong predictor of good outcome in the Chestnut Lodge borderlines (McGlashan, 1985). These advantages appeared to permit good occupational function despite handicaps, or, in the case of unusual attractiveness in females, to secure the attention of helpful persons who otherwise might not have endured the interpersonal turbulence.

Other factors outside the realm of traditional diagnosis that affect the life course include likeableness and self-discipline. The latter is compromised in many borderlines, hampering the development both of vocational and avocational skills. Cultural factors must also be considered. Admixture of schizotypal traits may be more noticeable in Swedish than in American patients with BPD. The suicide rate in borderlines will be a function, in part, of the general suicide rate in one's country: higher (than in the U.S.) in Hungary, Sweden, and Denmark; lower in Italy and Norway. Cohort effects may be discernible as well: Drug abuse was low in borderline patient samples before 1964; it has been higher ever since. Cocaine abuse has been particularly prevalent in the United States since 1980; it was less so earlier. The interaction of cocaine with BPD is more devastating than that of marijuana. The suicide rate in our country has been rising steadily over the past three decades for persons in their 20s (Solomon and Murphy, 1984); presumably this phenomenon affects the rates observed in borderline patients in various epochs.

The value of follow-up studies of borderlines is greatly enhanced by a high trace rate. So many variables affect outcome that even strong similarities between traced and untraced patients along conventional diagnostic/demographic lines cannot justify generalizations about the untraced group. Reliance upon mailed questionnaires tends to preselect respondents who are better integrated, more established in their community, and more cooperative with the requests of the research team. This factor may account for the finding that the schizophrenics in Plakun's study enjoyed outcomes nearly equal to those of the borderlines— a finding at variance with the Chestnut Lodge and Psychiatric Institute-500 studies. A certain proportion of borderline patients (about 10 percent in the Psychiatric Institute-500) will track counterintuitively; that is, their life course over the long term will be much more favorable or much worse than their initial evaluators had prognosticated. Thus, if 20 borderlines out of 200 remain to be traced, we can speculate that two or three will show a surprising result. But we cannot predict *which* patients will track in this unexpected way. In all likelihood, borderlines would exhibit greater unpredictability than would most other groups of patients. The very impulsivity and lability by which BPD is defined implies the sort of sensitive dependence upon the conditions of the moment, characteristics of "chaotic" systems (Gleick, 1987), such as the weather, that complicate enormously our efforts at prediction in any given case. Whereas good luck and bad luck cause little deviation in the life path of better integrated persons, a chance meeting with a supportive member of an "Anonymous" group may rescue a self-destructive borderline from serious substance abuse, while in another a love affair turned sour will precipitate suicide.

SUMMARY

Follow-up studies of patients in the borderline domain carried out before 1980 were, for the most part, small in scope, unsystematic, and either used diagnostic labels other than borderline or used nonreproducible criteria. A number of the studies during the present decade have used operational criteria, and were based on large numbers and high trace rates. Most of this work has concentrated on hospitalized patients.

Averaging the results from these studies permits one to outline several common life course patterns among formerly hospitalized patients with BPD by DIB or by *DSM-III* criteria. Typically, after a hospitalization during the patients' late teens or early twenties, they will continue to show major impairment in work, social, and close personal spheres, so that at two- or five-year follow-up they can scarcely be distinguished *functionally* from schizophrenic patients of similar age. Some 3 to 10 percent will already have committed suicide. As the BPD patients enter their 30s, 8 to 10 years after the index admission, many will begin to break out of their previously oscillating and poorly functioning course, to settle upon higher and steadier ground. This mellowing often correlates with the establishment of a reasonably harmonious sexual relationship, especially one in which there is little pressure to raise children. McGlashan's observations suggest (1985, p. 82) that good heterosexual adjustment premorbidly predicts better outcome in a borderline patient. A smaller portion of borderlines will achieve stability via renunciation of all efforts to achieve intimacy, settling instead for a lonelier but less stormy life. Though many former patients will mellow to the point where BPD can no longer be diagnosed (impulsivity diminishes; self-damaging acts cease; anger lessens . . .), a brittleness usually remains: Certain stresses (especially loss through rejection, divorce, or death of a significant other) can still precipitate transitory or at times protracted decompensation.

As many as two-thirds of the BPD patients will, in 8 to 10 years or more, eventually do "well" (usually with social success lagging behind the occupational, especially in the males), showing only minimal symptoms. These successes should not blind the clinicians to the still severely impaired portion, where BPD is still readily diagnosable and the life course still perilous.

A wide variety of factors contribute to the ultimate outcome. Some augur well: self-discipline, talent, likeableness, attractiveness, high I.Q.; others, poorly: substance abuse, aggressivity, parental victimization via incest or cruelty, having all eight BPD criteria, antisociality. So vast is the array of these factors and their combinations and interactions that, in relation to any given borderline patient, the art of prediction can only be refined with further study, never perfected. The next generation of studies should concentrate on *prospective* design, taking advantage of what has already been learned from the retrospective studies.

The follow-up studies thus far reported shed little light on the efficacy of specific forms of psychotherapy for patients with BPD. Large series with randomized or otherwise controlled research designs capable of testing a variety of treatment strategies have not been carried out for this patient group. With respect to hospitalized borderlines, it would appear that sanctuary and long-term support, especially during the critical third decade, are the key therapeutic elements (Stone, 1987a). Exploratory therapy is useful in selected patients; in others, a rehabilitative model concentrating on supportive therapy, along with training in vocational and leisure time activities, will be more appropriate. Given the reasonably good prognosis for the majority of hospitalized BPD patients, presumably the outlook for those who never require hospital/residential treatment is at least as good, if not better.

REFERENCES

Akiskal HS: Subaffective disorders: dysthymic, cyclothymic and bipolar II disorders in the "borderline" realm. Psychiatr Clin North Am 1981; 4:25–46

Akiskal HS, Chen SE, Davis GC, et al: Borderline: an adjective in search of a noun. J Clin Psychiatry 1985; 46:41–48

American Psychiatric Association: Diagnostic and Statistical Manual of Mental Disorders, Third Edition (DSM-III). Washington, DC, American Psychiatric Association, 1980

Bleuler M: Die schizophrenen Geistesstörungen im Lichte langjähriger Kranken-und Familiengeschichten. Stuttgart, Georg Thieme Verlag, 1972

Cahill T: Buried Dreams: Inside the Mind of a Serial Killer. New York, Bantam Books, 1980

Carpenter WT, Gunderson JG: Five year follow-up comparison of borderline and schizophrenic patients. Compr Psychiatry 1977; 18:567–571

Carpenter WT, Strauss JS, Bartko J: Flexible system for the diagnosis of schizophrenia. Science 1973; 182:1275–1278

Carpenter WT, Gunderson JG, Strauss JS: Considerations of the borderline syndrome: a longitudinal comparative study of borderline and schizophrenic patients, in Borderline Personality Disorders. Edited by Hartocollis P. New York, International Universities Press, 1977

Ciompi L, Müller C: Lebensweg und Alter der Schizophrenen. Berlin, Springer, 1976

Cleckley H: The Mask of Sanity, 5th ed. St. Louis, Mosby, 1976

Colson DB, Allen JG: Organic brain dysfunction in difficult-to-treat psychiatric hospital patients. Bull Menninger Clinic 1986; 50:89–98

Colson DB, Allen JG, Coyne L, et al: Profiles of difficult psychiatric patients. Hosp Community Psychiatry 1986; 37:720–724

Endicott J, Spitzer RL, Fleiss JL, et al: The Global Assessment Scale. Arch Gen Psychiatry 1976; 33:766–771

Gidro-Frank L, Peretz D, Spitzer R, et al: A five year follow-up of male patients hospitalized at Psychiatric Institute. Psychiatr Q 1967; 41:1–35

Gleick J: Chaos. New York, Viking Press, 1987

Grinker RR, Werble B: The Borderline Patient. New York, Jason Aronson, 1977

Grinker RR, Werble B, Drye RC: The Borderline Syndrome. New York, Basic Books, 1968

Gunderson JG, Singer MT: Defining borderline patients: an overview. Am J Psychiatry 1975; 132:1–10

Gunderson JG, Carpenter WT, Strauss JS: Borderline and schizophrenic patients: a comparative study. Am J Psychiatry 1975; 132:1257–1264

Hoch PH, Polatin P: Pseudoneurotic forms of schizophrenia. Psychiatr Q 1949; 23:248–276

Hoch PH, Cattell JP, Strahl MD, et al: The course and outcome of pesudoneurotic schizophrenia. Am J Psychiatry 1962; 119:106–115

Hollingshead AB, Redlich FC: Social Class and Mental Illness. New York, John Wiley & Sons, 1958

Holm K, Hundevadt E: Psykiatrisk pasient—episode eller livsform? En etterundersøkelse. Tidsskr. Norske Laegeforen 1976; 96:1131–1135

Holm K, Hundevadt E: Borderline states: prognosis and psychotherapy. Br J Med Psychol 1981; 54:335–340

Hurt S: Symptom clusters within DSM borderline personality disorder. Paper presented at 1st International Congress of Personality Disorders, August 4th, 1988

Kernberg OF: Borderline personality organization. J Am Psychoanal Assoc 1967; 15:641–685

Kety SS, Rosenthal D, Wender P, et al: Mental illness in the biological and adoptive families of adopted schizophrenics, in Transmission of Schizophrenia. Edited by Rosenthal D, Kety SS. Oxford, Pergamon Press, 1968

Kolb LC: A neuropsychological hypothesis explaining post-traumatic stress disorders. Am J Psychiatry 1987; 144:989–995

Kotila L, Lönnquist J: Adolescents who make suicide attempts repeatedly. Acta Psychiatr Scand 1987; 76:386–393

Kroll JL, Carey KS, Sines LK: Twenty-year follow-up of borderline personality disorder: a pilot study, in IVth World Congress of Biological Psychiatry, vol. VII. Edited by Stragass C. New York, Elsevier, 1985

Kullgren G, Renberg E, Jacobsson L: An empirical study of borderline personality disorder and psychiatric suicides. J Nerv Ment Dis 1986; 162:328–331

Leyton E: Compulsive Killers. New York, New York University Press, 1986

Luborsky L: Clinician's judgment of mental health. Arch Gen Psychiatry 1963; 9:407–417

Masterson J, Costello J: From Borderline Adolescent to Functioning Adult. New York, Brunner/Mazel, 1980

McGlashan TH: The prediction of outcome in borderline personality disorder: part V of the Chestnut Lodge follow-up study, in The Borderline: Current Empirical Research. Edited by McGlashan TH. Washington, DC, American Psychiatric Press, Inc., 1985

McGlashan TH: The Chestnut Lodge follow-up study, III: long-term outcome of borderline personality disorder. Arch Gen Psychiatry 1986a; 43:20–30

McGlashan TH: Schizotypal personality disorder: Chestnut Lodge follow-up study, VI: long-term follow-up perspectives. Arch Gen Psychiatry 1986b; 43:329–334

McGlashan TH: Borderline personality disorder and unipolar affective disorder. J Nerv Ment Dis 1987; 175:467–473

Nyman AK: Nonregressive schizophrenia: clinical course and outcome. Acta Psychiatr Scand 1978; (Suppl) 272:1–143

Paris J, Brown R, Nowlis D: Long-term follow-up of borderline patients in a general hospital. Compr Psychiatry 1987; 28:530–535

Perry JC: Depression in borderline personality disorder: lifetime prevalence at interview and longitudinal course of symptoms. Am J Psychiatry 1985; 142:15–21

Perry JC, Cooper SH: Psychodynamics, symptoms and outcome in borderline personality disorders and bipolar type II affective disorder, in The Borderline: Current Empirical Research. Edited by McGlashan TH. Washington, DC, American Psychiatric Press, Inc.

Plakun EM, Burkhardt PE, Muller JP: 14-year follow-up of borderline and schizotypal personality disorders. Compr Psychiatry 1985; 26:448–455

Pope HG, Jonas JM, Hudson JI, et al: The validity of DSM-III borderline personality disorder. Arch Gen Psychiatry 1983; 40:23–30

Solomon MI, Murphy GE: Cohort studies in suicide, in Suicide in the Young. Edited by Sudak HS, Ford AB, Rushforth NB. Boston, J Wright/PSG Inc., 1984

Spitzer RL, Endicott J, Gibbon M: Crossing the border into borderline personality and borderline schizophrenia. Arch Gen Psychiatry 1979; 36:17–24

Stern A: Psychoanalytic investigation and therapy in the borderline group of neuroses. Psychoanal Q 1938: 7:467–489

Stone MH: Psychotherapy of borderline patients in light of long-term follow-up. Bull Menninger Clinic 1987a; 51:231–247

Stone MH: Systems for defining a borderline case, in The Borderline Patient, vol. I. Edited by Grotstein J, Solomon M, Lang J. Hillsdale, NJ, The Analytic Press, 1987b

Stone MH: Individual psychotherapy with incest victims. Psychiatr Clin North Am (in press, a)

Stone MH: Long-Term Follow-Up of Borderline Patients: The P.I.-500. New York, Guilford Press (in press, b)

Stone MH: Long-term outcome of borderline patients with narcissistic personality disorder. Psychiatr Clin North Am (in press, c)

Stone MH, Stone DK, Hurt SW: Natural history of borderline patients treated by intensive hospitalization. Psychiatr Clin North Am 1987; 10:185–206

Stone MH, Hurt SW, Stone DK: The P.I.-500: long-term follow-up of borderline in-patients meeting DSM-III criteria, I: global outcome. Journal of Personality Disorders 1988; 1:291–298

Tucker L, Bauer SF, Wagner S, et al: Long-term hospitalization of borderline patients: a descriptive outcome study. Am J Psychiatry 1987; 144:1443–1448

Wallerstein R: Forty-Two Lives in Treatment. New York, Guilford Press, 1986

Werble B: Second follow-up study of borderline patients. Arch Gen Psychiatry 1980; 23: 3–7

Woolcott P: Prognostic indicators in the psychotherapy of borderline patients. Am J Psychotherapy 1985; 39:17–29

Afterword

by John G. Gunderson, M.D.

Borderline personality disorder has moved a long way from its beginnings as a poorly defined, idiosyncratically employed catchall term for difficult patients who didn't fit into existing categories. The contributions of such people as Kernberg (1967), Masterson (1971), Kety and colleagues (1968), and Grinker and associates (1968) in the 1960s provided incentives, stimulus, and models for the era of research and more ambitious treatments that occurred in the 1970s. That decade saw a shift of interest away from the boundary between borderline personality and schizophrenia and culminated with the inclusion of borderline personality disorder in *DSM-III*. A great deal of the literature since 1980 has concerned itself with the boundary of borderline personality and affective disorders. These studies have increasingly suggested that it may be nonspecific and conclusively have shown that it is not simple. As carefully documented by Soloff, particularly important has been the overall failure for antidepressants to have widespread, unique, or dramatic effects in resolving borderline psychopathology. Equally important, as noted by Stone, have been the many follow-up studies that have failed to show that persons diagnosed as having borderline personality subsequently develop typical major affective disorders. Certainly the studies on pathogenesis, most notably the family history and biological marker studies, support theories that point to some biogenetic overlap with affective disorders, but show the overlap is neither uniform nor unique. By no means is the border between borderline personality and affective disorders one which can be ignored or considered unimportant; it is a border, however, which seems to be similarly complicated for patients with other forms of serious personality disorder. The many diagnostic studies reviewed by Widiger and Frances give recognition to and illustrate the salience of a broad variety of comorbid Axis I conditions.

Whereas a first generation considered borderline personality as a possible variant of schizophrenia and a second generation became more concerned with the linkage to affective disorders, there is now growing interest in the boundary between borderline personality disorder with other types of personality disorder. Here, too, there are interesting biogenetic and therapeutic suggestions of an overlap with adjacent categories such as antisocial, histrionic, narcissistic, and schizotypal. Whereas the relationship to narcissistic personality has most captured the attention of psychoanalysts, the relationship to the latter—that is, schizotypal personality disorder—has gained a disproportionate amount of research attention. Studies of description and genetics have both pointed toward the distinctiveness of these personality types. Even studies of course and pharmacological response have supported a separation. The possible relationship to the other types of personality disorder, such as antisocial, histrionic, and even narcissistic, have been discovered almost incidentally. They have not received the research attention that they should, and it is hoped that they will by the time the next review on borderline personality is written.

Though the testimonials by distinguished psychoanalytically oriented clinicians as described by Adler lack the credibility of controlled research, they have been sufficiently persuasive to have stimulated much more interest in treatment. This interest has also been encouraged by the follow-up studies described by Stone. These studies establish that, if they survive, many borderline patients achieve reasonable social and interpersonal stability. This finding is very hopeful by showing that the usual, less ambitious, and limited treatments that help patients overcome crises may be more useful than previously known.

Within the treatment literature, the current reviews repeatedly point to two trends: In one of these, greater heterogeneity of response to any one modality is being found; and in the second trend, greater specificity of modality is being sought. The current practice of pharmacotherapy is complicated: Soloff notes that clinicians must recognize that selection of a drug is tied to differences in a particular borderline patient's phenomenology which affects the drug selection, and must also recognize the highly variable responsiveness of borderline patients to the various types of pharmacologic agents. These complications provide a clear incentive for future studies to define these subgroups and to explain the reasons for their differential responsiveness. These studies also provide a model that should be deployed with respect to the psychosocial interventions for patients with borderline personality disorder. Future attention will be needed to define the subgroup for whom a long-term, expensive, exploratory psychotherapy by extensively trained specialists such as psychoanalysts is indicated. Despite the highly influential advocates for such treatment, the little evidence which exists suggests that its "curative" effects are infrequent. Likewise, future research is needed to define those borderline patients who can engage in behavioral or cognitive treatments and the limits of what that form of treatment can be. Linehan notes that both the behavioral and cognitive efforts to treat borderline patients are in their earliest stage of development. Such efforts offer methods that specifically target problems seen in the first phase of treatment for most borderline patients. At the least, cognitive–behavioral strategies can be expected to be utilized more broadly and to bring an organizational rigor and specificity of effects to bear on the treatment of borderline patients that will be important for dynamic therapies to learn from and aspire to.

As a final caveat, it is exciting and encouraging to see so much energy being given to the study of a patient group that constitutes a high fraction of our "constituents" and who previously were relegated to a "wastebasket" status. There is no question that the term borderline personality disorder is now being used more uniformly and much more meaningfully. It is also clear that these patients' clinical care is being given more thoughtful and serious effort. Still there remain problems with defining the boundaries of this disorder (especially with other personality types) and problems with understanding its origins and course. Clearly it is time to move beyond retrospective reports of origins and beyond follow-up of retrospectively defined samples. It is to be hoped that continued refinement in our treatment methods can elevate the expected stabilization of functioning and relationships which now appears in 50 percent by 15 years. By the time of the third review on this subject, perhaps the rates will be closer to 75 percent by 5 years! We are still a long way from such goals.

REFERENCES

Grinker RR Sr., Werble B, Drye RC: The Borderline Syndrome: A Behavioral Study of Ego-Functions. New York, Basic Books, 1968

Kernberg OF: Borderline personality organization. J Am Psychoanalytic Assn 1967; 15:641–685

Kety SS, Rosenthal D, Wender PH, et al: The types and prevalence of mental illness in the biological and adoptive families of adopted schizophrenics, in The Transmission of Schizophrenia. Edited by Rosenthal D, Kety SS. Oxford, Pergamon Press Ltd, 1968

Masterson JF: Treatment of the Borderline Adolescent. New York, John Wiley and Sons, 1972

II

Child Psychiatry

II

Child
Psychiatry

Contents

Section II

Child Psychiatry
Foreword

by Jerry M. Wiener, M.D., Section Editor

This section of the annual *Review of Psychiatry* provides an update on the state of the art and of the science of six topics in child and adolescent psychiatry. Taken together they represent the core clinical categories and concerns of child psychiatry. Although not every important category could be encompassed (such as eating disorders, previously addressed in Volume 4 of this series, and substance use disorders), still, a familiarity with the conditions chosen will allow the practitioner to recognize, classify, and formulate a treatment approach to the large majority of children and adolescents presenting clinically with a psychiatric disorder.

In reading these chapters it is important to note the contribution initially of *DSM-III* and currently of *DSM-III-R* in describing these disorders and in allowing for largely reliable discriminated diagnoses. At the same time, the degree of overlap and covariance among several if not most of these conditions also is important to note. Examples of overlap include attention-deficit hyperactvity disorder with both conduct and mood disorders (including, in unusual circumstances, a bipolar disorder); severe mood disorders with schizophrenic disorders (especially in adolescents); of course the understanding of the many Axis I and Axis II disorders which can accompany, complicate, or be complications of mental retardation; and, finally, the relationship noted clinically between the anxiety and the mood disorders.

For each condition the authors discuss diagnosis using *DSM-III-R* criteria, and present what is known currently of epidemiology, etiologic concepts, comorbidity, and approaches to treatment.

In Chapter 7, Drs. Cantwell and Hanna take on perhaps the longest-established and certainly the most often reclassified disorder in child psychiatry—attention-deficit hyperactivity disorder. It is also the childhood disorder in which medication use was first established and is most widely utilized. And yet, as the chapter details, there are a multitude of still-to-be-answered research questions on subgroup classification, diagnostic specificity and comorbidity, etiology, pathophysiology, and, certainly, treatment and prognosis.

Anxiety disorders arising in childhood and adolescence were, for many years, in the theoretical and treatment domain of a developmentally oriented psychodynamic psychiatry. It is only quite recently that these conditions have attracted more research attention focusing on accurate description, epidemiology, biological aspects, and medication approaches to treatment. This is an exciting new area of discovery in the field, as is ably summarized by Drs. Leonard and Rapoport in Chapter 8.

In Chapter 9, the discussion of conduct disorders by Drs. Bailey and Egan reflects the heterogeneity and continually shifting conceptualizations of this collection of socially unacceptable behavior patterns. Here, too, we are learning more about subcategories and multiple etiologies in this quintessentially bio-psychosocial group of disorders.

Following the advent of antidepressants and a better understanding of affective disorders in adults, increasing clinical and research attention has been devoted to mood disorders in children and adolescents. We have come a long way from the time when childhood depression in a form similar to that found in adults was considered not to exist. In Chapter 10, Dr. Kashani and Mr. Sherman detail how much progress we've made and where we must continue to search for further answers in our attempt to understand mood disorders in children.

It is a particular pleasure, and, in some ways, a restitution, to include mental retardation in this section. For many reasons—social stigma, therapeutic pessimism, psychoanalytic priorities, institutionalization—mental retardation has been a group of functional and behavioral disorders long neglected by medicine, including child and adolescent psychiatry. In recent years a resurgence of interest in mental retardation reflects a lessening or a shift in all the factors identified above. It is particularly fitting that Drs. Szymanski, Rubin, and Tarjan are acknowledged for their expertise by coauthoring Chapter 11, for they are long-time tillers in a field considered unfertile by most of their colleagues.

Finally, Drs. Kestenbaum, Canino, and Pleak close this section with Chapter 12, reexamining the schizophrenic disorders of childhood and adolescence, including the continuing controversial question of their relationship to adult onset schizophrenia. Diagnostic criteria, questions of continuity or discontinuity among autism, pervasive developmental disorder, and childhood onset schizophrenia are explored, along with issues of etiologies and, as yet, insufficiently studied treatment approaches.

Each chapter stands alone to educate the reader on a particular category of disorder. At the same time, the chapters in this section resonate with similar themes and questions.

Chapter 7

Attention-Deficit Hyperactivity Disorder

by Dennis P. Cantwell, M.D., and Gregory L. Hanna, M.D.

This overview of the attention-deficit hyperactivity disorder (ADHD) will include various classification schemes and subtypes proposed for the disorder and give an outline of the core symptom pattern. Associated symptomatology that is often present in children with these disorders will be discussed, along with disorders that overlap with or may mimic the presence of ADHD. After a brief discussion of epidemiology we will discuss possible etiologic factors. We will then discuss natural history and outcome of the syndrome and end with a discussion of assessment and management.

CLINICAL PICTURE

Attention-deficit hyperactivity disorder is a heterogeneous collection of disorders that have been studied as well as any clinical syndrome in child psychiatry.

Probably the earliest conceptualization of this syndrome was that of "brain damage." Early studies, particularly of those children who developed encephalitis in the epidemic of 1917 and 1918, described a behavioral residual which included difficulties in motor activity, attention, and impulse control. Terms such as the "brain damage syndrome" and the "brain damage behavior syndrome" were coined to describe this clinical picture (Cantwell, 1975a).

It is true that children with brain damage have elevated rates of psychiatric disorder compared to children who do not have evidence of brain damage (Rutter et al, 1970). However, there is no unique clinical picture which develops in childhood as a result of brain damage.

A later term, "minimal brain damage," implied that the behavioral picture alone was enough to indicate the presence of subtle brain damage which could not be determined by more traditional measures (Cantwell, 1975a).

The term "minimal brain dysfunction" reflected the idea that there must be some functional rather than structural abnormality in the brain (Clements, 1966).

The "hyperkinetic reaction of childhood" was the official term in the *Diagnostic and Statistical Manual of Mental Disorders, Second Edition (DSM-II)* (American Psychiatric Association, 1968). Related terms included the "hyperactive child syndrome" (Cantwell, 1975a). Both of these terms are behaviorally oriented and do not imply any etiology, but do suggest that one symptom pattern (the motor activity) is more important than others.

In the *Diagnostic and Statistical Manual of Mental Disorders, Third Edition (DSM-III)* (American Psychiatric Association, 1980), the term was changed to "Attention Deficit Disorder," with the subtypes of Attention Deficit Disorder with Hyperactivity, Attention Deficit Disorder without Hyperactivity, and Attention Deficit Disorder Residual State. With the recent publication of the *Diagnostic and*

Statistical Manual of Mental Disorders, Third Edition, Revised (DSM-III-R) (American Psychiatric Association, 1987), the terminology has changed again. The primary term is "Attention-deficit Hyperactivity Disorder" (ADHD), listed as one of the "Disruptive Behavior Disorders," with an "Undifferentiated Attention Deficit Disorder" listed under "Other Disorders of Infancy, Childhood, or Adolescence." Table 1 lists the subtypes and criteria for these disorders in *DSM-III* and *DSM-III-R*.

The essential features according to *DSM-III* include a developmentally inappropriate short attention span, impulsivity, and hyperactivity. The core symptoms outlined in Table 1 for the three subtypes in *DSM-III* are recognized as being relatively common in other child psychiatric disorders and can indeed occur in normal children at various times. Thus, *DSM-III* added two other inclusion criteria for the diagnosis: an age of onset criterion and a duration criterion. The addition of these two inclusion criteria, in addition to the cross-sectional symptom pattern above, makes it less likely that one is dealing with an episodic condition that may present cross-sectionally somewhat like ADHD.

The *DSM-III* criteria were a major advance in outlining specific explicit behavioral criteria that must be present in three core clinical areas and also advanced the idea that this was an early onset condition that tends to be relatively chronic, although symptoms may vary in intensity. *DSM-III* also added certain exclusion criteria, outlined in Table 1.

DSM-III-R represents a marked change from *DSM-III*. First, there is only one subtype—Attention-deficit Hyperactivity Disorder (ADHD). The Residual State and Attention Deficit without Hyperactivity have been eliminated.

The *DSM-III* category is monothetic: Certain specific symptoms must be present for the diagnosis to be made. The *DSM-III-R* category is a polythetic category. There are 14 symptoms listed as characteristic of ADHD. *Any* 8 have to be present for at least 6 months. The permutations and combinations of any 8 out of 14 ensures a very heterogeneous clinical picture.

Polythetic categories tend to be broader than monothetic categories, leading to probable increased reliability of diagnosis. However, whether this change will lead to increased predictive validity and other forms of validity is a question for future research. Some of the 14 symptoms are thought to be characteristic of hyperactivity, some of attention, and some of impulsivity. But in contrast to *DSM-III*, symptoms in all three areas need not be present for the diagnosis to be made.

The text of *DSM-III-R* describes the core features of the disorder in a somewhat richer fashion than was done in *DSM-III*. Nevertheless, the descriptions are remarkably similar. *DSM-III-R* points out that there is some age specificity to the clinical picture, such that preschool children generally have more gross motor overactivity and frequent shifting from one activity to another as the signs of inattention and impulsivity.

In older children and in adolescents gross motor activity is less likely to be prominent, and excessive fidgeting and restlessness are more likely to be prominent. The manifestations of inattentiveness and impulsivity in older children and adolescents may be seen in the failure to complete tasks or instructions or in the performance of homework in a careless and slap-dash fashion. *DSM-III-R* also points out that in adolescents, impulsivity may be displayed in social activities such as joy-riding instead of doing homework. Obviously, age appro-

Table 1. Diagnostic Criteria for Attention Deficit Disorder: *DSM-III* versus *DSM-III-R*

DSM-III

Attention Deficit Disorder with Hyperactivity

The child displays, for his or her mental and chronological age, signs of developmentally inappropriate inattention, impulsivity, and hyperactivity. The signs must be reported by adults in the child's environment, such as parents and teachers. Because the symptoms are typically variable, they may not be observed directly by the clinician. When the reports of teachers and parents conflict, primary consideration should be given to the teacher reports because of greater familiarity with age-appropriate norms. Symptoms typically worsen in situations that require self-application, as in the classroom. Signs of the disorder may be absent when the child is in a new or a one-to-one situation.

The number of symptoms specified is for children between the ages of eight and ten, the peak age range for referral. In younger children, more severe forms of the symptoms and a greater number of symptoms are usually present. The opposite is true of older children.

A. **Inattention.** At least three of the following:
   (1) often fails to finish things he or she starts
   (2) often doesn't seem to listen
   (3) easily distracted
   (4) has difficulty concentrating on schoolwork or other tasks requiring sustained attention
   (5) has difficulty sticking to a play activity

B. **Impulsivity.** At least three of the following:
   (1) often acts before thinking
   (2) shifts excessively from one activity to another
   (3) has difficulty organizing work (this not being due to cognitive impairment)
   (4) needs a lot of supervision
   (5) frequently calls out in class
   (6) has difficulty awaiting turn in games or group situations

C. **Hyperactivity.** At least two of the following:
   (1) runs about or climbs on things excessively
   (2) has difficulty sitting still or fidgets excessively
   (3) has difficulty staying seated
   (4) moves about excessively during sleep
   (5) is always "on the go" or acts as if "driven by a motor"

D. Onset before the age of seven.

E. Duration of at least six months.

Table 1. Diagnostic Criteria for Attention Deficit Disorder: *DSM-III* versus *DSM-III-R* (*continued*)

F. Not due to Schizophrenia, Affective Disorder, or Severe or Profound Mental Retardation.

Attention Deficit Disorder without Hyperactivity

All of the features are the same as these of Attention Deficit Disorder with Hyperactivity except for the absence of hyperactivity; the associated features and impairment are generally milder. Prevalence and familial pattern are unknown.

Attention Deficit Disorder, Residual Type

A. The individual once met the criteria for Attention Deficit Disorder with Hyperactivity. This information may come from the individual or from others, such as family members.

B. Signs of hyperactivity are no longer present, but other signs of the illness have persisted to the present without periods of remission, as evidenced by signs of both attentional deficits and impulsivity (e.g., difficulty organizing work and completing tasks, difficulty concentrating, being easily distracted, making sudden decisions without thought of the consequences).

C. The symptoms of inattention and impulsivity result in some impairment in social or occupational functioning.

D. Not due to Schizophrenia, Affective Disorder, Severe or Profound Mental Retardation, or Schizotypal or Borderline Personality Disorders.

DSM-III-R

Attention-deficit Hyperactivity Disorder

Note: Consider a criterion met only if the behavior is considerably more frequent than that of most people of the same mental age.

A. A disturbance of at least six months during which at least eight of the following are present:

   (1) often fidgets with hands or feet or squirms in seat (in adolescents, may be limited to subjective feelings of restlessness)
   (2) has difficulty remaining seated when required to do so
   (3) is easily distracted by extraneous stimuli
   (4) has difficulty awaiting turn in games or group situations
   (5) often blurts out answers to questions before they have been completed

Table 1. Diagnostic Criteria for Attention Deficit Disorder: *DSM-III* versus *DSM-III-R* (*continued*)

---

(6) has difficulty following through on instructions from others (not due to oppositional behavior or failure of comprehension), e.g., fails to finish chores

(7) has difficulty sustaining attention in tasks or play activities

(8) often shifts from one uncompleted activity to another

(9) has difficulty playing quietly

(10) often talks excessively

(11) often interrupts or intrudes on others, e.g., butts into other children's games

(12) often does not seem to listen to what is being said to him or her

(13) often loses things necessary for tasks or activities at school or at home (e.g., toys, pencils, books, assignments)

(14) often engages in physically dangerous activities without considering possible consequences (not for the purpose of thrill-seeking), e.g., runs into street without looking

Note: The above items are listed in descending order of discriminating power based on data from a national field trial of the *DSM-III-R* criteria for Disruptive Behavior Disorders.

B. Onset before the age of seven.

C. Does not meet the criteria for a Pervasive Developmental Disorder.

Criteria for severity of Attention-deficit Hyperactivity Disorder:

Mild: Few, if any, symptoms in excess of those required to make the diagnosis and only minimal or no impairment in school and social functioning.

Moderate: Symptoms or functional impairment intermediate between "mild" and "severe."

Severe: Many symptoms in excess of those required to make the diagnosis and significant and pervasive impairment in functioning at home and school and with peers.

---

priate manifestations of hyperactivity, inattentiveness, and impulsivity must be taken into account when the disorder is being considered in an adult patient.

In addition to the core defining symptoms of the disorder, there are associated symptoms which are relatively common, including extreme lability of mood and temper tantrums, a low frustration tolerance, decreased self-esteem, and problems with academic achievement. The social disinhibition that often characterizes interpersonal relationships both with peers and with adults is often one of the more significant problems that these children face (Cantwell, 1984).

Children with this syndrome probably have more motor perceptual and motor coordination problems than children without the syndrome and may have more nonlocalizing neurological signs, often described as "soft" neurological signs in the literature (Shaffer et al, 1983). They also may have more minor physical anomalies (Rapoport et al, 1974) than children without this syndrome. However, none of these are characteristics of all children with the disorder and are not part of the core symptom pattern.

RELATED DISORDERS

Most of what we know about the clinical picture of the ADHD syndrome comes from studies of boys. In addition, there have been boys who have Attention Deficit Disorder with Hyperactivity. Much less is known about the clinical picture in girls and about the clinical picture of Attention Deficit Disorder without Hyperactivity. Carlson's review (1986) of the available literature concluded that the ADD without Hyperactivity subtype differs from the ADD with Hyperactivity subtype in behavior (aggression–conduct, social relationships, affective symptomatology, and impulsivity) (Berry et al, 1985; Edelbrock et al, 1984; King and Young, 1982; Lahey et al, 1985), and cognitive/learning differences (Carlson et al, in press; Maurer and Stewart, 1980; Sergeant and Scholten, 1985).

The study by Berry and colleagues (1985) suggests that both boys and girls with Attention Deficit Disorder with Hyperactivity demonstrate attentional, behavioral, and cognitive impairments. However, the children without the hyperactivity subtype demonstrated deficits along an attentional/cognitive axis. Management problems in antisocial behavior were correlates of the with-hyperactivity subtype, and these investigators found that increased impulsivity was not associated with attentional deficits in the absence of hyperactivity.

Berry and colleagues (1985) also demonstrated some significant findings that differentiated boys and girls. In those children who had ADD with Hyperactivity, the girls were characterized by more severe cognitive impairments. This was particularly true in the area of language function. The girls with ADD with Hyperactivity were younger at the time that they were referred for evaluation and also came from families of lower socioeconomic status. Boys with ADD with Hyperactivity were more likely to demonstrate disruptive uncontrolled behavior. In children with ADD without Hyperactivity, the girls had poorer self-esteem and were older than the boys with ADD without Hyperactivity at the time of first referral. Girls in both groups, with and without Hyperactivity, were more likely to be rejected by their peers than boys. Berry and colleagues concluded that girls with Attention Deficit Disorder were probably under-diagnosed and under-identified. They also suggested that cognitive deficits play the most prominent role in the identification of girls, but overt disruptive behavior disturbances are more likely to lead to referral for boys.

In addition to the associated symptoms noted above, many of these children present with other disorders that quite often overlap with the syndrome. When these disorders are present in their full form, they should be considered separate diagnoses.

The related disorders listed in Table 2 are Axis I and Axis II disorders that may co-occur with ADHD. These disorders may also be present on their own, with some episodic symptoms of ADHD. Thus, they may also mimic ADHD.

A careful differential diagnosis is called for. These issues are discussed more fully in Cantwell and Baker (1988) and Cantwell (1984).

Oppositional disorder and conduct disorders are two conditions that commonly co-occur with ADHD. Their presence suggests a poor prognosis for children with ADHD (Barkley, 1982; Loney, 1983; Stewart et al, 1981). Satterfield and Schell (1984) suggest that there may be underlying neurophysiological differences between ADHD children who do and do not develop conduct disorder. These two conditions may occur on their own and may mimic ADHD.

Tic disorders and Tourette's syndrome may also co-occur with ADHD. A substantial number of Tourette's syndrome patients give a history of ADHD in their early years (Cohen et al, 1985). Stimulant medication may precipitate tics, which may disappear when the medication is withdrawn, or may precipitate Tourette's syndrome, which does not disappear after the medication is withdrawn.

Pica is an eating disorder in which the inedible substances that may be ingested may contain lead. Such subclinical lead poisoning may lead to motor hyperactivity and mimic ADHD (Needleman et al, 1979).

Anxiety disorders and mood disorders are episodic problems in which there may be symptoms of inattentiveness, impulsivity, and motor activity that occur while the children are manifesting anxiety symptomatology and/or mood symptomatology. While anxiety and mood disorders less commonly overlap with ADHD than the disruptive behavior disorders, some studies (Carlson and Cantwell, 1982; Kovacs et al, 1984; Wender et al, 1981) suggest that these diagnoses may overlap with ADHD as well. Weinberg and Brumback (1976) have presented data suggesting that some children with an ADHD-like picture may be demonstrating a prepubertal manifestation of bipolar disorder which becomes more clear as the children get older. However, it should be noted that bipolar illness in prepubertal children is rare.

Children with schizophrenia with an onset in the prepubertal age range may also present with symptoms of attentional impairment (Asarnow and Sherman, 1984). These children do not necessarily demonstrate motoric overactivity and impulsivity, and their characteristic clinical picture generally does not present much difficulty in differential diagnosis.

Table 2.   Disorders Possibly Associated with ADHD

Axis One Disorders	Axis Two Disorders
Oppositional defiant disorder	Mental retardation
Conduct disorder	Pervasive developmental disorder
Tic disorders	Academic skills disorders
Tourette's syndrome	Language and speech disorders
Pica	Axis Three Conditions
Mood disorders	Neurologic disorders (i.e., seizure
Anxiety disorders	disorder, brain trauma)
Schizophrenia with childhood onset	Physical disorders (i.e., hyperthyroidism, pinworm infection)

Finally, adjustment disorders may present episodically with symptoms of ADHD which should resolve with time.

Many Axis II developmental disorders co-occur with ADHD. The mentally retarded have relatively high rates of ADHD (Aman, 1983), although the nature of their attention deficit may be qualitatively different from the attention deficit in the nonretarded. Likewise, children with pervasive developmental disorder, including infantile autism, may have a co-occurring ADHD syndrome (Greenhill, 1985). Children with academic skills disorders and speech and language disorders also have ADHD as a common co-occurring condition (Cantwell and Baker, in press b). Speech and language disorders and academic skills disorders are often seen alone or overlapping with each other without a true ADHD concomitant diagnosis in many cases with episodic difficulties with attentional problems, so that they mimic ADHD (Cantwell and Baker, in press b; Douglas, 1980).

Table 2 also indicates that various neurologic problems and various physical disorders may either overlap with or mimic ADHD. These are discussed more fully by Herskowitz and Rosman (1982).

EPIDEMIOLOGY

Shaywitz and his colleagues (personal communication, 1987) have reviewed prevalence studies in the pre-*DSM-III* era and in the *DSM-III* era. They conclude that despite the many difficulties in the studies, prevalence rates of ADHD in the school age population range between 10 and 20 percent when the studies use rating scales that are broadly similar and when teachers are the source of information. When parents are the source of information, prevalence rates may be higher. Some studies present prevalence rates much lower, in the 3 to 5 percent range, and are generally those that require the subject to be diagnosed by a professional. All the prevalence studies suggest that the ADHD syndrome is anywhere from two to four times more common in boys. Nevertheless, Shaywitz points out that underidentification of girls may be a significant problem. Their data suggest that ADD without hyperactivity occurs with a prevalence rate of approximately 25 percent of the prevalence of ADD with hyperactivity. Their suggestion is that boys may be identified more with this disorder than girls because girls may present somewhat differently, with primarily cognitive and language deficits and less in the way of physical aggression and acting out behavior.

In their own study of 445 children, which is an epidemiologic longitudinal study following children from kindergarten to the third grade, Shaywitz and his colleagues have found an overall prevalence rate of 23 percent for the ADD syndrome using *DSM-III* criteria (personal communication, 1987)

Etiology and Pathophysiology

There are numerous methodological problems in the study of the causes of a syndrome as heterogeneous as ADHD. As noted above, the inclusion criteria for ADHD have changed over the years, which probably has increased the variability and decreased the replicability of findings. Moreover, many of the abnormalities observed in ADHD are nonspecific or are confounded with other disorders such as conduct disorder. Even when a potential causal factor is associated reliably with ADHD, it appears in only a minority of those with the diagnosis. Thus, it is unlikely that a single etiological process will be demonstrated in ADHD. Instead, Rapoport and Quinn (1975, p. 41) have presented a more plausible perspective: "The symptoms of hyperactivity and impulsivity are most probably a final common means by which a variety of congenital, toxic, and environmental influences may be expressed." The literature on the etiology and pathophysiology of this disorder has been reviewed by Whalen (1983), Weiss and Hechtman (1986), Zametkin and Rapoport (1986, 1987a, 1987b), and Sokol and colleagues (1987).

Family Genetic Factors

Evidence from family history studies and adoption studies suggest that there is a significant genetic contribution to ADHD. Initially, two studies found that significantly more fathers and uncles of hyperactive children than of control children probably had been hyperactive as children themselves (Cantwell, 1972; Morrison and Stewart, 1971). These studies also found a high prevalence of sociopathy, alcoholism, and hysteria in the parents of hyperactive children but not in the parents of controls. In subsequent studies of adopted hyperactive children, a high prevalence of sociopathy, alcoholism, and hysteria was found in the biological parents but not in the adoptive parents (Cantwell, 1975b; Morrison and Stewart, 1973). In two more recent studies, ADHD with conduct disorder in children was linked with antisocial personality disorder, substance abuse, and somatization disorder in parents; however, ADHD without conduct disorder in children was not associated with any parental disorder (Lahey et al, 1988; Stewart et al, 1980). These findings are consistent to some extent with those of Biederman and colleagues (1987), who found that a spectrum of antisocial disorders and unipolar depression aggregated in the first degree relatives of ADHD boys with either conduct disorder or oppositional disorder, whereas the rates of these disorders were roughly equivalent in the first degree relatives of ADHD boys without conduct disorder or oppositional disorder and the first degree relatives of normal boys. In contrast to the previous studies, the rate of alcoholism in fathers was not increased in either ADHD subgroup.

These studies suggest that ADHD and conduct disorder are separate disorders that are caused by variables that result in familial patterns of transmission across generations. Thus, the genetic contribution to these disorders will have to be examined by studies with greater methodological rigor. For example, no adoption study has been done that differentiated between ADHD and conduct disorder with explicit diagnostic criteria and that blindly assessed relatives. In addition, no multigenerational family study has been done to determine whether ADHD and conduct disorder segregate independently across generations.

Sibling and twin studies also give some support to the notion of a genetic contribution to ADHD. Full siblings of hyperactive children were found to show more hyperactive behavior than did half-siblings (Safer, 1973). In two studies, there was greater similarity of activity level in the first year of life beween monozygotic twins than between dizygotic twins (Rutter et al, 1963; Torgersen and Kringlen, 1978). Parent ratings of hyperactivity in an older series of 186 same-sexed twins indicated a substantial hereditary component (Willerman, 1973). Nonetheless, these studies did not assess the genetic component of a clearly defined syndrome.

Neurophysiology

Many studies of ADHD have attempted to demonstrate physiological abnormalities in several ways—including cardiovascular and pulmonary measures, skin conductance and resistance, electroencephalographic recordings, and stature. Most studies of cardiac and electrodermal variables have found no differences between hyperactive and normal children in resting levels of autonomic activity (Montagu, 1975; Zahn et al, 1975; Ferguson et al, 1976; Barkley and Jackson, 1977). Some studies have suggested that ADHD children might be slower than normal in responding to environmental stimuli and may show less than normal levels of responding once stimulated (Zahn et al, 1975; Porges et al, 1975). Other studies have not found such differences (Ferguson et al, 1976; Barkley and Jackson, 1977). In an important review of this literature, Douglas (1983) stressed that the nature of the task and the incentive value of the reinforcers in the task have a significant impact on measures of arousal, inhibition, attention, impulsivity, and performance. She concluded that ADHD children may show both underarousal and overarousal depending on a variety of circumstances, and that the primary problem is a dysregulation of arousal.

Overall, most studies have found that ADHD children have an increased frequency of EEG abnormalities when compared to normal controls (Capute et al, 1968; Wikler et al, 1970). But a few studies have found no differences in EEG abnormalities in hyperactive children when compared to either normal controls or nonhyperactive emotionally disturbed children (Eeg-Olofsson, 1970; Werry et al, 1972). Many studies have noted a high incidence of diffuse nonspecific EEG changes and of extensive slow EEG activity in ADHD children (Capute et al, 1968; Satterfield et al, 1974; Grunewald-Zuberbier et al, 1975). In a series of 75 hyperactive children, the most consistent abnormality was the absence of an age appropriate number of well-organized alpha waves (Shetty, 1973). In addition, hyperactive children have difficulties with attenuation of alpha waves, which presumably reflects a decreased capacity to disattend to redundant events (Milstein et al, 1969; Fuller, 1977). Despite these differences, none of the abnormalities are specific to the ADHD syndrome.

All of the above abnormalities have been described as immature patterns and interpreted as representing delayed maturation of the central nervous system (CNS) in ADHD children. This hypothesis is supported by the increased normalization of EEGs in ADHD children with increasing age, particularly in late adolescence (Hechtman et al, 1978). Whether these abnormalities correlate with one or more of the core ADHD symptoms or with one of the clinical problems often associated with ADHD—such as learning disorder or aggression—is unknown at this time.

Neurochemistry

Most neurochemical studies have found no significant differences between ADHD children and normal controls. Two independent laboratories found that ADHD children excreted less MHPG (3-methoxy-4-hydroxyphenylglycol) than did normal controls (Shekim et al, 1983; Yu-cun and Yu-feng, 1984). No differences were found, however, by two other independent studies (Rapoport et al, 1978; Wender et al, 1971). Noradrenergic dysregulation is suggested by differences between ADHD children and normal subjects in the response of plasma norepinephrine to orthostatic challenge (Mikkelson et al, 1981), but this finding has not been replicated. Most drugs that are effective in the treatment of ADHD appear to alter measures of noradrenergic functioning that correlate with clinical improvement (Donnelly et al, 1986; Shekim et al, 1983; Zametkin et al, 1985a, 1985b). This is currently the strongest piece of evidence implicating a noradrenergic dysfunction in ADHD. Nonetheless, comparisons of clinically effective and clinically ineffective drugs have eliminated any single neurotransmitter hypothesis about ADHD (Zametkin and Rapoport, 1986, 1987a, 1987b).

Perinatal Stresses

Studies of perinatal problems have yielded complex and inconsistent findings. After a comprehensive examination of ADHD and normal children, Minde and colleagues (1968) were struck more by the similarities than by the differences between the two groups in rates of pregnancy problems, delivery complications, low birth weight, and neonatal diseases. In the prospective study done on the island of Kauai, perinatal stress was predictive of intelligence at age 10. But there was no relationship between these risk factors and school achievement, hyperactivity, and aggression (Werner et al, 1971). In summarizing the results of their 10-year follow-up study, the authors concluded that "ten times more children had problems attributed to the effects of a poor environment than to the effects of serious perinatal stress" (p. 134). In contrast, two studies have suggested a link between maternal smoking during pregnancy and overactive, impulsive behavior in children (Denson et al, 1975; Nichols and Chen, 1981). This factor remains to be examined carefully in future studies.

Lead, Sugar, and Food Additives

Several studies have concluded that lead levels below those previously considered toxic may contribute to cognitive and behavioral problems in school-age children (de la Burde and Choate, 1975; Smith et al, 1983; Needleman et al, 1979; Winneke, 1983). The intellectual deficits are small, but the finding is well replicated by different groups. The association between lead levels and ADHD symptoms is more uncertain. Perhaps the best evidence is provided by Needleman and colleagues (1979), who compared children with high and low lead dentine levels, and found that teachers rated those with high lead levels as more distractible, impulsive, and easily frustrated than those with low lead levels.

Although many parents and teachers are convinced that sugar ingestion adversely affects the academic and social behavior of ADHD children, little evidence supports a relationship between sugar ingestion and behavioral deterioration in this group. Three recent studies found no evidence for the notion that sugar causes or exacerbates ADHD symptoms (Wolraich et al, 1985, 1986; Milich and Pelham, 1986). One explanation for this misperceived association is that hyperactive children have difficulty in modulating their behavior in a changing environment, which is required when shifting from a snack or party period to the structured demands of classwork (Milich and Pelham, 1986). In addition to sugar, food additives have been examined for their effects on the behavior of ADHD children. Again, there is no compelling evidence that the behavior of hyperactive children in general is harmed by food additives or improved by special diets (Weiss et al, 1980; Kavale and Forness, 1983).

Psychosocial Stresses

A variety of studies suggest that the development of behavior and learning problems depends not only on the severity of biological deficits, but on environmental factors such as family adaptability and tolerance, psychological and socioeconomic assets, and stressful life events. An ecological perspective is supported by longitudinal studies of temperament (Thomas et al, 1968) and by evidence that social factors can compensate for early biological risk factors such a perinatal stress or low birth weight (Werner and Smith, 1977). Follow-up studies have shown that the severity and persistence of ADHD symptoms in early childhood are associated with lower socioeconomic status, ongoing family stress and disruption, and a conflicted mother–child relationship (Campbell et al, 1986; Paternite et al, 1980; Richman et al, 1982). Similarly, Loney and colleagues (1981) found that initial aggressiveness and family correlates of aggression such as parental hostility and punitive child-rearing practices are related to adolescent outcome measures of aggressiveness, delinquency, and school performance. Finally, Hechtman and associates (1984a) found that socioeconomic status and family mental health are predictors of adult outcome measures of educational achievement, work success, emotional adjustment, and drug abuse.

NATURAL HISTORY AND OUTCOME

The large number of published studies of the outcome of the ADHD syndrome have been reviewed by Weiss and Hechtman. The interested reader is referred to their seminal book (Weiss and Hechtman, 1986) for their very detailed descriptions of the various outcome studies. There are methodologic issues which may affect the outcome reported in various studies. These have been reviewed by Cantwell (1984).

Adolescent Outcome

The published data on adolescent outcome suggest that there is a general tendency for core ADHD symptoms to improve with time. Nevertheless, some core symptoms are still present in 50 to 80 percent of adolescent populations in various reported studies (Cantwell, 1985; Weiss, 1985). The way these core symptoms are manifested in adolescence may differ substantially from their presentation in childhood due to developmental changes. Conduct disorder and antisocial behavior is a common adolescent outcome. Twenty-five to 55 percent of various samples have been described as having serious problems with antisocial behavior in adolescence (Cantwell, 1985; Weiss, 1985; Weiss and Hechtman, 1986).

Some studies suggest that substance abuse (both alcohol and other drugs) is a common adolescent outcome, but others do not (Weiss, 1985). Gittelman's data (Gittelman et al, 1985) are important in that they suggest the persistence of core ADHD symptoms is almost necessary for antisocial behavior to develop. Moreover, of those who develop substance abuse, most if not all had pre-existing symptoms of conduct disorder and antisocial behavior.

Serious academic problems are also present in a significant number of adolescents. These include poor school achievement, repetition of grades, not completing high school, being less likely to attend college, and persistence of learning disabilities (Weiss and Hechtman, 1986; Cantwell, 1985). Low self-esteem, poor peer relationships, and demoralization syndromes are also common (Stewart et al, 1981), but there is a controversy as to whether there are increased rates of major depressive disorder, dysthymic disorder, and, possibly, bipolar disorder (Cantwell, 1985; Weiss, 1985; Weiss and Hechtman, 1986; Wender et al, 1981).

Adult Outcome

Less is known about adult outcome simply because fewer children have been followed into adult life. Employment behavior is not necessarily rated as abnormal by employers (Weiss and Hechtman, 1986). Nevertheless, there does seem to be an increased frequency of job changes, and some studies suggest that the social class level of the jobs are below those obtained by non-ADHD siblings and by the fathers of ADHD children, suggesting a possible downward drift in social class (Borland and Heckman, 1976).

Core symptoms of ADHD are reported to persist in 10 to 40 percent of various adult samples (Cantwell, 1985). Antisocial personality and substance abuse are also reported with increased frequency (Loney, 1983). Whether other personality disorders (such as borderline) or the episodic dyscontrol syndrome (Hartocollis, 1968) are more frequent in adults with ADHD is still questionable. Likewise, whether the ADHD syndrome may predispose to the schizophrenic spectrum disorders in adult life is also controversial.

Wender and colleagues (1981) report that a common outcome in his adult samples is a rather unique form of mood disturbance beginning in childhood with ups and downs, and progressing into adolescence and adult life with increasing periods of downs and a lower frequency of ups. Twenty-one out of 26 of his adult patients had such a "dysphoric" disorder, which Wender feels is different from major depressive disorder and dysthymic disorder.

Wender is also one of the few who have studied adults to suggest that anxiety disorder may be a common outcome (Wender et al, 1981). However, his sample contained an excess number of females in adult life compared to the number of females seen in childhood. Emotional lability also tends to be commonly reported in the adult samples, although this may be more part of the core symptomatology in adult life rather than a secondary complication (Garfinkel, 1986).

Mannuzza and Gittelman (1984) have systematically studied girls in childhood and followed them over time, and their data suggest that the adolescent outcome of girls with the ADHD syndrome is not significantly different from the outcome of boys with this disorder. It is not worse, but it is not better.

ASSESSMENT

As described in previous sections, the diagnosis of ADHD is based primarily on clinical information derived from a comprehensive evaluation of the child and the family, educational, and social environments. Collaboration with other physicians, psychologists, and educators is necessary for an accurate diagnosis and effective treatment. Because the core symptoms of ADHD are often present in other childhood neuropsychiatric syndromes, the diagnosis is to some extent a diagnosis of exclusion; exclusion criteria were discussed previously in the section on the clinical picture. Several sources of information, from different caregivers and settings, are necessary to establish the diagnosis. Thus, the evaluation should include detailed interviews of the child and the parents, as well as completed parent and teacher rating scales, to further assess the severity of ADHD symptoms and other behavioral difficulties. Table 3 lists some standard assessment instruments.

When interviewing the parents, it is important to consider developmental changes in the child's symptomatology. Because of the potential genetic and psychological implications of psychiatric disorders in the relatives, a detailed family history should be obtained during the parent interviews. In particular, the parents should be questioned about a family history of ADHD, learning disorder, conduct disorder, sociopathy, alcoholism, and substance abuse. Since the interview with the child occurs in a relatively confined and novel setting, it

Table 3. Summary of Assessment Instruments

Structured Psychiatric Interviews
  Diagnostic Interview for Children and Adolescents
    (DICA: Herjanic and Campbell, 1977)
  Kiddie-Schedule for Affective Disorders and Schizophrenia
    (K-SADS: Puig-Antich and Chambers, 1978)
  Diagnostic Interview Schedule for Children
    (DISC: Costello et al, 1984)

Behavior Rating Scales
  Child Behavior Checklist (parent and teacher report forms)
    (Achenbach and Edelbrock, 1983)
  Conners Parent Rating Scale—Revised
    (Goyette et al, 1978)
  Conners Teacher Rating Scales—Revised
    (Goyette et al, 1978)
  ADD-H Comprehensive Teacher Rating Scales
    (ACTeRS: Ullmann et al, 1984)

Neurological Examinations
  Neurological Examination for Subtle Signs
    (NESS: Denkla, 1985)
  Special Neurological Examination
    (Peters et al, 1975)

Psychometric Tests
  Wide Range Achievement Test
    (WRAT: Jastak and Jastak, 1965)
  Bender-Gestalt (Bender, 1938)
  Vineland Social Maturity Scales (Doll, 1953)
  Wechsler Intelligence Scale for Children—Revised
    (WISC-R: Kaufman, 1979)
  Illinois Test of Psycholinguistic Ability
    (ITPA: Kirk et al, 1968)

may be difficult to observe in the office the problems that the child may have with inattention, impulsivity, and overactivity (Sleator and Ullman, 1981). Interview techniques with ADHD children which may elicit these symptoms were described by Cantwell (1975).

Several structured psychiatric interviews for children and adolescents have been developed which can be used to confirm the diagnosis of ADHD and to screen for other psychiatric disorders. These interviews have separate schedules for parents and children. Because ADHD children usually underestimate the extent of their disruptive behavior, both schedules should be used. Structured diagnostic interviews for children and adolescents were examined in a special section of the *Journal of the American Academy of Child and Adolescent Psychiatry* (September, 1987). Recent advances in the assessment of ADHD were reviewed by Barkley (1987a).

Child behavior checklists and rating scales have become an essential part of the evaluation and diagnosis of ADHD. Obtaining parent and teacher rating scales, as well as any school reports or previous psychometric testing, prior to the first interview can facilitate the clinician's evaluation. Several rating scales now have excellent normative data and excellent reliability and validity. These include the parent and teacher versions of the Child Behavior Checklist (CBCL) by Achenbach and Edelbrock (1983). They have the practical advantages of simplicity, easy use by different observers, and a computer coded format that makes the data readily available. Nonetheless, the categories of childhood disorders generated by the CBCL are general (broad-band) so that other techniques are required to assign more refined (narrow-band) diagnoses to individual children. Moreover, the rate of misclassification of ADHD by parent and teacher rating scales is sufficiently high to preclude using them alone to make either clinical or research diagnoses (Lahey et al, 1987).

Barkley (1987b) provided a systematic and critical review of the rating scales currently used in the assessment of childhood behavior disorders. A special feature of *Psychopharmacology Bulletin* (Vol. 21, No. 4, 1985) presented the rating scales and assessment instruments used in pediatric psychopharmacology. Included in this issue was a review of the computerized cognitive tests which may prove to be clinically useful in the diagnosis and assessment of treatment response in ADHD (Swanson, 1985).

The physical examination is usually normal in children with ADHD. Nevertheless, a physical and neurological examination may be necessary to eliminate other conditions that may mimic or exacerbate ADHD. Measures of height and weight, along with descriptions of appearance and overall maturation, are important.

Visual and auditory acuity should be clinically assessed and, if questionable, followed by referral for further evaluation. Minor physical anomalies and soft neurological signs are increased in ADHD (Rapoport et al, 1974; Shaffer et al, 1983). But they are not specific to this syndrome and are not required for the diagnosis. Since there are no laboratory findings specific to ADHD, other laboratory tests should be done only to evaluate other suspected disorders.

Because of the patterns of comorbidity described above, educational testing and speech/language testing are often crucial in a comprehensive examination. Clinicians can evaluate, for example, academic achievement with the Wide Range Achievement Test, visual-motor skills with the Bender-Gestalt test, and social competence with the Vineland Social Maturity Scales. Children who are not doing well academically, especially those who are functioning significantly below the level that is expected by their age and intelligence, may need to be referred for more specific testing for developmental disorders. The limitations of psychological tests for differential diagnosis in child psychiatry have been discussed by Gittelman (1980).

TREATMENT

Stimulants and some other medications have been the most common treatment of ADHD in North America. This syndrome, however, usually consists of numerous deficits of multifactorial origin for which no single treatment is completely effective. Consequently, other treatments are necessary to optimize the functioning of ADHD children so that multimodal treatment has become the recommendation for most children with this disorder. Components of this treatment will vary from child to child, but generally will be selected from the following: parent involvement and education about the syndrome, parent management training, environmental manipulation, remedial or special education, social skills training, cognitive–behavioral therapy, individual and family psychotherapy, and medication.

Drug Treatments

Approximately 75 percent of children with ADHD respond to one or more of the stimulants. Moreover, the statistical superiority of the stimulants over placebo in the treatment of this syndrome is unequivocal (Cantwell and Carlson, 1978; Kavale, 1981). Consequently, the major issue in the treatment of an ADHD child is to determine whether a stimulant trial is indicated and whether there is a response to any of the stimulants. Table 4 presents clinical guidelines for a stimulant trial.

Since global clinical improvement from stimulants is no longer in doubt, recent studies have attempted to determine the more subtle clinical effects of these drugs on social interactions, academic performance, and long-term outcome. Numerous other studies have examined the potentially deleterious effects of stimulants on learning, memory, and growth. Finally, medications other than the standard stimulants have been investigated as treatments for ADHD. The recent literature on the pharmacotherapy of ADHD was reviewed by Gittelman-Klein (1987).

Several studies found that methylphenidate treatment of the ADHD child enhances cooperation between mother and child, reduces the mother's intrusive behavior, increases the mother's positive responses to the child, and increases compliance to maternal commands (Barkley et al, 1984, 1985). Similarly, other studies found that when hyperactive children are treated with methylphenidate, teachers are less controlling, less disciplining, and have less intense interactions with the children (Whalen et al, 1980, 1981).

Several studies showed that off-task behavior in the classroom is normalized by methylphenidate (Pelham et al, 1980, 1985). Similar results have been obtained in experimental classrooms (Whalen et al, 1979). In addition, controlled naturalistic studies of treated ADHD children have shown normalization of motor activity (Porrino et al, 1983) and of classroom behaviors such as noncompliance and interference (Abikoff and Gittelman, 1985).

Until recently, it was generally thought that stimulants had no impact on cognitive deficits or the acquisition of academic skills. Douglas and colleagues (1986), however, found that a low dose of methylphenidate (0.3 mg/kg) improved output, accuracy, efficiency, and learning acquisition in ADHD children. In addition, Pelham and colleagues (1985) found a linear relationship between methylphenidate dose and academic achievement as well as improved classroom behavior. Similarly, Rapport and associates (1988) found significant task behavior, and teacher's ratings of children's self-control. These studies raise doubts about the methodological rigor of earlier studies that stressed the lack of stimulant effects on classroom learning and performance.

Whether successful stimulant treatment of ADHD in childhood leads to a higher level of adaptive functioning in adolescence and adulthood is an important clinical question which has been addressed by several studies. For example, Hechtman and associates (1984b) compared adults who had received at least three years of continuous methylphenidate treatment in childhood with those who had not received such treatment. The formerly treated group was doing better in adulthood than those who had not been treated. In particular, the treated group had fewer car accidents, fewer problems with aggression, less

Table 4.   Clinical Guidelines for Stimulant Trials

---

(1) History of ADHD with no history of Tourette's syndrome

(2) Parent interviews and child psychiatric examination

(3) Parent and teacher ratings at baseline and periodically during treatment, with a decrease in scores of approximately 40 percent or more indicating a good response

(4) Measures of height, weight, resting pulse, and blood pressure at least four times a year

(5) Complete blood count with differential once a year

(6) Blood chemistries (including sodium, potassium, chloride, carbon dioxide, SGPT, SGOT, CPK, LDH, BUN, creatinine, glucose, phosphorus, cholesterol, total protein, uric acid) once a year

(7)
Stimulant:	single dose:	total daily dose:
Methylphenidate	0.25–1.0 mg/kg	5–80 mg/d
Dextroamphetamine	0.15–0.5 mg/kg	2.5–40 mg/d
Pemoline	0.5–2.0 mg/kg	18.75–112.5 mg/d

(8) Side-effects
common: insomnia, anorexia, abdominal distress, headaches
rare: dysphoria, tics, growth suppression, psychosis

(9) Periodic withdrawal to assess continuing need for medication

(10) Careful records of medication dispensing

psychiatric treatment, better social skills, and higher educational achievement than did the untreated group. Similarly, Loney and colleagues (1981) found that exposure to stimulants in childhood was positively associated in adolescence with better parent ratings, less police contact for alcohol and drug use, and less drunken driving. In contrast, Charles and Schain (1981) compared children who had received methylphenidate for an extended period of time with those who had not, and found that length of treatment was not associated with behavioral or scholastic outcome. Overall, it appears that effective stimulant treatment decreases the risk for alcohol and drug abuse later in life, which is important for those parents who are concerned about treating their children with a controlled substance.

These studies were naturalistic in that the treatment groups were self-selected and were not under experimental control. The evidence from such studies is therefore suggestive rather than definitive of a causal relationship. Because random assignment to either treatment or placebo groups for years is prohibited by both clinical and ethical considerations, information on long-term treatment effects will have to be gleaned from such naturalistic studies.

One follow-up study found that conduct disorder in adolescence occurred almost exclusively in youngsters with persisting ADHD (Gittelman et al, 1985). Clinical observations and research findings support the notion that stimulants are effective over long spans of time into adolescence and adulthood (Varley, 1983; Wender et al, 1985). This suggests that successful stimulant treatment during adolescence and even adulthood may be helpful in modifying the natural history of ADHD. Outcome may not be significantly affected, however, unless drug therapy is combined with other treatments (Satterfield et al, 1981).

The potentially deleterious effects of stimulants on learning, memory, and growth have been examined in numerous studies. A few conclusions can be drawn, but many questions remain. An early study of the effects of various stimulant dosages suggested that a high dose optimally improved social behavior but impaired cognitive performance (Sprague and Sleator, 1977). During the last 10 years, several studies have found limited evidence for a dissociation in the effects of stimulants on cognition and behavior and no evidence that treatment impairs some aspects of learning (Pelham et al, 1985; Rapport et al, 1988). There have been two reports of state-dependent learning during methylphenidate treatment (Swanson and Kinsbourne, 1976). Several other studies have failed to replicate this finding (Stephans et al, 1984; Steinhausen and Kreuzer, 1981). Finally, prospective studies suggest that cumulative stimulant dosage is associated with a decrement in growth velocity during childhood, but that the growth spurt compensates for this decrement, leaving adult height uncompromised (Hechtman et al, 1984b; Mattes and Gittelman, 1983).

Because methylphenidate and amphetamine have a short duration of action and occasionally produce significant side effects, other medications have been tested during the last 10 years for the treatment of ADHD. Comparisons of standard methylphenidate and sustained-release methylphenidate indicate that the sustained-release form is significantly less effective than the standard form on several measures of disruptive behavior, and that only a minority of children respond as well to the sustained-release form as to the standard form (Pelham et al, 1987). Similar results were obtained with magnesium pemoline in that the clinical effects are not as good as with the standard stimulants and the time of onset is somewhat delayed (Conners and Taylor, 1980). Its longer activity is inconsistent across children and is consequently unreliable. In short, sustained release methylphenidate and pemoline are potentially useful for children with severe rebound from the standard stimulants and for children unable to take more than one daily dose; but, in general, they do not appear to be as clinically effective as the standard stimulants.

Other medications have been investigated in an attempt to find alternatives to the standard stimulants and to test various pharmacological hypotheses about ADHD. Two monoamine oxidase inhibitors—tranylcypromine and clorgyline—were found to be effective in the treatment of ADHD. Moreover, they were thought without direct comparisons to be comparable to the stimulants in their efficacy (Zametkin et al, 1985b). Because of the necessity of maintaining a restricted diet, however, this class of medications is not practical for the treatment of most children and adolescents with ADHD. Pliszka (1987) has reviewed the evidence demonstrating that imipramine is not as effective as the stimulants, but that imipramine or another tricyclic antidepressant may be the drug of choice for children with ADHD and an associated anxiety or depressive disorder. In two open trials, desipramine was found to be safe and effective in the treatment of children and adolescents with ADHD (Gastfriend et al, 1985; Biederman et al, 1986). In contrast to previous studies, a total daily dose above 3.0 mg/kg was often used. Finally, clonidine was compared with placebo in a crossover design which yielded promising, yet inconclusive, results (Hunt et al, 1985). This medication may have some advantages over other medications in treating ADHD with an associated tic disorder, as well as having theoretical interest because of its unusual neuropharmacological action.

Psychosocial Treatments

Every component of a multimodal treatment for ADHD is dependent upon parental involvement and education about their child's disorder. Parents should be informed about the disorder—including its natural course, possible etiologic factors, and likely prognosis with and without treatment—in common descriptive terms. The literature indicates that children usually do not outgrow this disorder but rather grow into other problems. Thus, it is a disservice to tell parents that their child will develop normally without specific intervention. However, parents should be informed about the probability of different outcomes without suggesting that the condition is intractable. *The Hyperactive Child, Adolescent, and Adult* (Wender, 1987) is an excellent source of information and advice for parents of ADHD children.

All parents can be given some practical suggestions for the daily management of an ADHD child. One example is the importance of avoiding stressful situations known to cause difficulty, overstimulation, and excessive fatigue. Almost all parents can be taught the general principle of structuring the child's environment so that there are regular routines and proper limits set on the child's behavior. Specific problems—such as temper tantrums or fighting with siblings and others—can be the focus of individual sessions with the parents. Motivated parents without severe psychopathology themselves can be taught behavior management techniques so that they can be equipped to handle oppositional and defiant behavior as it arises. Barkley (1987c) has advocated group parent training in child management skills because it appears to be the most cost-effective method for managing the heavy caseload of disruptive behavior disorders in most child guidance clinics, and because it provides a potentially supportive network for the parents. Periodic retraining of parents usually is required in the long-term management of ADHD. *Living with Children* (Patterson and Gillon, 1968) summarizes these techniques and is written for parents.

The core symptoms of ADHD—inattention, impulsivity, and overactivity—are unlikely to respond to individual or group therapies alone. Yet there are some emotional and behavioral problems that appear to arise secondary to this syndrome which may be ameliorated by psychotherapy. These problems include low self-esteem, demoralization, distorted perceptions of social situations, and withdrawal from peers and adults. Gardner (1973) has written extensively about psychotherapeutic techniques for ADHD children with these problems.

Individual tutoring, remedial education, special education, and other forms of education or cognitive training are often necessary for ADHD children because of the academic failure engendered by this syndrome and because of the specific developmental disorders associated with it. Effective special education programs may be the most difficult treatment modality to find through the public school system. Special education teachers usually are trained in behavior modification techniques, and their behavioral program must be coordinated with the home behavioral program. Behavioral programs may be coupled also with cognitive techniques which emphasize self-monitoring, self-control, and altering internal self-messages (Cameron and Robinson, 1980).

As described above, some parents of ADHD children suffer from alcoholism, drug abuse, and other psychiatric disorders. While these parents can be involved in the child's treatment, they usually should be referred for individual therapy. If the child is stressed by a dysfunctional family which fails to respond to appropriate individual therapies, a more comprehensive family therapy is indicated.

The common expectation has been that a combination of pharmacologic and psychotherapeutic interventions would provide the optimal treatment for ADHD. The follow-up studies of combined treatments by Satterfield and colleagues (1981) support this prediction. Systematic studies of this prediction have been done by combining methylphenidate with behavior modification, with parent training in behavior management, and with cognitive training (see Gittelman-Klein, 1987, for a review).

The largest study comparing methylphenidate alone to methylphenidate combined with a behavior modification program at school and at home found that the combination treatment group was rated significantly better by teachers than the methylphenidate-alone group (Klein, 1986). However, direct classroom observations did not corroborate the teachers' evaluations. In a study that compared methylphenidate alone to methylphenidate combined with parent training, no significant advantage was found by adding parent training to medication (Firestone et al, 1981). Similarly, two studies showed that a combination of methylphenidate and cognitive training was no more effective than methylphenidate alone (Brown et al, 1985; Abikoff and Gittelman, 1985a). Finally, one study compared the effects of cognitive–behavioral therapy and methylphenidate on anger control in ADHD boys in verbally provocative situations (Hinshaw et al, 1984). Methylphenidate reduced the intensity of the boys' behavior but did not significantly increase either global or specific measures of self-control. Cognitive–behavioral therapy was more successful in enhancing both general self-control and the use of specific coping strategies. Again, however, there was no advantage in the combination of the two treatments.

REFERENCES

Abikoff H, Gittelman R: Hyperactive children treated with stimulants: is cognitive training a useful adjunct? Arch Gen Psychiatry 1985a; 42:953–961

Abikoff H, Gittelman R: The normalizing effects of methylphenidate on the classroom behavior of ADDH children. J Abnormal Child Psychology 1985b; 13:33–44

Achenbach TM, Edelbrock CS: Manual for the Child Behavior Checklist and Revised Child Behavior Profile. Burlington, VT, 1983

Aman MG: Psychoactive drugs in mental retardation, in Treatment Issues and Innovations in Mental Retardation. Edited by Matson JL, Andrasik F. New York, Plenum Press, 1983

American Psychiatric Association: Diagnostic and Statistical Manual of Mental Disorders, Second Edition (DSM-II). Washington, DC, American Psychiatric Association, 1968

American Psychiatric Association: Diagnostic and Statistical Manual of Mental Disorders, Third Edition (DSM-III). Washington, DC, American Psychiatric Association, 1980

American Psychiatric Association: Diagnostic and Statistical Manual of Mental Disorders, Third Edition, Revised (DSM-III-R). Washington, DC, American Psychiatric Association, 1987

Asarnow RF, Sherman T: Studies of visual information processing in schizophrenic children. Child Development 1984; 55:249–261

Barkley R: Guidelines for defining hyperactivity in children: attention deficit disorder with hyperactivity, in Advances in Clinical Psychology, Vol. 5. Edited by Lahey BE, Kazdin AB. New York, Plenum Press, 1982.

Barkley RA: The assessment of attention deficit-hyperactivity disorder. Behavioral Assessment 1987a; 9:207–233

Barkley RA: Child behavioral rating scales and checklists, in Assessment and Diagnosis in Child Psychopathology. Edited by Rutter M, Tuma AH, Lann S. New York, Guilford Press, 1987b

Barkley RA: Training Parents to Manage Behavior Problem Children. New York, Guilford Press, 1987c

Barkley RA, Jackson TL: Hyperkinesis, autonomic nervous system activity, and stimulant drug effects. J Child Psychol Psychiatry 1977; 18:347–357

Barkley RA, Karlsson J, Strzelecki E, et al: Effects of age and Ritalin dosage on the mother–child interactions of hyperactive children. J Consult Clin Psychol 1984; 52:750–758

Barkley RA, Karlsson J, Pollard S, et al: Developmental changes in the mother–child interactions of hyperactive boys: effects of two dose levels of Ritalin. J Child Psychol Psychiatry 1985; 26:705–715

Bender L: A Visual Gestalt Test and Its Clinical Use. New York, American Orthopsychiatric Association Research Monograph, 1938

Berry CA, Shaywitz SE, Shaywitz BA: Girls with attention deficit disorder: a silent minority? A report on behavioral and cognitive characteristics. Pediatrics 1985; 76:801–809

Biederman J, Gastfriend DR, Jellinek MS: Desipramine in the treatment of children with attention deficit disorder. J Clin Psychopharmacol 1986; 6:359–363

Biederman J, Munir K, Knee D: Conduct and oppositional disorder in clinically referred children with attention deficit disorder: a controlled family study. J Am Acad Child Adolesc Psychiatry 1987; 26:724–727

Borland H, Heckman H: Hyperactive boys and their brothers: a 25-year follow-up. Arch Gen Psychiatry 1976; 23:669–676

Brown RT, Wynne ME, Medenis R: Methylphenidate and cognitive therapy: a comparison of treatment approaches with hyperactive boys. J Abnorm Child Psychol 1985; 13: 69–87

Cameron MI, Robinson VM: Effects of cognitive training on academic and on-task behavior of hyperactive children. J Abnorm Child Psychol 1980; 8:405–419

Campbell SB, Breaux AB, Ewing LJ, et al: Correlates and predictors of hyperactivity and aggression: a longitudinal study of parent-referred problem preschoolers. J Abnorm Child Psychol 1986; 14:217–234

Cantwell DP: Psychiatric illness in the families of hyperactive children. Arch Gen Psychiatry 1972; 27:414–417

Cantwell DP (Ed): The Hyperactive Child: Diagnosis, Management, Current Research. New York, Spectrum Publications, 1975a

Cantwell DP: Genetics of hyperactivity. J Child Psychol Psychiatry 1975b; 16:261–264

Cantwell DP: Pharmacotherapy of ADD in adolescence: what do we know, where should we go, how should we do it? Psychopharmacol Bull 1985; 21:251–257

Cantwell, DP: Attention deficit and associated childhood disorders, in Contemporary Directions in Psychopathology. Edited by Millon T, Klerman GL. New York, Guilford, 1984

Cantwell DP, Baker L: Issues in the classification of child and adolescent psychopathology. J Am Acad Child Adolesc Psychiatry 1988; 27:521–533

Cantwell DP, Baker L: Language and language disorders. New York, Oxford University Press (in press)

Cantwell DP, Carlson GA: Stimulants, in Pediatric Psychopharmacology: The Use of Behavior Modifying Drugs in Children. Edited by Werry JS. New York, Brunner/Mazel, 1978

Capute AJ, Niedermeyer EF, Richardson F: The electroencephalogram in children with minimal cerebral dysfunction. Pediatrics 1968; 41:1104–1114

Carlson CL: Attention deficit disorder without hyperactivity, in Advances in Clinical Child Psychology, vol. 9. Edited by Lahey B, Kazdin A. New York, Plenum, 1986

Carlson CL, Lahey BB, Neeper R: Direct assessment of the cognitive correlates of attention deficit disorders with and without hyperactivity, Journal of Behavioral Assessment and Psychopathology (in press)

Carlson GA, Cantwell DP: Suicidal behavior and depression in children and adolescents. J Am Acad Child Psychiatry 1982; 21:361–368

Charles L, Schain R: A four-year follow-up study of the effects of methylphenidate on the behavior and academic achievement of hyperactive children. J Abnorm Child Psychol 1981; 9:495–505

Clements S: Minimal Brain Dysfunction in Children. NINDB Monograph No. 3. Washington, DC, U.S. Public Health Service, 1966

Cohen DJ, Leckman JF, Shaywitz BA: The Tourette syndrome and other tics, in The Clinical Guide to Child Psychiatry. Edited by Shaffer D, Ehrhardt AA, Greenhill LL. New York, Free Press, 1985

Conners CK, Taylor E: Pemoline, methylphenidate, and placebo in children with minimal brain dysfunction. Arch Gen Psychiatry 1980; 37:922–930

Costello AJ, Edelbrock CS, Dulcan MM, et al: Report of the NIMH Diagnostic Interview Schedule for Children (DISC). Washington, DC, National Institute of Mental Health, 1984

de la Burde B, Choate MS; Early asymptomatic lead exposure and development at school age. J Pediatr 1975; 87:475–481

Denkla MB: Revised neurological examination for subtle signs. Psychopharmacol Bull 1985; 21:773–800, 1985

Denson R, Nanson JL, McWatters MA: Hyperkinesis and maternal smoking. Canadian Psychiatric Association Journal 1975; 205:188–205

Doll E: Measurement of social competence, in Manual for the Vineland Social Maturity Scale. Princeton NJ, Educational Testing Service, 1953

Donnelly M, Zametkin AJ, Rapoport JL, et al: Treatment of hyperactivity with desipramine: plasma drug concentration, cardiovascular effects, plasma and urinary catecholamine levels, and clinical response. Clin Pharmacol Ther 1986; 39:72–81

Douglas VI: Self-control techniques: higher mental process in hyperactive children; implications for training, in Treatment of Hyperactive and Learning Disordered Children—Current Research. Edited by Knights RM, Bakker DJ. Baltimore, MD, University Park Press, 1980

Douglas VI: Attentional and cognitive problems, in Developmental Neuropsychiatry. Edited by Rutter M. New York, Guilford Press, 1983

Douglas VI, Barr RG, O'Neill ME, et al: Short term effects of methylphenidate on the cognitive, learning and academic performance of children with attention deficit disorder in the laboratory and the classroom. J Child Psychol Psychiatry 1986; 27:191–211

Edelbrock C, Costello AJ, Kessler MD: Empirical corroboration of the attention deficit disorder. J Am Acad Child Psychiatry 1984; 23:285–290

Eeg-Olofsson O: The development of the electroencephalogram in normal children and adolescents from the age of 1 through 21 years. Acta Paediatrica Scandinavica 1972; 208(Suppl):1–46

Ferguson HB, Simpson S, Trites RL: Psychophysiological study of methylphenidate responders and nonresponders, in Neuropsychology of Learning Disorders. Edited by Knights RK, Bakker DJ. Baltimore, MD, University Park Press, 1976

Firestone P, Kelly MJ, Goodman JT, et al: Differential effects of parent training and stimulant medication with hyperactives. J Am Acad Child Psychiatry 1981; 20:135–147

Fuller PW: Computer estimated alpha attenuation during problem solving in children with learning disabilities. Electroencephalography and Clinical Neurophysiology 1977; 42:148–156

Gardner RA: Psychotherapy of the psychogenic problems secondary to minimal brain dysfunction. International Journal of Child Psychotherapy 1973; 2:224–256

Garfinkel BD: Recent developments in attention deficit disorder. Psychiatric Annals 1986; 16:11–15

Gastfriend DR, Biederman J, Jellinek MS: Desipramine in the treatment of attention deficit disorder in adolescents. Psychopharmacol Bull 1985; 21:144–145

Gittelman R: The role of psychological tests for differential diagnosis in child psychiatry. J Child Psychiatry 1980; 19:413–438

Gittelman R, Manuzza S, Shenker R, et al: Hyperactive boys almost grown up, I: psychiatric status. Arch Gen Psychiatry 1985; 42:937–947

Gittelman-Klein R: Pharmacotherapy of childhood hyperactivity: an update, in Psychopharmacology: The Third Generation of Progress. Edited by Meltzer H. New York, Raven Press, 1987

Goyette CH, Conners CK, Ulrich F: Normative data on Revised Conners Parent and Teacher Rating Scales. J Abnorm Child Psychol 1978; 6:221–236

Greenhill LL: The hyperkinetic syndrome, in The Clinical Guide to Child Psychiatry. Edited by Shaffer D, Ehrhardt AA, Greenhill LL. New York, Free Press, 1985

Grunewald-Zuberbier E, Grunewald G, Rasche A: Hyperactive behavior and EEG arousal reactions in children. Electroencephalography and Clinical Neurophysiology 1975; 38:149–159

Hartocollis P: The syndrome of minimal brain dysfunction in young adult patients. Bull Menninger Clin 1968; 32:102–114

Hechtman L, Weiss G, Metrakos K: Hyperactive individuals as young adults: current and longitudinal electroencephalographic evaluation and its relationship to outcome. Canadian Medical Association Journal 1978; 118:919–923

Hechtman L, Weiss G, Perlman T, et al: Hyperactives as young adults: initial predictors of adult outcome. J Am Acad Child Psychiatry 1984a; 23:250–260

Hechtman L, Weiss G, Perlman T: Young adult outcome of hyperactive children who received long-term stimulant treatment. J Am Acad Child Psychiatry 1984b; 23:261–269

Herjanic B, Campbell W: Differentiating psychiatrically disturbed children on the basis of a structured interview. J Abnorm Child Psychol 1977; 5:127–134

Herskowitz J, Rosman NP: Pediatrics, Neurology, and Psychiatry—Common Ground. New York, Macmillan, 1982

Hinshaw SP, Henker B, Whalen CK: Self-control in hyperactive boys in anger-inducing situations: effects of cognitive-behavioral training and of methylphenidate. J Abnorm Child Psychol 1984; 12:55–77

Hunt RD, Minderaa RB, Cohen DJ: Clonidine benefits children with attention deficit disorder and hyperactivity: report of a double-blind placebo-crossover therapeutic trial. J Am Acad Child Psychiatry 1985; 24:617–629

Jastak JF, Jastak SR: The Wide Range Achievement Test (manual). Wilmington, Del, Guidance Associates, 1965

Kaufman AS: Intelligent Testing with the WISC-R. New York, John Wiley & Sons, 1979

Kavale K: The efficacy of stimulant drug treatment for hyperactivity: a meta-analysis. Journal of Learning Disabilities 1981; 15:280–289

Kavale K, Forness S: Hyperactivity and diet treatment: a meta-analysis of the Feingold hypothesis. Journal of Learning Disabilities 1983; 16:324–330

King C, Young RD: Attentional deficits with and without hyperactivity: teacher and peer perceptions. J Abnorm Child Psychol 1982; 10:483–495

Kirk SA, McCarthy JJ, Kirk WD: The Illinois Test of Psycholinguistic Abilities, revised edition. Champaign, IL, University of Illinois, 1968

Klein RG: Paper presented at the annual meeting of the American College of Neuropsychopharmacology, Washington, DC, December 1986

Kovacs M, Feinberg TL, Crouse-Novak MA, et al: Depressive disorders in childhood, I: a longitudinal prospective study of characteristics and recovery. Arch Gen Psychiatry 1984; 41:229–237

Lahey BB, Schaughency EA, Strauss CC, et al: Teacher ratings of attention problems in children experimentally classified as exhibiting attention deficit disorders with and without hyperactivity. J Am Acad Child Psychiatry 1985; 24:613–616

Lahey BD, McBurnett K, Piancentini JC, et al: Agreement of parent and teacher rating scales with comprehensive clinical assessments of attention deficit disorder with hyperactivity. Journal of Psychopathology Behavioral Assessment 1987; 9:429–439

Lahey BB, Piancentini JC, McBurnett K, et al: Psychopathology in the parents of children with conduct disorder and hyperactivity. J Am Acad Child Adolesc Psychiatry 1988; 27:163–170

Loney J: Research Diagnostic Criteria for childhood hyperactivity, in Childhood Psychopathology and Development. Edited by Guze SB, Earls FJ, Barrett JE. New York, Raven Press, 1983

Loney J, Kramer J, Milich R: The hyperkinetic child grows up: predictors of symptoms, delinquency, and achievement at follow-up, in Psychosocial Aspects of Drug Treatment for Hyperactivity. Edited by Gadow KD, Loney J. Boulder, CO, Westview Press, 1981

Mannuzza S, Gittelman R: The adolescent outcome of hyperactive girls. Psychiatric Research 1984; 13:19–29

Mattes JM, Gittelman R: Growth of hyperactive children on maintenance regimen of methylphenidate. Arch Gen Psychiatry 1983; 40:317–321

Maurer RG, Stewart MA: Attention deficit without hyperactivity in a child psychiatry clinic. J Clin Psychiatry 1980; 417:232–233

Mikkelson E, Lake CR, Brown GL, et al: The hyperactive child syndrome: peripheral sympathetic nervous system function and the effect of d-amphetamine. Psychiatry Research 1981; 4:157–169

Milich R, Pelham WE: Effects of sugar ingestion on the classroom and playgroup behavior of attention deficit disordered boys. J Consult Clin Psychol 1986; 54:714–718

Milstein V, Stevens J, Sachdev K: Habituation of the alpha attenuation response in children and adults with psychiatric disorders. Electroencephalography and Clinical Neurophysiology 1969; 26:12–18

Minde K, Webb G, Sykes D: Studies on the hyperactive child, VI: prenatal and perinatal factors associated with hyperactivity. Dev Med Child Neurol 1968; 10:355–363

Montagu JD: The hyperkinetic child: a behavioural electrodermal and EEG investigation. Dev Med Child Neurol 1975; 17:299–305

Morrison JR, Stewart MA: A family study of the hyperactive child syndrome. Biol Psychiatry 1971; 3:189–195

Morrison JR, Stewart MA: The psychiatric status of legal families of adopted hyperactive children. Arch Gen Psychiatry 1973; 3:888–891

Needleman HL, Guncoe C, Leviton A, et al: Deficits in psychologic and classroom performance of children with elevated dentine lead levels. N Engl J Med 1979; 300:689–695

Nichols PL, Chen T: Minimal Brain Dysfunction: A Prospective Study. Hillsdale, NJ, Lawrence Erlbaum, 1981

Paternite CE, Loney J, Langhorne JE: Relationships between symptomatology and SES-related factors in hyperkinetic/MBD boys, in Hyperactive Children: The Social Ecology of Identification and Treatment. Edited by Whalen CK, Henker B. New York, Academic Press, 1980

Patterson GR, Gillon ME: Living with Children. Champaign, IL, Research Press, 1968

Pelham WE, Schnedler RW, Bologna NC, et al: Behavioral and stimulant treatment of hyperactive children: a therapy study with methylphenidate probes in a within subject design. J Appl Behav Anal 1980; 13:221–236

Pelham WE, Bender ME, Caddell J, et al: Methylphenidate and children with attention deficit disorder. Arch Gen Psychiatry 1985; 42:948–952

Pelham WE, Sturges J, Hoza J, et al: Sustained release and standard methylphenidate effects on cognitive and social behavior in children with attention deficit disorder. Pediatrics 1987; 80:491–501

Peters JE, Romine JS, Dykman RA: A special neurological examination of children with learning disabilities. Dev Med Child Neurol 1975; 17:63–78

Pliszka SR: Tricylic antidepressants in the treatment of children with attention deficit disorder. J Am Acad Child Psychiatry 1987; 26:127–132

Porges SW, Walter GF, Korb RJ, et al: The influence of methylphenidate on heart rate and behavioral measures of attention in hyperactive children. Child Dev 1975; 46:727–733

Porrino LJ, Rapoport JL, Behar D, et al: A naturalistic assessment of the motor activity of hyperactive boys, II: stimulant drug effects. Arch Gen Psychiatry 1983, 40:688–693

Puig-Antich J, Chambers WJ: The Schedule for Affective Disorder and Schizophrenia for School-Aged Children. New York, New York State Psychiatric Institute, 1978

Rapoport JL, Quinn PO: Minor physical anomalies (stigmata) and early developmental deviation. International Journal of Mental Health 1975; 4:29–44

Rapoport JL, Quinn PO, Lamprecht F: Minor physical anomalies and plasma dopamine-beta-hydroxylase activity in hyperactive boys. Am J Psychiatry 1974; 121:386–389

Rapoport J, Mikkelsen EJ, Ebert MH, et al: Urinary catecholamine and amphetamine excretion in hyperactive and normal boys. J Nerv Ment Dis 1978; 66:731–737

Rapport MD, Stoner G, DuPaul GJ, et al: Attention deficit disorder and methylphenidate: a multilevel analysis of dose-response effects on children's impulsivity across settings. J Am Acad Child Adolesc Psychiatry 1988; 27:60–69

Richman N, Stevenson J, Graham PJ: Pre-school to School: A Behavioural Study. London, Academic Press, 1982

Rutter M, Korn S, Birch HG: Genetic and environmental factors in the development of "primary reaction patterns." British Journal of Sociology and Clinical Psychology 1963; 161–173

Rutter M, Graham P, Yule W: A Neuropsychiatric Study in Childhood. Philadelphia, J.B. Lippincott, 1970

Safer DJ: A familial factor in minimal brain dysfunction. Behav Genet 1973; 3:175–186

Satterfield JH, Schell AM: Childhood brain function differences in delinquent and non-delinquent hyperactive boys. Electroencephalogr Clin Neurophysiol 1984; 57:199–207

Satterfield JH, Cantwell DP, Saul RE, et al: Intelligence, academic achievement, and EEG abnormalities in hyperactive children. Am J Psychiatry 1974; 133:391–395

Satterfield JH, Satterfield BT, Cantwell DP: Three-year multimodal treatment study of 100 hyperactive boys. J Pediat 1981; 98:650–655

Sergeant JA, Scholten CA: On data limitations in hyperactivity. J Child Psychol Psychiatry 1985; 26:111–124

Shaffer D, O'Conner PA, Shafer SQ, et al: Neurological "soft signs": their origins and significance for behavior, in Developmental Neuropsychiatry. Edited by Rutter M. New York, Guilford 1983

Shekim WO, Javaid J, Dans JM, et al: Urinary MHPG and HVA excretion in boys with attention deficit disorder and hyperactivity treated with d-amphetamine. Biol Psychiatry 1983; 18:707–714

Shetty T: Some neurologic, electrophysiologic and biochemical correlates of the hyperkinetic syndrome. Pediatric Annals 1973; 29:29–38

Sleator EK, Ullmann RK: Can the physician diagnose hyperactivity in the office? Pediatrics 1981; 67:13–17

Smith M, Delves T, Lansdown R, et al: The effects of lead exposure on urban children. The Institute of Child Health/Southampton Study. Dev Med Child Neurol 1983; 25:(Suppl 47)1–54

Sokol MS, Campbell M, Goldstein M, et al: Attention deficit disorder with hyperactivity and the dopamine hypothesis: case presentations with theoretical background. J Am Acad Child Adolesc Psychiatry 1987; 26: 428–433

Sprague R, Sleator E: Methylphenidate in hyperkinetic children: differences in dose effects on learning and social behavior. Science 1977; 198:1274–1276

Steinhausen H, Kreuzer E: Learning in hyperactive children: are there stimulant-related and state-dependent effects? Psychopharmacology 1981; 74:389–390

Stephans R, Pelham WE, Skinner R: The state-dependent and main effects of pemoline and methylphenidate on paired-associate learning and spelling in hyperactive children. J Consult Clin Psychol 1984; 52:104–113

Stewart MA, de Blois CS, Cummings C: Psychiatric disorder in the parents of hyperactive boys and those with conduct disorder. J Child Psychol Psychiatry 1980; 21:283–292

Stewart MA, Cummings C, Singer S, et al: The overlap between hyperactive and unsocialized aggressive children. J Child Psychol Psychiatry 1981; 22:23–45

Structured diagnostic interviews for children and adolescents. J Am Acad Child Adolesc Psychiatry 1987; 26:611–675

Swanson JM: Measures of cognitive functioning appropriate for use in pediatric psychopharmacological research studies. Psychopharmacol Bull 1985; 21:887–890

Swanson JM, Kinsbourne M: Stimulant-related state-dependent learning in hyperactive children. Science 1976; 192:1354–1357

Thomas A, Chess S, Birch HG: Temperament and Behavior Disorders in Children. New York, University Press, 1968

Torgersen AM, Kringlen E: Genetic aspects of tempermental differences in infants: their cause as shown through twin studies. J Am Acad Child Psychiatry 1978; 17:433–434

Ullmann RK, Sleator EK, Sprague RL: A new rating scale for diagnosis and monitoring of ADD children. Psychopharmacol Bull 1984; 20:160–164

Varley C: Effects of methylphenidate in adolescents with attention deficit disorder. J Am Acad Child Psychiatry 1983; 22:351–354

Weinberg WA, Brumback RA: Mania in childhood: case studies and literature review. American Journal of Diseases in Children 1976; 130:380–385

Weiss B, Williams JH, Margen S, et al: Behavioral responses to artificial food colors. Science 1980; 207:1487–1489

Weiss G: Follow-up study on outcome of hyperactive children. Psychopharmacol Bull; 21:169–177

Weiss G, Hechtman LT: Hyperactive Children Grown Up. New York, Guilford Press, 1986

Wender PH: The Hyperactive Child, Adolescent and Adult. New York, Oxford University press, 1987

Wender P, Epstein RS, Kopin IJ, et al: Urinary monoamine metabolites in children with minimal brain dysfunction. Am J Psychiatry 1971; 127:1411–1415

Wender PH, Reimherr FW, Wood DR. Attention deficit disorder ('minimal brain dysfunction') in adults. Arch Gen Psychiatry 1981; 38:449–456

Wender PH, Reimherr FW, Wood D, et al: A controlled study of methylphenidate in the treatment of attention deficit disorder, residual type, in adults. Am J Psychiatry 1985; 142:547–552

Werner EE, Smith RS: Kanai's Children Come of Age. Honolulu University of Hawaii Press, 1977

Werner EE, Bierman JM, French FE: The Children of Kauai: A Longitudinal Study from the Prenatal Period to Age Ten. Honolulu, University Press of Hawaii, 1971

Werry JS, Minde K, Guzman A, et al: Studies on the hyperactive child, VII: neurological status compared with neurotic and normal children. Am J Orthopsychiatry 1972; 42:441–451

Whalen CK: Hyperactivity, learning problems, and the attention deficit disorders, in Handbook of Child Psychopathology. Edited by Ollendick T, Hersen M. New York, Plenum Press, 1983

Whalen CK, Henker B, Collins BE, et al: A social ecology of hyperactive boys: medication effects in structured classroom environments. J Applied Behav Anal 1979; 12:65–81

Whalen CK, Henker B, Dotemoto S: Methylphenidate and hyperactivity: effects of teaching behaviors. Science 1980; 208:1280–1282

Whalen CK, Henker B, Dotemoto S: Teacher response to the methylphenidate (Ritalin) versus placebo status of hyperactive boys in the classroom. Child Dev. 1981; 52:1005–1014

Wikler A, Dixon JR, Parker JB: Brain function in problem children and controls: psychometric, neurological, and electroencephalographic comparison. Am J Psychiatry 1970; 127:634–645

Willerman L: Activity level and hyperactivity in twins. Child Dev 1973; 44:288–293

Winneke G: Neurobehavioral and neurophsychological effects of lead, in Lead versus Health: Sources and Effects of Low Level Lead Exposure. Edited by Rutter M, Russell JR. Chichester, England, R. Wiley, 1983

Wolraich ML, Milich R, Stumbo P, et al: Effects of sucrose ingestion on the behavior of hyperactive boys. J Pediatr 1985; 106:675–681

Wolraich ML, Stumbo P, Milich R, et al: Dietary characteristics of hyperactive and control boys and their behavioral correlates. J Am Diet Assoc 1986; 86:500–504

Yu-cun A, Yu-feng W: Urinary 3-methoxy-4-hydroxy-phenylglycol sulfate excretion in seventy-three school children with minimal brain dysfunction syndrome. Biol Psychiatry 1984; 19:861–870

Zahn TP, Abate F, Little BC, et al: Minimal brain dysfunction, stimulant drugs and autonomic nervous system activity. Arch Gen Psychiatry 1975; 32:381–387

Zametkin AJ, Rapoport JL: The pathophysiology of attention deficit disorder with hyperactivity: a review, in Advances in Clinical Child Psychology. Edited by Lahey BB, Kazdin AE. New York, Plenum Press, 1986

Zametkin AJ, Rapoport JL: Neurobiology of attention deficit disorder with hyperactivity: where have we come in 50 years? J Am Acad Child Adolesc Psychiatry 1987a; 26:676–686

Zametkin AJ, Rapoport JL: Noradrenergic hypothesis of attention deficit disorder with hyperactivity: a critical review, in Psychopharmacology: The Third Generation of Progress. Edited by Meltzer HY. New York, Raven Press, 1987b

Zametkin AJ, Karoum F, Linnoila M, et al: Stimulants, urinary catecholamines and indoleamines in hyperactivity: a comparison of methylphenidate and dextroamphetamine. Arch Gen Psychiatry 1985a; 42:251–255

Zametkin AJ, Rapoport JL, Murphy DL, et al: Treatment of hyperactive children with monoamine oxidase inhibitors, I: clinical efficacy. Arch Gen Psychiatry 1985b; 42:962–969

Zametkin AJ, Rapoport JL, Murphy DL, et al: Treatment of hyperactive children with monoamine oxidase inhibitors, II: plasma and urinary monoamine findings after treatment. Arch Gen Psychiatry 1985c; 42:969–973

Chapter 8

Anxiety Disorders in Childhood and Adolescence

by Henrietta L. Leonard, M.D., and Judith L. Rapoport, M.D.

DIAGNOSIS OF THE ANXIETY DISORDERS IN CHILDHOOD AND ADOLESCENCE

An increasing interest in the anxiety disorders in childhood is related to the recognition that anxiety disorders are far more common than previously had been believed, and to the recent surge of research on the biology of anxiety. Certain anxiety diagnoses, once thought present only in adults, now are known to occur at a much earlier age. However, methodology lags behind interest. Few studies document the reliability of diagnosis, prevalence, risk factors, and/or the efficacy of interventions in childhood. While this chapter focuses on the last three years' research, several excellent reviews have covered earlier work (Beeghly, 1986; Gittelman, 1986).

DSM-III-R *Diagnosis and Childhood Anxiety Disorders*

A number of changes were made in the diagnostic criteria for anxiety disorders in the transition from the *Diagnostic and Statistical Manual of Mental Disorders, Second Edition (DSM-II)* to the *Diagnostic and Statistical Manual of Mental Disorders, Third Edition, Revised (DSM-III-R)*. Table 1 lists the *DSM-III-R* anxiety diagnoses. Generalized anxiety disorder, social phobia, obsessive compulsive disorder, and post-traumatic stress disorder underwent the most significant changes.

Table 1. *DSM-III-R* Anxiety Disorders

I. Anxiety Disorders of Childhood or Adolescence
    Separation Anxiety Disorder
    Avoidant Disorder of Childhood or Adolescence
    Overanxious Disorder

II. "Adult" Anxiety Disorders
    Panic Disorder with/without Agoraphobia
    Agoraphobia without History of Panic Disorder
    Social Phobia
    Simple Phobia
    Obsessive Compulsive Disorder
    Post-traumatic Stress Disorder
    Generalized Anxiety Disorder
    Anxiety Disorder Not Otherwise Specified

In *DSM-III-R*, generalized anxiety disorder can now be diagnosed in those under 18 years of age. The definition contains more somatic items and fewer cognitive ones, but still requires unrealistic or excessive worry; for example, about academic, athletic, and social performance.

The definition of social phobia is expanded and clarified, such that now the avoidant behavior must either interfere with occupational functioning, social activities, and/or personal relationships, or there must be marked distress about having the fear. For individuals under 18, the disturbance cannot meet the criteria for avoidant disorder of childhood or adolescence. However, in adults, the diagnosis of both social phobia and avoidant personality can be made. This discrepancy between rules for diagnosis of children and adults may prove problematic.

The diagnosis of obsessive compulsive disorder is more clearly defined but, most important, other Axis I diagnoses, including schizophrenia, are no longer exclusionary. If another Axis I disorder is present, however, the content of the obsession must be unrelated to it; for example, the guilty ruminative thoughts in the presence of a major depression. Tourette's syndrome also can now be a coexisting diagnosis.

DSM-III-R criteria for post-traumatic stress disorder have been made more age-appropriate, as they allow for the repetitive play in young children in which themes or aspects of the trauma are considered "reexperiencing" the traumatic event. In young children, the loss of recently acquired developmental skills such as toilet training or language skills is considered equivalent to the adult symptom of numbing of general responsiveness.

CHILDHOOD ANXIETY DISORDERS. The anxiety diagnoses listed in Table 1 are specifically designated for children: separation anxiety disorders, avoidant disorder of childhood or adolescence, and overanxious disorder. In actuality, the distinction between separation anxiety disorder and overanxious disorder may not be so clear. Note also that school refusal may be a symptom of separation anxiety or of a phobia. (See the section Separation Anxiety Disorder for further discussion.)

There are few systematic clinical data on children diagnosed with separation anxiety disorder or overanxious disorder. Recently, Last and colleagues (1987b) reported an investigation of 91 children referred to an anxiety clinic. Sixty-nine children (76 percent) met *DSM-III* criteria for either separation anxiety disorder (N = 22), overanxious disorder (N = 26), or, interestingly, both separation anxiety disorder and overanxious disorder (N = 21). The authors achieved high reliability in making the *DSM-III* diagnoses of separation anxiety disorder and overanxious disorder (kappa = 0.81). They point out the parallels with high comorbidity of the anxiety disorders in the adult population, suggesting that separation anxiety disorder and overanxious disorder may be the childhood equivalents of agoraphobia and generalized anxiety disorder, respectively.

Separation anxiety disorder and overanxious disorder children differed on both demographic characteristics and patterns of comorbidity. Ninety-one percent of the separation anxiety disorder children were prepubertal, whereas overanxious disorder children were more frequently post-pubertal. Children diagnosed with both separation anxiety disorder and overanxious disorder were younger than children diagnosed with overanxious disorder, but were slightly older than children diagnosed with separation anxiety disorder, leading to the hypothesis that separation anxiety disorder may be a precursor to the development of overanxious disorder. Overanxious disorder is more common in higher socio-economic groups, and separation anxiety disorder is more common in lower socioeconomic groups. The separation anxiety disorder group contained more girls than boys (unlike the equal sex ratio described in *DSM-III-R*), whereas the overanxious disorder group contained an equal sex distribution (in agreement with *DSM-III-R*). Children with overanxious disorder were significantly more likely to receive the coexisting diagnosis of simple phobia or panic disorder, perhaps representing a parallel with adult anxiety disorders, whereas one-third of adult patients with generalized anxiety disorder also meet *DSM-III* criteria for panic disorder. One-third of the children in the study by Last and colleagues (1987b) also met *DSM-III* criteria for major depression. Although the demographic data may in part reflect referral bias, they support the *DSM-III* (and *DSM-III-R*) distinction between separation anxiety disorder and overanxious disorder.

"ADULT" ANXIETY DISORDERS THAT CAN BE DIAGNOSED IN CHILDHOOD. In the "adult" diagnoses listed in Table 1, none specifically excludes children. Post-traumatic stress disorder and obsessive compulsive disorder have all been studied directly in children. Little is known about generalized anxiety disorder, panic disorder, social phobia, or agoraphobia in children, and it may well be that some anxiety symptoms come under one of the childhood anxiety disorders, for example, overanxious disorder or generalized anxiety disorder.

It is only recently that the psychiatric literature has documented that the diagnosis of panic disorder may appropriately be made in children. In the first report of panic attacks in prepubertal children, Van Winter and Stickler (1984), both pediatricians, reported 7 cases with children ranging from 9 to 17 years of age (ages of children's onset 8, 9, 11, 12, 12, 13, and 16.) Herskowitz (1986), also a pediatrician, reported 4 cases with children aged 9 to 16, presenting with neurological symptoms as a manifestation of a panic attack. Vitiello and colleagues (1987) reported on 2 boys, ages 8 and 10 (one with mitral valve prolapse), meeting adult criteria for panic disorder. The authors suggest that some children with severe school phobia might, in fact, have primary panic disorder which antedates a phobic school avoidance. Moreau and colleagues (1988) found seven cases of panic disorder in 220 children studied for being at risk for depression. Diagnosis was made by structural diagnostic assessment (K-SADS) of mother and child with blind ratings by a child psychiatrist, based on all available information. These reports suggest that panic disorder does occur in children in a symptom pattern similar to that of adults.

Most data on the age of onset of psychiatric disorders are from retrospective recall of adult patients. For example, Thyer and colleagues (1985) reported the retrospective self-reports of 423 psychiatric outpatients seen at a university hospital-based psychiatric clinic. For each anxiety disorder, the ages of onset clustered in a consistent range. A mean age of onset of $15.7(\pm 8.5)$ years for social phobia; $16.1(\pm 13.0)$ years for simple phobia; $22.8(\pm 12.0)$ years for generalized anxiety disorder; $25.6(\pm 14.6)$ years for obsessive compulsive disorder; $26.6(\pm 11.5)$ years for panic disorder; and $26.3(\pm 9.1)$ years for agoraphobia with panic attacks and $27.5(\pm 7.8)$ years for agoraphobia *without* panic attacks. In spite of limitations of outpatient sampling and retrospective recall, it is convincing that all the disorders could and did occur in childhood, most consistently social phobia and simple phobia.

Others have found an even younger age of onset for panic disorder (Von Korff et al, 1985; Sheehan et al, 1981). The multisite National Institute of Mental Health Epidemiologic Catchment Area Program sampled 3,000 persons, aged 18 years or older. These retrospective reports showed a peak onset of 15 to 19 years of age for panic attacks (Von Korff et al, 1985). In the population examined in the study by Moreau and colleagues (1988) the age of onset of panic disorder ranged from 5 to 18 years with a mean of 10.4 years. Sheehan and associates (1981) and Anderson and co-workers (1984) reported ages of onset for the other anxiety disorders to be similar to those found by Thyer. In summary, there appear to be two peak ages of onset for the anxiety disorders; one in middle to late adolescence for simple and social phobias, and another in the middle 20s for generalized anxiety disorder and agoraphobia.

In one of the few controlled studies of preschoolers, a group of 27 4- to 6-year-old therapeutic nursery school children meeting *DSM-III* criteria for an anxiety disorder were compared to matched controls on measures of ego-resiliency, ego-control, and temperament (Wolfson et al, 1987). Interestingly, high aggression and depression scores were also found in the children with a predominant symptom of anxiety. Unfortunately, this heterogeneous group was not divided by the specific *DSM-III* subcategories (separation anxiety disorder, overanxious disorder, and adjustment disorder with anxious mood). In addition, kappas for interrater reliability were not reported for the specific anxiety diagnoses, but the authors did state that 3 of 3 raters agreed in the assignment of 21 of 25 children to the anxiety disorder group, and 2 of 3 raters agreed in the assignment of the remaining children.

In summary, while diagnostic refinement for anxiety disorder in childhood continues, there is increasing evidence for the existence of all the anxiety disorders in childhood and adolescence.

DEMOGRAPHICS AND CHARACTERISTICS OF THE ANXIETY DISORDERS

Prevalence

Few pediatric epidemiological studies exist for psychiatric diagnoses and fewer specifically for anxiety disorders. Anderson and colleagues (1987) studied *DSM-III* disorders in 792 11-year-old children from the general New Zealand population. The Diagnostic Interview Schedule for Children (DISC) was used with good interrater reliability (kappa of 0.86). The 1-year prevalence for anxiety disorders ranged from 3.5 percent for separation anxiety disorder, 2.9 percent for overanxious disorder, 2.4 percent for simple phobia, to 0.9 percent for social phobia. Most anxiety disorders had an over-representation of females, except for overanxious disorder with a male:female ratio of 1.7:1.

Comorbidity

Comorbidity is common in childhood anxiety; is the pattern similar to that of adults? Last and colleagues (1987e) examined 73 consecutive admissions to their outpatient anxiety disorder clinic for children and adolescents. Of the 24 children with a primary diagnosis of separation anxiety disorder, *one-third* received a concurrent diagnosis of overanxious disorder. The reverse was not true for the 11 children with a primary diagnosis of overanxious disorder. Only one case of separation anxiety disorder was found. This group was most likely to receive an additional diagnosis of either social phobia (one-third) or avoidant disorder (one-fourth).

The group with primary major depression often had a coexisting social phobia and/or overanxious disorder, suggesting a roughly equivalent prevalence of depressive disorders in anxiety disordered children, as is seen in adults (Barlow et al, 1986). Surprisingly, there was no clear-cut pattern of comorbidity for the social phobic (school) group. Last and co-workers conclude that overanxious disorder (the probable childhood "equivalent" of generalized anxiety disorder) is an independently occurring coexisting disorder in children, whereas in adults the generalized anxiety symptoms are more likely to be an associated feature of a different disorder.

Close links are seen between depression and anxiety in adults (Akiskal and McKinney, 1975). In children, just as in adults, there appears to be an intimate relationship between those diagnoses, although the extent of the overlap is not clearly understood. Four controlled studies have looked at this relationship in pediatric populations. Hershberg and colleagues (1982) compared 28 depressed children with 14 anxious ones and found that depressed children had some anxious symptoms and that the anxious children had some depressed symptoms, but they did not usually qualify for the second diagnosis. In contrast, Bernstein and Garfinkel (1986) (reviewed later in this chapter) found that 50 percent of chronic school refusers (N = 26) met *DSM-III* criteria for both anxiety and depression. Eighty-one percent of the 16 school refusers diagnosed as having an anxiety disorder showed a coexisting depression. Kolvin and associates (1984) found that 45 percent of 51 school phobics were also depressed. Strauss and co-workers (1988) studied the presence of depression in 106 anxiety disordered children and adolescents. Twenty-eight percent of the anxious children and adolescents met *DSM-III* criteria for a concurrent major depression. (Note that this study population spanned 5–17 years of age and contained a spectrum of all anxiety disorders.) Anxious children and adolescents with depression were older, had more severe anxiety symptomatology, and had different rates of obsessive compulsive disorder and agoraphobia than anxious children without major depression. Anxious children with depression received multiple diagnoses more frequently. The 28 percent comorbidity was lower than the 45 percent and 81 percent reported above, but is explained by the authors as due to methodological issues. (Strauss' patients had a broad range of anxiety disorders and a greater age range.) The authors stress the need for further studies to determine the effect of depression on the classification, treatment, and prognosis of anxiety disorders.

Geller and colleagues (1985) looked at the coexistence of anxiety and depression starting with a depressed population defined by the Kiddie-SADS. Of 59 5- to 16-year-old (prepubertal group N = 36, postpubertal group N = 23) with major depression, 86 percent of the prepubertal group and 47 percent of the postpubertal group met criteria for separation anxiety disorder. Interestingly, separation anxiety usually began after the onset of depression in both groups.

The New Zealand population study cited earlier (Anderson et al, 1987) also found a high degree of comorbidity of anxiety disorders and of those disorders with depression. Fifty-five percent of the disorders occurred in combination with one or more other disorders, and 45 percent occurred as a single disorder. Of the 59 anxious children, 23 had an additional diagnosis of attention deficit disorder, conduct disorder, or depression. This is important, as it extends the generality of the studies by Last and colleagues beyond clinically referred populations.

Therefore, in both the clinically referred and the general population, comorbidity appears common for the anxiety disorders. Why do some diagnoses have patterns of comorbidity and not others? For example, why might one-third of the separation anxiety disorder children have a concurrent overanxious disorder? Last and co-workers found a roughly equivalent prevalence of depressive disorders in anxiety disordered children as is seen in adults. This prevalence of a coexisting depression varies greatly from study to study, and the relationship is not clearly understood.

Risk Factors

The relationship between parental psychopathology and anxiety disorders in their offspring has been addressed in four controlled studies. Two approaches have been used: "top down" studies looked at parents with known anxiety and/or depression (and other psychiatric diagnoses) to see if there is any specificity in the disorders of their children; "bottom up" studies start with the child as the identified patient, and determine the parents' psychiatric status.

Weissman and colleagues (1984) studied children, ages 6 to 17, of adult probands with primary major depression, anxiety disorder, and matched normal controls. Unfortunately, minor children were not interviewed directly (information was obtained from a first-degree relative), and adults with anxiety disorder *alone* were not selected. Forty-two percent of the children having a parent with depression and panic disorder had some anxiety diagnosis (most frequently separation anxiety disorder), as did 27 percent of the children of a parent with depression and agoraphobia, 15 percent of offspring of parents with depression and generalized anxiety disorder, 21 percent of children of parents with depression alone, and 15 percent of depression and generalized anxiety disorder. Thus children's diagnoses tended roughly to follow those of their parents. The highest rate of anxiety disorder was found in children of a parent with depression plus panic disorder. Children of probands with depression and panic and/or agoraphobia had a higher rate of phobias. The number of years of exposure to parental illness and the age at exposure did not predict risk. It seems, therefore, that depression plus agoraphobia or panic disorder confers a particular risk for the child. Specificity of transmission is suggested by the greatest frequency of anxiety diagnosis in the children of probands with depression and panic. Panic disorder in the parents conferred more than a *threefold* risk of separation anxiety in the children.

Turner and colleagues (1987) also examined children of anxious and depressed adults in their clinic. Fifty-nine children from 7 to 12 years of age were interviewed by blind raters using the Anxiety Disorders Interview Schedule (kappa was 0.82). Sixteen were the children of an anxiety disordered parent (agoraphobia or obsessive compulsive disorder), 14 of a dysthymic disordered parent, 13 of parents with no identified psychiatric diagnosis, and 16 deemed normal based on semistructured interview. The children of an anxiety disordered parent were twice as likely to have a *DSM-III* anxiety disorder diagnosis than were children of dysthymic disorder parents, and were seven times more likely to have a *DSM-III* anxiety disorder diagnosis than were the children of normal parents. Despite the limitation of the study, their findings suggest that children of an anxiety disordered nondepressed parent are at greater risk.

Last and associates (1987c), in a "bottom up" study, evaluated lifetime psychiatric illness in mothers of anxious children. The Interview Schedule for Children was used for the child with kappas ranging from 0.64 to 1.00, and the Structured Clinical Interview for *DSM-III* was administered to the mothers, with overall agreement between the two rating clinicians of 86 percent. Mothers were rated by interviewers who were blind to the diagnosis of the child. A control group consisted of mothers of children with other psychiatric disturbance (that is, excluding anxiety and depression). Mothers of the children in the three anxiety groups (separation anxiety disorder, overanxious disorder, and separation anxiety disorder plus overanxious disorder) had a *highly* significant life-time rate of anxiety compared to mothers of controls (p = .005). Eighty-three percent of the mothers of the anxious children had a life-time history of an anxiety disorder. Rates of affective disorders for mothers of anxious children were also higher than for controls, although those differences were not statistically significant. Surprisingly, a higher rate of affective disorders was *not* found in the mothers of the anxious children. Slightly more than one-half of the mothers (57 percent) of the anxious children had an anxiety disorder at the same time that their children were being evaluated. Mothers of children with both overanxious disorder and separation anxiety disorder had the highest percentage of themselves having two or more diagnoses, including two or more anxiety diagnoses. Forty-one percent of the mothers of the children with overanxious disorder plus separation anxiety disorder had a history of a simple phobia. While several studies have pointed out that children of anxious adults are at risk for developing anxiety disorders, this is the first controlled study, starting with the child, that shows such a high incidence of anxiety disorders in the mother. Authors caution that it is unclear whether this relationship among anxiety disorders is specific to the mother–child dyad.

Do mothers of anxious children report a history of a *childhood* anxiety disorder, and, if so, is it the same type of disorder as that diagnosed in their child? Last and colleagues (1987d) studied the relationship between mothers and their children for *childhood* anxiety disorders. Sixty-four children with separation anxiety disorder and/or overanxious disorder (N = 21 separation anxiety disorder, N = 26 overanxious disorder, N = 17 separation anxiety disorder plus overanxious disorder) and 33 children with nonanxiety psychiatric diagnoses served as controls. Mothers completed a Childhood History Questionnaire for separation anxiety disorder and overanxious disorder that was scored by a blind rater. Mothers of overanxious disorder children were more likely to have had a diagnosis of overanxious disorder *as a child* than were the mothers of separation anxiety disorder children or of controls (p = .01). This high concordance suggests that children with overanxious disorder are manifesting the specific type of childhood anxiety disorder that their mothers had. Surprisingly, the same relationship was not found for separation anxiety disorder; there was no significant difference in the prevalence of separation anxiety disorder in the mothers of children with separation anxiety disorder, overanxious disorder, or controls. Why might there be a specific relationship between mothers and children for overanxious disorder but not for separation anxiety disorder? Last and colleagues (1987d) hypothesized that symptoms of overanxious disorder may be easier to recall than those of separation anxiety disorder, or that the six-month criteria for overanxious disorder made it more "memorable" than the two-week criteria for separation anxiety disorder.

"Behavioral inhibition to the unfamiliar" is a well defined early temperamental characteristic that is prevalent in young children of parents with agoraphobia and panic disorder (Kagan et al, in press). Biederman and co-workers (1988) studied the psychopathological correlates of behavioral inhibition in 30 4- to 7-year-old "children-at risk" (parents with psychiatric disorders) and in 41 epidemiologically derived children. Assessments of the children were done blindly using structured interviews (DICA-P) with the mothers. In the "children-at-risk" sample, the "inhibited children" (n = 18) had a significantly higher rate of *DSM-III* diagnoses (77.8 vs. 41.7 percent, $p < 0.05$) and overanxious disorder (27.8 vs. 0.0 percent, $p < 0.05$) than the "noninhibited" (n = 12) group. The behaviorally inhibited children had higher rates of all diagnosable disorders, including anxiety disorders (33.3 vs. 8.3 percent) and affective disorders (22.2 vs. 0.0 percent) than the uninhibited group. Unlike the "children-at-risk" group, the epidemiological sample had diagnoses primarily limited to anxiety disorders (45 percent for the "inhibited" vs. 26 percent for the "uninhibited"). Biederman and colleagues (1988) conclude that "behavioral inhibition to the unfamiliar" in children is a risk factor for psychopathology, specifically for anxiety disorders.

NEW RESEARCH ON SPECIFIC ANXIETY DISORDERS

Post-traumatic Stress Disorder in Children

There are no controlled studies of post-traumatic stress disorder in children. However, there is unusual interest in this subject, and some clinical descriptive studies are quite suggestive.

Terr (1983) followed up 25 of the 26 Chowchilla school-bus kidnapping victims four years after the incident. Even four to five years later, every child exhibited a post-traumatic stress response. Terr felt that several features of these children distinguished their post-traumatic stress disorder from that of adults. Children did not exhibit full/partial amnesia, "psychic numbing," flashbacks, nor a deterioration in school performance. On the other hand, post-traumatic play and reenactment was common, time skew was frequent, and they believed their futures would be limited. Brief psychiatric intervention that had taken place 5–13 months after the trauma clearly did not prevent symptoms at follow-up. Symptom severity correlated with family pathology, the child's prior vulnerabilities, and community bonding. Terr's thesis is that children are not more flexible than adults following psychic trauma.

Terr (1986) later studied 20 children who had suffered psychic trauma prior to age 5. Twenty-eight to 36 months of age appears to be the cut-off for recall by verbal memory. Trauma prior to this age can be recalled as behavioral memories, while verbal memories require conscious awareness.

One highly relevant controlled study compared 15 post-traumatic stress disorder Vietnam veterans with 11 veterans who were being seen for medical treatment at the VA who did *not* meet criteria for post-traumatic stress disorder (van der Kolk, 1985). The subjects who developed post-traumatic stress disorder after fighting in Vietnam had been *adolescents* while in combat. The veterans with post-traumatic stress disorder had developed intense attachments to other soldiers in their unit, which had been disrupted by their buddies' deaths. If replicated, this is an important finding.

Separation Anxiety Disorder

Separation anxiety disorder has come under special scrutiny because of the apparent relationship between separation anxiety in childhood and agoraphobia in adulthood, and because of the heterogeneity of school refusal syndromes.

Gittelman and Klein (1984) reviewed the probable relationship between separation anxiety and agoraphobia. Included in the evidence is the finding that the offspring of adults with agoraphobia and panic disorder are more likely to have separation anxiety than other children (Weissman et al, 1984). Agoraphobic women had a greater rate of separation anxiety as children than did women with other anxiety disorders. Unfortunately, however, there are no prospective follow-up studies of children with separation anxiety disorder into adulthood to see if they are at greater risk for agoraphobia. It is not clear, for example, whether severity of adult agoraphobia correlates with a history of separation anxiety in childhood.

"School refusal," although not a *DSM-III-R* diagnosis, clearly is an observed entity. Those children most often fall into the diagnoses of separation anxiety disorder, simple phobia (for school), or depression. Last and colleagues (1987a) compared 48 children with separation anxiety disorder to 19 children with phobic disorder of school. They explained that difficulty in attending school can stem from separation problems *or* from excessive fear about something about the school itself. Not all children with separation anxiety disorder exhibit school refusal, and not all children with school phobia manifest separation anxiety. Their data support this distinction between groups.

Children with separation anxiety disorder were more likely to be female (69 percent versus 27 percent in school phobics), prepubertal, from families with lower socioeconomic backgrounds, and have other *DSM-III* diagnoses (92 percent versus 63 percent) than the school phobics. Mothers of separation anxiety disordered children had a four-fold greater incidence of an affective disorder than did mothers of school phobic children. Age of intake also differed such that children with separation anxiety were younger than the school phobics. The authors believe that these findings support the *DSM-III* criteria for distinguishing these diagnoses.

British studies have also noted different subgroups of the school phobics. Kolvin and co-workers (1984) described a "depressed" group and a "residual school refusal" group which differ on suicidal thoughts, loss of energy, dysphoric mood, and initial insomnia. Although clinically distinct, they speculate as to whether the groups are actually on a spectrum of severity of depression.

Bernstein and Garfinkel (1986) studied the role of depression and anxiety in chronic school refusers. The 15 males and 11 females (mean age 13.7 years) showed considerable overlap between affective and anxiety disorders. Sixty-nine percent met criteria for depression, 62 percent met criteria for anxiety, and 50 percent met criteria for both. Not surprisingly, patients meeting criteria for both disorders were the most symptomatic. Severe anxiety and depression may be as difficult to distinguish in children as in adults.

Obsessive Compulsive Disorder

Obsessive compulsive disorder (OCD) appears in children in virtually the same form as in adults (Rapoport, 1986). In children and adolescents the differential diagnosis would include a major depression (either with or without psychotic symptoms) with obsessional features, anorexia nervosa/bulimia, Tourette's syndrome, pervasive developmental disorder, autism, severe anxiety disorder with obsessional features, schizophrenia, and phobias. With these other diagnoses the thoughts are often not described as ego dystonic, and therefore distinguishable from obsessive compulsive disorder. Young children may have trouble identifying thoughts and behaviors as ego dystonic. However, the anorexic/bulimic's obsessive preoccupation with weight, food, and calorie counting may resemble the intensity of the thoughts and behaviors of obsessive compulsive disorder. Although not clearly understood, an association between anorexia nervosa and obsessive compulsive disorder may be present. The stereotypes of children with autistic and pervasive developmental disorder bear superficial resemblance to obsessive compulsive disorder rituals but lack ego-dystonicity and are even reassuring to the patient. The comorbidity of obsessive compulsive disorder with Tourette's syndrome is well documented, although these patients may exhibit only *features* of obsessive compulsive disorder (Frankel et al, 1986). Families of Tourette's syndrome patients have an increase in the incidence of obsessive compulsive disorder (Pauls et al, 1985).

The only large epidemiological study of obsessive compulsive disorder done with adolescents was conducted by Columbia University with over 5,000 high school students 12 to 22 years of age. The population consisted of all those available from an entire county in New Jersey. Flament and colleagues (in press) found a point prevalence of 0.35 percent for obsessive compulsive disorder in this unselected population. While much greater than any previously reported, this is probably an underestimation, and the weighted prevalence estimate is closer to one percent.

The largest systematically studied group of obsessive compulsive disorder children and adolescents was carried out at the Child Psychiatry Branch of the National Institute of Mental Health (NIMH). The 70 children studied had a mean age of onset of 10.2 years, with 7 of the patients having onset at less than 7 years of age. Males have an earlier age of onset at 9.8 years of age, versus 11.0 years for the females. Males outnumber females by more than 2:1, although this ratio is most striking in the younger age groups. There is a positive family history in about 20 percent of directly interviewed first degree relatives. Three of seven of the earliest onset cases had a parent with obsessive compulsive disorder. Father/son pairs predominate (N = 10), but two mother/son, two mother/daughter, and three father/daughter affected pairs are also documented.

Most children experience a single obsession or compulsion at the onset, continue this for months or years, and gradually shift to another. At least three-quarters of patients have had a period of excessive washing. Obsessive sexual thoughts are uncommon in children but likely in adolescence. With the AIDS epidemic, it is increasingly common for an adolescent to present with this as his primary obsessive thought, providing a rationale for excessive rumination and washing rituals. Associated diagnoses were present in 74 percent of the patients, with major depression (23 percent), overanxious disorder (16 percent), and simple phobia (17 percent) being the most common. Motor tics were found in 20 percent of the patients, occurring most frequently in males, younger patients, and those with family members with obsessive compulsive disorder. Fewer than 20 percent of the obsessive compulsive disorder patients met criteria for the adult definition of obsessive compulsive personality disorder, suggesting a discontinuity between state and trait.

Follow-up data on the children and adolescents with obsessive compulsive disorder are limited. Twenty-five of the first 27 obsessive compulsive disorder patients (93 percent) in the NIMH project were reevaluated 2–5 years later (Flament et al, in press). Only 7 (28 percent) of the patients received no psychiatric diagnosis at follow-up. Of the 17 (68 percent) of the original patients who still qualified for the diagnosis of obsessive compulsive disorder, only 5 (20 percent) had obsessive compulsive disorder as their only diagnosis. The remaining 12 had one or more additional diagnoses, most commonly depressive disorder (recurrent, unipolar depression) and/or an anxiety disorder, including generalized anxiety, social phobia, and separation anxiety. This outcome was surprisingly poor for all the patients, and there were virtually *no* predictors of outcome at follow-up, including baseline symptoms, severity, or initial clomipramine response! A second follow-up study, after more intensive intervention with all treatment modalities, is now underway.

A number of neurobiological studies of obsessive compulsive disorder are underway. A "serotonergic hypothesis" of obsessive compulsive disorder is based primarily on response to clomipramine, whose main pharmacological effect in vitro is the selective inhibition of serotonin reuptake into presynaptic nerve terminals (Hamberger and Tuck, 1973). Lithium and L-tryptophan, which presumably increase serotonergic function, may augment clomipramine response (Rasmussen, 1984). (For a review of the serotonergic theory see Zohar and Insel, 1987.) Evidence supporting neuroanatomic abnormalities, more specifically in the basal ganglia, include the association between obsessive compulsive disorder and Tourette's syndrome, postencephalitic Parkinson's disease, abnormalities on PET scans (Baxter et al, 1987) and CT scans (Luxenberg et al, 1988), and association of obsessive compulsive disorder with Sydenham's chorea (Swedo et al, 1987). Evidence for neuroendocrine disturbance includes the higher incidence of onset of obsessive compulsive disorder at puberty for females, the exacerbation of symptoms at menses, the precipitation of obsessive compulsive disorder postpartum (S. Rasmussen, personal communication, 1987), and the usefulness of antiandrogens for some cases of obsessive compulsive disorder (Casas et al, 1986; Swedo, in press). Similarities between obsessive compulsive disorder rituals and animal grooming behaviors have led to an intriguing speculation about the underlying etiology and the unleashing of a "fixed action pattern" in these children (Swedo, in press).

Two controlled studies of clomipramine treatment of children and adolescents with obsessive compulsive disorder found clomipramine (mean dose 141 mg/day) significantly better than placebo in a 5-week placebo controlled crossover study (Flament et al, 1985, 1987). Seventy-five percent of the children and adolescents had a moderate to marked improvement; 16 percent were unchanged. In general, the drug was well tolerated and had a side effect profile similar to that expected with any tricyclic antidepressant. Improvement was generally not seen until week three. Drug response could not be predicted from any baseline measure, including mode or age of onset, symptom pattern, duration or severity of illness, or age. Pretreatment platelet serotonin concentration correlated significantly with clinical response to clomipramine. (A high pretreatment level of platelet serotonin was a strong predictor of a favorable clinical outcome.)

To ensure a truly double-blind study by using an active comparison drug and to compare clomipramine with a standard antidepressant available on the market, a second double-blind crossover study was carried out comparing clomipramine and desmethylimipramine, a selective noradrenergic reuptake blocker (Leonard et al, 1988).

Thirty-two children and adolescents (22 female and 10 male), aged 8 to 19, with severe obsessive compulsive disorder have completed this ongoing study. Mean Hamilton scale of depression was 8.0 (± 4.8 range from 1–20).

Clomipramine was highly superior to desipramine in ameliorating obsessive compulsive symptoms. Surprisingly, desmethylimipramine produced little or no improvement and was not much more effective than the placebo had been in the study by Flament and colleagues. The average clomipramine dosage was again fairly low (157 ± 54 mg/day) with a range of 68–250 mg. Some clinical improvement could be seen at week three, and was statistically significantly at weeks four and five. This clomipramine–desmethylimipramine comparison replicates for children the efficacy and specificity of clomipramine in obsessive compulsive disorder that has been reported in adults.

DRUG TREATMENT

Antidepressant Trials

There are few published controlled studies for pharmacological treatment of any of the childhood and adolescent anxiety disorders. Since 1971, when imipramine was shown superior to placebo for school phobia (Gittelman-Klein, 1971), few others have sought to replicate or extend the finding. Berney and colleagues (1981) did not find that low dose clomipramine (ranging from 40 mg/day for 9-year-olds to 75 mg/day for 14-year-olds) was superior to placebo in a double-blind trial of school phobics. Neither study excluded depressed children, and Berney did not distinguish between the separation anxiety child and the school phobic child. A double-blind study is currently underway comparing the efficacy of behavior therapy with placebo to behavior therapy with imipramine for children with separation anxiety or school phobic disorder, and excluding children with depressive disorders (C. Last, personal communication, 1988).

Benzodiazepines

Bernstein and associates (1987) compared alprazolam, imipramine, and placebo treatment of anxiety and depressive symptoms in an ongoing study of school phobics (aged 7 to 17). Subjects were assigned one of three groups: imipramine, alprazolam, or placebo. Individual psychotherapy and a graduated school reentry plan are used for all subjects. Preliminary findings with a sample size of 25 found that both medications were superior to placebo (p=0.05). There was a greater decrease of symptoms with alprazolam (dose 0.03 mg/kg) than with imipramine (dose 3 mg/kg) on the Anxiety Rating for Children.

There are no controlled studies on the use of high-potency benzodiazepines in children and adolescents. Biederman (1987), who first reported on the use of clonazepam for panic-like symptoms, gave three prepubertal children 0.5–3 mg of clonazepam with reduction of symptoms and no adverse effects. Interestingly, each child also met criteria for either separation anxiety disorder or overanxious disorder, and the clinical presentation was consistent with adult-type panic symptoms either with or without agoraphobia. As Biederman cautions, however, a certain positive pharmacologic response should not be used as a diagnostic validator.

Antipsychotics

Antipsychotics are not indicated for childhood anxiety disorders. However, an interesting finding with this class of drugs deserves special mention. School phobia has been noted to *develop* in Tourette's patients on haloperidol or pimozide. Linet (1985) coined the term "neuroleptic separation anxiety syndrome," and this phenomenon, now reported several times, might provide some clue to the underlying pathophysiology of this disorder.

PSYCHODYNAMIC, COGNITIVE, AND BEHAVIORAL TREATMENT

Psychodynamic, cognitive, and behavior modification psychotherapy clearly have an important role in the treatment of anxiety disorders. In reviewing the most recent research studies, one finds a surprising lack of empirical data with these specific treatment modalities. Most of the literature consists of single-case studies which demonstrate the effectiveness of certain techniques or of behavioral treatment series.

Blagg and Yule (1984) published one of the few controlled group comparison studies. These authors systematically applied their behavioral treatment to a treatment series of 30 school refusers in Britain. The outcome was compared to a group of 16 hospitalized children who attended a psychiatric unit and hospital school and to a third group of 20 who received psychotherapy and home tutoring. All 66 cases satisfied the school-refusal diagnostic criteria, but no selection or random allocation to treatment groups took place. The authors acknowledged the difficulty in matching the three treatment groups. The three groups did differ significantly on mean age and subtype of the school refusal diagnosis, but not on sex or social class. The behavioral treatment group did significantly better (as measured by child returning to full-time school without further problems) at one year's outcome than either of the other two groups (p = 0.001). They concluded that behavior treatment is the treatment of choice for school refusal.

Ultee and colleagues (1982) studied 24 children, ages 5 to 10 years, who had a fear of swimming. The *in vitro* treatment group received four sessions of *in vitro* desensitization (gradual imaginal exposure to fear-evoking stimuli plus relaxation) followed by four sessions of *in vivo* desensitization (real-life exposure to fear-evoking stimuli plus relaxation). The *in vivo* group had eight sessions of gradual real exposure. The control group took part in the tests only. Better results were achieved by the desensitization *in vivo* than by the desensitization *in vitro* or by the control procedure (p<0.0005). They conclude that in the treatment of anxiety in children, the *in vivo* treatment is superior to the *in vitro* method, and that initial *in vitro* desensitization did not increase the efficacy of subsequent desensitization *in vivo*.

Mansdorf and Luken's (1987) report is included because of its complete treatment model for separation-anxious children exhibiting school phobia. The authors described a six-step cognitive–behavioral psychotherapy strategy for children and parents. Although the report described its success in only two children, it is unique enough to merit special attention here. Mansdorf and Luken's assessment consisted of a cognitive analysis of the child (regarding attending school and separating from parents), an environmental analysis (determining the consequences of refusal for the child), and a cognitive analysis of the parents (regarding parental beliefs concerning the child's problem and attitudes toward implementing strict measures of operant control). The intervention program consisted of cognitive self-instruction of the child (teaching the child to use coping self-statements), cognitive restructuring of the parents (presenting parents with their distorted beliefs concerning their child), and environmental restructuring (behavior techniques where reinforcement was based upon school attendance). They acknowledge that studies using more rigid designs must be done, but that this combination of operant and cognitive treatment for the child and adult is particularly successful.

The behavioral literature on the treatment of anxiety disorders in children is thoroughly reviewed by Wells and Vitulano (1984). Although the psychodynamic, cognitive, and behavioral psychotherapy interventions often are successful, clearly more empirical studies are called for.

SUMMARY

Anxiety disorders in childhood and adolescence are far more prevalent than had been thought, ranging from .4 percent for obsessive compulsive disorder (probably an underestimation) to 3.5 percent for separation anxiety disorder. Systematic studies of diagnosis, prevalence, risks, and treatment are few, but a number of parallels with adult anxiety disorders are emerging.

Changes in the diagnostic criteria of the anxiety disorders from *DSM-III* to *DSM-III-R* are an improvement in "tightening up" several of the diagnoses. Several studies support the diagnostic validity of separation anxiety disorder, overanxious disorder, and avoidant disorder. Technically, all the "adult" anxiety disorders diagnoses can be made in children; how generalized anxiety disorder and social phobia are distinguished in childhood is unclear. Are some childhood anxiety disorders the "equivalent" of the adult diagnoses? Is overanxious disorder the childhood equivalent of generalized anxiety disorder? Is separation anxiety disorder the childhood equivalent and/or precursor of adult agoraphobia? The long-term prospective studies which would answer these questions are lacking.

As with adults, comorbidity is common in childhood anxiety disorders; that is, one-third of a group of separation anxiety disorder children had a secondary diagnosis of overanxious disorder. In Anderson's (1984) New Zealand nonclinical population, 55 percent of the childhood psychiatric disorders (anxiety and nonanxiety) occurred in combination with one or more others. In children, just as in adults, there appears to be a close relationship between depression and anxiety. The actual percentage of comorbidity varies greatly from study to study (from a minimal percentage in Hershberg, 1982, to 81 percent in Bernstein and Garfinkel, 1986) and probably varies with the populations selected and the diagnostic schemes.

Both "bottom up" and "top down" studies find a link between anxiety disorders in children and their parents. Clearly, children are at greater risk for developing an anxiety disorder if a parent has that diagnosis (Turner and colleagues [1987] found it as high as seven times as likely than in children of normal parents) and that depression plus panic disorder may convey a particularly high risk (Weissman, 1984). There is evidence that children's diagnoses in general may follow that of the proband parent (Weissman, 1984); interestingly, overanxious disorder, but not separation anxiety disorder, showed a concordance (Last et al, 1987d), although it is not clear if this was due to methodological issues.

There are preliminary findings relevant to the treatment of and the prognosis in the childhood anxiety disorders. The post-traumatic stress disorder study found that children are not more flexible than adults following a psychic trauma, suggesting the need for controlled treatment trials to evaluate whether outcome is affected by earlier and more intensive intervention. The clomipramine trials in obsessive compulsive disorder provide one of the few controlled studies for psychopharmacological intervention in children and adolescents with an anxiety disorder. Clomipramine's specificity and efficacy is dramatic and compelling for what has been an intractable disorder. Ongoing controlled studies for the psychopharmacological treatment of childhood anxiety disorders have begun to focus on the relative merits of behavioral and drug treatment. Clearly, more systematic studies are required for all the treatment modalities. The results of these studies will prove particularly useful.

REFERENCES

Akiskal HS, McKinney WT: Overview of recent research in depression: integration of ten conceptual models into a comprehensive clinical frame. Arch Gen Psychiatry 1975; 32:285–305

American Psychiatric Association: Diagnostic and Statistical Manual of Mental Disorders, Third Edition (DSM-III). Washington, DC, American Psychiatric Association, 1980

American Psychiatric Association: Diagnostic and Statistical Manual of Mental Disorders, Third Edition, Revised (DSM-III-R). Washington, DC, American Psychiatric Association, 1987

Anderson DJ, Noyes R, Crowe RR: A comparison of panic disorder and generalized anxiety. Am J Psychiatry 1984; 141:572–575

Anderson JC, Williams S, McGee R, et al: DSM-III disorders in preadolescent children. Arch Gen Psychiatry 1987; 44:69–76

Barlow DH, DiNardo PA, Vermilyea JA, et al: Co-morbidity and depression among the anxiety disorders: issues in diagnosis and classification. J Nerv Ment Dis 1986; 174:63–72

Baxter L, Phelps M, Massiotti J, et al: Local cerebral glucose metabolic rates of obsessive compulsive disorder compared to unipolar depression and normal controls. Arch Gen Psychiatry 1987; 44:211–218

Beeghly JHL: Anxiety and anxiety disorder in childhood, in Treating Anxiety Disorders. Edited by Munoz RA. San Francisco, Jossey-Bass, 1986

Berney T, Kolvin I, Bhate SR, et al: School phobia: a therapeutic trial with clomipramine and short-term outcome. Br J Psychiatry 1981; 138:110–118

Bernstein GA, Garfinkel BD: School phobia: the overlap of affective and anxiety disorders. J Am Acad Child Psychiatry 1986; 25:235–240

Bernstein G, Garfinkel B, Borchardt C: Imipramine versus alprazolam for school phobia. Paper presented at the annual meeting of the American Academy of Child and Adolescent Psychiatry, Washington, DC, Oct. 1987

Biederman J: Clonazepam in the treatment of prepubertal children with panic-like symptoms. J Clin Psychiatry 1987; 48:38–41

Biederman J, Rosenbaum JF, Kagan J: Psychiatric correlates of behavioral inhibition in clinical and epidemiologic samples of young children. Paper presented at the 141st annual meeting of the American Psychiatric Association, Montreal, Canada, May 1988

Blagg NR, Yule W: The behavioral treatment of school refusal—a comparative study. Behav Res Ther 1984; 22:119–127

Casas ME, Alvarez P, Duro C, et al: Antiandrogenic treatment of obsessive compulsive neurosis. Acta Psychiatr Scand 1986; 73:221–222

Flament MF, Rapoport JL, Berg CJ, et al: Clomipramine treatment of childhood obsessive-compulsive disorder: a double-blind controlled study. Arch Gen Psychiatry 1985; 42:977–983

Flament MF, Rapoport JL, Murphy DL, et al: Biochemical changes during clomipramine treatment of childhood obsessive-compulsive disorder. Arch Gen Psychiatry 1987; 44:219–225

Flament MF, Whitaker A, Rapoport JL, et al: Obsessive compulsive disorder in adolescence: an epidemiological study. J Am Acad Child Adolesc Psychiatry (in press)

Frankel M, Cummings JL, Robertson MM, et al: Obsessions and compulsions in Gilles de la Tourette's syndrome. Neurology 1986; 36:378–382

Geller B, Chestnut EC, Miller MD, et al: Preliminary data on DSM-III associated features of major depression disorders in children and adolescents. Am J Pschiatry 1985; 142:643–644

Gittelman R (Ed): Anxiety Disorders of Childhood. New York, Guilford Press, 1986

Gittelman-Klein R, Klein DF: Controlled imipramine treatment of school phobia. Arch Gen Psychiatry 1971; 25:204–207

Gittelman R, Klein DF: Relationship between separation anxiety, panic and agoraphobic disorders. Psychopathology 1984; 17:56–65

Hamberger B, Tuck JR: Effect of tricyclic antidepressants on the uptake of noradrenaline and 5-hydroxytryptamine by rat brain slices incubated in buffer of human plasma. Eur J Clin Phamacol 1973; 229–235

Hershberg SG, Carlson GA, Cantwell DP, et al: Anxiety and depressive disorders in psychiatrically disturbed children. J Clin Psychiatry 1982; 43:358–361

Herskowitz J: Neurologic presentations of panic disorder in childhood and adolescence. Dev Med Child Neurol 1986; 26:617–623

Kagan J, Reznick JS, Snidman N: The biology and psychology of behavioral inhibition in young children. Child Dev (in press)

Kolvin I, Berney TP, Bhate S: Classification and diagnosis of depression in school phobia. Br J Psychiatry 1984; 145:347–357

Last CG, Francis G: School phobia. Advances in Clinical Psychology (in press)

Last CG, Francis G, Hersen M, et al: Separation anxiety and school phobia: a comparison using DSM-III criteria. Am J Psychiatry 1987a; 144:653–657

Last CG, Hersen M, Kazdin AE, et al: Comparison of DSM-III separation anxiety and overanxious disorders: demographic characteristics and patterns of comorbidity. J Am Acad Child Adolesc Psychiatry 1987b; 26:527–531

Last CG, Hersen M, Kazdin AE, et al: Psychiatric illness in mothers of anxious children. Am J Psychiatry 1987c; 144:1580–1583

Last CG, Philips JE, Statfeld A: Childhood anxiety disorders in mothers and their children. Child Psychiatry and Development 1987d; 18:103–112

Last CG, Strauss CC, Francis G: Comorbidity among childhood anxiety disorders. J Nerv Ment Dis 1987e; 175:726–730

Leonard HL, Swedo S, Rapoport JL, et al: Treatment of childhood obsessive compulsive disorder with clomipramine and desmethylimipramine: a double-blind crossover comparison. Psychopharmacol Bull 1988; 24:93–95

Linet LS: Tourette syndrome, pimozide, and school phobia: the neuroleptic separation anxiety syndrome. Am J Psychiatry 1985; 142:613–615

Luxenberg JS, Swedo SE, Flament MF, et al: Neuranatomic abnormalities in obsessive-compulsive disorder detected with quantitative x-ray computed tomography. Am J Psychiatry 1988; 145:1089–1093

Mansdorf IJ, Luken E: Cognitive-behavioral psychotherapy for separation anxious children exhibiting school phobia. J Am Acad Child Adolesc Psychiatry 1987; 26:222–225

Moureau D, Warner VS, Weissman MM: Panic disorder in children: does it exist? Paper presented at the 141st annual meeting of the American Psychiatric Association, Montreal, Canada, May 1988

Pauls DL, Towbin KE, Leckman JF, et al: Gilles de la Tourette's syndrome and obsessive-compulsive disorder: evidence supporting a genetic relationship. Arch Gen Psychiatry 1986; 43:1180–1182

Rapoport JL: Annotation, child obsessive-compulsive disorder. J Child Psychol Psychiatry 1986; 27:285–289

Rasmussen SA: Lithium and tryptophan augmentation in clomipramine-resistant obsessive-compulsive disorder. Am J Psychiatry 1984; 143:317–322

Sheehan DV, Sheehan KE, Minichiello WE: Age of onset of phobic disorders: a reevaluation. Compr Psychiatry 1981; 22:544–553

Strauss CC, Last CG, Hersen M, et al: Association between anxiety and depression in children and adolescents with anxiety disorders. J Abnorm Child Psychol 1988; 16:57–68

Swedo SE: Rituals and releasers: an ethological model of OCD, in Obsessive Compulsive Disorder in Children and Adolescents. Edited by Rapoport JL. Washington, DC, American Psychiatric Press Inc. (in press)

Swedo SE, Rapoport JL, Cheslow DL, et al: Increased incidence of obsessive compulsive symptoms in patients with Sydenham's chorea. Paper presented at the annual meeting of the American Academy of Child and Adolescent Psychiatry, Washington DC, October, 1987

Terr L: Chowchilla revisited: the effects of psychic trauma four years after a school bus kidnapping. Am J Psychiatry 1983; 140:1543–1550

Terr L: What happens to early memories of trauma? A study of twenty children under age 5 at the time of documented traumatic events. Paper presented at the 139th annual meeting of the American Psychiatric Association, Washington, DC, 1986

Thyer B, Parrish RT, Curtis GC, et al: Ages of onset of DSM-III anxiety disorders. Comp Psychiatry 1985; 26:113–122

Turner SM, Beidel DC, Costello A: Psychopathology in offspring of anxiety disorders patients. J Consult Clin Psychol 1987; 55:229–235

Ultee CA, Griffioen D, Schellekens J: The reduction of anxiety in children: a comparison of the effects of systematic desensitization in vitro and systematic desensitization in vivo. Behav Res Ther 1982; 20:61–67

van der Kolk BA: Adolescent vulnerability to PTSD. Psychiatry 1985; 48:365–370

Van Winter JT, Stickler GB: Panic attack syndrome. J Pediatrics 1984; 105:661–665

Vitiello B, Behar D, Wolfson S, et al: Panic disorder in prepubertal children. Am J Psychiatry 1987; 144:525–526

Von Korff MR, Eaton WW, Keyl P: Epidemiology of panic attacks and panic disorder. Results from 3 community surveys. Am J Epidemiology 1985; 122:970–981

Weissman MM, Leckman JE, Merikangas KR, et al: Depression and anxiety disorders in parents and children. Arch Gen Psychiatry 1984; 41:845–852

Wells K, Vitulano L: Anxiety disorders in children, in Behavioral Theories and Treatment of Anxiety. Edited by Turner SM. New York, Plenum Press, 1984

Wolfson J, Fields JH, Rose SA: Symptoms, temperament, resilency, and control in anxiety disordered preschool children. J Am Acad Child Adolesc Psychiatry 1987; 26:16–22

Zohar J, Insel TR: Obsessive compulsive disorder: psychobiological approaches to diagnosis, treatment, and pathophysiology. Biol Psychiatry 1987; 22:667–687

Chapter 9

Conduct Disorders

by George W. Bailey, M.D., and James H. Egan, M.D.

Violent, aggressive crime committed by adults has reached staggering rates in this country. Adults who lie, rob, maim, murder, lack remorse, and cannot sustain consistent employment or interpersonal relationships are the most frequent perpetrators. These antisocial adults are a well known population to psychiatrists, the courts, and the coroner.

Children and adolescents who lie, steal, fight, run away, destroy property, violate rules, and defy authority also are familiar to child and adolescent psychiatrists, the courts, and the coroner. In 1981, youths younger than 18 constituted 18.4 percent of the arrests for violent crimes and 38.7 percent for crimes against property. More alarming, children 15 years or younger accounted for approximately 5 percent of arrests (Lewis, 1986). These childhood and adult behaviors are intimately linked (Robins, 1966, 1979; Olweus, 1979; Henn et al, 1980).

The literature on conduct disorders in children is voluminous; the issue is extensively reported with many excellent reviews (for example, Quay, 1986; Kazdin, 1987). This chapter provides an overview and an update of current knowledge about conduct disorders, and points to areas in which research is still needed.

DEFINITION AND DELINEATION OF THE PROBLEM

Antisocial behavior (Kazdin, 1987b) broadly refers to any behavior that involves a violation of social rules or aggressive acts against others. Antisocial behavior in children includes such activities as physical aggression, theft, vandalism, firesetting, lying, truancy, oppositional/noncompliant behavior, and defiance of authority.

Controversy continues regarding almost every aspect of the conduct disorders. The term includes a broad range of behaviors which may occur in varying combinations, there is no identified etiology, and identification is descriptive and involves clinical judgment. Therefore there is no complete consensus on definition, classification, etiology, diagnosis, treatment, or outcome of antisocial behaviors in children at this time.

CLASSIFICATION AND DIAGNOSIS

There are three major classification systems:

1. The *Diagnostic and Statistical Manual of Mental Disorders, Third Edition, Revised (DSM-III-R)* (American Psychiatric Association, 1987).

The authors wish to express their appreciation to Dr. Karen C. Wells for her advice and assistance in the preparation of this chapter.

2. The World Health Organization Multiaxial Classification (Rutter et al, 1969, 1975b).
3. The International Classification of Diseases (ICD-9) (1979).

Of these, and in spite of controversy about its usefulness and validity in this category (Rutter and Shaffer, 1980), *DSM-III-R* is the official and by far the most widely used classification system for psychopathologic disorders in North America (Quay, 1986).

The *Diagnostic and Statistical Manual of Mental Disorders, Third Edition (DSM-III)* (American Psychiatric Association, 1980) delineated four specific subtypes of conduct disorder based on the presence or absence of adequate object relations and aggressive antisocial behavior. These four included undersocialized-aggressive; socialized-aggressive; undersocialized-nonaggressive, and socialized-nonaggressive.

In *DSM-III-R*, this four-group subtyping was changed, reportedly because it lacked clinical utility and was at variance with research findings. The revised subtyping continues to reflect a consistent major research distinction—the presence or absence of socialization. In the new subtyping, the aggression dimension remains intact.

In *DSM-III-R*, conduct disorder is one of three subcategories classified under disruptive behavior disorders. Along with attention-deficit hyperactivity disorder (ADHD) and oppositional-defiant disorder, this group represents a category characterized by socially disruptive behaviors that generally are more distressing to others than to the children who have them. There is a significant degree of covariance among the three.

The essential diagnostic feature of conduct disorder is a persistent pattern of conduct that infringes on the basic rights of others and violates major age-appropriate societal norms or rules. Aggressive acts are the predominant way in which the rights of others are violated. Although there may be considerable overlap in symptomatology between conduct disorder and oppositional-defiant disorder, the conduct problems, particularly including aggression, are significantly more pervasive and serious in the former.

The revised criteria comprise a single index of symptoms, in part selected to better identify young children with the disorder. The diagnostic criteria for conduct disorder include a list of 13 behaviors. Three or more of the following must be present for at least six months: fighting, lying, stealing, truancy from home or school, destruction of property (including fire-setting and breaking and entering), forced sexual activity, and physical cruelty to people or animals. In addition, there are criteria to determine if the disorder is mild, moderate, or severe.

The three subtypes in *DSM-III-R* roughly correspond to types noted in *DSM-III*. The group type is the most common and corresponds to the earlier socialized-nonaggressive type. The discriminating feature is that the conduct problems occur predominantly in group activities with peers. A difference from *DSM-III* is that aggression may or may not be present in this type.

The *DSM-III-R* solitary aggressive type correlates with the *DSM-III* undersocialized-aggressive type and involves aggressive physical activity directed toward adults and peers. The discriminating variable is that the child initiates this activity as a solitary rather than as a group activity.

A final group, the undifferentiated type, is for children and adolescents with a mixture of clinical features that cannot be classified as either of the other two. Although this is a residual group, it may be more common than the other two (American Psychiatric Association, 1987).

If another of the disruptive behavior disorders or any additional mental disorders coexist (as examples, learning, language, or anxiety disorders), these should be diagnosed in addition.

Associated Features

Children with antisocial behavior are also more likely to have academic deficiencies manifested by poor grades, low achievement level, and specific skill deficits—especially in reading (Glueck and Glueck, 1968; Bachman et al, 1978; Sturge, 1982). Children high in aggressiveness or other antisocial behavior show poor social skills and rejection by peers (Behar and Stewart, 1982; Carlson et al, 1984).

Table 1. *DSM-III-R* Diagnostic Criteria for Conduct Disorders

A. A disturbance of conduct lasting at least six months, during which at least three of the following have been present:

    (1) has stolen without confrontation of a victim on more than one occasion (including forgery)

    (2) has run away from home overnight at least twice while living in parental or parental surrogate home (or once without returning)

    (3) often lies (other than to avoid physical or sexual abuse)

    (4) has deliberately engaged in fire-setting

    (5) is often truant from school (for older person, absent from work)

    (6) has broken into someone else's house, building, or car

    (7) has deliberately destroyed others' property (other than by fire-setting)

    (8) has been physically cruel to animals

    (9) has forced someone into sexual activity with him or her

    (10) has used a weapon in more than one fight

    (11) often initiates physical fights

    (12) has stolen with confrontation of a victim (e.g., mugging, purse-snatching, extortion, armed robbery)

    (13) has been physically cruel to people

B. If 18 or older, does not meet criteria for Antisocial Personality Disorder.

Reprinted from American Psychiatric Association: Diagnostic and Statistical Manual of Mental Disorders, Third Edition, Revised (DSM-III-R). Washington, DC, American Psychiatric Association, 1987. Reprinted by permission.

EPIDEMIOLOGY

Conduct disorder is generally accepted as the most prevalent form of specific childhood disorder. In addition, it is predominantly a male disorder (Gilbert, 1957; Robins, 1981).

The epidemiology of the disorder is far from clear. First, the true prevalence of conduct disorder is difficult to estimate given different criteria and variations in rates for children of different ages, sexes, socioeconomic classes and geographical locales (Quay, 1986).

Second, many past studies (including some as recent as 1986) failed to differentiate between the undersocialized and the socialized varieties of conduct disorders (Quay, 1986).

Third, as has been noted, other common childhood disorders often covary with conduct disorders; in particular, the hyperactivity spectrum and learning disorders. These and other issues confound the findings and interpretation of epidemiologic studies.

In spite of the above, there are many epidemiologic studies in the literature that share common findings. A brief review of selected studies follows.

Studies agree that aggressive conduct problems in children are ubiquitous. Studies have looked separately at children who have been clinically referred and those in the general population. Between one-third and two-thirds of these children who are clinically referred are referred because of aggressive and antisocial behaviors (Quay, 1986; Chamberlain and Patterson, 1985).

General population studies concur with these commonly cited prevalence findings. In general population studies on 10- and 11-year-olds in Britain, the prevalence for conduct disorder for both sexes was 4 percent in rural (Rutter et al, 1970, 1975a) and 8 percent in urban settings (Graham, 1979). In both of Rutter's studies (1970 and 1975), conduct disorder was three times more prevalent in boys than girls and, at an overall rate of 6.8 percent for psychiatric disorders, was the most prevalent disorder noted.

Within a total rate of 12 percent for all psychiatric disorders in Australia, Glow (1984) reported a combined urban/suburban, male/female rate of 4 percent for conduct disorders. Similar to the studies by Rutter and colleagues, the rate for boys was twice that for girls.

ETIOLOGIC CONSIDERATIONS

Conduct disorders are excellent examples of conditions reflecting a biopsychosocial determination. Recent research has added significantly to the current understanding and conceptualization of conduct disorders.

Genetic and Biologic Issues

Genetic influences in conduct disorders are evidenced by family, adoptee, and twin studies. For example, many studies involving parents and offspring suggest significant genetic contributions to adult criminal behavior (Mednick and Christiansen, 1977; Bohman et al, 1982; Gabrielli and Mednick, 1983). Still unresolved, however, is whether conduct disorder in children and adolescents is inevitably followed by criminality in adults (Quay, 1986).

Adoption studies suggest a strong interplay between genetic and environmental factors. Hutchings and Mednick (1974, 1977) reported that adopted away offspring of criminal fathers were more likely to be antisocial than adopted children of noncriminal fathers. In addition, children with both criminal biologic and criminal adoptive fathers were reported at greatest risk.

Twin studies by O'Connor and colleagues (1980) compared parental ratings of identical and fraternal twins on problems relating to socialization. On eight factor analytically derived scales, they found statistically significant higher intra-class correlations for identical than for fraternal twins. In addition, this statistical significance held true for those scales considered related to conduct disorder (bullying, restlessness, and school problems).

It is important to note that these studies, although promising, are preliminary and, as yet, inconclusive. Based on current data, there is no direct evidence for a genetic contribution to the etiology of conduct disorders (Quay, 1986).

Issues related to genetic studies involve investigations on temperament. Researchers have identified a pattern of infant and early child behavior often labeled as "difficult" (Thomas et al, 1968). A link between this temperamental variable and later conduct disordered symptomatology is intriguing to consider. Plomin (1983), however, reports that temperament in infancy is not significantly associated with later problems and that, although the "difficult" temperamental cluster does predict behavioral outcomes at statistically significant levels, the clinical utility of this association remains undetermined.

Studies on brain chemistry and behavior also attempt to understand the etiology of aggressive conduct disorders. To date these have been preliminary, but also promising. One example is the work of Rogeness and colleagues (1982) who compared socialized conduct disorder, undersocialized conduct disorder, and normal control children on four biochemical factors: dopamine-beta-hydroxylase, catechol-o-methyl transferase, monoamine oxidase, and serotonin. The undersocialized conduct disorder group had significantly lower dopamine-beta-hydroxylase activity than either the socialized conduct disorder or the control group. The socialized group had higher catechol-o-methyl transferase and there were no differences in either monoamine oxidase or serotonin. A later study by the same group using a larger sample (Rogeness et al, 1984) confirmed the relationship between low plasma levels of dopamine-beta-hydroxylase and undersocialized conduct disorders.

Efforts to correlate physiology and conduct disorders also have yielded preliminary studies. Examples include studies on heart rate (Raine and Venables, 1984a), galvanic skin response (Borkovec, 1970; Raine and Venables, 1984b), and electroencephalography (Lewis et al, 1982). As yet, there are no conclusive findings.

Psychologic

Although biologic and constitutional factors appear important in the etiology of conduct disorders, the psychologic component remains a central feature, especially in terms of current management. Any comprehensive attempt to evaluate and manage conduct disorders must include an understanding of the typical motivations, defense mechanisms and maneuvers, styles of interpersonal behavior, and psychodynamic issues that characterize this group of children and adolescents.

Psychoanalysts have attempted to understand the unconscious mechanisms that underlie deviant behavior. Examples include Aichhorn's description of the "defective superego" (1935), Grossbard (1962) pointing to the "ego deficiencies" that contribute to deviant behavior, and Johnson and Szurek's (1952) description of the concept of "superego lacunae" in which children tended to act out the unconscious antisocial wishes of their parent.

It is important to keep in mind that, along with biologic and social factors, personal and psychodynamic factors contribute to conduct disorders.

Social

The sociological and experiential aspects of conduct disorders have been extensively studied and have yielded the most helpful conceptual and treatment perspectives. Various aspects of a child's social environment and experiences may affect the development of antisocial behavior.

Low socioeconomic status has been correlated with the development of antisocial behavior in children (Robins, 1966; Rutter et al, 1970). However, several researchers (Robins 1979; Hetherington et al, 1982; Wells and Forehand, 1985) have concluded that processes within the family, rather than socioeconomic status per se, are more important etiologic determinants. These include less education, limited use of available resources, poor parenting and social coping skills, limited employment success, and marital discord.

Social learning theorists have emphasized imitation of an antisocial, aggressive, or criminal model as a major factor in the development of antisocial behavior in children (Bandura and Walters, 1963; Berbavitz, 1962). Evidence also supports an interaction between imitation, genetic susceptibility, and adverse family factors. Hutchings and Mednick (1974) found that a son is more likely to be criminal when both his biological and adoptive fathers are criminal than when criminality is present in only one father.

Parental psychopathology and the development of antisocial behavior in children has been studied. Maternal anxiety, irritability, and depression may be particularly important in the development of conduct problems (Hetherington et al, 1982; Patterson, 1982). These same factors also predict the mothers' negative view of their children (Forehand et al, 1982) and whether they remain in treatment (McMahon et al, 1981).

Patterson's (1980) MMPI studies of mothers revealed elevations on psychopathic deviate, hypomania, and schizophrenia scales for undersocialized (aggressive or nonaggressive) children, and elevations on scales indicating depression, rigidity, and social introversion for mothers of socialized aggressive or oppositional children.

Irritability in fathers also correlates with conduct disorder in children. Patterson (1982), however, found that paternal irritability has less relative importance than maternal irritability because the fathers of conduct disordered children are often inadequate, emotionally distant, and participate minimally in child rearing.

Paternal MMPI studies (Johnson and Lobitz, 1974) also reveal significant correlation between psychopathic deviate, hypomania, and schizophrenia in fathers and deviance in their children.

Parental psychopathology, substance abuse, criminal behavior by the father, marital discord, father absence, harsh inconsistent punishment practices, and poor supervision are commonly associated with antisocial behavior in children (Kazdin, 1987b; Rutter and Giller, 1983).

Several investigators have shown the protective aspects of a good relationship with one parent who is consistent in discipline and affection. This serves to potentially counterbalance the effects of a poor relationship or negative attitude of the other parent (Hetherington et al, 1982; O'Leary, 1984).

Patterson (1982) describes the development and treatment of conduct disorders through the dynamics of the "coercive family process." According to his studies, coercion occurs when deviant behavior by the child is supported or directly reinforced by a parent. This process leads to a loop of negative reinforcement of both child and parental behaviors. Disrupting this paradigm has lead to a method of treatment (see Treatment section).

ASSESSMENT

In addition to a psychiatric evaluation, mental status, and neurological examinations, the most common assessment methods for conduct disorders include behavioral checklists, self-report scales, and direct observation (Quay, 1986).

Behavior Checklists

Behavior checklists are completed by parents, teachers, and/or other caretakers. Several checklists or rating scales are available, including the Revised Behavior Problem Checklist (Quay, 1983), the Conners' Teacher (Conners, 1969) and Parent Rating Scales (Goyette et al, 1978), and the Louisville School Behavior Checklist (Miller, 1972). All these rating scales show adequate test–retest reliability and internal consistency (Boyle and Jones, 1985). Table 2 is an example of the Conners' Teacher Rating Scale.

Self-report Scales

Current data on the use of self-report instruments are limited (Quay, 1986) and the instruments themselves are problematic. In order to complete such questionnaires, the child must be able to read and process written information. Children with conduct disorders often have significant reading or language difficulties, making a self-report questionnaire difficult unless read to them. Also, conduct disordered symptomatology are expressions of externalized behavior that children either deny, project, or fail to endorse as problems.

Behavioral Observations

Structured observational schemes are useful to observe and measure behavior of aggressive children both qualitatively and quantitatively (Patterson, 1982). Currently, structured observational schemes are primarily research tools. Their utility as clinical tools for practitioners is undetermined.

DIFFERENTIAL DIAGNOSIS

Psychiatric conditions from psychosis to adjustment disorders may present with antisocial behaviors. It is important to avoid premature closure on diagnosing a conduct disorder because of the multiple causes, dynamics, and motivations for antisocial behavior. Thoughtful differential diagnosis is critical because antisocial behavior may obscure potentially more treatable conditions. In addition, many of the disturbances noted below may occur in association with conduct disorder. As noted earlier, if other disorders are present, both diagnoses should be made (American Psychiatric Association, 1987).

Attention-deficit Hyperactivity Disorder (ADHD)

Conduct disordered symptomatology and hyperactivity may be intimately intertwined (Prinz et al, 1981; Werry et al, 1987). Symptoms common to both include excess motor activity, restlessness, inattention, distractibility, and impulsivity. Hyperactivity as a behavioral characteristic often is associated with the undersocialized conduct disorder dimension.

Table 2. Conduct Disorder and Asocial Factors from the 39-item Conners' Teacher Rating Scale

IV. Listed below are descriptive terms of behavior. Place a check in the column which best describes this child. ANSWER ALL ITEMS.

Observation	Degree of Activity			
	Not at All	Just a Little	Pretty Much	Very Much
Classroom Behavior				
15. Quarrelsome				
16. Mood changes quickly and drastically				
17. Acts "smart"				
18. Destructive				
19. Steals				
20. Lies				
21. Temper outbursts, explosive, and unpredictable behavior				
Group Participation				
22. Isolates himself from other children				
23. Appears to be unaccepted by group				
25. No sense of fair play				
27. Does not get along with opposite sex				
28. Does not get along with same sex				
29. Teases other children or interferes with their activities				
Attitude Toward Authority				
31. Defiant				
32. Impudent				
36. Stubborn				
38. Uncooperative				

Adapted from Conners CK: A teacher rating scale for use in drug studies with children. Am J Psychiatry 1969; 126:884–888.

Studies of children with diagnosed conduct disorder have identified large subgroups (up to 75 percent) who are motorically overactive and aggressive (Stewart et al, 1981; Prinz et al, 1981). Nonclinic population studies also identify a high correlation between conduct disordered behavior and hyperactivity (Sandberg et al, 1980; Prinz et al, 1981).

Follow-up studies have shown that a significant number of children with ADHD develop conduct and substance use disorders as adolescents (Cantwell, 1985; Gittelman et al, 1985). In looking further at this reported link, Satterfield and colleagues (1987) compared predelinquent ADHD boys treated with stimulant medication and multimodal treatment. Their findings suggest that multimodal treatment may be an effective approach to preventing the progression from ADHD to conduct disorder.

Careful delineation of the presence of one or both disorders is critical in terms of management because ADHD is eminently more treatable than conduct disorder.

Oppositional-Defiant Disorder

This diagnostic entity is the other major syndrome of aggressive behavior in childhood. The essential features are disobedience and provocative opposition to authority figures, primarily the parents, but including teachers and others. The oppositional behavior includes temper tantrums, argumentativeness, stubbornness, noncompliance, and violation of minor rules. When major societal rules are broken, opposition-defiant disorder is ruled out and the diagnosis of conduct disorder is made (American Psychiatric Association, 1987).

Affective Disorders

A relationship has been demonstrated between conduct disorder and depression in adolescents (Chiles et al, 1980); in prepubertal children (Puig-Antich, 1982); and in both children and adolescents (Marriage et al, 1986). Carlson and Cantwell (1980) found a similar co-occurrence, but in addition, showed that primary affective disorder is distinguishable from conduct disorder based largely on history. In their study, the conduct disordered children had histories of more chronic and severe antisocial behaviors and the onset of conduct problems followed the onset of the primary affective symptoms.

No studies as yet examine the relationship between conduct disorder and bipolar disorder in children. The episodic nature of the hyperactivity and affective instability, plus a positive family history for affective disorder (especially bipolar illness), assists in making such a distinction.

Personality Disorders

There is an association between severe childhood antisocial behavior and adult antisocial personality disorder (Robins, 1970). This association is less clear for other types of personality disorders.

Children with conduct disorders, however, often exhibit features of specific personality disorders, in particular borderline personality organization and marked narcissistic features. In addition, most antisocial and conduct disordered children utilize projection as a major defense and are prone to paranoid ideations. These personality traits often appear to be ingrained, stable over time, and unrelated to a specific phase of development or environmental conditions.

TREATMENT

Kazdin (1987b) has published an excellent review of the treatment of antisocial behavior in children. He noted what many who attempt to treat these children have known: "To date, little in the way of effective and empirically established treatment is available." He, like others who work with these children and their families, are undaunted by the current pessimistic view of treatment. There are promising treatment options under investigation. The following is an overview of current treatment modalities.

Pharmacologic

The literature provides no definitive guidelines for pharmacologic management. Pharmacologic treatment, when used, should be only one part of a comprehensive treatment plan.

There is no specific medication for the treatment of conduct disorder. However, medication that affects carefully delineated target symptoms may be a helpful adjunct to other treatment modalities. The target symptoms that may respond to medication are aggressivity, self-injurious behavior, and hyperactivity.

Chlorpromazine, haloperidol, and lithium have proved effective in treating the aggression, hyperactivity, and explosive affect in conduct disordered children. Chlorpromazine, however, produces sedation whereas lithium and haloperidol do not (Campbell et al, 1982).

In a large, well designed study on carefully diagnosed children with undersocialized aggressive conduct disorders, Campbell and colleagues (1984) found both haloperidol and lithium carbonate better than placebo for reducing aggression. Lithium was preferable to haloperidol because of less effect on cognition and more safety regarding tardive dyskinesia. Based on these findings, a trial of lithium is warranted in a seriously undersocialized aggressive conduct disorder as part of an overall management plan.

Stimulant medications are effective in aggressive conduct disorders with concurrent ADHD (Werry et al, 1975). There is no evidence that stimulants are useful in uncomplicated conduct disorders.

When concurrent depressive symptoms are present, tricyclic antidepressants may be useful. Puig-Antich (1982) reported preliminary benefit in using tricyclic antidepressants in children with features of both disorders; however, studies using tricyclics for conduct disorders alone are lacking.

Conduct disordered children may have associated epileptiform conditions that contribute to their aggression (Monroe, 1973). Diphenylhydantoin (Looker and Connors, 1970) and carbamazepine (Rivinus, 1982) have been studied. There is no clear basis for treating aggressive conduct disorders with anticonvulsants in the absence of a clinical seizure disorder with or without EEG abnormalities. Those with seizure disorders should receive appropriate anticonvulsants and if their aggressive behavior improves, this is an added benefit.

Psychosocial

The efficacy of individual psychotherapy in all its forms has not been demonstrated (Kazdin, 1987b). As mentioned previously, however, this does not preclude the importance of a psychodynamic understanding of the child and family.

Behavior therapy may be useful, particularly in the management of aggressive and self-injurious behavior. Individual social skills training, contingency management, and token economies are the common forms of behavioral treatment (Kazdin, 1987b).

Attempts to treat antisocial behavior by family therapy using traditional methods does not sufficiently alter the maladaptive behavior (Kazdin, 1987). One form of family therapy, functional family therapy (Alexander and Parsons, 1973; Alexander et al, 1976), has shown preliminary efficacy. Functional family therapy is a blend of behavioral, systems, and cognitive–behavioral principles that attempts to clarify the functional role that conduct problems play within the family and to alter maladaptive family communication and interaction. The few outcome studies available (Alexander and Parsons, 1973; Klein et al, 1977) show promise.

Parent Training

Parent management training has many proponents. Patterson, in particular, has provided considerable research on this form of treatment and has demonstrated it to be especially promising. He and his colleagues (Patterson et al, 1975, 1982; Patterson, 1982) have focused on altering what are called coercive parent–child interactions in the home that foster aggressive child behavior and distinguish families with antisocial children.

There are various formats for parent management training; however, generally all involve direct training procedures for parents that teach them how to interact differently with their child. For example, Forehand and McMahon (1982) utilize a progressive series of structured interactions (attending, rewarding, differential ignoring, issuing proper commands and "time out" from social reinforcement) that are taught directly to parents. These alter the pattern of parent–child interchange so that prosocial rather than coercive behaviors are reinforced and supported within the family.

Controlled outcome studies support the efficacy of this treatment approach as reflected on measures of child behavior at home and at school (Patterson, 1982; Fleischman, 1981).

Problem-Solving Social Skills Training

Another promising treatment approach is cognitive–behavioral problem-solving social skills training. This focuses on cognitive processes and deficits in the child that mediate maladaptive interpersonal behavior (Kendall and Braswell, 1985). Problem-solving social skills training studies have shown that altering the child's cognitive processes can favorably alter behaviors at home and at school (Kendall and Braswell, 1985; Lochman et al, 1984).

Parent management training, which is parent directed, appears effective by altering the interactions of aggressive children in and out of the home; whereas problem-solving social skills training, which is child-directed, may provide the child with the tools to alter his or her own behavior. Kazdin and colleagues (1987) evaluated the effectiveness of combining parent management training and problem-solving social skill training on an inpatient population of conduct disordered children. Posttreatment and follow-up at one year showed that children in the combined parent management training–problem-solving social skills training group showed significantly less aggressive and externalizing behavior at home and at school, more prosocial behavior, and better overall adjustment than did the control group. He cautioned, however, that this inpatient study was preliminary and lacks data for extrapolation to outpatient populations.

COURSE AND PROGNOSIS

Olweus (1979) reviewed the stability of aggression in boys from studies between 1935 and 1978 and found that aggression at ages 8 to 9 correlates with aggression observed 10 to 14 years later.

Richman and colleagues (1982) rated children's conduct-disordered behavior using parent questionnaires at ages three, four, and eight years. One-third of those with manifest conduct problems showed continuity of the behaviors from age three to age eight. The highest degree of continuity was demonstrated among those judged to be moderately to severely disturbed. They concluded that for boys the behavioral characteristics of a conduct disorder at age three are associated with the diagnosed disorder at age eight.

Robins has conducted the best known studies linking childhood behaviors to adult outcomes (Robins, 1966, 1979). In a summary of her work in 1979, she reported that adult antisocial behavior is best predicted by the variety and combinations of childhood antisocial behaviors rather than by any particular behavior, and that childhood behaviors are better predictors than family variables. In addition, in spite of the important role that childhood antisocial behaviors play in forecasting adult antisocial behavior, most antisocial children do not grow up to be severely antisocial adults (Robins, 1979; Farrington, 1978). She added, however, that among those who did not grow up to become severely antisocial, very few were completely free of antisocial behaviors as adults. There was no distinction between the socialized and undersocialized types in Robins' work.

A 1980 study by Henn and co-workers (1980) on institutionalized youths did compare adult outcomes with the two types (socialized and undersocialized). Three groups were studied: undersocialized aggressive, undersocialized nonaggressive, and socialized. The socialized group did better while incarcerated (that is, they spent less time incarcerated, had earlier age of discharge, and had fewer returns to the institution). The two undersocialized groups remained incarcerated longer and were more likely to be arrested later for an adult crime.

Two facts are clear about outcome. Without treatment, conduct disordered behavior, in particular aggression, persists across time and the long-term prognosis for these children is poor (Wells and Forehand, 1985).

CONCLUSIONS AND REFLECTIONS

The current status of conduct disorder is not substantially different from what has been presented in multiple previous reports. Conduct disorder remains the most common psychiatric disorder in childhood and affects more boys than girls. It is one of our most costly disorders in terms of morbidity, mortality, and effects on families, schools, communities, and mental health systems.

There appears to be a significant increase in the frequency, severity, and pervasiveness of conduct disorder symptoms in children. There are long inpatient and outpatient waiting lists and a seemingly endless line of boys and increasingly more girls with antisocial behavior.

Even when an adequate diagnostic assessment is completed and recommendations are made, significant practical problems remain. Shortened hospital stays are mandated by current reimbursement policies and there is a frustrating lack of adequate and appropriate foster care, day treatment, and residential facilities for the appropriate disposition of these children and their families.

Often the parents (many of whom are single parents) are themselves emotionally and socioeconomically disadvantaged. Many lack the physical and emotional reserves and resources to adequately deal with their conduct disordered children.

While parent management training and problem-solving social skills training are promising as treatment modalities, making these understandable and applicable to many of these children, their families, and communities represents significant problems. Having adequate reimbursable time, staff, and facilities to teach and implement these highly structured skills is another major need.

Future directions should include increased efforts in prevention, early recognition, and intervention of dysfunctional families and conduct disordered children.

More emphasis on psychodynamic understanding in psychiatric training programs and further refinement of the biological correlates of brain–behavior interactions are needed.

Studies that differentiate between the socialized and undersocialized groups and their outcomes as well as a continued search for new and further refinement of promising treatment options are badly needed. Additional community resources to deal with these children are an absolute necessity.

REFERENCES

Aichhorn A: Wayward Youth. New York, Viking Press, 1935

Alexander JF, Parson BV: Short-term behavioral intervention with delinquent families: impact on family process and recidivism. J Abnorm Psychol 1973; 81:219–225

Alexander JF, Barton C, Schiavo RS, et al: Systems-behavioral intervention with families of delinquents: therapeutic characteristics, family behavior, and outcome. J Consult Clin Psychol 1976; 44:656–664

American Psychiatric Association: Diagnostic and Statistical Manual of Mental Disorders, Third Edition (DSM-III). Washington, DC, American Psychiatric Association, 1980.

American Psychiatric Association: Diagnostic and Statistical Manual of Mental Disorders, Third Edition, Revised (DSM-III-R). Washington, DC, American Psychiatric Association, 1987

Bachman JG, Johnston LD, O'Malley PM: Delinquent behavior linked to educational attainment and post-high school experiences, in Colloquium on the Correlates of Crime and the Determinants of Criminal Behavior. Edited by Otten L. Arlington, MA, Mitre, 1978

Bandura A, Walters RH: Social Learning and Personality Development. New York, Holt, Rinehart & Winston, 1963

Behar D, Stewart MA: Aggressive conduct disorder of children. Acta Psychiatr Scand 1982; 65:210–220

Berbavitz L: Aggression: A Social Psychological Analysis. New York, McGraw-Hill, 1962

Bohman AL, Cloninger CR, Sigvardsson S, et al: Predisposition to petty criminality in Swedish adoptees, I: genetic and environmental heterogeneity. Arch Gen Psychiatry 1982; 39:1233–1241

Borkovec TD: Autonomic reactivity to sensory stimulation in psychopathic, neurotic and normal adolescents. J Consult Clin Psychol 1970; 35:217–222

Boyle MH, Jones SC: Selecting measures of emotional and behavioral disorders of children for use in the general population. J Child Psychol Psychiatry 1985; 26:137–159

Campbell M, Cohen IL, Small AM: Drugs in aggressive behavior. J Am Acad Child Psychiatry 1982; 21:107–117

Campbell M, Perry R, Green WH: The use of lithium in children and adolescents. Psychosomatics 1984; 25:95–106

Cantwell DP: Hyperactive children have grown up. Arch Gen Psychiatry 1985; 42:1026–1028

Carlson CL, Lahey BB, Neeper R: Peer assessment of the social behavior of accepted, rejected, and neglected children. J Abnorm Child Psychol 1984; 12:189–198

Carlson G, Cantwell D: Unmasking masked depression in children and adolescents. Am J Psychiatry 1980; 137:945–949

Chamberlain P, Patterson GR: Conduct disorders: aggressive behavior in middle childhood, in The Clinical Guide to Child Psychiatry. Edited by Shaffer D, Ehrhardt AA, Greenhill LL. New York, Free Press, 1985

Chiles J, Miller M, Cox G: Depression in an adolescent delinquent population. Arch Gen Psychiatry 1980; 37:179–183

Commission on Professional and Hospital Activities: The International Classification of Diseases, Clinical Modifications, Ninth Revision. Ann Arbor, Edward Bro, 1979

Conners CK: A teacher rating scale for use in drug studies with children. Am J Psychiatry 1969; 126:884–888

Farrington DP: The family background of aggressive youths, in Aggression and Antisocial Behavior in Childhood and Adolescence. Edited by Hersov LA, Berger AL, Shaffer D. London, Pergamon, 1978

Fleischman, MJ: A replication of Patterson's "Intervention for Boys with conduct problems." J Consult Clin Psychol 1981; 49:343–351

Forehand R, McMahon RT: Helping the Noncompliant Child: A Clinician's Guide to Parent Training. New York, Guilford Press, 1982

Forehand R, Wells KC, McMahon RJ, et al: Maternal perceptions of maladjustment in clinic-referred children: an extension of earlier research. Journal of Behavior Assessment 1982; 4:145–151

Gabrielli WF, Mednick SA: Genetic correlates of criminal behavior. American Behavioral Scientist 1983; 27:59–74

Gilbert GM: A survey of "referral problems" in metropolitan child guidance centers. J Clin Psychol 1957; 13:37–42

Gittelman R, Mannuzza S, Shenker R, et al: Hyperactive boys almost grown up. Arch Gen Psychiatry 1985; 42:937–947

Glow RA: Classroom behaviour problems. An Australian normative study of the Conners teacher rating scale. Unpublished manuscript, 1984, cited in Psychopathological Disorders of Childhood, third edition. Edited by Quay HC, Werry JS. New York, Wiley, 1986

Glueck S, Glueck E: Delinquents and non-delinquents in perspective. Cambridge, MA, Harvard University Press, 1968

Goyette CH, Conners CK, Ulrich RF: Normative data on the Revised Conners Parent and Teacher Rating Scales. J Abnorm Child Psychol 1978; 6:211–236

Graham P: Epidemiological studies, in Psychopathological Disorders of Childhood, second edition. Edited by Quay HC, Werry JS. New York, Wiley, 1979

Grossbard H: Ego deficiency in delinquents. Am J Orthopsychiatry 1962; 43:171–178

Henn FA, Bardwell R, Jenkins RL: Juvenile delinquency revisited. Arch Gen Psychiatry 1980; 37:1160–1163

Hetherington EM, Cox M, Cox CR: Effects of divorce on parents and children, in Nontraditional Families. Edited by Lamb M. Hillsdale, NJ, Erlbaum, 1982

Hutchings B, Mednick SA: Registered criminality in the adoptive and biologic parents of registered male adoptees, in Genetics, Environment and Psychopathology. Edited by

Mednick SA, Schulsinger F, Bell P, et al. Amsterdam, North-Holland/American Elsevier, 1974

Hutchings B, Mednick SA: Criminality in adoptees and their adoptive and biological parents, in Biosocial Bases of Criminal Behavior. Edited by Mednick S, Christiansen KO. New York, Gardner Press, 1977

Johnson AM, Szurek SA: The genesis of antisocial acting out in children and adults. Psychoanal Q 1952; 21:323

Johnson SM, Lobitz GK: The personal and marital adjustment of parents as related to observed child deviance and parenting behavior. J Abnorm Child Psychol 2:192–207, 1974

Kazdin AE: Conduct Disorder in Childhood and Adolescence. Newbury Park, CA, Sage, 1987a

Kazdin AE: Treatment of antisocial behaviors in children: current status and future directions. Psychol Bull 1987b; 102:187–203

Kazdin AE, Esvelt-Dawson K, French NH, et al: Effects of parent management training and problem-solving training combined in the treatment of antisocial child behavior. Am Acad Child Adolesc Psychiatry 1987; 26:416–424

Kendall PC, Braswell L: Cognitive-Behavioral Therapy for Impulsive Children. New York, Guilford Press, 1985

Klein NC, Alexander JF, Parson BV: Impact of family systems intervention on recidivism and sibling delinquency: a model of primary prevention and program evaluation. J Consult Clin Psychol 1977; 45:469–474

Lewis DO: Conduct disorders, in Psychiatry. Edited by Michels R, Cavener JO, Brodie K, et al. Philadelphia, Lippincott, 1986

Lewis DO, Pincus JH, Shanok SS, et al: Psychomotor epilepsy and violence in a group of incarcerated adolescent boys. Am J Psychiatry 1982; 139:882–887

Lochman JE, Burch PR, Curry JF, et al: Treatment and generalization effects of cognitive-behavioral and goal setting interventions with aggressive boys. J Consult Clin Psychol 1984; 52:915–916

Looker A, Conners CK: Diphenylhydantoin in children with severe temper tantrums. Arch Gen Psychiatry 1970; 23:80–89

Marriage K, Fine S, Moretti M, et al: Relationship between depression and conduct disorder in children and adolescents. J Am Acad Child Psychiatry 1986; 25:687–691

McMahon RJ, Forehand R, Griest DL, et al: Who drops out of therapy during parent behavioral training? Behavior Counseling Quarterly 1981; 1:79–85

Mednick SA, Christiansen KO (Eds): Biosocial bases of criminal behavior. New York, Gardner Press, 1977

Miller LC: School Behavior Checklist: an inventory of deviant behavior for elementary school children. J Consult Clin Psychol 1972; 38:138–144

Monroe RK: Anticonvulsants in the treatment of aggression. J Nerv Ment Dis 1973; 160:119–126

O'Connor M, Foch T, Sherry T, et al: A twin study of specific behavioral problems of socialization as viewed by parents. J Abnorm Child Psychol 1980: 8:189–199

O'Leary KD: Marital discord and children: problems, strategies, methodologies and results, in Children in Families Under Stress. Edited by Doyle A, Gold D, Moskowitz DS. New Directions for Child Development, #24. San Francisco, Jossey-Bass, 1984

Olweus D: Stability of aggressive reaction patterns in males: a review. Psychol Bull 1979; 86:852–875

Patterson GR: Mothers: The Unacknowledged Victims. Monographs of the Society for Research in Child Development. 45:Serial 186, 1980

Patterson GR: Coercive Family Process. Eugene, OR, Castalia, 1982

Patterson GR, Reid JB, Jones RR, et al: A Social Learning Approach to Family Intervention, vol 1. Eugene, OR, Castalia, 1975

Patterson GR, Chamberlain P, Reid JB: A comparative evaluation of a parent-training program. Behavior Therapy 1982; 13:638–650

Plomin R: Childhood temperament, in Advances in Clinical Child Psychology. Edited by Lahey BB, Kazdin AE. New York, Plenum, 1983

Prinz RJ, Connor PA, Wilson CC: Hyperactive and aggressive behaviors in childhood: intertwined dimensions. Journal for Research in Crime and Delinquency 1981; 1:33–37

Puig-Antich J: Major depression and conduct disorder in prepuberty. J Am Acad Child Psychiatry 1982; 21:118–128

Quay HC: A dimensional approach to behavior disorders. The Revised Behavior Problem Checklist. School Psychol Rev 1983; 12:244–249

Quay HC: Conduct disorders, in Psychopathological Disorders of Childhood, 3rd ed. Edited by Quay HC, Werry JS. New York, Wiley, 1986

Raine A, Venables PH: Electrodermal nonresponding, antisocial behavior, and schizoid tendencies in adolescents. Psychophysiology 1984a; 21:424–433

Raine A, Venables PH: Tonic heart rate levels, social class and antisocial behaviour in adolescents. Biological Psychology 1984b; 18:123–132

Richman N, Stevenson J, Graham PJ: Pre-school to School: A Behavioral Study. London, Academic Press, 1982

Rivinus TM: Psychiatric effects of the anti-convulsant regimens. J Clin Psychopharmacol 2:162–165, 1982

Robins LN: Deviant Children Grown Up. Baltimore, Williams & Wilkins, 1966

Robins LN: The adult development of the antisocial child. Seminars in Psychiatry 1970; 2:420–434

Robins LN: Sturdy childhood predictors of adult outcome replication from longitudinal studies, in Stress and Mental Disorder. Edited by Barrett JE, Rose RM, Klerman GL. New York, Raven Press, 1979

Robins LN: Epidemiological approaches to natural history research: antisocial disorders in children. J Am Acad Child Psychiatry 1981; 20:566–680

Rogeness GA, Hernandez JM, Macedo CA, et al: Biochemical differences in children with conduct disorder socialized and undersocialized. Am J Psychiatry 1982; 139:307–311

Rogeness GA, Hernandez JM, Macedo CA, et al: Clinical characteristics of emotionally disturbed boys with very low activities of dopamine-beta-hydroxylase. J Am Acad Child Psychiatry 1984; 23:203–208

Rutter M, Giller H: Juvenile Delinquency: Trends and Perspectives. New York, Penguin Books, 1983

Rutter M, Shaffer D: A step forward or a step backward in terms of the classification of child psychiatric disorders? J Am Acad Child Psychiatry 1980; 19:371–394

Rutter M, Lebovici S, Eisenberg L, et al: A tri-axial classification of mental disorders in childhood. J Child Psychol Psychiatry 1969; 10:41–61

Rutter M, Tizard J, Whitmore K: Education, Health and Behavior. London, Longmans, 1970

Rutter M, Cox A, Tupling C, et al: Attainment and adjustment in two geographical areas, I: Prevalence of psychiatric disorder. Br J Psychiatry 1975a; 126:493–509

Rutter M, Shaffer D, Shepherd M: A multi-axial classification of child psychiatric disorders. Geneva, World Health Organization, 1975b

Sandberg ST, Wieselberg M, Shaffer D: Hyperkinetic and conduct problem children in a primary school population: some epidemiologic considerations. J Child Psychol Psychiatry 1980; 21:293–311

Satterfield JH, Satterfield BT, Schell AM: Therapeutic interventions to prevent delinquency in hyperactive boys. J Am Acad Child Adolesc Psychiatry 1987; 26:56–64

Stewart MH, Cummings C, Singer S, et al: The overlap between hyperactive and unsocialized aggressive children. J Child Psychol Psychiatry 1981; 22:35–45

Sturge C: Reading retardation and antisocial behavior. J Child Psychol Psychiatry 1982; 23:21–31

Thomas A, Chess S, Birch HG: Temperament and Behavior Disorders in Children. New York, New York University Press, 1968

Wells KC, Forehand R: Conduct and oppositional disorders, in Handbook of Clinical Behavior Therapy with Children. Edited by Bornstein PH, Kazdin AE. Homewood, IL, Dorsey Press, 1985

Werry JS, Aman MG, Lampen E: Haloperidol and methylphenidate in hyperactive children. Acta Paediatr Scand 1975; 42:26–40

Werry JS, Reeves JC, Elkind GS: Attention deficit disorder, conduct, oppositional, and anxiety disorders in children, I: a review of research on differentiating characteristics. J Am Acad Child Adolesc Psychiatry 1987; 26:2:133–143

Chapter 10

Mood Disorders in Children and Adolescents

by Javad H. Kashani, M.D., F.R.C.P.(C), and
Daniel D. Sherman, M.A.

The first volume in the *Review of Psychiatry* series devoted a section to child and adolescent depression (Grinspoon, 1982). By this time, the field included the pioneering work of Cytryn and McKnew (1972), Malmquist (1971), and Poznanski and Zrull (1970), giving impetus to the constructs of childhood and adolescent depression. More recently, substantive reviews continue to organize the expanding empirical literature while highlighting areas in need of research (Digdon and Gotlib, 1985). By all appearances, the explosive growth of the field will continue, necessitating periodic reviews of the literature as represented by the present chapter.

According to the *Diagnostic and Statistical Manual of Mental Disorders, Third Edition (DSM-III)* (American Psychiatric Association, 1980), the relationship between mood and affect is analogous to that between climate and weather. As a result, affect can be conceptualized as state-like, whereas mood is better described as trait-like. Because we are more interested in the existence of a pervasive and sustained syndrome rather than transient, nonpervasive states of "depression," it seemed natural to use mood disorders as an important component of the title of this chapter.

This review covers issues related to classification, the etiology and/or maintenance of depression, and a discussion of epidemiology. Recent research is addressed, illustrating the co-occurrence of other disorders with depression. Following a rationale for the application of a developmental perspective to child and adolescent mood disorders, a reference to treatment concludes the chapter.

CLASSIFICATION

The classification and diagnostic criteria for mood disorders in children continue to be controversial and unsettled, but advancing through research. In 1970, Ling and colleagues proposed inclusion and exclusion criteria. Their criteria were later refined by Weinberg and co-workers (1973), which subsequently became one of the better known standards for diagnosing childhood depression. Weinberg's criteria did not include pervasive anhedonia, but did consider lowered self-esteem as an essential symptom. In addition, Weinberg excluded psychomotor retardation, suicidal ideation, and guilt as qualifying symptoms. However, social withdrawal, somatic complaints, and changes toward school were included. Poznanski (1979) added the essential criteria of nonverbal dysphoria and social

The authors thank Elizabeth B. Weller, M.D., for her comments on the manuscript.

withdrawal, but chose not to consider appetite disturbances or psychomotor agitation as qualifying symptoms.

Other investigators who proposed and developed classifications included McConville (1973), Philips (1979), and Cytryn and McKnew (1972); the latter's classification included a) an acute condition with mild family psychopathology in a child who was previously well adjusted; b) chronic depression in a child who had premorbid problems and at least one depressed parent; c) masked depression (that is, depression that was masked by other childhood symptomatology and was associated with family psychopathology). Cytryn and colleagues (1980) later recommended that the concept of masked depression be abandoned in favor of *DSM-III* criteria for childhood depression. Likewise, while Research Diagnostic Criteria (Feighner et al, 1972) was previously used by some investigators, it too gradually was supplanted by *DSM-III*.

Poznanski and associates (1985) compared four sets of diagnostic criteria: RDC, *DSM-III*, the Weinberg, and the Poznanski criteria. They found a consensus for three symptoms among all four sets of criteria: sleep disturbance, fatigue, and cognitive impairment. The authors concluded that the major disagreement among the four sets of criteria in their study resulted from the interviewers' rating of dysphoric mood. Specifically, while the interviewers' rating of dysphoric mood was based upon the child's nonverbal affect, the child and parent verbally denied the presence of dysphoria.

The *Diagnostic and Statistical Manual of Mental Disorders, Third Edition, Revised (DSM-III-R)* (American Psychiatric Association, 1987) subclassifies mood disorders into bipolar and depressive disorders. There are two types of bipolar disorders: 1) bipolar disorder with the presence of at least one manic episode; and 2) cyclothymia, with numerous, alternating episodes of both hypomania and depressive symptoms (Table 1).

There are also two types of depressive disorders: 1) major depression, which minimally requires a two-week duration; and 2) dysthymia, which requires at least a one-year duration for children and adolescents.

Little empirical work exists on bipolar disorders in children and adolescents. This lack is particularly apparent in the cyclothymia literature (Klein et al, 1985). However, the presence of bipolar disorders in children is increasingly acknowledged. While clear-cut mania is rarely seen in children, the disorder is likely underdiagnosed in adolescents (Casat, 1982). Because children suffering from bipolar disorder or attention-deficit hyperactivity disorder share the symptoms of overactivity, distractibility, and decreased attention span, these disorders should be distinguished from each other.

The changes found in *DSM-III-R* are admittedly for the better. The requirement of impaired functioning serves as one illustration of this improvement. Unlike the overinclusiveness of the 1980 version, *DSM-III-R* requires that the degree of impairment interfere with social and occupational (school) functioning. Second, *DSM-III* required a minimum of one-week duration (unless hospitalization was involved) of elevated, expansive, or irritable mood for a diagnosis of mania. In contrast, *DSM-III-R* is less restrictive for mania because it excludes the time requirement. Third, *DSM-III-R* requires that the depressive behavior represent a significant departure from baseline functioning.

Overall, *DSM-III-R* provides stricter inclusion criteria than did *DSM-III*. However, unlike *DSM-III*, the revised version does not require the presence of special criteria for the diagnosis of depression in preschoolers. To illustrate, *DSM-III* accepts sad facial expression as an equivalent for depressed mood, while *DSM-III-R* neither grants this allowance nor any special set of criteria for children under age six (Table 2).

A number of investigators have questioned *DSM-III* for neglecting consideration of the developmental issues involved (Cichetti and Schneider-Rosen, 1986; Rutter, 1986a) in mood disorders. To amend these shortcomings, some researchers (for example, Carlson and Garber, 1986) have proposed alternatives to *DSM-III*. Cantwell (1983) suggested that the essential *DSM-III* criteria remain the same, albeit with the addition of age-specific symptoms. This approach requires validation through future developmental studies.

ETIOLOGY: THEORETICAL MODELS

It is unlikely that any one model of causation accounts for childhood and adolescent unipolar depression in its entirety. Instead, the various models make both unique and overlapping contributions to a final common pathway (Akiskal and McKinney, 1975). In this section, we will review the major approaches to both the etiology and maintenance of child and adolescent unipolar depression. These

Table 1. Overall Classification Differences Between *DSM-III* and *DSM-III-R*

DSM-III	*DSM-III-R*
Affective Disorders	Mood Disorders

I. Major Affective Disorders
   A. bipolar disorder
      1. mixed
      2. manic
      3. depressed
   B. major depression
      1. single episode
      2. recurrent
	I. Bipolar Disorders
	   A. bipolar disorder
	      1. mixed
	      2. manic
	      3. depressed
	   B. cyclothymia
	   C. bipolar disorder NOS

II. Other Specific Affective Disorders
   A. cyclothymic disorder
   B. dysthymic disorder (or depressive neurosis)
	II. Depressive Disorders
	   A. major depression
	      1. single episode
	      2. recurrent
	   B. dysthymia (depressive neurosis)
	      specify: primary or secondary type
	      specify: early or late onset
	   C. depressive disorder NOS

III. Atypical Affective Disorder
   A. atypical bipolar disorder
   B. atypical depression	

Table 2. Differences in *DSM-III* and *DSM-III-R* Criteria for Mania, Major Depressive Disorder, and Dysthymic Disorder

DSM-III	*DSM-III-R*
I. Mania	
B. Duration of at least one week (or any duration if hospitalization is necessary)	B. No duration requirement
C. When the affective syndrome is absent, the clinical picture is dominated by neither of the following: 1. preoccupation with mood-incongruent delusions or hallucinations 2. bizarre behavior	D. The delusions or hallucinations *can* exist but not for longer than two weeks. Also, the reference to bizarre behavior has been deleted.
D. Not superimposed on either schizophrenia, schizophreniform disorder, or a paranoid disorder.	E. Not superimposed on schizophrenia, schizophreniform disorder, delusional disorder, or psychotic disorders NOS.
E. No mention of the impact of antidepressant treatment upon mood disorder is made.	F. Somatic antidepressant treatment (e.g., drugs, ECT) that apparently precipitates a mood disturbance should *not* be considered an organic etiologic factor.
II. Major Depressive Disorder	
B. Requires satisfaction of at least four of eight criteria.	A. Requires satisfaction of at least five of nine criteria.
B. No mention of irritable mood as a substitute criterion for children or adolescents.	A. Allows irritable mood as a substitute criterion for depressed mood in children and adolescents.
B. In children under six, hypoactivity substitutes for psychomotor agitation or retardation and signs of apathy substitute for loss of interest or pleasure in usual activities.	A. No mention of substitute criteria for children under six.
B. When the affective syndrome is absent, the clinical picture is dominated by neither of the following: 1. preoccupation with mood-incongruent delusions or hallucinations 2. bizarre behavior	C. The delusions or hallucinations *can* exist but not for longer than two weeks. Also, the reference to bizarre behavior has been deleted.

Table 2. Differences in *DSM-III, DSM-III-R* Criteria for Mania, Major
Depressive Disorder, and Dysthymic Disorder (*continued*)

DSM-III	*DSM-III-R*
D. Not superimposed on either schizophrenia, schizophreniform disorder, or a paranoid disorder.	D. Not superimposed on schizophrenia, schizophreniform disorder, delusional disorder, or psychotic disorder **NOS.**
III. Dysthymia (Depressive Neurosis)	
A. No mention of irritable mood as a substitute criterion for children or adolescents.	A. Allows irritable mood as a substitute criterion for depressed mood in children and adolescents.
B. The depressive symptoms can be separated by intervals lasting no longer than a few (i.e., 3) months at a time.	C. The depressive symptoms can be separated by intervals lasting no longer than two months at a time.
D. Requires satisfaction of at least 3 of 13 criteria.	B. Requires the satisfaction of at least two of six criteria. Criteria 4, 6, 7, 8, 9, 10, 12, and 13 from *DSM-III* are deleted. Criteria 1 (poor appetite or over-eating) is new in *DSM-III-R.*
E. No explicit reference to excluding a manic or hypomanic episode is made.	E. Requires that the patient has never had a manic or unequivocal hypomanic episode.
F. Requires that dysthymia superimposed on a pre-existing mental disorder must be distinguished from the patient's usual mood.	G. Requires that organic contributors to the etiology and maintenance of dysthymia (e.g., prolonged administration of antihypertensive medication) be ruled out.

approaches include the biochemical, genetic, psychodynamic, cognitive distortion, social skills deficits, learned helplessness, self-control, and family systems approaches. While less developed than the unipolar depression literature, the literature on bipolar illness will also receive attention.

Biological Models

NEUROTRANSMITTER APPROACH. In 1959, Everett and Toman proposed that catecholamines and serotonin have an important role in mood disorders. Later, the tenets of the catecholamine hypothesis evolved into the permissive hypothesis of affective disorders. According to the permissive hypothesis, depression is associated with low levels of both serotonin and norepinephrine. The permissive hypothesis represents one biological model underpinning pharmacologic treatment. However, the mechanism of tricyclic action in children remains unknown. Cytryn and colleagues (1974) reported that urinary metabolite changes in affectively disordered children are somewhat age dependent. The authors reported no differences in norepinephrine or vanillylmandelic acid excretion.

Generally speaking, the sensitivity and specificity of biological correlates in childhood depression are moderate. In addition, these markers are largely of the "state" not "trait" variety. That is, the markers are abnormal during the depressive episode and then return to normal during nondepressed states.

NEUROENDOCRINE MARKERS (Cortisol Secretion).   The hypersecretion of cortisol and early escape from dexamethasone suppression is a state marker for child and adolescent depression. The data on the usefulness of the dexamethasone suppression test (DST) with children are increasingly supportive. Using 6- to 12-year-old inpatients with major depressive disorder, Weller and colleagues (1984) found a 70 percent sensitivity and 93 percent specificity of the DST. However, the study lacked normal and nondepressed psychiatric controls. In a later controlled study, Weller and co-workers (1985) used the combined results of an 8:00 A.M. cortisol suppression index (CSI) and a 4:00 P.M. DST to achieve a 94 percent sensitivity and 75 percent specificity. Thus, when combined, the DST and CSI adequately differentiate prepubertal depressives from a heterogeneous group of psychiatric controls and a normal control sample. However, the specificity of the technique in differentiating subtypes of prepubertal depression (that is, major depressive disorder, dysthymic disorder) has not been examined.

SLEEP ARCHITECTURE (Sleep EEG).   Polysomnography does yield markers for major depressive disorder in adults. However, these findings cannot be extrapolated to major depressive disorder in prepubertal children (Ryan and Puig-Antich, 1985). Instead, evidence for maturational effects among prepubertal depressives indicates that the sleep electroencephalogram (EEG) is an age-sensitive marker. They hypothesize that attenuated first rapid eye movement (REM) period latency in prepubertal major depressives during depression-free states normalizes during depression. Thus, shortened first REM period latency may either represent a marker of trait or a marker of past depression. Therefore, sleep EEG might represent a "trait" marker for prepubertal depression. Additional research is required to determine whether the sleep EEG also represents a marker for depression in adolescents (Puig-Antich, 1986).

GENETIC APPROACH.   With qualifications, research supports the role of genetic transmission in the etiology of depression. For instance, Tsuang (1978) reported an average monozygotic twin concordance rate of 76 percent for mood disorders, 19 percent for dizygotic twins, and 67 percent concordance for monozygotic twins reared apart. However, the high average monozygotic concordance rate is perhaps mitigated by the likelihood that monozygotic twins develop in environments of greater similarity than dizygotic twins.

Puig-Antich (1980) reported a .42 lifetime morbidity risk for major depressive disorder in first degree relatives over 16 years of age. Because the morbidity risk for adults with major depressive disorder is .30, it has been assumed, reasonably, that prepubertal major depressives carry a heavier pathogenic loading than adults. However, the additional use of segregation and threshold models is required to test genetic hypotheses.

BIPOLAR DISORDER.   There is widespread evidence that bipolar illness occurs in families. Like unipolar depression, the specific role played by genetic factors remains unclear. For instance, while the wide range of bipolar morbid risk estimates among first degree relatives is partially explained by method variance, it also is possible that these estimates are affected by genetic heterogeneity (Strober et al, in press, a).

Because of the possibility of genetic heterogeneity, research has focused upon the relationship between age of onset of the illness and the degree of familial transmission. Studies by Dwyer and DeLong (1987) and by Strober, Morrell, and colleagues (in press, b) reported unexpectedly high lifetime prevalence rates of affective illness in the relatives of children and adolescent probands. A conclusion consistent with these findings is that early onset bipolar illness indicates a genetic diathesis of greater severity than later onset illness.

Psychological Models

PSYCHODYNAMIC. According to psychodynamic theorists, the loss of an ambivalently loved object causes anger to be turned inward. Depression is thought to be the result of this anger. This model is not supported by an empirical literature. The work of Bibring (1965) represents a second psychodynamic approach to the etiology of depression. According to Bibring, depression results from one's lack of ability to achieve one's ego ideals. A third psychodynamic approach to depression has been called an "object loss" model. Akiskal and McKinney (1975) reviewed the evidence for two posits of this approach, only one of which carries direct implications for childhood depression. According to the second posit, object loss in early childhood places an individual at risk for the development of depression in adulthood. However, if one assumes that the loss of a parent during childhood is the most traumatic object loss, then there is little support for this second posit because parental death during childhood does not carry etiologic significance in adult depression. For an additional discussion on the psychodynamics of depression, the reader is referred to the work of Bemporad (1978).

It is noteworthy that many of the following studies in the "psychological approaches" section rely upon what Eisenberg (1986) calls "psychometric depression." "Psychometric depression" defines depression by the use of cutting scores on measures of symptom severity. On the other hand, "clinical depression" is assessed via structured or semi-structured interviews keyed to *DSM-III* criteria. While some researchers assume that adolescents diagnosed by paper and pencil (psychometric) measures are clinically equivalent to adolescents diagnosed via clinical interviews, additional research is required to justify this assumption. Otherwise, using the label "depressed" to describe these two forms of depression when there is a low correspondence between these forms of "psychometric depression" and "clinical depression" may add confusion to the literature.

LIFE STRESS MODEL. According to the adult literature, antecedent life events most likely carry a facilitating, or maintaining, rather than an etiological relationship with depression. Moreover, as mentioned in the previous section, the empirical literature does not support an etiological link between parental death during childhood and later adult depression. Nevertheless, it remains plausible that parental separation or discord may supply a foundation for childhood depression. Furthermore, at least one study has reported that preschoolers with depressive symptomatology come from families who reported more stressful life events than appropriate controls (Kashani et al, 1986).

COGNITIVE DISTORTION MODEL. According to Beck (1976), maladaptive cognitions regarding the self, one's experiences (the world), and the future constitute what he terms the "cognitive triad." Beck proposes that a maladaptive developmental history might evolve from one that does not prepare the child for failure or one that overly sensitizes the child to failure. In theory, this developmental history leads to the formation of the cognitive triad, which results in hopelessness, helplessness, and depression.

Studies indicating the alteration of mood and psychometric depression via cognitive manipulations lend support that is consistent with Beck's formulation. Additional evidence that depressives report heightened sensitivity to the quality of negative and neutral experiences also supports Beck. Finally, depressives have been shown to distort their perceptions (or at least their reported perceptions) of the world by underestimating their receipt of high frequency feedback relative to nondepressives.

However, contrary data suggest that cognitive manipulations produce their effects through experimental demand. That is, the cues present in the experimental situation enable subjects to ascertain reasonably the experimental hypotheses and to alter their behavior so as to perform in accordance with these cues. Moreover, while Beck proposes that depressives overestimate the occurrence of negative self-evaluation, another literature indicates that depressives are actually more accurate in their judgments of negative self-relevant stimuli than nondepressives (Coyne and Gotlib, 1983).

In sum, it appears that support for the cognitive theory remains inconsistent. Moreover, it is not clear whether the existing support reflects the causes, co-effects, or consequences of depression. With this caveat in mind, the child literature does support the existence of the cognitive triad. First, the self-concepts of depressed children differ from those of nondepressed children (for example, Strauss et al, 1984). Second, a study lacking normal controls found that depressed inpatient children exhibit negative biases in their world views (Asarnow et al, 1987). Third, a negative view of the future has been reported in a clinic sample meeting *DSM-III* criteria for major depressive disorder and in children with depressive symptomatology (Kazdin et al, 1983b). Thus, it appears that depressed children do manifest the cognitive distortions outlined in Beck's cognitive triad. However, what remains unknown is the extent to which these cognitive "distortions" are rooted in a depressing environment, and the extent to which they are secondary to other causes (such as anger, guilt, and criticism turned against the self).

In the future, it would be interesting to examine whether a set of depressed children and adolescents perceive themselves and their environments more accurately than their nondepressed counterparts. Moreover, it is possible that, compared to depressed children, some nondepressed children manifest cognitive distortions by overestimating their abilities and their control over their environments.

SOCIAL SKILLS DEFICITS. According to this model, a reduction in the quality or quantity of social reinforcement causes or at least maintains depression. For instance, Lewinsohn and Hoberman (1982) hypothesize that social skills deficits lead to receipt of a low rate of response-contingent positive reinforcement, and the low response-contingent positive reinforcement causes depression. However, Youngren and Lewinsohn (1980) note that empirical support for this hypothesis is lacking. In addition, they report that the social skills deficits may be secondarily, rather than causally, related to depression.

There exists both supportive and disconfirming evidence for the role of social skills deficits in the etiology and/or maintenance of childhood depression. Examples of the former include lower peer ratings of depressed children's popularity, and lower teacher ratings of depressed children's social competence. Using multiple informants (child, peer, teacher), Reaven (1986) found that the constructs of social withdrawal, social competence, and negative social behavior predicted childhood depression. However, the study did not address the question of etiology.

Kaslow and colleagues (1984) report that indirect support for the etiological status of social skills deficits derives from the use of social skills training to treat childhood depression. Nevertheless, an intervention need not possess etiological status to carry therapeutic efficacy.

Disconfirming evidence comes from studies that relied heavily upon self-report measures. Consequently, it is possible that these measures assessed children's perceptions of how one ought to behave rather than how children themselves actually behave.

In sum, while the empirical literature indicates that focusing upon social skills deficits appears beneficial, many studies lack the inclusion of a nondepressed control group. Moreover, the reliance upon self-report measures of "psychometric depression," rather than upon structured diagnostic interviews, erodes the generalizability of these studies to clinic populations.

LEARNED HELPLESSNESS. According to the original formulation of learned helplessness theory (Seligman, 1975), the experience of uncontrollable events leads to the expectation that one lacks the ability to control future outcomes. This expectation of no control results in what have been termed "helplessness deficits," which assume the form of a) motivational, b) cognitive, and c) emotional deficits. As with many developing theories, shortcomings of the original model soon became apparent and a reformulation was proposed (Abramson et al, 1978).

The reformulated theory married attribution theory with what was then, for the most part, an animal model extrapolated to humans. The reformulation represents a cognitive diathesis model applied to depression. According to the reformulation, the explanation that one gives for outcomes modulates expectancies for future outcomes and, thus, for one's reactions to the outcomes. To illustrate, if an individual experiences a bad outcome and if his or her explanatory style invokes internal, stable, and global causes, then that person is at risk for depression. Consequently, explanatory style alone is insufficient to produce learned helplessness deficits.

Using a community school sample of 8- to 13-year-old children with depressive symptoms, Seligman and colleagues (1984) found that children with depressive symptoms were more likely than the "nondepressed" to endorse internal, stable, and global explanations for bad events. The authors also reasoned that because mothers' attributional style (but not fathers') correlated with the styles and symptoms of their children, the child may learn the attributional style or the depressive symptoms from the mother and, subsequently, child and mother may maintain each other's depressive styles.

Nolen-Hoeksema and co-workers (1986) again relied upon a community school sample of "psychometrically depressed" children, this time with ages ranging from 8 to 11 years. Maladaptive explanatory style was found to correlate with concurrent "depression" and to predict later depression. Furthermore, the predictive power of explanatory style was neither due to its being a symptom of "depression" nor to the influence of earlier depression on explanatory style. It is noteworthy that an attempt recently has been made to cast the "helplessness" theory of depression as a "hopelessness" theory of depression (Alloy et al, 1988).

In future research, the learned helplessness account of childhood depression will profit from longitudinal designs extending beyond one year. Moreover, the research should include a sample of clinically depressed children and adolescents to investigate the correspondence between "psychometric depression" and clinical depression in childhood and adolescence.

SELF-CONTROL.   Kanfer's (1970) seminal work on self-control underpins Lynn Rehm's model of depression (Rehm, 1977). According to the self-control model of depression, depressives are deficient in at least one of the following areas: 1) self-monitoring; 2) self-evaluation; and 3) self-reinforcement. Deficits in these three areas may take the form of: 1) the selective focusing of attention upon negative events; 2) the focusing of attention upon immediate rather than upon delayed consequences of one's actions; 3) the setting of unrealistic and unattainable performance criteria; 4) the misattribution of personal success and failure; 5) an insufficient amount of self-reinforcement; and 6) excessive self-punishment.

Cole and Rehm (1986) tested the third, fifth, and sixth implications of the model from a family systems perspective. The results indicated that mothers of depressed adolescents do reward less. In addition, high standard-setting distinguished depressed clinic children from nondepressed clinic children but not from normal controls. No other predictions received support.

FAMILY SYSTEMS APPROACH.   While published in 1949, the work of Dewey and Bentley remains influential today. According to these authors, transactional models represent the highest level of scientific inquiry, whereas models at the level of self-action (that is, self-control, cognitive distortion, and so on) as the sole explanations of a construct (that is, childhood depression) are to be rejected by a sophisticated science. The family systems approach is a transactional approach that provides a contextual means of viewing depression in children, adolescents, and adults. Thus, unlike diagnostic taxonomies that attempt to classify children as having pathology located within themselves, general systems theory views childhood depression as a behavior maintained by various interacting systems and subsystems.

One implication of systems theory is that both etiology and early childhood history lose their importance in suggesting intervention. Instead, treatment focuses upon the aspects of system functioning that maintain or make the depression necessary for the system. For instance, Minuchin (1974) has defined two broad classes of symptoms. The implication of a *system-maintained symptom* for childhood depression is that the various systems and subsystems of which the child is a member maintain the depression. On the other hand, a *system-maintaining symptom* means that the childhood depression functions to maintain the family system. For example, by directing the parents' attention away from their marital difficulties and toward his behavior, the depressed child may unintentionally function to decrease marital strife.

Coyne (1976) was one of the first researchers to explicate the role of the family in the *maintenance* of depression. Since that time, numerous researchers have investigated the links between various aspects of systemic function and childhood depression. The aforementioned work of Cole and Rehm (1986) serves as one example of this research. Future research would benefit from the use of direct observations of parent–child relations in order to reveal the sequential nature of these reciprocal interactions. Moreover, because of the differences between these groups, subtypes of child and adolescent depression should be studied separately, rather than combined as a whole.

EPIDEMIOLOGY

In this section, sex- and age-related demographic data are reviewed in both general population and clinically referred samples. We include general population studies because they provide normative child data on the spectrum of psychopathology among individuals who may never be referred to clinicians.

Age

We are unaware of the existence of any published data applying *DSM-III* criteria to samples of infants.

PRESCHOOLERS.   The last few years have witnessed major advances in the understanding of depression within this age group. Through the use of adult diagnostic criteria (Kashani et al, 1984; Kashani and Carlson, 1987), these studies provide substantial evidence for the existence of major depressive disorder in preschoolers as young as three years of age. Kashani and colleagues (1983, 1986) reported on two samples of preschoolers from the general population in which there was only one depressed child among 350 preschoolers (0.3 percent). In another comprehensively evaluated, clinically referred sample of 1,000 preschoolers, only 9 (less than 1 percent) met the adult criteria for major depressive disorder (Kashani and Carlson, 1987). Based upon these results, the authors concluded that the diagnosis of depressive disorder using adult criteria represents an infrequent finding in preschool-age children.

Prepubertal

The frequency of major depressive disorder in this age group has been studied both in the general population and in clinically referred samples. Using two independent, nonreferred samples, Kashani and co-workers found that about 1.8 percent of the prepubertal children in New Zealand (1983) and 1.9 percent of those in the United States (1979) met *DSM-III* criteria for major depressive disorder. Shifting to inpatient child psychiatry samples, Kazdin and colleagues (1983a) found 15 percent of their sample to be depressed. Similarly, Kashani and co-workers (1982) reported 13 percent of their referred sample to be depressed.

Adolescents

A recent study by Kashani and associates (1987) utilized structured interviews with community sample adolescents ranging in age from 14 to 16 years. The authors reported a prevalence of major depressive disorder in this age group which was more than twice that found among prepubertal children. In addition to satisfying *DSM-III* criteria for major depressive disorder, 4.7 percent of the adolescents were judged to be dysfunctional and in need of treatment. The finding that depression increases with age from childhood through adolescence has also been reported by Rutter (1986b), who found that the number of 14-year-olds with depressive disorder was thrice that of 10-year-olds.

As one might expect, the frequency of major depressive disorder for hospitalized adolescents is much greater than it is in community settings. To illustrate, Robbins and colleagues (1982) reported major depressive disorder in about 28 percent of the adolescents in their sample.

Sex

The frequency of depression in prepubertal children has been reported to be similar in both males and females. However, with increasing age, the prevalence of both depressive symptoms and depressive disorders becomes greater in girls than in boys (Kashani et al, 1987; Rutter, 1986a). While the reason for this is not yet clearly understood, several explanations have been proposed. Among them are biological factors (that is, sex-specific hormonal changes and rates of sexual maturity) and social factors (Rutter, 1986b).

In summary, although epidemiology is in part concerned with the frequency of occurrence of a given disorder, the consideration of demographic variables (that is, age, sex) yields important information. However, the main thrust of the epidemiology of mood disorders involves the constant surveillance of age- and/or sex-specific factors, as well as other variables that contribute to the development and/or maintenance of mood disorders.

COMORBIDITY

The development of the structured interview in adult and child psychiatry has improved the reliability and validity of psychiatric diagnosis in numerous ways. For instance, the use of structured interviews diminishes both information and criterion variance, which results in improved standardization. In addition, the breadth of the structured interview enables the gathering of a wide variety of data across diverse behavioral domains. Consequently, the ability to reliably and validly diagnose additional disorders increases. Furthermore, the use of the structured interview, both clinically and in research, has aided in the diagnosis of disorders that otherwise would have been missed unless they represented the foci of specific scientific inquiry.

Using structured interviews keyed to *DSM-III* criteria, researchers recently have identified the coexistence of psychiatric disorders in both children and adolescents. For instance, Orvaschel et al. (1987) reported the coexistence of depression and attention deficit disorder in the children of parents with unipolar depression. The authors also reported that, based upon the parental history, attention deficit disorder preceded the onset of depression (Orvaschel, 1987). Carlson and Cantwell (1980) reported similar results. Although attention deficit disorder in depressed children and adolescents has been thought by some authors to be a precursor of mania in later life (Strober et al, in press, b), the significance of this comorbidity remains unclear.

In recent years, numerous studies (Chiles et al, 1980; Puig-Antich, 1982) have supported the coexistence of conduct disorder with depression. For instance, an uncontrolled study by Puig-Antich (1982) reported that about one-third of his sample of boys fitting Research Diagnostic Criteria for major depressive disorder also fit the *DSM-III* criteria for conduct disorder. Furthermore, he noted the disappearance of conduct disorder in depressed children treated with antidepressants and concluded that the conduct disorder was superimposed on a pre-existing depression. Opposed to this conclusion is the work of Kovacs and her colleagues (1984). These researchers reported that conduct disorder preceded, rather than followed, the onset of depression. Because of these conflicting findings, firm conclusions cannot be drawn at this time.

The most frequently occurring comorbidity has been reported for depression and anxiety. For instance, Kovacs and colleagues (1984) reported that 33 percent of the depressed children in their sample had a coexisting anxiety disorder. This frequency of comorbidity has also been reported by other authors (Ryan et al, 1987; Kashani et al, 1987).

The question as to which condition is primary and which is secondary is presently unanswerable. However, data presented by Stavrakaki and co-workers (1987) indicate that while younger anxious children are not concurrently depressed, older depressed children are concurrently anxious. Stavrakaki and colleagues hypothesized that anxiety develops first with depression later superimposed on the anxiety symptoms.

Seligman (1975) has reported two stages of response to situations involving loss, danger, or threat with both infrahuman and human samples. According to Seligman, the subject initially responds to danger with anxiety, which disappears after the threatening condition is brought under control. However, if the threat persists, the anxiety also persists. In future situations where the individual perceives a continuing inability to control the danger, depression results. The depression is said to stem from the loss of control over reinforcing factors and the ensuing learned helplessness.

Most of the studies cited above involve *DSM-III* Axis I dignoses. This state of affairs is probably due to the fact that most of the structured interviews for children and adolescents are based upon Axis I rather than Axis II criteria. Although not as numerous, there are a few studies that include *DSM-III* Axis II diagnoses. For instance, McManus et al. (1984) found that 25 percent of an inpatient adolescent sample with a diagnosis of borderline personality had a coexisting major depression.

In conclusion, the study of comorbidity adds to our knowledge base and improves patient care. Treating one disorder while remaining ignorant of a co-occurring disorder is suboptimal. Instead, the treatment plan should consider the whole person by sampling across numerous behavioral domains and by utilizing different theoretical approaches in order to maximize patient care.

DEVELOPMENTAL PERSPECTIVES

The question of whether adult diagnostic criteria are applicable to the diagnosis of depression in children and adolescents continues to interest clinical researchers. There is evidence that depression exists in a wide age range (that is, from preschool age through preadolescence and into adulthood). However, it is questionable whether the capability for feeling and expressing depressive symptoms among these age groups remains constant. Because of this, several authors advocate a model of child and adolescent depression based on developmental theory. For instance, Cicchetti and Schneider-Rosen (1986) argue that children of different ages and diverse developmental stages have unique life experiences and consequently are not likely to manifest symptomatology in the same way as adults who no longer experience the rapidly changing, multifaceted developmental dynamics of preadulthood. Instead, they propose that preadults experience depressive symptomatology in a wide variety of age-appropriate and developmentally specific ways.

Garber (1984) recommends identifying age-appropriate signs and symptoms that take into account the individual's level of functioning in the cognitive, affective, and social domains. She also notes that the developmental approach does not recommend abandoning the symptom-complex approach to diagnosis. Instead, a developmental approach urges the clinical researcher to look beyond the symptom-complex by: 1) identifying phase-specific manifestations of childhood depression and eliminating age-appropriate symptoms; 2) broadening symptom definitions in order to encompass phenomenologically relevant developmental differences; and 3) enlarging the diagnostic perspective through the inclusion of new categories (that is, level of adaptation and competence).

Rutter (1986a) notes that children are developing individuals and not small adults. Consistent with this notion is his recommendation that researchers investigate age-dependent variations in susceptibility to stress, which he feels might account for differing depression prevalence rates across age groups. Differing prevalence rates across age groups are indicative of these variations in stress susceptibility. Moreover, Rutter stresses the importance of identifying manifestations of depression at various age levels from psychosocial, cognitive, and biological perspectives.

Carlson and Garber (1986) proposed some changes in the diagnostic process to reflect this developmental perspective. They noted that aside from dysphoric mood, *DSM-III* criteria for major depressive disorder give equal weight to the remaining eight depressive signs/symptoms. Therefore, they suggest a more complex set of diagnostic rules comprising a three-tiered process.

The first tier encompasses a set of core indicators. This group of signs/symptoms is hypothesized to occur with equal frequency in all age groups. Because a certain number of these core indicators would be necessary, but insufficient for a diagnosis of depression, the first tier appears similar to the current *DSM-III/DSM-III-R* structures.

The second set of indicators is comprised of depressive signs/symptoms which rarely occur in children. Extreme guilt is an example of a second tier indicator. If present, each indicator would be counted as a depressive sign/symptom. If absent, the diagnosis of depression is not necessarily precluded.

The third set of indicators includes those signs/symptoms which are highly associated with childhood depression (such as social withdrawal), but are not among those essential symptoms required by *DSM-III-R*. However, if these symptoms are present, they are included among the required number of symptoms for depression. Therefore, by carrying different weights, the presence (or absence) of various depressive symptoms contributes to the formation of a diagnostic format of greater flexibility than the one in current use.

In a recent study, Ryan and colleagues (1987) studied depressed children and adolescents who were referred to their clinic. The authors recommended that some symptoms which are not core symptoms of depression in *DSM-III* (i.e., somatic complaints, social withdrawal) be considered for inclusion among the diagnostic criteria for this age group.

It appears that age-appropriate symptom manifestations are crucial to these developmental considerations. Carlson and Garber (1986) state that there is not much difference between depression in adolescents and adults. However, they do suggest that modification of the adult criteria becomes necessary with decreasing age. Accordingly, the cognitive and verbal expression abilities of the preschooler necessitate a modification in the methods of data collection. For instance, the use of multiple sources of information, and the utilization of toys and play to elicit age-appropriate depressive symptomatology, will help gear the assessment toward the child's level of functioning (Kashani and Carlson, 1987).

TREATMENT

Treatment issues are especially important because of the relationship between mood disorders and suicide. It should be clear from the foregoing review that the two major approaches—biological and psychological—to the treatment of child and adolescent mood disorders generally lack support for their etiological status. The systems approach does not concern itself with questions regarding etiology. Instead, it focuses upon the maintenance of depression. However, from the treatment outcome literature, it appears that the lack of empirical support for a theoretical model does not prevent the related intervention from carrying therapeutic efficacy.

It is important to note that studies involving children and adolescents utilize different definitions of clinical improvement. Thus, it remains possible that pharmacologic interventions bring clinical improvement of depressive symptoms to the relative neglect of enhanced performance in the interpersonal, school, and family realms. In addition, it is recommended that use of these agents be limited to clinical depression. Moreover, because of the delay between drug trial initiation and the onset of clinical response, pharmacological agents should be used cautiously when the risk of suicide is great.

While tricyclic antidepressants appear effective in treating childhood depression when therapeutic blood plasma levels are maintained (Preskorn et al, 1982), it remains unclear whether this therapeutic effect surpasses the placebo effect (Puig-Antich et al, 1987). Moreover, no relationship between drug plasma level and clinical response has been obtained in adolescent samples. There is evidence of greater lethality among DST nonsuppressors who attempt suicide than in suppressors.

The research on monoamine oxidase inhibitors (MAOIs) in childhood depression is methodologically flawed. MAOI trials with children suffering from major depressive disorder do not yet exist. Like studies using tricyclics, studies involving MAOIs have not explored their impact upon children's academic performance. As an aside, it is possible that the DST will be useful as a state marker for monitoring treatment response to pharmacological agents.

While there is support for the efficacy of lithium in the treatment of cyclic behavioral disorders that mimic bipolar illness (Davis, 1979; DeLong, 1978) and in the treatment of *DSM-III* diagnosed mania in prepubertal children (Varanka et al, in press), this support is tentative. To date, few double-blind placebo controlled studies exist. An additional, often overlooked problem, is that of lithium resistance in adolescents. Moreover, data from long-term studies are presently nonexistent.

While useful for heuristic purposes, psychodynamic approaches with children are, for the most part, unsupported by an empirical literature. This may prove problematic in an era when cost effectiveness and documented treatment efficacy determine treatment selection.

The antecedent life stress approach with children has received considerably less research attention than the approach has with adults. One suggestion for future child and adolescent research is to study antecedent life stress and coping in response to stress as a dynamic, unfolding process, rather than as a static unitary event or as an aggregation of stresses.

Beck's cognitive theory has benefited from outcome research in which his cognitive therapy has initially surpassed imipramine treatment for psychometrically depressed adults (Rush et al, 1977). Finding the same with a group of clinically depressed children would contribute substantially to the outcome literature.

While the social skills approach appears important in at least the maintenance of child and adolescent depression, we were not able to locate controlled outcome research utilizing this treatment approach with either children or adolescents. In addition to the promise of this approach, it is conceivable that the concomitant use of pharmacological agents might further enhance treatment efficacy.

The work of Seligman and his colleagues indicates that both clinic and nonclinic samples of children employ explanatory styles similar to those of clinic and nonclinic adult inpatients. Moreover, children's explanatory styles have shown stability over the course of one year (Nolen-Hoeksema et al, 1986). An implication of Seligman's cognitive diathesis model is that attribution retraining (Dweck, 1975) can be used to correct explanatory styles known to precipitate psychometric depression. Outcome studies employing attribution retraining using clinically depressed, clinically nondepressed, and nonclinic children and adolescents would benefit this line of research.

As partially tested by Cole and Rehm (1986), the self-control model of depression has received limited support. However, it is possible that their use of a 10-minute laboratory sample of family interaction was inadequate to capture the naturalistic (that is, home) interactions of family members. As a result, the model's efficacy as a basis for treatment remains unclear. What is clearer is that Cole and Rehm (1986) chose to partially test the model from a family systems perspective.

According to family systems theory, child and adolescent depression is best viewed as part of the social context in which the symptomatology exists. Because the pathological behavior is inextricably intertwined with the family system, family therapy is the treatment of choice. Frequently, therapy involves the restructuring of family dynamics to decrease the functional utility of the depression. While preliminary support exists for the nonspecific contribution of child-reported family relations to childhood depression, this research is in its infancy. The use of sequential analyses in the home environment will benefit future research. No outcome studies on the efficacy of family therapy for the specific treatment of child or adolescent mood disorders were located for this review.

We have presented numerous approaches to both the etiology (and/or maintenance) and treatment of child and adolescent mood disorders. At this stage a brief reflection on the broad theoretical assumptions in the field is appropriate. While models that locate pathology within the individual continue to receive considerable research attention, an emphasis upon the reciprocal exchange between person and environment shows that child and adolescent depression researchers are becoming increasingly sophisticated in their conceptualization of psychopathology. While transactional approaches currently take the form of family systems theory, there is no reason to expect that other approaches need remain unidirectional. For instance, it is plausible to propose that once the mechanism(s) by which tricyclics work to alleviate childhood depression is (are) revealed, these mechanisms will also prove to be transactional in nature. Moreover, transactional approaches are highly compatible with developmental approaches that are only of late receiving more adequate research attention.

It is thought-provoking to glance several decades into the future. Perhaps during that time, what experimental-clinical researchers now conceptualize as the result of inputs into a final common pathway will then occupy a more central position in a transactional approach to the developmental psychopathology of mood disorders.

REFERENCES

Abramson LY, Seligman MEP, Teasdale JD: Learned helplessness in humans: critique and reformulation. J Abnorm Psychol 1978; 87:4974

Alloy LB, Abramson LY, Metalsky GI, et al: The hopelessness theory of depression: attributional aspects. Br J Clin Psychol 1988; 27:5–21

Akiskal HS, McKinney WT: Overview of recent research in depression. Arch Gen Psychiatry 1975; 32:285–305

American Psychiatric Association: Diagnostic and Statistical Manual of Mental Disorders, Third Edition (DSM-III). Washington, DC, American Psychiatric Association, 1980

American Psychiatric Association: Diagnostic and Statistical Manual of Mental Disorders, Third Edition, Revised (DSM-III-R). Washington, DC, American Psychiatric Association, 1987

Asarnow JR, Carlson GA, Guthrie D: Coping strategies, self-perceptions, hopelessness, and perceived family environments in depressed and suicidal children. J Consult Clin Psychol 1987; 55:361–366

Beck AT: Cognitive Therapy and the Emotional Disorders. New York, International Universities Press, 1976

Bemporad J: Psychodynamics of depression and suicide in children and adolescents, in Severe and Mild Depression. Edited by Arieti S, Bemporad J. New York, Basic Books, 1978

Bibring E: The mechanism of depression, in Affective Disorders. Edited by Greenacre P. New York, International Universities Press, 1965

Cantwell DP: Depression in childhood: clinical picture and diagnostic criteria, in Affective Disorders in Childhood and Adolescence: An Update. Edited by Cantwell DP, Carlson GA. New York, Spectrum Publications, 1983

Carlson GA, Cantwell DP: Unmasking masked depression in children and adolescents. Am J Psychiatry 1980; 137:445–449

Carlson GA, Garber J: Developmental issues in the classification of depression in children, in Depression in Young People: Developmental and Clinical Perspectives. Edited by Rutter M, Izard CE, Read PB. New York, Guilford Press, 1986

Casat CD: The under- and over-diagnosis of mania in children and adolescents. Compr Psychiatry 1982; 23:552–559

Chiles JA, Miller ML, Cox GB: Depression in an adolescent delinquent population. Arch Gen Psychiatry 1980; 37:1179–1184

Cicchetti D, Schneider-Rosen K: An organizational approach to childhood depression, in Depression in Young People: Developmental and Clinical Perspectives. Edited by Rutter M, Izard CE, Read PE. New York, Guilford Press, 1986

Cole DA, Rehm LP: Family interaction patterns and childhood depression. J Abnorm Child Psychol 1986; 14:297–314

Coyne JC: Toward an interactional description of depression. Psychiatry 1976; 39:28–40

Coyne JC, Gotlib IH: The role of cognition in depression: a critical appraisal. Psychol Bull 1983; 94:472–505

Cytryn L, McKnew DH: Proposed classification of childhood depression. Am J Psychiatry 1972; 129:2

Cytryn L, McKnew DH, Logue M, et al: Biochemical correlates of affective disorders in children. Arch Gen Psychiatry 1974; 31:659–661

Cytryn L, McKnew DH, Bunney WE: Diagnosis of depression in children: a reassessment. Am J Psychiatry 1980; 137:22–25

Davis RE: Manic depressive variant syndrome of childhood: a preliminary report. Am J Psychiatry 1979; 136:702–705

DeLong GR: Lithium carbonate treatment of select behavior disorders suggesting manic-depressive illness. J Pediatr 1978; 93:689–694

Dewey J, Bentley AF: Knowing and the known. Boston, Beacon Press, 1949

Digdon N, Gotlib IH: Developmental considerations in the study of childhood depression, in Developmental Review, vol. 5. Troy, MO, Academic Press, Inc., 1985

Dweck CS: The role of expectations and attributions in the alleviation of learned helplessness. J Pers Soc Psychol 1975; 31:674–685

Dwyer JT, DeLong GR: A family history study of twenty probands with childhood manic-depressive illness. J Am Acad Child Adolesc Psychiatry 1987; 26:176–180

Eisenberg L: When is a case a case?, in Depression in Young People: Developmental and Clinical Perspectives. Edited by Rutter M, Izard CE, Read PB. New York, Guilford, 1986

Everett GM, Toman JEP: Mode of action of rauwolfia alkaloids and motor activity, in Biological Psychiatry, vol. 1. Edited by Masserman JH. New York, Grune and Stratton, 1959

Feighner JP, Robins E, Guze SB, et al: Diagnostic criteria for use in psychiatric research. Arch Gen Psychiatry 1972; 26:56–73

Garber J: The developmental progression of depression in female children, in Childhood Depression, no. 26. Edited by Cicchetti D, Schneider-Rosen K. San Francisco, Jossey-Bass, 1984

Grinspoon L (Ed): Psychiatry 1982: American Psychiatric Association Annual Review, vol. 1. Washington, DC, American Psychiatric Press, Inc, 1982

Kanfer FH: Self-monitoring: methodological limitations and clinical applications. J Consult Clin Psychol 1970; 35:148–152

Kashani JH, Carlson GA: Seriously depressed preschoolers. Am J Psychiatry 1987; 144:348–350

Kashani J, Ray JS: Depressive symptoms among preschool-age children. Child Psychiatry Hum Dev 1983; 13:233–238

Kashani J, Simonds JF: The incidence of depression in children. Am J Psychiatry 1979; 136:1203–1205

Kashani JH, Cantwell DP, Shekim WO, et al: Major depressive disorder in children admitted to an inpatient community mental health center. Am J Psychiatry 1982; 139:671–672

Kashani J, McGee RO, Clarkson SE, et al: Depression in a sample of 9-year-old children. Arch Gen Psychiatry 1983; 40:1217–1222

Kashani JH, Ray JS, Carlson GA: Depression and depression-like states in preschool-age children in a child development unit. Am J Psychiatry 1984; 141:1397–1402

Kashani JH, Holcomb WR, Orvaschel H: Depression and depressive symptomatology in preschool children from the general population. Am J Psychiatry 1986; 143:1138–1143

Kashani JH, Carlson GA, Beck NC, et al: Depression, depressive symptoms, and depressed mood among a community sample of adolescents. Am J Psychiatry 1987; 144:931–934

Kaslow NJ, Rehm LP, Seigel AW: Social-cognitive and cognitive correlates of depression in children. J Abnorm Psychol 1984; 12:605–620

Kazdin AE, French NH, Unis AS, et al: Assessment of childhood depression: correspondence of child and parent ratings. J Am Acad Child Psychiatry 1983a; 22:157–164

Kazdin AE, French NB, Unis AS, et al: Hopelessness, depression and suicidal intent among psychiatrically disturbed inpatient children. J Consult Clin Psychol 1983b; 51:504–510

Klein DN, Depue RA, Slater JF: Cyclothymia in the adolescent offspring of parents with bipolar affective disorder. J Abnorm Psychol 1985; 94:115–127

Kovacs M, Feinberg TL, Crouse-Novak M, et al: Depressive disorders in childhood. Arch Gen Psychiatry 1984; 41:643–649

Lewinsohn PM, Hoberman HM: Depression, in International Handbook of Behavior Modification and Therapy. Edited by Belluk AS, Heren M, Kazdin AE. New York, Plenum Press, 1982

Ling W, Oftedal G, Weinberg W: Depressive illness in childhood presenting as severe headache. Am J Dis Child 1970; 120:122–124

Malmquist CP: Depressions in childhood and adolescence (first of two parts). N Engl J Med 1971; 284

McConville BJ, Boag LC, Purohit AP: Three types of childhood depression. Canadian Psychiatric Association Journal 1973; 18

McManus M, Alessi NE, Grapentine WL, et al: Psychiatric disturbance in serious delinquents. J Am Acad Child Psychiatry 1984; 23:602–615

Minuchin S: Families and Family Therapy. Cambridge, MA, Harvard University Press, 1974

Nolen-Hoeksema S, Girgus JS, Seligman MEP: Learned helplessness in children: a longitudinal study of depression, achievement, and explanatory style. J Pers Soc Psychol 1986; 51:435–442

Orvaschel H, Ye W, Walsh-Allis G: Comorbidity of ADD and depression in children at risk for affective disorder. Paper presented at the 34th annual meeting of the American Academy of Child and Adolescent Psychiatry. Washington, DC, October 1987

Philips I: Childhood depression: interpersonal interactions and depressive phenomena. Am J Psychiatry 1979; 136:511–515

Poznanski E, Zrull JP: Childhood depression: clincal characteristics of overtly depressed children. Arch Gen Psychiatry 1970; 23:8–15

Poznanski E, Cook S, Carroll B: A depression rating scale for children. Pediatrics 1979; 64:442–450

Poznanski E, Mokros HB, Grossman J, et al: Diagnostic criteria in childhood depression. Am J Psychiatry 1985; 142:1168–1173

Preskorn SH, Weller EB, Weller RA: Depression in children: relationship between plasma imipramine levels and response. J Clin Psychol 1982; 43:450–453

Puig-Antich J: Affective disorders in childhood. Psychiatr Clin North Am 1980; 3:403–424

Puig-Antich J: Major depression and conduct disorder in prepuberty. J Am Acad Child Psychiatry 1982; 21:118–128

Puig-Antich J: Psychobiological markers: effects of age and puberty, in Depression in Young People: Developmental and Clinical Perspectives. Edited by Rutter M, Izard CE, Read PB. New York, Guilford Press, 1986

Puig-Antich J, Perel JM, Lupatkin W, et al: Imipramine in prepubertal major depressive disorders. Arch Gen Psychiatry 1987; 44:81–89

Reaven N: Depression and social functioning in children. Unpublished doctoral dissertation, University of Missouri–Columbia, 1986

Rehm LP: A self-control model of depression. Behavior Therapy 1977; 8:787–804

Robbins DR, Alessi NE, Cook SC, et al: The use of the research diagnostic criteria for depression in adolescent psychiatric inpatients. J Am Acad Child Psychiatry 1982; 21:251–255

Rush AJ, Beck AT, Kovacs M, et al: Comparative efficacy of cognitive therapy and pharmacotherapy in the treatment of depressed outpatients. Cognitive Therapy and Research 1977; 1:17–37

Rutter M: Depressive feelings, cognitions, and disorders: a research postscript, in Depression in Young People: Developmental and Clinical Perspectives. Edited by Rutter M, Izard CE, Read PB. New York, Guilford Press, 1986a

Rutter M: Child psychiatry: The interface beween clinical and developmental research. Psychol Med 1986b; 16:151–169

Ryan ND, Puig-Antich J: Affective illness in adolescence, in the American Psychiatric Association Annual Review, vol. 5. Edited by Frances AJ, Hales RE. Washington, DC, American Psychiatric Press, Inc., 1986

Ryan ND, Puig-Antich J, Ambrosini P, et al: The clinical picture of major depression in children and adolescents. Arch Gen Psychiatry 1987; 44:854–861

Seligman MEP: Helplessness: On Depression, Development and Death. San Francisco, Freeman and Company, 1975

Seligman MEP, Peterson C, Kaslow NJ, et al: Attributional style and depressive symptoms among children. J Abnorm Psychol 1984; 93:235–238

Stavrakaki C, Vargo B, Boodoosingh L, et al: The relationship between anxiety and depression in children: rating scales and clinical variables. Can J Psychiatry 1987; 32:433–439

Strauss CC, Forehand R, Frame C, et al: Characteristics of children with extreme scores on the children's depression inventory. J Clin Child Psychol 1984; 13:227–231

Strober M, Hanna G, McCracken J: Bipolar illness, in Handbook of Child Psychiatric Diagnosis. Edited by Last C, Hersen M. New York, John Wiley & Sons (in press, a)

Strober M, Morrell W, Burroughs J, et al: A family study of bipolar I disorder in adolescence: early onset of symptoms linked to increased familial loading and lithium resistance. J Affective Disord (in press, b)

Tsuang MT: Genetic counseling for psychiatric patients and their families. Am J Psychiatry 1978; 135:1465–1475

Varanka TM, Weller EB, Weller RA, et al: Lithium treatment of prepubertal manic children with psychotic features. J Affective Disord (in press)

Weinberg WA, Rutman J, Sullivan L, et al: Depression in children referred to an educational diagnostic center: diagnosis and treatment. J Pediatr 1973; 83:1065–1072

Weller EB, Weller RA, Fristad MA, et al: The dexamethasone suppression test in hospitalized prepubertal depressed children. Am J Psychiatry 1984; 141:290–291

Weller RA, Weller EB, Fristad MA, et al: A comparison of the cortisol suppression index and the dexamethasone suppression test in prepubertal children. Am J Psychiatry 1985; 142:1370–1372

Youngren MA, Lewinsohn PM: The functional relationship between depression and problematic interpersonal behavior. J Abnorm Psychol 1980; 89:333–341

Chapter 11

Mental Retardation

by Ludwik S. Szymanski, M.D., I. Leslie Rubin, M.D., and George Tarjan, M.D.

Mental retardation is a term used to characterize the level of intellectual as well as adaptive functioning of an individual. It does not say anything about etiology, pathogenesis, prognosis, or management. Despite its rather nonspecific and relatively unsubstantial phenomenology, it is a powerful, emotion-laden term, for both the individual and society. For these reasons it becomes vital to understand clearly the appropriate use of this term, the context in which it may be used, its implications for the patient and the family, its long-term management, and what it means in terms of the roles of the physician, particularly the psychiatrist.

The field of mental retardation has progressed considerably in the past three decades, as demonstrated in four main areas. First, we have gained an understanding of the cause of many cases of mental retardation, due to discoveries of the pathogenesis of various syndromes associated with it. Second, some of these syndromes can now be treated or prevented. Third, attitudes toward retarded persons and the care given to them have changed dramatically, from neglect and segregation in custodial facilities to active treatment, education and integration in the community. Fourth, and most relevant for mental health professionals, is the increased understanding that retarded persons are at risk for the same kinds of mental disorders as those encountered in the general population, and concomitant advances in the techniques of diagnosis and treatment of these disorders.

PSYCHIATRY, MENTAL RETARDATION, AND SOCIETY

The care of retarded children dates to the beginnings of psychiatry as a medical profession. The French physician Jean-Marc-Gaspard Itard described the treatment of Victor, the famous "wild boy of Aveyron," who was a severely deprived child, affected with spasmodic movements, apparently exhibiting self-stimulatory behaviors, with poor attention and poor ability for interpersonal relationships (Lane, 1976). Today he might meet the criteria for a pervasive developmental disorder with mental retardation. Itard's student, Edouard Seguin, devoted his professional life to the education of retarded children. His follower, Dr. Samuel Gridley Howe, was the first to establish programs for retarded children based on principles of education, family living, and mainstreaming in the society. The American Association for Mental Deficiency evolved from the organization started in 1876 by psychiatrists who were superintendents of schools for retarded persons.

The relationship of psychiatry to mental retardation reflects both the evolution of society's attitudes toward mentally retarded persons and the evolution of psychiatry as a profession. Through most of the years between the era of Howe and our time, psychiatrists gradually stopped serving retarded children. This reflected society's changing view of the retarded child from one who was educable but needing to be protected, to one who was a potential source of criminality, moral debasement, and from whom the society needed protection by involuntary segregation in custodial institutions and even by sterilization. Second, psychiatrists' perceived professional roles with the retarded children evolved from the initial role of humanistic educator, diagnostician, and therapist, to neuropathologist, diagnostician, and administrator. With the advent of a psychoanalytic orientation, which considered intact cognition, language, and insight as prerequisite for therapeutic success, the retarded children became less a focus of psychiatric attention. The first half of the 20th century, called a "tragic interlude" (Donaldson and Menolascino, 1977), was characterized by the mass institutionalization of retarded persons, with psychiatrists functioning as diagnosticians and administrative "gatekeepers" for the institutions. While mental retardation continued to be considered a province of child psychiatry, the psychiatrists became more and more ignorant of the subject. In a 1975 survey by the American Academy of Child Psychiatry, only about one-half of child psychiatry training programs included mental retardation related topics in their curricula. In textbooks the emphasis was given to the minute delineation of phenotypical features of mental retardation syndromes (although a psychiatrist rarely needed to diagnose them, such diagnoses usually being made by a pediatrician).

On the other hand, rarely anything was mentioned about the existence, much less about the diagnosis and treatment, of mental disorders in retarded children. Philips (1966) pointed out three then-prevalent misconceptions about mentally retarded children (which are still encountered today): first, that their behavior is a function of the retardation, rather than of interpersonal relationships; second, that emotional disorders of retarded children are different in kind; and third, that their maladaptive behavior patterns are the result of organic brain damage. Woodward and colleagues (1970) pointed out the psychiatrist's obsession with classifying children's disorders into organic and nonorganic. The psychiatrists were still considered the experts in the diagnosis of mental retardation, usually done on the basis of IQ alone. Such diagnosis was necessary for placement in an institution or in special classes. Deprived, poor, and non-English-speaking immigrant children tested low, and thus often would be classified as retarded (Sarason and Doris, 1979), while mildly retarded middle class children would often be considered as having a neurotically based learning block, a "need not to know," and would receive long term psychotherapy to improve their IQ.

In the 1960s society's attitudes toward mentally retarded persons started to change as the result of the work of parents' groups, the initiative of President Kennedy, and landmark court decisions on the right of these persons to education and treatment. The concept of normalization developed in Scandinavia (Wolfensberger, 1972) stated that mentally retarded persons should be given opportunities in everyday life that are as close to usual ways of life as possible. This has been interpreted as the right to live in circumstances that are most normal and least restrictive. The current standards of care for retarded children include the right to live in a family environment and, at present, retarded children are rarely put in institutions. Their families obtain a variety of supports and if they still cannot provide for the child's needs, placement with specially trained foster parents or adoptive parents increasingly are becoming available.

The Public Law (PL) 94–142 and state laws that followed established the right of all retarded children to public education and necessary services. The PL 99–457 of 1987 requires the states to develop early intervention services for handicapped children from birth to three years, and mandates free public education and services for handicapped children from age three.

Retarded adults are now provided with services to enable them to live in the community, with their families or in group homes, and to be gainfully employed or occupied in day programs according to their abilities. Individuals from institutions are being placed in the community (deinstitutionalized) as the facilities for them become available, including residences and programs for those that are both mentally retarded and mentally disturbed (Kiernan and Morrison, 1983; Kiernan and Stark, 1986).

THE CONCEPT AND DEFINITION OF MENTAL RETARDATION

While mental retardation has been historically referred to as an illness or disease, it differs from the usual concept of a disease. Similar to mental disorders, it is a behavioral syndrome (Spitzer and Williams, 1985) with symptoms of sufficient severity to be associated with distress or dysfunction. It differs from most mental disorders in that it is not characterized by the presence of abnormal behaviors but by normal behaviors being below a level considered normal for the age by the particular culture. Thus, on one level mental retardation is a social phenomenon reflecting societal expectations for a person's behavior at that particular age and setting. The diagnosis of significant retardation is less dependent on cultural values, however, since in virtually all cultures the presence of basic skills such as self-care and communication is expected (except in very young children). When the functional deficiencies are of a milder degree, the individual might or might not be labeled mentally retarded, depending on the extent to which these deficiencies are an obstacle to adaptive functioning. In addition, there may be the symptoms and signs of an underlying disorder (if such is present), which has caused brain dysfunction of a degree that a diagnosis of mental retardation is warranted.

The current diagnostic criteria for mental retardation in the *Diagnostic and Statistical Manual of Mental Disorders, Third Edition, Revised (DSM-III-R)* (American Psychiatric Association, 1987) are based essentially on the 1973 revision of the definition developed by the American Association on Mental Deficiency (Grossman, 1983). Briefly, these criteria require the following:

A. Significantly subaverage intellectual functioning, defined as an IQ of 70 or below (or based on clinical judgment in infants).
B. Concurrent deficits in adaptive functioning relative to the person's age and cultural expectations.
C. Onset before the age of 18.

The current definition is tridimensional and requires that all three criteria be met. Mental retardation is further subclassified into mild, moderate, severe, and profound, depending on the IQ level (Grossman, 1983; American Psychiatric Association, 1987). Each has certain developmental characteristics (Table 1).

Table 1. Developmental Characteristics

Degree of Retardation	Preschool 0–5 years	School Age 6–20 years	Adult 21 years and older
Mild			
I.Q. 50–55 to 70; 85% of all retarded persons.	Often not diagnosed until later age.	Learns academic pre-vocational skills with some special training.	Lives and works in the community. May not be easily identified as retarded.
Moderate			
I.Q. 35–40 to 50–55; 10% of all retarded persons.	Fair motor development. Can learn to talk and care for basic needs.	Learns functional academic skills and can be independent in familiar surroundings.	Performs semi-skilled work under sheltered conditions. May achieve competitive employment.
Severe			
I.Q. 20–25 to 35–40; 3–4% of all retarded persons.	Slow motor development and some communication skills. May have physical handicaps.	Can talk or learn to communicate. Cares for personal needs.	Can contribute to self-maintenance with supervision in work and living situations.
Profound			
I.Q. 20–25 or less; 1–2% of all retarded persons.	Overall responsiveness is minimal. Often has secondary physical handicaps.	Motor development is slow. Can be taught basic self-care skills.	Some communication skills. Cares for basic needs and performs highly structured work activities.

Adapted, with permission, from What Everyone Should Know About Mental Retardation. Greenfield, MA, Channing L. Bete Co., Inc., 1979

The definition and classification of mental retardation is still unsettled. Zigler et al (1984) and Hodapp and Zigler (1986) maintain that mental retardation is an innate characteristic of an individual. They proposed to define it by the measure of intelligence alone, excluding social adaptation as a part of the definition, since some mentally retarded individuals, as defined by the IQ, nevertheless can achieve a successful adaptation.

EPIDEMIOLOGY OF MENTAL RETARDATION

Estimates of the prevalence of mental retardation have changed through the years, reflecting above all the changes in the definition of mental retardation, as well as the research methodology that is used. Traditionally, a prevalence of about three percent of the general population was accepted (President's Committee on Mental Retardation, 1970; Grossman, 1973). The cutoff of two standard deviations below the population mean on the IQ distribution curve will also yield an estimate of about three percent prevalence. However, the current definition of mental retardation is based not only on measures of intellectual functioning but also on the adaptive behavior level. Mercer (1973) demonstrated that results of psychological testing could be misleading if the tests were not standardized according to the cultural background of the tested population. Based on Mercer's results, Tarjan and colleagues (1973) estimated the prevalence of mental retardation to be about one percent. Baird and Sadovnick (1985) identified a cohort of retarded persons in British Columbia on the basis of being recipients of specialized services, and estimated the overall prevalence to be 7.7 per 1,000 population. Usually the more severe the degree of retardation, the earlier the diagnosis is made: partly because the developmental delay is more global and more obvious, and partly because associated physical handicaps are more frequent and obvious. Mildly retarded children often are not diagnosed until school age, when they start failing in academic subjects. Some individuals in the upper range of mild mental retardation later may acquire good vocational and self-help skills, become independent, and thus will not qualify for the diagnosis of mental retardation, despite IQ scores below 70.

THE CONCEPT OF MENTAL RETARDATION AS A MANIFESTATION OF CNS DYSFUNCTION

Cognitive abilities can be thought of as only one of the functions of the central nervous system (CNS). Therefore, mental retardation can be seen as a manifestation of CNS dysfunction (Rubin, 1989), and the etiology of mental retardation examined in the context of various causes of brain dysfunction. The spectrum of these etiological factors includes hereditary and genetic, physical, chemical, infectious, traumatic, degenerative, vascular, neoplastic, and other influences. An insult to the CNS can lead to disruption in any one or several of CNS functions. If the elements related to cognitive functioning are affected to a sufficient degree, the clinical syndrome of mental retardation will result. Similarly, disorders of motor function that result are termed cerebral palsy. More often than not, the pathogenic process will affect more than one CNS function. Each of the disturbances that results may contribute to the individual's disability, leading to a variety of associated conditions.

As a rule, the more severe the causative pathogenic process, the more significant the insult to the brain, and the more severe the degree of resulting retardation, with greater chance for other systems to be affected. As a result, the

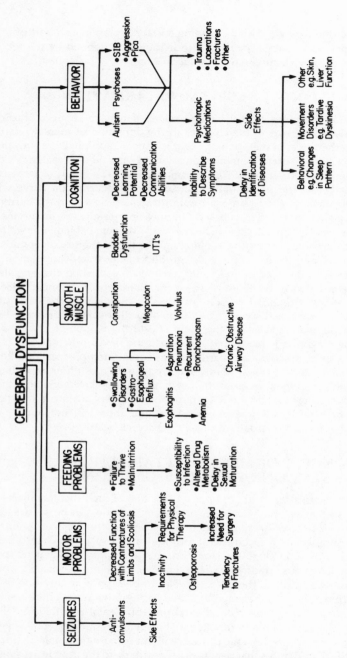

Figure 1. Schematic representation of some manifestations of CNS dysfunction. Reported from Rubin IL: Management of children and adults with severe and profound central nervous system dysfunction, in Developmental Disabilities: Delivery of Medical Care for Children and Adults. Edited by Rubin IL, Crocker AC. Philadelphia, Lea and Febiger, 1989.

more severe the mental retardation, the more frequent are the associated conditions and handicaps (Hagberg and Kyllerman, 1983; Rubin, 1989) (Table 2).

CLASSIFICATION OF ETIOLOGIES OF MENTAL RETARDATION

Table 3 represents the etiologies of mental retardation as seen in patients assessed at the Developmental Evaluation Clinic of The Children's Hospital, Boston (Crocker and Nelson, 1983; Crocker, Personal Communication, 1988). These have been classified according to the chronology of their occurrence. Approximately one-third of all causes are of identifiable prenatal origin and approximately one-third are of undetermined etiology. It should be kept in mind that in many situations several causative mechanisms are operating and determine the final outcome—the level of the retardation and of the functional handicap, even if one mechanism has been primary. Frequently the psychosocial and environmental factors complicate the retardation arising from pre- or perinatal causes. Psychosocial factors have been identified as the single most significant factor in predicting the outcome of low birth weight infants, both in terms of morbidity and mortality (Rubin, 1983; Moser, 1983).

ESTABLISHING AN ETIOLOGICAL DIAGNOSIS

Evaluation of etiology takes place in two main contexts. In the first, the child already has been identified as functioning in the mentally retarded range and is referred to the clinician to determine the cause of this developmental delay. In the second, the child is brought to the attention of the clinician for a condition which may have mental retardation as one of its manifestations and which may emerge only at a "later stage. This situation arises, for example, in the systematic follow up of "high risk" infants, where the likelihood of mental retardation complicating the child's life is greater than in the general population (Rubin,

Table 2. Rates of Associated Handicaps in Swedish School Age Children with Mental Retardation

	Percent handicapped by IQ level	
Handicap	Under 50	50 to 70
Cerebral palsy	21	9
Epilepsy	37	12
Hydrocephalus	5	2
Severe impairment of hearing	8	7
Severe impairment of vision	15	1
One or more associated neurologic handicap	40	24

Adapted from Hagberg B, Kyllerman M: Epidemiology of mental retardation—a Swedish survey. Brain Dev 5:441–449, 1983

1989), or when an infant or child is diagnosed as having a physical, biochemical, or other disorder in which mental retardation is a possible feature.

In either situation a comprehensive history and examination are needed: the difference resting in the focus or objective and, therefore, in the nature of questions asked and the aspects of the physical examination that will be emphasized.

Obtaining Historical Information

The purpose of history-taking is to try to identify the time of the possible CNS insult, to determine the causative factor, and to obtain a description of development and current functioning. While interviewing the parents it is also important to clairfy whether they harbor, or may develop, guilt feelings related to the child's condition. The interview may include, already at this stage, support and counseling to address these feelings. Another important issue is to determine whether there is a risk for recurrence of the mental retardation in this family.

The history should include:

Table 3. Diagnostic Classification

Patients seen at the Developmental Evaluation Clinic, The Children's Hospital, Boston (N = 2841), who ranged from borderline intelligence to profound retardation.

I. *Hereditary Issues*	5%
Inborn errors of metabolism (e.g., Tay-Sachs disease)	
Other single gene abnormalities	
Chromosomal aberrations (translocations, fragile-x)	
Polygenic familial syndromes	
II. *Early Alterations of Embryonic Development*	32%
Chromosomal changes (e.g., Down's syndrome)	
Prenatal influence syndrome (e.g., toxins)	
III. *Other Pregnancy and Perinatal Problems*	11%
Fetal malnutrition/placental insufficiency	
Perinatal problems (e.g., prematurity, hypoxia)	
IV. *Acquired Childhood Diseases*	4%
Infections (e.g., meningitis, encephalitis)	
Cranial trauma	
Other (e.g., cardiac arrest)	
V. *Environmental and Behavioral Problems*	18%
(Commonly combined with other handicaps)	
Psychosocial deprivation	
Severe parental mental illness	
Severe mental illness of the child	
VI. *Unknown Causes*	30%

Source: Crocker AC: Personal communication (1988)

1. A relevant family history, and the construction of a genetic family tree, with particular emphasis on developmental, learning, behavioral, medical, and other disorders (Meryash, 1989).
2. A pregnancy history, including ease or difficulty in becoming pregnant, previous pregnancies, details of the pregnancy in question, differences between this and other pregnancies, intake of medications, alcohol and substance abuse, smoking, and illnesses while pregnant (Golden and Rubin, 1983).
3. The details of birth, including duration and nature of labor and delivery, birth weight, gestational age (or duration of pregnancy), Apgar scores, and perinatal complications, if any. It is important to remember that it may be necessary to be specific in the questioning as well as to ask more general and open-ended questions (Rubin, 1983).
4. The developmental history of the child, with an emphasis on the acquisition of motor skills (such as sitting, crawling, walking), language development, nonverbal communication, and other developmental milestones.
5. The social and emotional development, including such elements as eye contact, cuddliness, sleep patterns, feeding habits, elimination, and interaction with parents, siblings, and peers.
6. The ability to learn, whether this be self-help or academic skills, and the learning rate and style.
7. A general health history.

The Physical Examination

The following are the more important areas that should be assessed during the physical examination:

1. The general behavior and demeanor of the child and the quality of interaction with the family or caregivers and with the examiner.
2. The physical features and whether they are in any way striking or unusual as to suggest a specific syndrome; for example, Down syndrome. If they do not obviously suggest a diagnosis but raise a suspicion, then referral to a clinical geneticist is warranted (Meryash, 1989).
3. The neurological status, with particular emphasis on functional level. Among others, the following areas should be addressed: gross motor functioning (such as walking, running, climbing); fine motor skills (such as pencil grasp); and coordination skills (such as hopping on one foot, rapid alternating movements of hand and fingers).
4. A general examination to explore the possibility of involvement of other organ systems. General nutritional status and growth parameters are important. From a functional point of view it is important to assess whether vision and hearing are intact. Formal visual and auditory screening by an ophthalmologist and audiologist, respectively, may be required.

Other Investigations

At this stage the preliminary diagnostic formulation probably will have emerged. On the basis of the longitudinal developmental history and other data it should also be possible to determine whether the disorder of development is of a fixed, fluctuating, or progressively deteriorating nature (Figure 2). This is important in determining the diagnosis and helping to determine the prognosis and the approach to management.

On the basis of the clinical data obtained so far, one should determine whether further investigation should focus predominantly on neurological elements (and include tests such as the electroencephalogram [EEG], computed tomography [CT] scan, magnetic resonance imaging [MRI]), whether it should follow a more biochemical course (with amino acid determination, mucopolysaccharide screen), whether a prenatal infection of the TORCH group (toxoplasmosis, rubella, cytomegalovirus, herpes) is suspected (requiring antibody titers), or whether a more detailed dysmorphological study and chromosomal analysis are needed.

Conclusion of the Evaluation

Having established an etiological diagnosis, which is possible only in approximately 70 percent of the cases (Table 3), or at a least general diagnostic classification, it then becomes important to determine what medical, psychiatric, educational, and other interventions are necessary. The treatment and habilitation plan should be as comprehensive as necessary (Szymanski and Crocker, 1989). It is essential to discuss the findings extensively with the family, to assess their reaction to the diagnosis (both of the etiology and of the mental retardation itself), and to provide them with support and follow-up as needed.

Psychological Testing

For diagnostic purposes the intellectual level is assessed by means of individually administered psychological tests. Their accuracy may be influenced by cultural factors, the child's cooperation, and the presence of motor, sensory and other handicaps; thus proper tests must be carefully selected, administered, and interpreted by well trained and experienced psychologists. In general, the older or more handicapped the child, the more the tests are reliably predictive of future performance. Tests used with infants assess psychomotor development, and they yield not numerical IQ, but a developmental quotient. For infants the *DSM-III-R* definition of mental retardation accepts the clinical judgment of the presence of subaverage intellectual functioning; but when more objective measurement is needed, the Bayley Scales of Infant Development are the most widely used. For preschoolers, the Stanford-Binet Scale is the most popular. For retarded, nonverbal children the Merrill-Palmer Scale and Leiter International Performance Scale, which assess performance rather than verbal skills, are often used. For older children and adults, the Wechsler Intelligence Scale for Children–Revised and Wechsler Adult Intelligence Scale–Revised are the most popular. They yield numerical IQs, reflecting performance, verbal, and full scale scores. There are many instruments used to assess adaptive functioning, the Vineland Social Maturity Scale being the most popular. With more verbal, retarded persons, projective tests are valuable in assessing personality and psychopathology.

A REVIEW OF SELECTED DIAGNOSTIC GROUPS

Hereditary Disorders

These disorders are of preconception in origin and include at least four major subgroups:

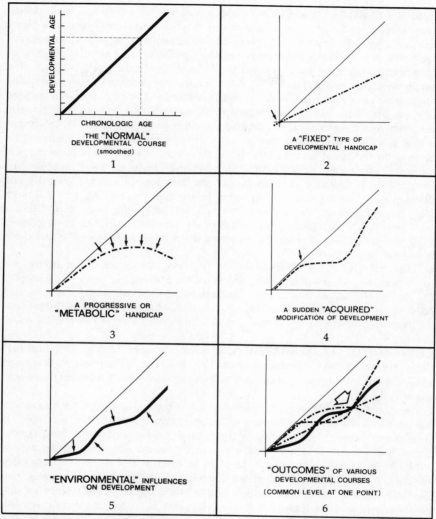

Figure 2. Schematic representation of patterns of developmental disorders. (1) Normal developmental course. (2) "Fixed" type of developmental disorder which has its origins in the pre- and perinatal periods and is nonprogressive. (3) "Metabolic" type of disorder of development wherein the manifestations of the underlying process (for example, Tay-Sachs disease) occur after birth and evolve into a progressively deteriorating course. (4) "Acquired" developmental disorder: the curve represents normal development up to a point of insult (arrow) to the CNS. There is a spectrum of potential courses after this point, depending on the type and severity of the insult. (5) "Environmental" disorder of development: demonstrates a fluctuating course which may represent periods of stress (arrows pointing down) alternating with periods of nurturance and/or positive intervention (arrows pointing up). (6) Outcomes: the convergence (large arrow) of the various developmental courses diagrammatically represents the point when the clinician becomes aware of the developmental disorder and attempts to elucidate the etiology, treatment plan, and prognosis.

INBORN ERRORS OF METABOLISM. Among this group are those conditions which generally have a genetic defect of an autosomal recessive type. Examples include Tay-Sachs disease, phenylketonuria (PKU), and mucopolysaccharidoses. These disorders have as their pathological basis the absence of an enzyme, resulting in a deficiency of the desired end-point product of a biochemical process, and an accumulation of another product in excessive quantities, which has a destructive effect on the organism. The clinical manifestations of these disorders will obviously be specific to each, but have in common the tendency to a progressively debilitating course (Figure 2). With PKU, treatment is now possible through the dietary restriction of phenylalanine, preventing the damage to the brain and mental retardation that would otherwise occur. Of interest is the recent progress in understanding "maternal PKU" (Lenke and Levy, 1980). Young women with the genetic disorder of PKU, but who did not develop retardation because of an appropriate diet in early life, will still have high blood levels of phenylalanine, which will affect the brain of the fetus, resulting in severe retardation, even though the child does not have genetic PKU. However, the fetus can be protected if the mother resumes the diet prior to becoming pregnant.

OTHER SINGLE GENE DISORDERS. Among this group of conditions are those which have an autosomal or sex-linked recessive inheritance; for example, the group of phakomatoses, most commonly neurofibromatosis and tuberous sclerosis, which have an autosomal dominant inheritance, as well as the muscular dystrophies. They may be associated with varying degrees of mental retardation.

CHROMOSOMAL ABERRATIONS. In this category are the chromosomal disorders which have a hereditary basis. An example is the translocation form of Down syndrome, which accounts for approximately four percent of this disorder.

The Fragile-x syndrome is another condition belonging to this group, which has gained considerable attention in recent years (Hagerman et al, 1983). It involves a "fragile" site, actually a constriction, at the end of the long arm of the x chromosome, which is a marker, rather than the site of the actual defect. While at first females were considered to be carriers and males the only ones affected, it is now known that approximately two-thirds of carrier females may have clinical manifestations, including retardation (usually mild), learning disabilities, and various mental disorders (Reiss et al, 1988). In some cases the carrier female inherited the Fragile-x from a clinically nonaffected father. The phenotypical characteristics include long face, large ears, and macroorchidism in males. Affected males are usually functioning within the severe to mild mental retardation range. In some, a characteristic behavioral pattern is seen, including self-stimulation, irritability, anxiety, and a short attention span. There are reports of an association of this syndrome with autism, although there is no agreement on this finding.

POLYGENIC FAMILY SYNDROMES. This is a less well defined group of retardation syndromes occurring in families, with varying and multiple manifestations.

Early Alterations of Embryonic Development

In this group are two major categories:

CHROMOSOMAL DISORDERS. Although chromosomal disorders originate prior to conception, their effects become manifest during embryonic development. The most notable in this group is Down syndrome (Pueschel et al, 1985). This is the most common of recognized syndromes that have mental retardation as a manifestation, mostly in the moderate or mild range. Its overall incidence is about 1:1,000 of live births, increasing with maternal (and to a lesser degree paternal) age. Its physical phenotype is well known and indeed these individuals have been considered the stereotype of mental retardation. There are many congenital and acquired conditions that are associated with Down syndrome, including congenital heart defects, abnormalities of the gastrointestinal tract, atlantoaxial instability, hypothyroidism, eye abnormalities, and hearing deficits. Advances in diagnosis and treatment, as well as a more positive view of these individuals, have made medical care more available and have improved their life span dramatically.

Neuropathological changes characteristic of Alzheimer's disease have been described in middle age, but not necessarily accompanied by clinical dementia. These are discussed later in this chapter. The advances in knowledge of this disorder, coupled with an increased public acceptance (largely due to efforts of groups such as Down syndrome Congress), have led to major changes in the management of this condition. In the past, parents were advised routinely to institutionalize an affected baby; at the present such practices are not accepted and individuals with Down syndrome live, and adapt well, in the community.

PRENATAL INFLUENCE SYNDROMES. Many factors can influence the development of the fetus (Golden and Rubin, 1983). Their impact on brain development depends on both the nature of the insult (such as viral-congenital rubella, chemical-fetal alcohol syndrome) and on the timing of the insult. The earlier in fetal life the insult occurs, the more severe are its effects. The insults that occur later in gestation will have more subtle effects, the most common of which are the disorders of neuronal migration. Many syndromes have been described, characterized by various malformations and retardation of varying severity.

Perinatal Factors

These include conditions that arise in later pregnancy (for example, fetal malnutrition secondary to placental insufficiency) and those which relate to the birth and immediate neonatal period (Rubin, 1983; Golden and Rubin, 1983; Rubin, 1989). The most common example is the low birth weight infant who may have experienced respiratory distress requiring assisted ventilation, with a 50 percent likelihood of an intraventricular hemorrhage.

Acquired Childhood Diseases

In this category are those conditions which cause some degree of brain damage, whether the agent is infectious (such as meningitis), chemical (lead toxicity), traumatic, or asphyxial (associated with a cardiac arrest). The consequences of these insults often can be severe.

Environmental and Behavioral Problems

This is the most vaguely defined category, often referred to in the past as "nonorganic," reflecting an inability to demonstrate brain pathology by currently available means, rather than its absence. The retardation in these cases is generally milder in nature and more prevalent in lower socioeconomic groups. These psychosocially deprived children are often at risk for other hazards: malnutrition, trauma, and lead poisoning; thus, multiple etiological factors may be involved. These hazards are increased if the parent suffers from severe mental illness, while developmental delays are more frequent in their offspring (Marcus et al, 1985).

Unknown Causes

As already mentioned it is not always possible to establish an etiological diagnosis. In some of these cases there is evidence for several possible pathogenic influences, but their roles and significance are unclear. In others no causative factors can be found by currently available diagnostic techniques. In most of these cases the etiology can be presumed to be of prenatal origin.

PERSONALITY DEVELOPMENT IN MENTALLY RETARDED PERSONS

Developmental Crises and Adaptation

EARLY CHILDHOOD. There is no special feature common to all mentally retarded infants. Development and behavior will depend on the degree of retardation and on associated physical handicaps that may be present, as well as on environmental and other factors. However, certain patterns and distortions of development have been described as common in retarded infants and young children. The development of the attachment and affectional behaviors may be delayed (Klaus and Kennell, 1976; Emde and Brown, 1978; Cicchetti and Sroufe, 1978; Hagamen, 1980; Hanzlik and Stevenson, 1986). Stone and Chesney (1978) found disturbances in behaviors such as eye contact, social smiling, and social vocalizing. These infants might be over- or understimulated by their parents and may respond with withdrawal or irritability (Szymanski, 1983). Associated handicaps, particularly in sensory systems, may further affect the development of a child's interpersonal attachments.

SCHOOL AGE. The major factor determining the adaptation of school-aged retarded children has been the availability of appropriate early education. Public Law (PL) 94–142, guaranteeing public education for all handicapped children, has been a milestone in this respect. Besides usual preacademic or academic subjects, the programs now include instruction in self-help, social, communication, motor, and other skills, as well as specialized therapies (such as speech and occupational). However, school attendance exposes retarded children to certain stresses as well: the need to separate from parents, to develop self-control, a degree of independence, and to follow social conventions. Except for the very retarded, these children are well aware of their failures and parental disappointment. Varieties of behavioral compensatory and defense mechanisms may appear, ranging from passivity and withdrawal to aggression (Szymanski, 1983). There is still no agreement on the merits of integrating retarded and nonretarded children (mainstreaming) in the classroom. Some studies indicate that mainstreamed children are better accepted socially, while others find that integrated children are more often rejected, or that the acceptance largely depends on the child's behavior and competence (review by Corman and Gottlieb, 1978; Bak and Siperstein, 1987).

ADOLESCENCE. Adolescence is even more stressful for retarded than for nonretarded persons, as the former must cope with the fact of the permanence of the handicap (Szymanski, 1980; Szymanski and Crocker, 1989). Due to the cognitive delay, particularly egocentricity, and difficulties in abstract thinking, even mildly retarded adolescents are often immature, poorly accepted by nonretarded peers, overprotected by their parents, and socially isolated. Behavioral maladaptive defenses may include withdrawal, dependency, acting out, and "pseudoadolescence." Virtually all (except the most retarded who focus on auto-eroticism) have concerns about sexuality, which are usually unanswered, since sexuality education, although very effective, is still not common. Misconceptions still persist of retarded persons as oversexed or asexual. Due to progress in the field of human rights, sterilization on parental request is not an option now. However, with proper education (focusing on strengths and teaching skills which lead to success), sexuality training, social and other opportunities, retarded adolescents can adapt and function well (within their limitations) with no more, or even fewer behavioral problems, compared to nonretarded adolescents.

Personality Development

There are many misconceptions about the personality patterns of retarded persons: that they are a homogenous group with a typical personality pattern, defined by brain damage and by mental age; that they do not suffer from the "usual" mental disorders; and that adaptation depends solely on IQ (Philips, 1966; Szymanski and Crocker, 1989). In fact, retarded persons do not have a "typical" personality, although certain features are commonly seen: concreteness; dependency on routine; irritability and anxiety resulting primarily from experiences of failure and society's rejection (Wills, 1983, Szymanski and Crocker, 1989); "outerdirectness" (Zigler and Balla, 1977); a dependency, often fostered by caregivers. Behaviors linked to underlying mental retardation syndromes might be seen: anxiety and hyperactivity in Fragile x syndrome or self-injurious biting in Lesh Nyhan syndrome. However, the most important determinants of personality patterns are environmental influences, and they, together with the cognitive level, determine a person's adaptation.

MENTAL DISORDERS IN RETARDED PERSONS

Mentally retarded persons suffer the same mental disorders as nonretarded ones, although the clinical manifestations may be modified by the presence of retardation and associated handicaps, primarily affecting communication and verbal skills (Szymanski, 1980). Most prevalence studies suffer from two major problems: inconsistent use of diagnostic criteria for mental retardation and for mental disorders; and selected study cohorts (although some focused on random populations). In the classic Isle of Wight study (Rutter et al, 1970), emotional disorders were four to five times more frequent in retarded than in nonretarded children. In a retrospective study by Koller and colleagues (1983) of the total population of retarded persons born in a city in England within a 5-year period, 61 percent were reported as having a behavioral disorder in childhood. Gostason (1985) assessed a representative cohort of retarded persons in Sweden, between 20 and 60 years old, and reportedly used *DSM-III* diagnostic criteria. Thirty-three percent of the mildly retarded, 71 percent of the more seriously retarded, and 23 percent of controls were given at least one *DSM-III* diagnosis. Lund (1985) diagnosed a psychiatric disorder in 27.1 percent of a representative sample of retarded adults in Denmark. In other studies of referred or otherwise selected populations, the prevalence of mental disorders was also high: Chess and Hassibi (1970), 60 percent; Philips and Williams (1975), 87 percent; Corbett and colleagues (1975), 43 percent; Szymanski (1987), 74 percent of mildly/moderately and 42 percent of severely/profoundly retarded children.

THE PSYCHIATRIC DIAGNOSTIC EVALUATION OF RETARDED PERSONS

Szymanski (1980) reviewed studies on psychiatric diagnosis of retarded persons and described the principles of diagnostic assessment. History—which is generally provided by the caregivers—must be detailed and must review the patient's total functioning and behaviors, not only those about which the caregivers complain. The history should be interpreted in the context of environmental factors, including management by the caregivers and their motivation, as well as by the availability of vocational, recreational, and other opportunities. A specific behavioral description of the presenting symptoms should be obtained, rather than the caregivers' interpretation or value judgment ("he is aggressive") accepted. The reasons for referral at this point should be understood. Typically, these patients are referred because they are disturbing to others rather than because they are disturbed. With support and reassurance (but not paternalizing) most retarded persons are cooperative and open. Verbal interviewing has to be adapted to the usually concrete level of the patient's communication. Nonverbal techniques such as activities, play, and detailed behavioral observation are important as well. The assessment should be done in a comprehensive context, considering the patient's associated handicaps, background, education, and life experiences. The environmental factors (such as management by the caregivers) should be considered, both those that cause and those that maintain the symptoms. Thus, the symptoms should not be taken at face value; for example, hearing "voices" may represent an imaginary friend resulting from boredom and not from hallucinations.

Szymanski and Crocker (1989) described four ways in which clinical symptoms may be affected in retarded persons: by the developmental level; by the communication skills being too low for verbalizing emotions (such as depression); by life experiences and opportunities (in an understaffed institution aggression might be the way to secure staff attention); and by a coexisting physical disorder (for example, hypothyroidism common in Down syndrome may present as depression).

A REVIEW OF SELECTED MENTAL DISORDERS

In retarded persons, just as in nonretarded ones, the diagnostician should assess whether the presenting symptoms are a part of a major mental disorder. No behavioral pattern is typical for mental retardation. While some retarded persons are aggressive, most are not. Diagnosing diverse behavioral manifestations as part of mental retardation does not make sense and, in fact, such a category (the *DSM-III* fifth digit of the code for Mental Retardation) has been eliminated in the *DSM-III-R*. A diagnosis of a major mental disorder is not justified in all cases where disturbed behavior exists. In some cases other categories can be used, such as stereotypy/habit disorder for major self-injurious behaviors. Because of space constraints, only the major mental disorders as they occur in retarded persons will be reviewed here.

Psychotic Disorders

The diagnosis of psychosis in mentally retarded persons is often difficult and confusing to psychiatrists. Starting as early as Kraepelin (Reid, 1972) behaviors such as manneristic movements of retarded persons were considered by some as diagnostic of psychosis, while others did not think that retarded persons could have genuine schizophrenia. Reid (1972) and Heaton-Ward (1977) felt that the feasibility of diagnosis of schizophrenia in retarded persons and particularly of its subtypes would depend on the level of language present. The modern view is that retarded persons may have the same psychotic disorders as nonretarded ones, and that they can be diagnosed by the usual criteria. In nonverbal persons hallucinations might be sometimes inferred from observable behavior, but often the *DSM-III* category of "psychotic disorders not otherwise classified (atypical psychosis)" must be used. Of the recent studies, using varying criteria, Reid (1980) diagnosed psychosis in 8 percent of children studied; Eaton and Menolascino (1982) diagnosed psychosis in 24 of 168 patients; Gostason (1985) diagnosed psychosis in 4 of 51; and Szymanski (1987), using *DSM-III* criteria, diagnosed psychosis in 17 percent of mildly/moderately and 30 percent of severely/profoundly retarded patients.

Mood Disorders

While in the earlier literature there was controversy over whether retarded persons could suffer from depression (Gardner, 1967), such cases had been reported (review by Sovner and Hurley, 1983). Szymanski and Biederman (1984) feel that depression in this population has been grossly underdiagnosed and untreated. Eaton and Menolascino (1982) did not diagnose depression in their patients, while Gostason (1985) diagnosed atypical depression in one of 75 mildly retarded adults. On the other hand, Szymanski (1987), using *DSM-III* criteria, diagnosed a depressive disorder in 14 percent of mildly/moderately retarded children and 13 percent of adults. He stressed that the diagnosis may depend largely on behavioral and vegetative symptoms, since if there are insufficient speech skills the verbalizations of dysphoria and low self-image may be absent. The *DSM-III-R* permits reporting of depressed mood by either the patient *or* by outside observers. The differential diagnosis may include dementia (Szymanski and Biederman, 1984; Szymanski and Crocker, 1989), reaction to a move (such as "relocation syndrome" (Cochran et al, 1977), reaction to a loss of an important caregiver in a profoundly retarded adult similar to a reactive attachment disorder of infancy, and a medical disorder such as hypothyroidism (for which patients with Down syndrome are somewhat more at risk). Manic episodes occur in retarded persons as well (Rivinus and Harmatz, 1979) and the manifestations, like those in depression, will depend on the level of functioning, with behavioral symptoms presenting in nonverbal individuals.

Pervasive Developmental Disorders

These will only be mentioned here, since they are discussed in detail elsewhere in this volume. It is well known now that pervasive developmental disorder and retardation frequently coexist, since a majority of children with infantile autism are also mentally retarded. Some behaviors in these two disorders are similar, such as self-stimulation. However, the essential features, particularly the deficits in interpersonal relatedness and the quality of the language deficits, are quite different. Psychosis is not infrequently diagnosed in older children and adults with residual autism if a comprehensive history has not been obtained. On the other hand, these individuals can develop a psychosis later in life, superimposed on the residual autism.

Organic Mental Syndromes and Disorders

These diagnoses should be made only if the presence of brain dysfunction and its causative relationship to the behavioral/emotional manifestations can be demonstrated (Lipowski, 1980; Szymanski and Crocker, 1985). While mental retardation, particularly of a more severe degree, is obviously related to a brain dysfunction—even if that cannot always be documented by currently available measures—it does not mean that all disturbed behaviors of a retarded person are directly related to such dysfunction. Among these disorders, Alzheimer's disease recently has received considerable attention because of the association with Down syndrome. While most of these adults over 40 appear to have neuro-pathological changes of the Alzheimer type, they are usually not associated with clinical dementia until a later age (review by Cutler et al, 1985). Depression in these persons is not infrequently misdiagnosed as dementia, with destructive effects, since they will not receive the appropriate treatment and their caregivers may "give up" on them.

MANAGEMENT OF MENTAL DISORDERS IN RETARDED PERSONS

General Principles

Szymanski and Crocker (1989) have delineated seven steps in developing a treatment program for these individuals: comprehensive diagnostic assessment; assessment of whether an intervention is needed; assessment of factors causing and maintaining the problems; choice of treatment modalities; delineation of treatment goals; setting a follow-up mechanism; and respecting a retarded patient's rights. Mentally retarded persons who also have a mental disorder usually have multiple handicaps. Thus, they need multiple services and, to be effective, the treatment plan should be comprehensive, providing both treatment for the particular mental disorder as well as general support, education, and training. Various treatment approaches may have to be used concurrently.

Psychotherapies

The basic techniques of psychotherapy are applicable to retarded persons, as had been noticed early by Yepsen (1952). Since then, many reports on psychotherapy with retarded persons have been published (reviews by Jakab, 1970, and Szymanski, 1980). As in diagnostic interviewing, both verbal and nonverbal approaches are used. The verbal approaches have to be adapted to the patient's verbal capacities and generally should be concrete and structured, directive, but empathetic without being condescending. The therapists should have the capacity to be flexible and use themselves as role models. Acquisition of insight is not the goal, but, rather, amelioration of emotional distress and developing better coping strategies. Individual, group, and multiple family group therapy (Szymanski and Kiernan, 1983) are used.

Rational Use of Psychotropic Medications

Multiple reports exist on various aspects of these drugs in "the retarded." However, there are no basic differences in their use with retarded and nonretarded persons, and in both cases the same principles of sound medical practice should be employed. If the drug's action is affected, it is not by the retardation per se but by the underlying mental retardation syndrome. As in general psychiatry, the drugs should be used for treatment of a mental disorder and not to eliminate single behaviors, even though target behaviors may be used to monitor the drugs' effectiveness. However, these drugs should not be used just because an objectionable behavior exists. For instance, aggressive behavior in response to command hallucinations, and superficially similar aggression aimed to secure a caregiver's attention, should be treated differently. Unfortunately, through the years these drugs, primarily antipsychotics, have been abused through wholesale prescribing to retarded persons to induce docility and compliance, usually for the caregivers' convenience (review by Rivinus, 1980). Before drugs are used, less invasive alternatives should be considered. The drugs should not be used alone, but together with all other measures that are indicated. There is no evidence that polypharmacy is beneficial and probably it is often detrimental. Close monitoring of effectiveness per changes in predetermined target behaviors, as well as watching for adverse side effects, is necessary since retarded patients are rarely capable of reporting these themselves. The smallest effective doses should be used and periodic tapering of the medication is needed to document whether the treatment is still needed. Side effects which the patients cannot adequately describe and which produce a behavioral disturbance (such as akathisia) should not be confused with relapse of the basic disorder. Recently the considerable effects of antipsychotic medication withdrawal have been recognized (Gualtieri et al, 1986), and to minimize them the medication should be stopped in a very gradual and slow manner. Legal requirements in the particular state should be observed if the patient is incompetent to give informed consent for the treatment.

SUMMARY

Mental retardation is a nonspecific, generic term, denoting a group of people whose common denominator is a lowered level of cognitive and adaptive functioning. While it is not a discrete disease entity, it is conceptualized as an expression of brain dysfunction which may be due to one or several causative processes. As a group, mentally retarded persons are at higher than average risk for developing mental disorders, which can be recognized and treated. Provision of a full range of diagnostic and therapeutic mental health services to this population is an important responsibility of the psychiatric profession.

REFERENCES

Alvarez N: Neurological examination, in Comprehensive Management of Cerebral Palsy. Edited by Thompson GH, Rubin IL, Bilenker RM. New York, Grune & Stratton, 1983

Aman MG, Singh NN, Stewart AW, et al: The Aberrant Behavior Checklist: a behavior rating scale for the assessment of treatment effects. Am J Ment Defic 1985; 89:485–491

American Psychiatric Association: Diagnostic and Statistical Manual of Mental Disorders, Third Edition (DSM-III). Washington, DC, American Psychiatric Association, 1980

American Psychiatric Association: Diagnostic and Statistical Manual of Mental Disorders, Third Edition, Revised (DSM-III-R). Washington, DC, American Psychiatric Association, 1987

Anthony JC, Folstein M, Romanoski AJ, et al: Comparison of the lay interview schedule and a standardized psychiatric diagnosis. Arch Gen Psychiatry 1985; 42:667–675

Baird PA, Sadovnick AD: Mental retardation in over half-a-million consecutive live births: an epidemiological study. Am J Ment Defic 1985; 89:323–330

Bak JJ, Siperstein, GM: Effects of mentally retarded children's behavioral competence on nonretarded peers' behaviors and attitudes: toward establishing ecological validity in attitude research. Am J Ment Defic 1987; 92:31–39

Bear DM: Temporal lobe epilepsy—a syndrome of sensory-limbic hyperconnection. Cortex 1979; 15:537–584

Bear DM, Freeman R, Greenberg M: Behavioral alterations in patients with temporal lobe epilepsy, in Psychiatric Aspects of Epilepsy. Edited by Blumer D. Washington, DC, American Psychiatric Press, 1984

Campbell M, Green WH: Pervasive developmental disorders of childhood, in Comprehensive Textbook of Psychiatry. Edited by Kaplan HI, Sadock BJ. Baltimore, Williams & Wilkins, 1985

Cantor S: The Schizophrenic Child. Montreal, Eden Press, 1982

Cantwell DP, Russell AT, Mattison R, et al: A comparison of DSM-II and DSM-III in the diagnosis of childhood psychiatric disorders, I: agreement with expected diagnosis. Arch Gen Psychiatry 1979; 36:1208–1213

Chess S: Evolution of behavior disorders in a group of mentally retarded children. J Am Acad Child Psychiatry 1977; 16:5–18

Chess S, Hassibi M: Behavior deviations in mentally retarded children. J Am Acad Child Psychiatry 1970; 9:282–297

Cicchetti D, Sroufe A: An organizational view of affect: illustration from the study of Down's syndrome infants, in The Development of Affect. Edited by Lewis M, Rosenblum LA. New York, Plenum, 1978

Cochran W, Sran P, Varano G: The relocation syndrome in mentally retarded individuals. Ment Retardation 1977; 15:10–12

Conroy JW, Derr KE: Survey and Analysis of the Habilitation and Rehabilitation Status of the Mentally Retarded with Associated Handicapping Conditions. Washington, DC, D.H.E.W., 1971

Corbett JA, Harris E, Robinson R: Epilepsy, in Mental Retardation and Developmental Disabilities, vol. 7. Edited by Wortis J. New York, Brunner/Mazel, 1975

Corman L, Gottlieb J: Mainstreaming mentally retarded children: a review of the research, in International Review of Research in Mental Retardation. Edited by Ellis NR. New York, Academic, 1978

Crocker AC, Nelson RP: Mental retardation, in Developmental–Behavioral Pediatrics. Edited by Levine MD, Carey WB, Crocker AC, et al. Philadelphia, WB Saunders, 1983

Cushna B, Szymanski LS, Tanguay PE: Professional roles and unmet manpower needs, in Emotional Disorders of Mentally Retarded Persons. Edited by Szymanski LS, Tanguay PE. Baltimore, University Park Press, 1980

Cutler NR, Heston LL, Davies P, et al: Alzheimer's disease and Down's syndrome: new insights. Ann Intern Med 1985; 103:566–578

DeMyer MK, Hintgen JN, Jackson RK: Infantile autism reviewed: a decade of research. Schizophr Bull 1981; 7:388

Donaldson JY, Menolascino FJ: Past, current and future roles of child psychiatry in mental retardation. J Am Acad Child Psychiatry 1977; 3:352–374

Earl CJ: The primitive catatonic psychosis of idiocy. Br J Med Psychol 1934; 14:231–253

Eaton LF, Menolascino FJ: Psychiatric disorders in the mentally retarded: types, problems and challenges. Am J Psychiatry 1982; 139:1297–1303

Emde RN, Brown C: Adaptation to the birth of a Down's syndrome infant: grieving and maternal attachment. J Am Acad Child Psychiatry 1978; 17:299–323

Gardner WI: Occurrence of severe depressive reactions in the mentally retarded. Am J Psychiatry 1967; 124:142–144

Garrard SD, Richmond JB: Diagnosis in mental retardation and mental retardation without biological manifestations, in Medical Aspects of Mental Retardation. Edited by Carter CH. Springfield, IL, Charles C Thomas, Publisher, 1967

Golden NL, Rubin IL: Intrauterine factors, in Comprehensive Management of Cerebral Palsy. Edited by Thompson GH, Rubin IL, Bilenker RM. New York, Grune & Stratton, 1983

Gostason R: Psychiatric illness among the mentally retarded: a Swedish population study. Acta Psychiatr Scand (Suppl) 1985

Grossman HJ (Ed): Manual on Terminology and Classification in Mental Retardation. Washington, DC, American Association on Mental Deficiency, 1973

Grossman HJ (Editor): Classification in Mental Retardation. Washington, DC, American Association on Mental Deficiency, 1983

Gualtieri CT, Schroeder SR, et al: Tardive dyskinesia in young mentally retarded individuals. Arch Gen Psychiatry 1986; 43:335–340

Hagamen MB: Family adaptation to the diagnosis of mental retardation in a child and strategies of intervention, in Emotional Disorders of Mentally Retarded Persons. Edited by Szymanski LS, Tanguay PE. Baltimore, University Park Press, 1980

Hagberg B, Kyllerman M: Epidemiology of mental retardation—a Swedish survey. Brain Dev 1983; 5:441–449

Hagerman RJ, McKenzie McBogg P (Editors): The Fragile X Syndrome. Dillon, Colorado, Spectra Publishing Co., 1983

Hall RCW, Popkin MK, Devaul RA, et al: Physical illness presenting as psychiatric disease. Arch Gen Psychiatry 1978; 35:1315–1320

Hall RCW, Gardner ER, Stickney SK, et al: Physical illness manifesting as psychiatric disease, II. Arch Gen Psychiatry 1980; 37:989–995

Hanzlik JR, Stevenson MB: Interaction of mothers with their infants who are mentally retarded, retarded with cerebral palsy, or nonretarded. Am J Ment Defic 1986; 90:513–520

Heaton-Ward A: Psychosis in mental handicap. Br J Psychiatry 1977; 130:525–533

Helzer JE, Robins LN, McEvoy LT, et al: A comparison of clinical and diagnostic interview schedule diagnoses. Arch Gen Psychiatry 1985; 42:657–666

Hodapp RM, Zigler E: Reply to Barnett's comments on the definition and classification of mental retardation. Am J Ment Deficiency 1986; 91:117–119

Jacobson JW: New York's Needs Assessment and Developmental Disabilities: Preliminary Report (Technical Monograph No. 78–10). Albany, NY, O.M.R.D.D., 1979

Jakab I: Psychotherapy of the mentally retarded child, in Diminished People. Edited by Bernstein NR. Boston, Little, Brown & Co., 1970

Kazdin AE, Matson JL, Senatore V: Assessment of depression in mentally retarded adults. Am J Psychiatry 1983; 140:1040–1043

Kendell RE: DSM-III: a British perspective. Am J Psychiatry 1980; 137:1630–1631

Kendell RE: DSM-III: a major advance in psychiatric nosology, in International Perspectives on DSM-III. Edited by Spitzer RL, Williams JBW, Skodol AE. Washington, DC, American Psychiatric Press, 1983

Kiernan WE, Morrison P: Rehabilitation and habilitation of the adult, in Comprehensive Management of Cerebral Palsy. Edited by Thompson GH, Rubin IL, Bilenker RM. New York, Grune & Stratton, 1983

Kiernan WE, Stark JA (Editors): Pathways to Employment for Adults with Developmental Disabilities. Baltimore, Paul H. Brookes Publishing Co., 1986

Klaus MH, Kennell JH: Maternal-Infant Bonding. St. Louis, C.V. Mosby Co., 1976

Klerman GL: Diagnosis of psychiatric disorders in epidemiologic field studies. Arch Gen Psychiatry 1985; 42:723–724

Koller H, Richardson SW, Katz M, et al: Behavior disturbance since childhood among a 5-year birth cohort of all mentally retarded young adults in a city. Am J Ment Defic 1983; 87:386–395

Kolvin I: Psychoses in childhood—a comparative study, in Infantile Autism: Concepts, Characteristics and Treatment. Edited by Rutter M. Edinburgh, Churchill Livingstone, 1971

Lane H: The Wild Boy of Aveyron. Cambridge, MA, Harvard University Press, 1976

Lenke RR, Levy HL: Maternal phenylketonuria and hyperphenylalaninemia. N Engl J Med 1980; 303:1202

Lipowski ZJ: A new look at organic brain syndromes. Am J Psychiatry 1980; 137:674–678

Lund J: The prevalence of psychiatric morbidity in mentally retarded adults. Acta Psychiatr Scand 1985; 72:563–70

Malamud N: Neuropathology of organic brain syndromes associated with aging, in Aging and the Brain. Edited by Gaitz CM. New York, Plenum Press, 1972

Marcus J, Hans SL, Mednick SA, Schulsinger F, et al: Neurological dysfunctioning in offspring of schizophrenics in Israel and Denmark. A replication analysis. Arch Gen Psychiatry 1985; 42:753–761

Mattison R, Cantwell DP, Russell AT, et al: A comparison of DSM-II and DSM-III in the diagnosis of childhood psychiatric disorders, II: interrater agreement. Arch Gen Psychiatry 1979; 36:1217–1222

May JV: The dementia praecox–schizophrenia problem. Am J Psychiatry 1931; 11:401–446

Menolascino FJ: Emotional disturbance and mental retardation. Am J Ment Defic 1965; 70:248–256

Menolascino FJ: The facade of mental retardation. Am J Psychiatry 1966; 122:1227–1235

Menolascino FJ: Emotional disturbances in mentally retarded children. Am J Psychiatry 1969; 126:168–179

Menolascino FJ: Down's syndrome: clinical and psychiatric findings in an institutionalized sample, in Psychiatric Approaches to Mental Retardation. Edited by Menolascino FJ. New York, Basic Books, 1970

Menolascino FJ, Bernstein NR: Psychiatric assessment of the mentally retarded child, in Diminished People. Edited by Bernstein NR. Boston, Little, Brown, 1970

Mercer JR: Labeling the Mentally Retarded: Clinical and Social Systems Perspectives on Mental Retardation. Berkeley, University of California, 1973

Meryash D: Hereditary and genetic disorders, in Developmental Disabilities: Delivery of Medical Care for Children and Adults. Edited by Rubin IL, Crocker AC. Philadelphia, Lea & Febiger, 1989

Meryash DL, Szymanski LS, Gerald PS: Infantile autism associated with the Fragile x syndrome. J Autism Dev Disord 1982; 3:295–301

Moser H: Psychosocial mental retardation, in Comprehensive Management of Cerebral Palsy. Edited by Thompson GH, Rubin IL, Bilenker RM. New York, Grune & Stratton, 1983

O'Gorman G: Psychosis as a cause of mental defect. Journal of Mental Science 1954; 100:934–943

Philips I: Children, mental retardation and emotional disorder, in Prevention and Treatment of Mental Retardation. Edited by Philips I. New York, Basic Books, 1966

Philips I, Williams N: Psychopathology and mental retardation: a study of 100 mentally retarded children, I: psychopathology. Am J Psychiatry 1975; 132:1265–1271

President's Committee on Mental Retardation: The Six-Hour Retarded Child. Washington, DC, US Government Printing Office, 1970

Pueschel SM, Tingey C, Rynders JE, et al: New Perspectives on Down's Syndrome. Baltimore, Paul H. Brookes, 1985

Reid AH: Psychosis in adult mental defectives. Br J Psychiatry 1972; 120:205–212

Reid AH: Psychiatric disturbances in the mentally handicapped. Proceedings of the Royal Society of Medicine 1976; 69:509–512

Reid AH: Psychiatric disorders in mentally handicapped children: a clinical and follow-up study. J Ment Defic Res 1980; 24:287–298

Reiss S, Levitan GW, Szyszko J: Emotional disturbance and mental retardation: diagnostic overshadowing. Am J Ment Defic 1982; 86:567–574

Reiss AL, Hagerman RJ, Vinogradov S, et al: Psychiatric disability in female carriers of the fragile x chromosome. Arch Gen Psychiatry 1988; 45:25–30

Rivinus TM: Psychopharmacology and the mentally retarded patient, in Emotional Disorders of Mentally Retarded Persons. Edited by Szymanski LS, Tanguay PE. Baltimore, University Park Press, 1980

Rivinus TM, Harmatz JS: Diagnosis and lithium treatment of affective disorder in the retarded: five case studies. Am J Psychiatry 1979; 136:551–554

Ropper AH, Williams RS: Relationship between plaques, tangles and dementia in Down's syndrome. Neurology 1980; 30:639–644

Rubin IL: Perinatal factors, in Comprehensive Management of Cerebral Palsy. Edited by Thompson GH, Rubin IL, Bilenker RM. New York, Grune & Stratton, 1983

Rubin IL: Follow-up of high risk infants, in Developmental Disabilities: Delivery of Medical Care for Children and Adults. Edited by Rubin IL, Crocker AC. Philadelphia, Lea & Febiger, 1989

Rubin IL: Severe central nervous system dysfunction, in Developmental Disabilities: Delivery of Medical Care for Children and Adults. Edited by Rubin IL, Crocker AC. Philadelphia, Lea & Febiger, 1989

Russell AT: The mentally retarded emotionally disturbed child and adolescent, in Children with Emotional Disorders and Developmental Disabilities. Edited by Sigman M, Orlando, FL, Grune & Stratton, 1985

Russell AT, Tanguay PE: Mental illness and mental retardation: cause or coincidence? Am J Ment Defic 1981; 85:570–574

Russell AT, Cantwell DP, Mattison R, et al: A comparison of DSM-II and DSM-III in the diagnosis of childhood psychiatric disorders, III: multiaxial features. Arch Gen Psychiatry 1979; 36:1223–1226

Rutter M, Shaffer D: DSM-III: a step forward or back in terms of the classification of child psychiatric disorders? J Am Acad Child Psychiatry 1980; 19:371–394

Rutter M, Greenfeld D, Lockyer M: A five to fifteen year follow-up study of infantile psychosis, II: social and behavioral outcome. Br J Psychiatry 1967; 113:1183

Rutter M, Graham P, Yule W: A Neuropsychiatric Study in Childhood. London, Spastics International Medical Publications, 1970

Rutter M, Shaffer D, Shepherd M: A Multiaxial Classification of Child Psychiatric Disorders. Geneva, W.H.O., 1975

Sarason SB, Doris J: Educational Handicap, Public Policy, and Social History. New York, The Free Press, 1979

Senatore V, Matson JL, Kazdin AE: An inventory to assess psychopathology of mentally retarded adults. Am J Ment Defic 1985; 89:459–466

Shulman BH: Legal aspects of education for the handicapped, in Comprehensive Management of Cerebral Palsy. Edited by Thompson GH, Rubin IL, Bilenker RM. New York, Grune & Stratton, 1983

Sigelman CK, Budd EC, Spanhel CL, et al: When in doubt say yes: acquiescence in interviews with mildly retarded persons. Ment Retard 1981; 18:53–58

Sovner R, Hurley A: Do the mentally retarded suffer from affective illness? Arch Gen Psychiatry 1983; 40:61–67

Spitzer RL, Williams JBW: Classification of mental disorders, in Comprehensive Textbook of Psychiatry/IV. Edited by Kaplan HI, Sadock BJ. Baltimore, Williams & Wilkins, 1985

Stone NW, Chesney BH: Attachment behaviors in handicapped infants. Ment Retardation 1978; 16:8–12

Szymanski LS: Psychiatric diagnostic evaluation of mentally retarded individuals. J Am Acad Child Psychiatry 1977; 16:67–87

Szymanski LS: Psychiatric diagnosis of retarded persons, in Emotional Disorders of Mentally Retarded Persons. Edited by Szymanski LS, Tanguay PE. Baltimore, University Park Press, 1980

Szymanski LS: Emotional problems in a child with serious developmental handicap, in Developmental-Behavioral Pediatrics. Edited by Levine MD, Carey WB, Crocker AC, et al. Philadelphia, WB Saunders Co., 1983

Szymanski LS: Integrative approach to diagnosis of mental disorders in retarded persons, in Mental Retardation and Mental Health. Edited by Stark JA, Menolascino FJ, Albarelli MH, et al. New York, Springer-Verlag, 1988

Szymanski LS, Biederman J: Depression and anorexia nervosa of persons with Down's syndrome. Am J Ment Defic 1984; 89:246–251

Szymanski LS, Crocker AC: Mental Retardation, in Comprehensive Textbook of Psychiatry/IV. Edited by Kaplan HI, Sadock BJ. Baltimore, Williams & Wilkins, 1985

Szymanski LS, Crocker AC: Mental Retardation, in Comprehensive Textbook of Psychiatry/V. Edited by Kaplan HI, Sadock BJ. Baltimore, Williams & Wilkins, 1989 (in press)

Szymanski LS, Kiernan WE: Multiple family group therapy with developmentally disabled adolescents and young adults. Int J Group Therapy 1983; 33:521–534

Tanguay PE: Early infantile autism and mental retardation: differential diagnosis, in Emotional Disorders of Mentally Retarded Persons. Edited by Szymanski LS, Tanguay PE. Baltimore, University Park Press, 1980

Tanguay PE: Toward a new classification of serious psychopathology in children. J Am Acad Child Psychiatry 1984; 23:373–384

Tanguay PE, Szymanski LS: Training of mental health professionals in mental retardation, in Emotional Disorders of Mentally Retarded Persons. Edited by Szymanski LS, Tanguay PE. Baltimore, University Park Press, 1980

Tarjan G, Wright SW, Eyman RK, et al: Natural history of mental retardation: some aspects of epidemiology. Am J Ment Defic 1973; 77:369–379

Turner G, Brookwell R, Daniel A, et al: Heterozygous expression of x-linked mental retardation and the x chromosome marker (Frax) (927). N Engl J Med 1980; 303:662–664

Webster TG: Unique aspects of emotional development in mentally retarded children, in Psychiatric Approaches to Mental Retardation. Edited by Menolascino FJ. New York, Basic Books, 1970

Williams J: The multiaxial system of DSM-III: where did it come from and where should it go? I: its origins and critiques. Arch Gen Psychiatry 1985a; 42:175–180

Williams J: The multiaxial system of DSM-III: where did it come from and where should it go? II: empirical studies, innovations and recommendations. Arch Gen Psychiatry 1985b; 42:181–186

Willis F: Self esteem in the retarded, in Development and Sustenance of Self Esteem in Childhood. Edited by Mack J, Ablon S. New York, International Universities Press, 1983

Wise PH, Kotelchuck M, Wilson ML, et al: Racial and socioeconomic disparities in childhood mortality. N Engl J Med 1985; 313:360–366

Wolfensberger W: The Principle of Normalization in Human Services. Toronto, National Institute on Mental Retardation, 1972

Woodward KF, Jaffe N, Brown D: Early psychiatric intervention for young mentally retarded children, in Psychiatric Approaches to Mental Retardation. Edited by Menolascino FJ. New York, Basic Books, 1970

Yepsen LN: Counseling the mentally retarded. Am J Ment Deficiency 1952; 57:205–213

Zigler E, Balla D, Hodapp R: On the definition and classification of mental retardation. Am J Ment Deficiency 1984; 89:215–230

Zigler E, Balla D: Personality factors in the performance of the retarded. J Am Acad Child Psychiatry 1977; 16:19–37

Chapter 12

Schizophrenic Disorders of Childhood and Adolescence

by Clarice J. Kestenbaum, M.D., Ian A. Canino, M.D., and Richard R. Pleak, M.D.

This chapter focuses on a re-examination of the schizophrenic disorders of childhood and adolescence, including questions concerning the relationship between childhood and adult onset schizophrenia. What are the diagnostic criteria for both types? Is there a clinical syndrome specific to the adult who was diagnosed schizophrenic in childhood and, conversely, are there prodromal signs or symptoms manifested early in life by those individuals who become schizophrenic in adult life? Are the disorders, or subtypes of the disorders, continuous or discontinuous from childhood to adulthood?

DIAGNOSTIC CRITERIA (*DSM-III-R*)

The *Diagnostic and Statistical Manual of Mental Disorders* had in its first edition (*DSM*) and second edition (*DSM-II*) (American Psychiatric Association, 1952, 1968) a separate diagnosis for childhood schizophrenia. With the inclusion of the diagnosis of autism in the *Diagnostic and Statistical Manual of Mental Disorders, Third Edition* (*DSM-III*) and the *Diagnostic and Statistical Manual of Mental Disorders, Third Edition, Revised* (*DSM-III-R*) (American Psychiatric Association, 1980, 1987), the diagnosis of childhood schizophrenia was deleted, and *DSM-III-R* does not differentiate between childhood, adolescent, and adult onsets. There is now no lower limit on age of onset listed in either the criteria or the description of the illness, although *DSM-III-R* does note that onset occurs usually during adolescence or early adulthood (peak onset occurs between the ages of 15 and 24; Loranger, 1987). Thus, the diagnostic criteria for schizophrenia in *DSM-III-R* are identical for children and adults.

In *DSM-III-R* overt psychotic symptoms such as delusions, hallucinations, and disturbance of thought (for example, loosening of associations) must be present for the diagnosis of schizophrenia. Such symptoms may be more difficult to assess in the child than in the adult. Delusions and hallucinations must be differentiated from the child's fantasies, not always an easy task. A child may readily express wishes that are not delusional, but would appear to be if expressed by an adult. Hallucinations in children accompany a wide variety of disorders (Chambers, 1986) and are less specific for schizophrenia than when present in adults. Thought disorder is similarly difficult to assess in young children. Isolated findings such as bizarre responses to Rorschach stimuli or to Children's Thematic Apperception Test cards, while contributory, cannot be used alone to justify a diagnosis of schizophrenia. *DSM-III-R* also includes the caveat that these symptoms are not due to mental retardation (both diagnoses can coexist in an individual, provided the psychotic symptoms are not due to the retardation). Should mental retardation be present, the clinician must make the often difficult determination whether the degree of retardation is enough to cause the psychotic symptoms; although this determination may not significantly alter treatment, it will affect prognosis.

Deterioration from a previous level of functioning is another diagnostic criterion of schizophrenia in *DSM-III-R*. Again, this may be difficult to appreciate in the young child, although it may be most noticeable in the child's school performance and peer relations. Signs of the illness must be continuously present for six months, which may include this prodromal deterioration.

While the same diagnostic criteria for schizophrenia are used for children and adults in *DSM-III-R*, the manual does not take into account the differences in the assessment and manifestation of psychotic symptoms in the child.

SCHIZOPHRENIA IN CHILDHOOD: HISTORICAL VIEW

The concept of schizophrenia in childhood has a long and varied course. Disagreement regarding a psychodynamic versus an organic etiology goes back to the 1900s. DeSanctis's "dementia praecoccissima" and Heller's "dementia infantilis," originally considered early manifestations of schizophrenia, were, most likely, postencephalitic states leading to mental deficiency. Several clinical syndromes with overlapping symptomatology had often been confused by including them all under the rubric "childhood schizophrenia." Thus, Bender's childhood schizophrenia, Kanner's infantile autism, Mahler's symbiotic psychosis, and Bergman and Escalona's "unusually sensitive children," among others, were all assigned the label "childhood schizophrenia" (Kestenbaum, 1978). The two major clinical syndromes were those of Bender (1942) and Kanner (1943). Loretta Bender described childhood schizophrenia as a clinical entity occurring before puberty which "reveals pathology in behavior at every level and in every area of integration of patterning within the functioning of the central nervous system, be it vegetative, motor, perceptual, intellectual, emotional, or social." She viewed the disorder as based on a dysmaturation of the central nervous system (CNS), including a strong constitutional factor, often leading to onset within the first two years with uneven development, neurological soft signs, and motility disturbances (whirling, flapping), emotional instability, extreme anxiety, and a severe language disorder. The final clinical picture, she held, was determined by the age of onset and the level of maturation attained.

Early Infantile Autism

In 1943 Leo Kanner described 11 children whose symptoms of extreme disturbance occurred within the first two years of life and included aloneness and the desire for sameness, severe disturbance in language (echolalia, neologisms, reversal of pronouns), and profound withdrawal from people. He believed the disorder was nonorganic but noted that "these children have come into the world with innate inability to form the usual, biologically provided affective contact with people" (Kanner, 1943).

Kanner held that this syndrome of early infantile autism was an expression of schizophrenia in childhood. Psychogenic theories of autism which implicated the parents as causal agents were proposed by Kanner, among others. There continued to be confusion about overlapping syndromes (Goldfarb, 1961). A

Table 1. *DSM-III-R* Schizophrenia: Summary

A. Presence of characteristic psychotic symptoms in the active phase: either (1), (2), or (3) for at least one week. . . .
   1. two of the following
     a. delusions
     b. prominent hallucinations
     c. incoherence or marked loosening of associations
     d. catatonic behavior
     e. flat or grossly inappropriate affect
   2. bizarre delusions. . . .
     prominent hallucinations (auditory)

B. Functioning in . . . work, social relations and self care is markedly below the highest level achieved before onset . . . (or, when the onset is in childhood or adolescence, failure to achieve expected level of social development).

C. Schizoaffective Disorder and Mood Disorder with psychotic features have been ruled out. . . .

D. Continuous signs . . . for at least six months . . . (including) an active phase (of at least one week) . . . with or without a prodromal or residual phase . . . prodromal or residual symptoms:
   1. Marked social isolation or withdrawal
   2. Marked impairment in role functioning
   3. Markedly peculiar behavior
   4. Marked impairment in personal hygiene
   5. Blunted or inappropriate affect
   6. Digressive, vague, overelaborate, or circumstantial speech, or poverty of content of speech
   7. Odd beliefs or magical thinking . . . over-valued ideas, ideas of reference
   8. Unusual perceptual experiences
   9. Marked lack of initiative, interest, or energy.

E. It cannot be established that an organic factor initiated and maintained the disturbance.

F. If there is a history of Autistic Disorder, the additional diagnosis of schizophrenia is made only if prominent delusions or hallucinations are also present.

Classification of Course

   1. subchronic
   2. chronic
   3. subchronic with acute exacerbation
   4. chronic with acute exacerbation
   5. in remission
   6. unspecified

Table 1. *DSM-III-R* Schizophrenia: Summary (*continued*)

Types

295.2 Catatonic type
  1. catatonic stupor . . . or mutism
  2. catatonic negativism
  3. catatonic rigidity
  4. catatonic excitement
  5. catatonic posturing

295.1 Disorganization type
  A. Incoherence, marked loosening of associations, or grossly disorganized behavior
  B. Flat or grossly inappropriate affect
  C. Does not meet the criteria for catatonic type

295.3 Paranoid type
  A. Preoccupation with one or more systematized delusions with frequent auditory hallucinations related to a single theme
  B. None of symptoms noted under catatonic or disorganized type

295.9 Undifferentiated type
  A. Prominent delusions, hallucinations, incoherence, or grossly disorganized behavior
  B. Does not meet the criteria for paranoid, catatonic, or disorganized type

295.6 Residual type
  A. Absence of prominent delusions, hallucinations, incoherence, or grossly disorganized behavior
  B. Continuing evidence of the disturbance, as indicated by two or more of the residual symptoms listed in criterion D. of schizophrenia

From American Psychiatric Association: Diagnostic and Statistical Manual of Mental Disorders, Third Edition, Revised. Washington, DC, American Psychiatric Association, 1987

British working party formulated nine points which they felt distinguished the schizophrenic syndrome of childhood (Creak, 1961). These included: gross and sustained impairment of relationships with people; apparent unawareness of personal identity to a degree inappropriate to age; pathological preoccupation with particular objects or certain characteristics of them without regard to their accepted functions; sustained resistance to change in the environment and a striving to maintain or restore sameness; abnormal perceptual experience (in the absence of discernible organic abnormality); acute, excessive, and seemingly illogical anxiety as a frequent phenomenon; speech either lost or never acquired, or showing failure to develop beyond a level appropriate to an earlier age; distortion in motility patterns; and a background of serious retardation in which islets of normal, near normal, or exceptional intellectual function or skill may appear.

Barbara Fish (1975) concluded that gross impairment in human relationships and noncommunicative speech were the two symptoms both necessary and sufficient to make the diagnosis. These symptoms are now considered pathognomonic of autism and are not considered manifestations of schizophrenia in *DSM-III-R*.

Other workers used the age of onset of symptoms as a primary criterion in classification, dividing the group of children into those with onset between birth and age three; onset between three and five; and onset after five years. The late onset group is composed of children who manifest the symptoms associated with adult schizophrenia: formal thought disorder, hallucinations, and delusions. Kolvin et al (1971) and Rutter (1972) were influential in establishing infantile autism and schizophrenia as two distinct disease entitles. Bender (1942), as well as Fish (1975), however, continued to propose that infantile autism and schizophrenic disorder with childhood onset were the same pathological entity manifested by different symptoms according to age of onset and severity.

The end result of years of controversy is that in *DSM-III-R*, early forms of childhood psychoses are now subsumed under pervasive developmental disorder, with infantile autism considered the prototype of the developmental disorder, while the child with onset after age five is usually labeled schizophrenic.

Evidence for autism representing a group of disorders distinct from schizophrenia has been reviewed by Petty and colleagues (1984). Some indications for autism as a separate disorder include 1) earlier age of onset; 2) rarity of positive family history of schizophrenia; 3) low incidence (4.5/10,000) (Lotter, 1967) compared with approximately 1 percent for adult onset schizophrenia; and 4) prevalance of mental retardation. Yet follow-up studies (Howells and Guirguis, 1984) and clinical reports (Tanguay and Cantor, 1986) suggest that schizophrenia, usually of the poor prognosis nonremitting type, may develop in some individuals who fulfilled criteria for autism in childhood.

In summary, Green (1988) notes that the autistic children who subsequently meet criteria for schizophrenia possibly comprise a small etiologically distinct subgroup. This subgroup has a significant symptom overlap with infantile autism and a maturational inability to express those differentiating symptoms of schizophrenic disorder that require the more mature level of development present in older children.

ETIOLOGY AND RISK FACTORS

The concept of a basic core, unique to the schizophrenia syndrome, is not a new one. If valid, the schizophrenic core should consist of a set of measurable traits which would distinguish schizophrenia from other psychopathological conditions. These traits (which might include life-long manifestations of disordered thought, language, attention, and, secondarily, affect) should be detectable in schizophrenic individuals at all times independent of a psychotic or nonpsychotic state.

Several investigators have been convinced of the presence of a pathological core in schizophrenia, present from birth as an inherited predisposition, or genotype, that does not necessarily manifest itself by psychotic symptoms of delusions or hallucinations (Rado, 1956).

Despite enormous research efforts, to date no biological or neurophysiological markers (such as catecholamines, monoamine oxidase, abnormal eye tracking,

EEG evoked potentials, or DNA studies) have been implicated with certainty. Regarding current views on the strength of the genetic factor in schizophrenia and the mode of transmission, the likelihood is that for unmistakable cases, a genetic factor constitutes a necessary though not sufficient antecedent. The mode of transmission may be polygenic or may involve a single major locus gene. Heterogeneity involving a common neurobiological pathway is likely; currently high-risk studies are providing more definitive answers. Such studies offer a unique opportunity to examine the interaction of biological vulnerability and intrafamilial process (gene-environment interaction) which antedate and play a role in the development of schizophrenia.

Follow-Back Studies

Follow-back studies have attempted to trace the childhood records of adult schizophrenics. Watt (1972) found that a group of children later hospitalized for schizophrenia demonstrated school behavior different from other children. The school records of the schizophrenic group demonstrated that the index cases were clearly identifiable as deviant in childhood before they demonstrated any clear indications of psychotic disorganization. The patterns of maladjustment included gender differences: preschizophrenic boys demonstrated primary evidence of unsocialized aggression and secondary evidence of internal conflict, overinhibition, and depression; preschizophrenic girls demonstrated primary evidence of oversensitivity, conformity, and introversion. Other findings included the occurrence of a severe social stressor (for example, parental death) and organic handicaps (such as neurological deficits) among preschizophrenics. In a later study (Prentky et al, 1979), psychiatric symptom patterns of first hospital admission patients were correlated with childhood measures of social competence. Their results confirmed the hypothesis that low social competence is associated with withdrawal, thought disorder, and antisocial acting out. It would seem that chronic schizophrenics have a life-long history of biological deficits, low social competence, and maladaptation.

In accordance with the view that schizophrenia is a heterogeneous disorder with extreme variation in symptoms and course (Cloninger, 1987), Keefe and colleagues (1987) selected a subgroup of chronic schizophrenics for investigation. They compared a group of severely deteriorated male schizophrenics with a control group of chronic schizophrenics whose illness had been marked by remission alternating with exacerbations. After careful assessment of severity of symptoms (affective, positive and negative, negative sexual function, age of onset, and family history, among other variables), the results, consistent with other studies, suggested that "those patients with the most chronic deteriorated course are substantially unlike other schizophrenic patients." Poor outcome patients appeared to possess more core symptoms of schizophrenia, exhibited more negative symptoms and formal thought disorder than controls, and resembled the patients described by Prentky's group.

Prospective Studies

A number of prospective studies of children-at-risk for schizophrenia are underway. Risk figures indicate that the children of schizophrenics are at greater risk for developing schizophrenia than the population at large; approximately 13 percent for the child of one schizophrenic parent compared with 0.8–1 percent for the child with no schizophrenic parent (Gottesman and Shields, 1972). The longitudinal study permits the researcher greater objectivity through its reliance on a matched control sample, double blind ratings, and the passage of time in which to study incipient pathology. Mednick and Schulsinger (1968), two of the originators of the longitudinal approach to high-risk studies, believe that the offspring of schizophrenic mothers show a particular vulnerability to schizophrenic illness as a joint function of a) genetic loading and b) pregnancy and birth complications. This combined liability results in an infant who demonstrates a labile pattern of autonomic responsivity. Fish (1975) and Marcus and colleagues (1987) report a higher incidence of neurological "soft signs" in babies who later develop schizophrenic symptomatology. These include erratic and disorganized maturational patterns in activity and alertness, as well as autonomic instability.

Marcus and co-workers (1987) in the NIMH Israeli Kibbutz-City Study, followed the development of offspring of schizophrenic parents from middle childhood through early adulthood. A subgroup of 13 infants born to schizophrenic mothers showed clear neurobehavioral deficits often accompanied by poor social competence. The authors contend that schizophrenic illness involves constitutional factors whose expression can be observed as early as infancy.

In corroboration of this hypothesis, Heinrichs and Buchanan (1988) suggest that there is a higher prevalence of neurological abnormalities in the schizophrenics they studied compared to control subjects. Neurological abnormalities were shown to be correlated with bizarreness and distractibility, formal thought disorder, and cognitive impairment, more characteristic of chronic rather than acute course. The authors suggest that neurological abnormalities may predate the identifiable onset of the schizophrenic illness and predict a chronic, debilitating course. These findings have important implications in evaluating schizophrenia with early onset *before* the appearance of psychotic symptoms, for example, hallucinations and delusions.

Fish believes that a pandevelopmental retardation, or "pandysmaturation"—a transient dysregulation of motor, visual motor, and physical development noted between birth and two years—predicts vulnerability to later schizophrenia; the interaction of genetic and environmental factors may be implicated. A poor intrauterine environment would exemplify such a "constitutional" factor.

She described an acute paranoid schizophrenic decompensation in a 19-year-old male whose course she had followed from birth (Fish, 1986). The child of a schizophrenic mother, the boy demonstrated a "pandysmaturation" in infancy: He did not smile until four months of age, rocked, and was considered to have "odd affect." By six he was an "odd looking child," aggressive, hypersensitive, guarded, and suspicious. He was known to be cruel to animals (he cut off the legs of his pet turtle). Speech was reportedly slow, and affect flat. His fantasies and dreams were filled with death and violence. He was accident prone. He was diagnosed as having schizotypal personality disorder. At age 19 he became violent and disorganized; he heard voices and believed his mother was trying to kill him, and became preoccupied with homicidal and suicidal thoughts. At that time he was diagnosed paranoid schizophrenic. (Note that he would not meet the *DSM-III-R* criteria for schizophrenia until the final decompensation at age 19, while by other criteria he might have been labeled schizophrenic from childhood).

The New York High Risk Project

Erlenmeyer-Kimling (1976) and Erlenmeyer-Kimling and Cornblatt (1987), in describing the New York High Risk Project, noted that one of the primary aims of the project was the identification of early indicators of genetic liability to the development of schizophrenic disorders (as, for example, in attentional and informational processing).

It was assumed that a certain percentage of the study's children would experience psychotic decompensation in later life and that careful assessment of these children at regular intervals would reveal developing pathology and permit the identification of vulnerable individuals within the high-risk group. Two of the groups have been studied over a 16-year period beginning in 1971.

The study focuses on neurological, psychophysiological, psychiatric, psychological, and social measures. Because hypotheses regarding psychobiological dysfunction in adult schizophrenics suggest that schizophrenics may have difficulty processing stimuli, tests were selected to measure attentional dysfunction and distractibility in children of schizophrenic parents and two comparison groups. These included EEG measures of auditory and visual evoked potentials; and a variety of cognitive, attentional, and distractibility measurements, including the Continuous Performance Test (CPT) (Rutschmann et al, 1986) and the Attention Span Task (ATS).

Results demonstrated that attentional tasks, in particular, have been found to differentiate the high-risk group from the comparison groups (children of parents with affective disorder and parents without psychopathology). Consistent group differences were found on both the CPT and ATS. The high-risk subjects made significantly fewer correct responses and more random commission errors than the normal comparison group with and without distraction. As noted by Rutschmann and colleagues (1986), "only a subgroup of the high-risk group is at true genetic risk for schizophrenia while other members of the HR group have no increased genetic risks." The hypothesized dysfunctions assumed to be continuous with deficiencies observed in some adult schizophrenics may be present in all subjects with high-risk genotypes, or may only be present in truly "premorbid" subjects (that is, in subjects who will actually develop schizophrenia).

The high-risk subgroup which is deviant on the laboratory measures showed increasing overlap with the subjects who demonstrate subsequent behavior problems (Cornblatt and Erlenmeyer-Kimling, 1984). Thus, it seems that subjects showing early deficits on laboratory measures are becoming increasingly deviant behaviorally as they get older, a finding that supports the hypothesis that attentional dysfunctions serve as early predictors of later pathology. According to Rutschmann and colleagues (1986), there is an association between low performance for discriminability on the CPT in childhood and psychopathology in adolescence which "may be added as a tentative early indicator of subsequent psychopathology assumed to precede schizophrenia and related disorders."

By the end of the fourth testing period the mean age of group members of the original cohort was 20 and most of the subjects had entered the schizophrenia risk period. Of the 190 adolescents available for follow-up, 14 have been hospitalized for a psychiatric disorder [9 from the high-risk group, 4 from the psychiatric comparison, and 1 from the normal comparison group (Erlenmeyer-Kimling and Cornblatt, 1987)].

Those hospitalized for schizophrenia tended to have had lower IQ scores, particularly in the verbal subtests at the first testing, compared to the high-risk group as a whole (Erlenmeyer-Kimling et al, 1984). Most of the hospitalized subjects had poor Bender-Gestalt results, poor total scores on the pediatric neurological scores, and poor CPT scores. On the composite attentional indices (CPT, ATS, and WISC Digit Span), the hospitalized high-risk patients were among the worst performers on the composite score compared to the high-risk group as a whole. Moreover, the Global Assessment scores (GAS) administered during the initial evaluation were lower for the hospitalized high-risk subjects than for other subjects in a mean rating. The high-risk group contains a significantly (p<.004) greater percentage (27 percent) of subjects with composite attentional deviance scores than does the normal comparison (6 percent) or psychiatric comparison (11 percent) group (Erlenmeyer-Kimling and Cornblatt, 1987).

In summary, the data on the subjects who have been hospitalized or are in psychiatric treatment suggest a pattern for the high-risk subjects in which lower IQ (particularly verbal IQ) and poor performance on the Bender-Gestalt, neurological examination, and attentional indices at young ages may be indicative of later psychopathology.

PSYCHOBIOLOGICAL RESEARCH

Psychobiological research on schizophrenia in children and adolescents has largely been an extension of such research in adults. With the development of the vulnerability hypothesis (Zubin and Spring, 1977) and the work on populations at high risk for developing schizophrenia, investigators have looked for markers of vulnerability in individuals prior to onset (if any) of symptoms. Most of the psychobiological research done in the area of childhood/adolescent schizophrenia has been with samples of offspring of schizophrenics who are at relatively high risk for developing schizophrenia, rather than with the small number of youth who are already symptomatic. This research has focused primarily on cognitive and physiological measures, rather than on anatomic measures and determination of blood and cerebrospinal fluid components.

As noted previously, studies of children and adolescents at risk for schizophrenia have shown deficits in attention and responsiveness (Rutschmann et al, 1986; Nuechterlein and Dawson, 1984). High-risk children and adolescents have been found to have several possible vulnerability markers, including high electrodermal responsiveness to aversive stimuli, deviant smooth pursuit eye movements, attenuated P300 on evoked potentials, reduced alpha and heightened delta on EEG, and deficits in vigilance tasks, attention, and serial recall.

Asarnow and colleagues (1986) have attempted to delineate the specific CNS structures which mediate and form a biological substrate for the symptoms of the disorder and provide a basis for understanding how that substrate produces dysfunctions which eventuate in the cognitive impairments of childhood onset schizophrenia. They believe that information processing impairments may be associated with vulnerability to schizophrenic disorder. Disturbance in controlled attentional processes, they suggest, leads to communication deviance. The schizophrenic child appears vague, digressive, and is less likely to attend to a wide variety of cues.

Similar cognitive findings have been made in the few studies done in symptomatic youth. Carter and co-workers (1982) found that schizophrenic children are inferior to nonschizophrenic children on performance measures of the Wechsler Intelligence Scale for Children and the Primary Mental Abilities–Spatial Test, and on paired-associate learning tasks. However, most of their subjects fulfill the criteria for autism and not schizophrenia as defined by DSM-III. Selin and Gottschalk (1983) reported impaired abstraction and increased EEG abnormalities in schizophrenic adolescents.

In a rare report on metabolic measures in schizophrenic youth, Varma et al (1983) found that eight schizophrenic adolescents had increased serum glycosaminoglycans and protein-bound carbohydrates.

The state of psychobiological research in schizophrenic youth is preliminary. The above findings of psychophysiological abnormalities and deficits in attention, information processing, and performance point out the need and promise of future research in these areas.

CLINICAL CHARACTERISTICS AND DIFFERENTIAL DIAGNOSIS

Adolescent Onset

Differential diagnosis in adolescence is difficult, particularly in the acute phase of illness. Too often adolescent psychopathology has been labeled adolescent turmoil (Masterson, 1968) (identity disorder in DSM-III-R) until symptoms have become too florid to be considered "normal behavioral variants." Typical signs and symptoms of schizophrenic breakdown may include high levels of anxiety, incoherent speech (difficulty with the written and spoken word), overinclusive thinking, loss of concentration, preoccupation with inner thoughts, hallucinations, thought broadcasting, bizarre actions (that is, grimacing), and poor emotional control.

Even the most stringent set of criteria (Feighner et al, 1972) does not always differentiate manic from schizophrenic patients. The presence or absence of delusions and hallucinations is a frequent component of both disorders (Taylor et al, 1974). Paranoid ideation can be observed during a manic episode. Carlson and Strober (1978) described six cases of adolescents initially called schizophrenic who were subsequently rediagnosed having bipolar disorder. These patients exhibited symptoms of euphoric mood, verbosity, expansiveness, hypersexuality, irritability, aggressiveness, sleep loss in the manic phase, and anhedonia and vegetative symptoms in the depressed phase. The investigators considered the possibility that developmental issues masked the affective disorder.

Borderline personality disorder must also be considered when evaluating a psychotic adolescent. Borderline adolescents with abnormal sensitivity to hallucinogens cannot always be differentiated from schizophrenics where the precipitant to decompensation is illicit drug use.

Organic mental syndromes should always be considered. Rivinus and colleagues (1972) described 12 children whose deteriorating school performance and emotional instability antedated visual and postural symptoms from CNS pathology. Temporal lobe epilepsy may mimic schizophrenia or mania (Bear et al, 1985).

A multidimensional approach to assessment can avoid many pitfalls and help point to more accurate diagnosis. The diagnosis of premorbid personality is contributory, particularly when the diagnosis of schizoid or schizotypal personality has previously been established.

Childhood Onset

Differential diagnosis of childhood onset schizophrenia is difficult because of the lack of agreement among researchers regarding age of onset, severity, and symptoms which overlap with autism. Kydd and Werry (1982) noted that the onset may be insidious (80 percent, according to Green, 1988), prodromal over a few days or weeks, or fulminating. As noted earlier, Petty and co-workers (1984) and Tanguay and Cantor (1986) reported a few cases of schizophrenia developing subsequent to a diagnosis of autism. Epidemiological data are scanty but suggest that schizophrenia is rare before age five, that frequency is low (0.03 percent) (Steinburg, 1985), and that sex ratios before puberty are overwhelmingly male (Kolvin et al, 1971; Kydd and Werry, 1982).

Clinical descriptions abound (Bender, 1942; Vrono, 1973), although in these studies no attempt is made to distinguish schizophrenia from autism or organic psychoses. Kolvin and colleagues (1971) found that some classical schizophrenic symptoms were present in children with onset after age four: hallucinations, thought disorder, and blunting of affect (children with abnormal preoccupations, disinterest in people, stereotypy, echolalia, and overactivity were considered autistic). Hallucinations must be evaluated with care. Chambers (1986) documented a high incidence of auditory hallucinations in children with affective disorders, and Rothstein (1981) concluded that there is a high frequency of normal children who report hallucinations. In certain cultures hallucinations of a religious nature are commonly reported (Canino, 1985). Side effects of commonly used medications occasionally include hallucinations (Chambers, 1986)

Impairments in perceptual motor skills were noted by Bender (1942), Goldfarb (1961), Fish (1975), Rutter and Garmezy (1983), and attentional deficits by Asarnow and colleagues (1986). Goldfarb (1974) observed that in his longitudinal study of 40 schizophrenic children, all demonstrated impairment in human relationships, defects in personal identity, and excessive anxiety provoked by change and communication disturbance. (Most of these children, however, would be considered as fulfilling criteria for autism by *DSM-III-R*.) Children with neurological findings and abnormal EEGs increasingly are reported (Kolvin, 1971; Rutter, 1972). DeMeyer and colleagues (1981) and Cantor and co-workers (1982) have reported hypotonia (neuromuscular dysfunction) in the group of childhood schizophrenics with onset before age five.

Intellectual functioning is variable. While less impaired than autistic children, many schizophrenic children have been found to have mild to moderate retardation (Kolvin, 1971). In Green's sample (1988), IQ range was 65 to 125 with a mean of 86; language delays have been reported by Cantor and colleagues (1982), and Fish (1975).

Social and Emotional Features

Most clinical reports describe social withdrawal, moodiness, irrational fears, lack of empathy, disinhibition, and immaturity. Thus, peer relationships are severely compromised from early childhood; "neurotic-like" symptoms (phobias, obsessive compulsive behavior) must be carefully evaluated before making a diagnosis of schizophrenia.

EVALUATION

A careful history is essential before making a diagnosis with any degree of certainty. A full genetic history should be taken with careful attention to non-hospitalized family members who present bizarre or schizotypal features. The prenatal and early developmental history is particularly important in relation to speech and language, social relations, sleep patterns, and evidence of magical thinking. The child's reaction to death, separation, and trauma should be examined in detail. It is necessary to obtain medical and school reports. A thorough neurological examination including EEG should be obtained in every case to rule out, among other organic conditions, temporal lobe epilepsy. The mental status examination should be done in several sessions, particularly with an anxious child. A structured interview, used for assessment of psychosis in children, should be used in addition (Kiddie SADS) (Puig-Antich et al, 1983). Psychological evaluation should include projective tests as well as neuropsychological tests. An assessment of family functioning can help determine biosocial risk factors and treatment recommendations.

OUTCOME

Because of the lack of controlled studies of childhood schizophrenia, the dissimilarity of diagnostic criteria used, and the rarity of the illness, follow-up studies are, for the most part, unreliable and impressionistic. Outcome of adolescent-onset schizophrenia seems to fall into two groups: those who recover following an acute onset and those with continuing incapacity whose condition becomes chronic. Adolescents with high intelligence, normal EEG, and late onset have better outcomes, particularly if affective symptoms were present (Annesley, 1961). Wing (1976) observed that schizophrenic children follow a course similar to the adult disorder, namely that some have no further episodes, some relapse, and some remain chronically incapacitated, although he concluded that the average outcome compares unfavorably with other psychiatric disorders.

There are few outcome studies of childhood onset schizophrenia. Most of the follow-up studies (Eisenberg, 1956; Creak, 1961) describe the outcome in autistic children. Rutter (1972) stated that IQ had prognostic significance (children with IQ below 60 have a worse prognosis). Goldfarb (1974) selected 40 institutionalized school age schizophrenic children for a three-year longitudinal study and compared them with 65 normal children (many fulfilled criteria for autism). Forty variables were divided into two categories: characteristics which may be expected to improve solely on the basis of maturation, and characteristics which reflect primary influence of social and educational experience. There was impressive evidence of growth and change, communication, educational achievement, and social competence. They remained below levels attained by the normal comparison groups, however; those abnormalities which change the least were activity level and muscle tone, reflecting the "level of integrity of the schizophrenic child's nervous system."

More recently Eggers (1978) followed up 57 children first seen in childhood. Fifty-one percent were "improved," and 20 percent in complete remission at 15 year follow-up. Best outcome occurred with acute onset, good premorbid personality (outgoing, responsive), and well differentiated symptoms. Children with onset before age 10 had the worst outcome. Kydd and Werry (1982) confirmed these findings in their own follow-up study of schizophrenic children.

TREATMENT APPROACHES

The therapeutic modality adopted with schizophrenic children has more often reflected the therapist's theoretical bias as well as the heterogeneity of the childhood schizophrenic population (Cantor and Kestenbaum, 1986). Treatment modalities have ranged from individual psychotherapy, milieu therapy, family therapy, psychoeducational therapy, and a variety of paraverbal therapies, often with the addition of psychopharmacological interventions. Each schizophrenic child presents with a unique set of developmental strengths and vulnerabilities, different cognitive capacity, motivation, level of communication, and familial and educational experience.

Symptom expression and degree of dysfunction are variable so that individual personality traits, constitutional vulnerabilities, familial, and social–educational environment should be carefully assessed in order to institute an individualized comprehensive treatment approach; this might include supportive psychotherapy, educational planning, medication, and parental counseling (Kron and Kestenbaum, 1988).

In view of the fact that children and adolescents are still in the process of development and still strongly influenced by their environment, any treatment approach, be it on an outpatient or inpatient basis, should integrate the social, familial, psychodevelopmental, biological, and educational aspects of care with the day-to-day care of the child.

There are as yet few controlled studies concerned with treatment outcome in schizophrenic children. As noted previously, predictions of better outcome include acute onset, clear precipitants, good premorbid adjustment, and well differentiated symptomatology (Eggers, 1978).

Psychopharmacological Interventions

Despite the widespread use of neuroleptics in child and adolescent psychiatric patients, these medications are used predominantly for conduct problems rather than psychoses. Although the primary psychopharmacologic treatment of schizophrenia in youth is with neuroleptics, there are no controlled studies in the literature assessing the benefits of neuroleptics (or other medications) in schizophrenic children, and only a few in schizophrenic adolescents. Most reports lump together all childhood psychoses, including autism and schizophrenia, and thus the efficacy of psychotropic medications in childhood schizophrenia per se has not been well established.

Studies in adolescent schizophrenics with agents such as haloperidol, loxapine, thiothixene, thioridazine and molindone (Realmutto et al, 1984; Greenhill et al, 1985) suggest that neuroleptics lessen psychotic symptoms but cause significant sedation, dystonia, and extrapyramidal symptoms (EPS). Unfortunately, most such studies do not have large enough sample sizes or adequate descriptions of their patient samples to determine symptom duration (childhood or adolescent onset), the presence/absence of autistic symptoms, or the heterogeneity of the sample.

Due to the lack of any controlled studies in prepubertal schizophrenics, one is left to rely on clinical experience and small-sample case reports. Once again, many of the latter do not discriminate between schizophrenia and autism: if they do, the number of schizophrenic subjects is too small to permit conclusions. In general, investigators such as Campbell (1985) and O'Gorman (1965) indicate that even though some psychotic symptoms may be ameliorated, the efficacy of neuroleptics appears to be less than that with adults. This is particularly true of anergic and apathetic children who may become excessively sedated or get worse on neuroleptics, even at low doses (Campbell, 1985). Indeed, Campbell notes that neuroleptics in youth are most effective in lessening psychomotor excitement.

Recommendations for the use of neuroleptics in childhood schizophrenia are, by necessity, based on clinical reports and the experience of using these medications in nonschizophrenic children. Early initiation of neuroleptics in the course of psychotic symptoms may facilitate the child's ability to respond to other types of therapies and to educational remediation. No one neuroleptic or type of neuroleptic has clear-cut advantages over others. Higher potency neuroleptics such as haloperidol and trifluoperazine are less sedating and may have less associated cognitive impairment than lower potency drugs such as chlorpromazine and thioridazine. However, the risk of withdrawal and tardive dyskinesia may be greater, as may the incidence of dystonia, EPS, and akathisia. Generally, clinicians begin neuroleptic treatment with lower doses in children than in adults, primarily due to the increased susceptibility of children to EPS (for example, beginning haloperidol at 0.5 or 1 mg twice a day). Just as with adults, there is some controversy regarding concomitant initiation of antiparkinsonian agents with the neuroleptics to lessen the likelihood of EPS and dystonia (Campbell, 1985; Kydd and Werry, 1982), although many clinicians now will begin both together, especially with high potency neuroleptics. Due to the possibility of long-term and severe adverse affects such as tardive dyskinesia and neuroleptic malignant syndrome, short trials (several months) of neuroleptics and drug holidays are recommended, and the concurrent use of more than one neuroleptic is discouraged. Long-acting depot forms of neuroleptics are not generally used in children. Monitoring neuroleptic plasma levels in clinical treatment is felt to be of little value: the meaning of such levels in adults is not well established (Baldessarini et al, 1988), let alone in children where there has been no substantial research. In general, neuroleptic plasma levels are in the same range as in adolescents and adults.

Alternative drug treatments to neuroleptics in childhood/adolescent onset schizophrenia have not been sufficiently studied. Medications such as typical neuroleptics, lithium, anticonvulsants, antidepressants, and others have been too little used or reported on for any recommendations to be made as to their use in schizophrenic children or adolescents.

Psychosocial Intervention: Individual Psychotherapy

Psychotherapy with schizophrenic children has traditionally followed two main directions, "expressive" and "suppressive" (Escalona, 1964). Expressive therapy, derived from concepts inherent in the psychoanalysis of neurotic individuals, permits the expression of previously unconscious material, while suppressive therapy proceeds from a recognition of the fact that psychotic children have difficulty repressing experiences which in normal children would be outside awareness.

Mahler (1968) describes therapy with young schizophrenic children as necessitating "corrective symbiotic techniques." Berlin (1973) describes dynamically oriented strategies in his work with schizophrenic children. Cantor and Kestenbaum (1986; Kestenbaum, 1978) have suggested that the therapist function as an auxiliary ego and facilitator of sensory perceptions. They suggest a reality oriented treatment approach that helps develop better communication skills and more adaptive defenses.

Family Interventions

Current thinking reflects the complex transactions that occur in parent–child interactions (Sameroff et al, 1984). Increasingly children are seen as having unique biologically based traits that have a powerful effect on parenting behaviors throughout the various phases of the child's development. It often is difficult to determine when the child's symptoms are caused by parental dysfunctions or how much of the parental style results from the child's behavior. Studies of family factors that are believed to be stressful to vulnerable children have described communication deviance (Wynne et al, 1977) and "high expressed emotion" or negative affective climate (Vaughn and Leff, 1976) in these families.

Pre- and posttreatment comparisons of family intervention techniques with adolescent patients (Hogarty et al, 1986) demonstrated that when reductions of negative affect and a shift to low expressed emotion are accomplished, the relapse rate is significantly diminished. When family management techniques were combined with individual social skills training and medication, the relapse rate was 0 percent at one year follow-up.

Family intervention techniques include support, information, coping skills development, communication training, and, whenever possible, the active behavioral involvement of the family in the child's treatment.

Behavior Therapy

Behavioral approaches have been described with psychotic children and usually include parents and, in residential settings, clinical staff. Successful behavioral interventions have been reported in changing maladaptive social skills, speech problems, and cognitive difficulties (Yates, 1970). A variety of behavior therapy models have been described, from positive reinforcement techniques to aversive conditions for self-destructive or avoidance behaviors and bizarre motility patterns.

Depending on age, level of development, and severity of the symptoms, many approaches have been offered to complement the major treatment strategies with psychotic children and adolescents. In view of the focused approaches of these other therapies, the literature often does not differentiate clearly between autistic, schizophrenic, and emotionally disturbed children and adolescents. Ruttenberg and colleagues (1980), in a review of treatment approaches, include sensory motor integrative therapy, language therapy, play therapy, art therapy, and music therapy. They suggest that the best approach, nevertheless, is a multidisciplinary one that integrates learning theory, behavioral strategies, psychodynamic therapy, and, when necessary, medication. Recently, there has been an increasing interest in approaches that focus on interpersonal cognitive problem-solving deficits. Even though their utility has not been established formally, they have been implemented with emotionally disturbed boys in residential treatment centers (Elias, 1979). These interventions focus on the covert thinking processes which underlie effective social interactions in children.

CONCLUSION

It is obvious from the foregoing that schizophrenia in childhood and adolescence is still a complex and controversial syndrome. There seems little doubt that schizophrenia comprises a heterogeneous group of disorders with multiple factors involved in the genesis, course, and outcome. Advances in research methodology are helping to identify etiological subtypes and discern the schizophrenia genotype from its phenocopy. If, indeed, genetic error leads to biochemical endophenotype to neurophysiological endophenotype to abnormal behavior and social interaction (Meehl, 1972), core deficits in schizophrenic individuals should be studied prior to psychotic decompensation. We must have a multiaxial approach to examining data on various aspects of the disorder: symptoms, onset, etiology (predisposition, genetic loading), personality type, and precipitants, such as life events and social influences. We need to tap the biological determinants of behavior—"trait," rather than "state" disturbance, particularly the appearance of a premorbid trait which may be present in the non-ill family members of schizophrenic patients.

Subtype signs and symptoms pathognomonic of schizophrenia may exist in attenuated forms for years before individuals are hospitalized with acute breaks. These symptoms may disrupt social adjustment, marital states, and work competence (Strauss et al, 1974).

It may be that some individuals vulnerable to schizophrenia lack some central executive control functions that regulate the processing of information as demonstrated by the delay in language, lower verbal IQ, and attentional tests. The limitations in specific information processing capacities may lead to subsequent problems in socialization and later symptom formation (Cornblatt and Erlenmeyer-Kimling, 1984). For example, such deficits may result in a lack of empathy (sensitivity to the feelings of others), according to Asarnow et al (1986) and thus result in increasing social isolation as social skills progressively fall further behind.

In the case of the prepsychotic child, we cannot change an individual's constitutional predisposition, but early detection of the child-at-risk, or the already ill, can lead to early intervention which could minimize the degree of serious disturbance in adult life. We could ascertain which environments enhance and which diminish the likelihood of psychotic decompensation. Such environmental interventions may not prevent a decompensation in adult life, but the social, vocational, and academic skills thus acquired would shorten the course of the illness and give schizophrenic children sufficient adaptive equipment to help them cope successfully with their own vulnerability.

REFERENCES

American Psychiatric Association: Diagnostic and Statistical Manual of Mental Disorders, First Edition (DSM). Washington, DC, American Psychiatric Association, 1952

American Psychiatric Association: Diagnostic and Statistical Manual of Mental Disorders, Second Edition (DSM-II). Washington, DC, American Psychiatric Association, 1968

American Psychiatric Association: Diagnostic and Statistical Manual of Mental Disorders, Third Edition (DSM-III). Washington, DC, American Psychiatric Association, 1980

American Psychiatric Association: Diagnostic and Statistical Manual of Mental Disorders, Third Edition, Revised (DSM-III-R). Washington, DC, American Psychiatric Association, 1987

Annesley TP: Psychiatric illness in adolescence: presentation and prognosis. Journal of Mental Science 1961; 107:268–278

Asarnow R, Sherman T, Strondberg R: The search for the biological substrate of childhood onset schizophrenia. J Am Acad Child Psychiatry 1986; 25:601–604

Baldessarini RJ, Cohen BM, Teicher MH: Significance of neuroleptic dose and plasma level in the pharmacological treatment of psychoses. Arch Gen Psychiatry 1988; 45:79–91

Bear DM, Freeman B, Greenberg B: Behavioral alterations in patients with temporal lobe epilepsy, in Behavioral Aspects of Epilepsy. Edited by Blumer D. Washington, DC, American Psychiatric Press, 1985

Bender L: Childhood schizophrenia. The Nervous Child 1942; 1:138–140

Berlin I: Simultaneous psychotherapy with a psychotic child and both parents, in Clinical Studies in Childhood Psychosis. Edited by Szurek SA, Berlin IN. New York, Brunner/Mazel, 1973

Campbell M: Schizophrenic disorders and pervasive developmental disorders/infantile autism, in Diagnosis and Psychopharmacology of Childhood and Adolescent Disorders. Edited by Wiener JM. New York, John Wiley & Sons, 1985

Canino I: A comparison of symptoms and diagnoses in Hispanic and black children in an outpatient mental health clinic. J Am Acad Child Psychiatry 1985; 25:254–259

Cantor S, Evans J, Pearce J, et al: Childhood schizophrenia: present but not accounted for. Am J Psychiatry 1982; 139:758–762

Cantor S, Kestenbaum CJ: Psychotherapy with schizophrenic children. J Am Acad Child Psychiatry 1986; 25:623–630

Carlson GA, Strober M: Manic-depressive illness in early adolescence. J Am Acad Child Psychiatry 1978; 17:138–153

Carter L, Alpert M, Stewert SM: Schizophrenic children's utilization of images and words in performance of cognitive tasks. J Autism Dev Disord 1982; 12:279–293

Chambers WJ: Hallucinations in psychotic and depressed children, in Hallucinations in Childhood. Edited by Pilowsky D, Chambers WJ. Washington, DC, American Psychiatric Press, 1986

Cloninger RC: Genetic principles and methods in high risk studies of schizophrenia. Schizophr Bull 1987; 13:515–523

Cornblatt B, Erlenmeyer-Kimling L: Early attentional predictors of adolescent behavioral disturbances in children-at-risk for schizophrenia, in Children-At-Risk for Schizophrenia—A Longitudinal Perspective. Edited by Watt NI, Anthony EJ, Wynne L, et al. New York, Cambridge University Press, 1984

Creak M: Schizophrenic syndrome in childhood: report of a working party. Br J Psychiatry 1961; 109:84–89

Demyer MK, Hintgen IN, Jackson RK: Infantile autism reviewed: a decade of research. Schizophr Bull 1981; 7:388

Eggers C: Course and prognosis of childhood schizophrenia. Journal of Autism and Childhood Schizophrenia, 1978; 8:21–36

Eisenberg L, Kanner L: Early infantile autism: 1943–1955. Am J Orthopsychiatry 1956; 26:556–566

Elias MJ: Helping emotionally disturbed children through prosocial television. Exceptional Children 1979; 46:217–218

Erlenmeyer-Kimling L: A prospective study of children at risk for schizophrenia: methodological considerations and some preliminary findings, in Life History Research in

Psychopathology. Edited by Wirt R, Winokor G, Roff M. Minneapolis, University of Minnesota Press, 1976

Erlenmeyer-Kimling L, Cornblatt B: The New York high risk project—a follow-up report. Schizophr Bull 1987; 13:451–461

Erlenmeyer-Kimling L, Kestenbaum CJ, Bird H, et al: Assessment of the New York high risk subjects in a sample who are now clinically deviant, in Children At Risk for Schizophrenia—A Longitudinal Perspective. Edited by Watt NF, Anthony EJ, Wynne L, et al. New York, Cambridge University Press, 1984

Escalona S: Some considerations regarding psychotherapy with psychotic children, in Child Psychotherapy. Edited by Haworth MH. New York, Basic Books, 1964

Feighner JP, Robins E, Guze SB, et al: Diagnostic criteria for use in psychaitric research. Arch Gen Psychiatry 1972; 25:57–63

Fish B: Biological antecedents of psychosis in children, in The Biology of the Major Psychoses (Association for Research into Mental Disorders Publication No. 54). Edited by Freeman DX. New York, Raven Press, 1975

Fish B: Antecedents of an acute schizophrenic break. J Am Acad Child Psychiatry 1986; 25:595–600

Goldfarb W: Childhood Schizophrenia. Cambridge, MA, Harvard University Press, 1961

Goldfarb W: Growth and change of schizophrenic children: a longitudinal study. New York, John Wiley & Sons, 1974

Gottesman I, Shields J: Schizophrenia and genetics: a twin study vantage point. New York, Academic Press, 1972

Green WA: Pervasive developmental disorders, in Handbook of Clinical Assessment of Children and Adolescents. Edited by Kestenbaum CJ, Williams DT. New York, New York University Press, 1988

Greenhill LL, Soloman M, Pleak R, et al: Molindone hydrochloride treatment of hospitalized children with conduct disorder. J Clin Psychiatry 1985; 46:20–25

Heinrichs DW, Buchanan RW: A significance and meaning of neurological signs in schizophrenia. Am J Psychiatry 1988; 145:11–18

Hogarty GE, Anderson CM, Reiss DJ, et al: Family psychoeducation, social skills training, and maintenance chemotherapy, in the aftercare treatment of schizophrenia. Arch Gen Psychiatry 1986; 43:633–642

Howells JG, Guirguis WR: Childhood schizophrenia 20 years later. Arch Gen Psychiatry 1984; 41:123–128

Kanner L: Autistic disturbances of affective contact. The Nervous Child 1943; 2:217–250

Keefe RSE, Mohs RC, Losonczy MI, et al: Characteristics of very poor outcome schizophrenics. Am J Psychiatry 1987; 144:889–895

Kestenbaum CJ: Childhood psychosis: psychotherapy, in Handbook of Treatment of Disorders in Childhood and Adolescence. Edited by Wolman BE, Egan J, Ross AO. Englewood Cliffs, NJ, Prentice-Hall, 1978

Kolvin J, Ounsted C, Humphrey M, et al: Studies in the childhood psychosis, I–VI. Br J Psychiatry 1971; 1118:385–415

Kron L, Kestenbaum CJ: Children at risk for psychotic disorder in adult life, in Handbook of Clinical Assessment of Children and Adolescents. Edited by Kestenbaum CJ, Williams, DT. New York, New York University Press, 1988

Kydd RR, Werry JS: Schizophrenia in children under 16 years. J Autism Dev Disord 1982; 12:343–357

Loranger AW: Sex differences in age of onset of schizophrenia. Schizophr Bull 1987; 13:157–161

Lotter V: Epidemiology of autistic conditions in young children, I: prevalance. Soc Psychiatry 1967; 1:124–137

Mahler MS: On human symbiosis and the vicissitudes of individuation. New York, International Universities Press, 1968

Marcus J, Hans SL, Nagler S, et al: Review of the NIMH Israeli Kibbutz–city study and the Jerusalem infant development study. Schizophr Bull 1987; 13:425–438

Masterson J: The psychiatric significance of adolescent turmoil. Am J Psychiatry 1968; 124:1549–1554

Mednick SA, Schulsinger F: Some premorbid characteristics related to breakdown in children with schizophrenic mothers, in The Transmission of Schizophrenia. Edited by Rosenthal D, Kety SS. New York, Pergamon Press, 1968

Meehl PE: A critical afterword, in Schizophrenia and Genetics. Edited by Gottesman I, Shields J. New York, Academic Press, 1972

O'Gorman G: The psychoses of childhood: the schizophrenic syndrome, in Modern Perspective in Child Psychiatry. Edited by Howells JG. Springfield, IL, Charles C Thomas, 1965

Nuechterlein KH, Dawson ME: Information processing and attentional functioning in the developmental course of schizophrenic disorders. Schizophr Bull 1984; 10:160–203

Petty LF, Ornitz EM, Michelman JD, et al: Autistic children who become schizophrenic. Arch Gen Psychiatry 1984; 41:129

Prentky RA, Watt NF, Fryer JH: Longitudinal social competence and adult psychiatric symptoms at first hospitalization. Schizophr Bull 1979; 5:306

Puig-Antich J, Chambers WJ, Jabrinzi MA: The clinical assessment of current depressive episodes in children and adolescents: interview with parents and children, in Childhood Depression. Edited by Cantwell A, Carlson G. New York, Spectrum, 1983

Rado SC: Dynamics and classification of disordered behavior, in Psychoanalysis of Behavior: Collected Papers. New York, Grune & Stratton, 1956

Realmuto GM, Erickson WD, Yellin AM, et al: Clinical comparison of thiothixene and thioridazine in schizophrenic adolescents. Am J Psychiatry 1984; 141:440–442

Rivinus I, Jamson DL, Graham PJ: Childhood organic neurological disease presented as psychotic disorder. Arch Dis Child 1972; 50:115–119

Rothstein A: Hallucinatory phenomena in childhood: a critique of the literature. J Am Acad Child Psychiatry 1981; 20:623–635

Rutschmann J, Cornblatt B, Erlenmeyer-Kimling L: Sustained attention in children at risk for schizophrenia: findings with two visual continuous performance tests in a new sample. J Abnorm Psychol 1986; 14:365–385

Ruttenberg B, Angert A: Psychotic disorders, in Emotional Disorders in Children and Adolescents: Medical and Psychological Approaches to Treatment. Edited by Sholivar P, Bensen M, Blinder B. New York, SP Medical and Scientific Books, 1980

Rutter M: Childhood schizophrenia reconsidered. Journal of Autism and Childhood Schizophrenia 1972; 2:315–331

Rutter M, Garmezy N: Developmental psychopathology, in Handbook of Child Psychology, fourth edition. Edited by Mussen PH. New York, John Wiley & Sons, 1983

Sameroff AJ, Barocas K, Seifer R: The early development of children born to mentally ill women, in Children at Risk for Schizophrenia: A Longitudinal Perspective. Edited by Watt NF, Anthony EJ, Wynne LC, et al. New York, Cambridge University Press, 1984

Selin CL, Gottschalk LA: Schizophrenia, conduct disorder and depressive disorder: neuropsychological, speech sample and EEG results. Perceptual and Motor Skills 1983; 57:427–444

Steinburg D: Psychotic and other severe disorders in adolescence, in Child and Adolescent Psychiatry: Modern Approaches, 2nd edition. Edited by Rutter M, Hersov L. Oxford, England, Blackwell Scientific Publications, 1985

Strauss JS, Carpenter WT, Bartko JJ: Speculations on the processes that underlie schizophrenic symptoms and signs. Schizophr Bull 1974; 11:61–75

Tanguay PE, Cantor SL: Schizophrenia in children—introduction. J Am Acad Child Psychiatry 1986; 25:591–594

Taylor MA, Gaztanaga P, Abrams R: Manic-depressive illness and acute schizophrenia: a clinical family history and treatment response study. Am J Psychiatry 1974; 131:678–682

Varma R, Michos GA, Gordon BJ, et al: Serum glycoconjugates in children with schizophrenia and conduct and adjustment disorders. Biochem Med 1983; 30:206–214

Vaughn CE, Leff JP: The influence of family and social factors on the course of psychiatric illness: a comparison of schizophrenic and depressed neurotic patients. Br J Psychiatry 1976; 129:125–137

Vrono M: Schizophrenia in childhood and adolescence. International Journal of Mental Health 1973; 2:8–11

Watt NF: Longitudinal changes in the social behavior of children hospitalized for schizophrenia as adults. J Nerv Ment Dis 1972; 42:155

Wing JL: Early childhood autism: clinical, educational, and social aspects, 2nd edition. Oxford, Pergamon Press, 1976

Wynne LC, Singer MT, Bartko JJ, et al: Schizophrenics and their families: research on prenatal communication, in Developments in Psychiatric Research. Edited by Tanner JM. London, Hodder & Stoughton, 1977

Yates A: Behavior Therapy. New York, John Wiley & Sons, 1970

Zubin J, Spring B: Vulnerability—a new view of schizophrenia. J Abnorm Psychol 1977; 86:103–126

Afterword

by Jerry M. Wiener, M.D.

Each of these chapters raises similar issues and questions that are at the cutting edge of modern child and adolescent psychiatry. From perhaps the oldest (mental retardation) to the most recent (mood disorders) of the diagnostic categories in our field, there is a gathering momentum of research studies utilizing standardized diagnostic criteria from *DSM-III-R* and an increasingly sophisticated scientific methodology.

The discussions presented by this group of authors reflect a growing excitement in new findings about familiar disorders. From these chapters it is possible to identify the direction of the field over the next several years:

1. A progressive refinement of the diagnostic criteria for disorders arising in childhood and adolescence, including an expansion of field-tested reliability and validity studies in the development of *DSM-IV* and subsequent classifications.
2. The increasing importance of utilizing a developmentally oriented and truly biopsychosocial model for the understanding and treatment of these disorders. Both psychosocial and biologic models, when applied alone, prove reductionistic and insufficient for exploring etiology or treatment efficacy, although it is clear that the major gains of the near future will likely be made in understanding the biological aspects more than the psychosocial.
3. There is as yet no instrument more valuable or necessary than an empathic physician trained to perform a comprehensive diagnostic assessment that includes both the child or adolescent and the family, and who can then effect a comprehensive treatment plan that attends to all the important needs of the child and the resources of the family.

III

Alcoholism

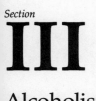
Contents

Section III
Alcoholism
Foreword
by Roger E. Meyer, M.D., Section Editor

Since the publication of the last special section on alcoholism in *Psychiatry Update: The American Psychiatric Association Annual Review, Volume III* (Grinspoon, 1984), there have been a number of major developments in research and clinical practice. The definition of alcohol dependence has been changed since the publication of the *Diagnostic and Statistical Manual of Mental Disorders, Third Edition (DSM-III)* (American Psychiatric Association, 1980). The new *Diagnostic and Statistical Manual of Mental Disorders, Third Edition, Revised* (American Psychiatric Association, 1987) *(DSM-III-R)* criteria for alcohol dependence are based largely on the earlier formulation of the alcohol dependence syndrome described in *International Classification of Diseases, Ninth Revision, Clinical Modification (ICD-9-CM)* (Commission on Professional and Hospital Activities, 1980), and in the paper by Edwards and Gross (1976). *DSM-III-R* encourages the diagnostician to classify severity of dependence; and alcohol abuse is offered as a residual category. *DSM-III* considered alcohol abuse and dependence to be discrete categories. The *DSM-III-R* criteria emphasize alcohol consumatory behavior, its primacy in relationship to other behavioral options, and impaired control over drinking behavior. *DSM-III* definitions of alcohol dependence emphasized tolerance and physical dependence—and failed to differentiate dependence from alcohol-related disabilities. While severe alcohol dependence should be accompanied by psychosocial disabilities, the latter are substantially influenced by culture, personality, and the presence of comorbid psychopathology.

Primarily three types of research have supported the validity and utility of measuring the severity of alcohol dependence (as described in the alcohol dependence syndrome). Studies on the symptom patterns of alcoholics in treatment using factor analytic (Skinner, 1982) and Guttmann Scaling techniques (Rounsaville et al, unpublished), as well as similar dependent symptom clusters in large cross-cultural cohorts (Babor et al, 1987), suggest a high degree of coherence of the symptom complex. One study, using Guttmann Scaling of data from a sample of Scottish alcoholics, failed to confirm that the seven elements of the alcohol-dependent syndrome could conform to a single dimension (Chick, 1980).

At least six studies have suggested that severity of dependence had prognostic significance in clinical populations (Polich et al, 1980; Opford et al, 1976; Vaillant, 1983; Skinner et al, 1982; Babor, in press; Heizer, 1985). In two studies (Heather et al, 1983; Litman et al, 1984), severity of dependence did not significantly predict the outcome. In general, studies in North America support the premise that a moderate drinking outcome is not possible for severely dependent alco-

---

This work was supported by the National Institute on Alcohol Abuse and Alcoholism Grant #5 P50 AA0350.

holics, whereas the two studies from the United Kingdom suggest that moderate drinking could be a stable outcome for some severely dependent drinkers. As a consequence of this work, research utilizing behavioral therapies to effect a moderate drinking outcome among alcoholics in treatment in the United States has been suspended, whereas such approaches are being applied to nondependent problem drinkers in the United States and to alcoholics in some treatment programs in the United Kingdom.

Finally, biobehavioral studies of alcoholic dependence in the laboratory suggest that dependent alcoholics (compared with controls) manifest autonomic arousal (increased skin conductance and heart rate) when presented with an alcoholic beverage stimulus (Hodgson et al, 1979; Kaplan et al, 1983; Kaplan et al, 1984; Kaplan et al, 1985; Laberg et al, 1986); manifest an increase in craving after a *priming* ethanol drink (Hodgson et al, 1979); are more likely to respond to placebo malt beverage as though it were real beer (where real beer and a malt beverage are administered under double-blind conditions) (Kaplan et al, 1983; Kaplan et al, 1984); and appear to show idiosyncratic hormonal responses to the stimulus presentation of a glass of beer and to the consumption of a placebo malt beverage (Morse et al, 1985; Dolinsky et al, 1987).

As described in Chapter 13, "Explanatory Models of Alcoholism," the alcohol dependence syndrome (and its offspring in *DSM-III-R*) represents a kind of biobehavioral reformulation of the disease concept of alcoholism. The latter was first elaborated by Benjamin Rush in 1790 (Rush, 1790), and it was emphasized in writings of 19th century physicians. It was most strongly advocated in the tenets of Alcoholics Anonymous and in the writings of E.M. Jellinek (Jellinek, 1960). Between 1962 and 1976, the disease concept came under attack by behavioral and social scientists, whose work raised many questions about the progressive nature of the disorder and the validity of concepts such as *loss of control* of drinking. Since 1976, the work of other behavioral and social scientists (and of clinicians) has led to a redefinition of alcohol dependence that appears to have clinical utility. Moreover, because it does not rely upon social consequences to define the disorder, it lends itself to the development of animal model analogs, which may lead to a better understanding of the biology of the disorder and to improved technologies for treatment and prevention.

Cloninger, Dinwiddie, and Reich, in Chapter 14, describe the status of genetics research in the alcohol field. Studies over the past three decades have highlighted the clustering of alcoholism within families and the possible genetic basis of that phenomenon. Studies in twins, half siblings, and adoptees generally support the genetic hypothesis; and studies that describe electrophysiological and pharmacogenetic differences between sons of alcoholics and controls suggest potential phenotypic markers of risk. Cloninger's own work has served to highlight the heterogeneity of alcoholism and suggests a genetic basis for that heterogeneity. Work in this area has proceeded to the point where molecular genetic strategies can be fruitfully applied to studies in extended family pedigrees. This work should lead to more precise markers of risk, as well as to a clearer understanding of the genetic factors associated with risk and the environmental factors that lead to the expression of the disorder.

Neurobiological research on the effects of acute and chronic alcohol administration has also become more sophisticated and relevant to the behavioral phenomena as elaborated in Chapter 15, "Neurobiology of Alcohol Action and

Alcoholism," by Dr. Floyd Bloom. This research should lead to a better understanding of the biology of alcohol intoxication, reinforcement, tolerance, physical dependence, and the syndrome of alcohol dependence. In the absence of specific ethanol *receptors*, research to explain the actions of alcohol on the brain had focused on the ability of ethanol to perturb general membrane functions *in vitro* (Goldstein, 1987; Taraschi et al, 1987), through its actions on the lipid component. It was postulated that acute alcohol administration had a disordering (or a *fluidizing*) effect on membrane lipids, whereas membranes from chronically ethanol-treated animals were more resistent to the fluidizing effects of alcohol. This was offered as an explanation of tolerance. As membranes became "more rigid" consequent to chronic ethanol administration, the maintenance of normal lipid structure would require the presence of ethanol. The latter was offered as a tentative explanation of physical dependence. Bloom highlights more recent *in vitro* biochemical essays, as well as cellular electrophysiological studies (and separate bodies of anatomic and neurochemical evidence), that offer a more specific pharmacological profile in which "it is the membrane-mounted proteins of selected subsets of neurons that are the main targets of pharmacologically relevant actions of alcohol." This latter analysis (compared with the lipid-focused hypothesis) is more compatible with ethanol's specific behavioral profile and with data that support important pharmacogenetic differences in strains of rats and mice, as well as in children of alcoholics. Bloom points out that single cell recordings suggest that some brain systems seem relatively insensitive to ethanol at high concentrations (for example, the cerebellar neurons), whereas the hippocampus, inferior olivary nucleus, and locus coeruleus show much greater sensitivity. In contrast to these studies, multiple investigations have failed to identify any consistent relationship between the content, synthesis, or catabolism of any neurotransmitter and the doses of alcohol required to produce intoxication. More promising studies comparing alcohol-preferring and alcohol-nonpreferring rats suggest a relationship between the serotonin content and alcohol-consuming behavior (Murphy et al, 1985, 1987). The hypothesis that ethanol exposure results in the production of monoamine-aldehyde condensation products in the central nervous system—which could explain the effects of alcohol and alcohol dependence—has not been validated, despite considerable research. Finally, Bloom highlights the controversy surrounding the effects of ethanol on the benzodiazepine–gamma amino-butyric acid (GABA) receptor complex. These issues are also addressed by Kranzler and Orrok in their report (Chapter 18) of the effects of the partial inverse agonist R15-4513 on ethanol intoxication in the rat and on chloride channel flux in synaptoneurosome preparations. At this writing, it is not clear whether GABAergic mechanisms play a role in some or all of the intoxicating effects of ethanol. Over the next five years, our understanding of the neurobiology of alcohol intoxication, reinforcement, tolerance, withdrawal symptoms, and dependence will be substantially advanced by the explosion of knowledge in neurobiology.

Issues of psychiatric comorbidity are considered at great length in Chapter 16, by Rounsaville and Kranzler. Comorbid psychiatric disorders may serve as risk factors for the development of alcoholism. Some psychiatric disorders may modify the course, symptom picture, and treatment response of alcoholic patients, while other psychiatric disorders appear to be a consequence of the alcoholism. With the introduction of *DSM-III* in 1980, a number of studies have served to highlight the high prevalance of comorbid psychiatric disorders in alcoholic patient populations. The presence of these conditions complicates response to traditional treatment modalities, highlighting the importance of psychiatry in the rehabilitation of many alcoholic patients.

Chapter 17, by Frances, Galanter, and Miller, describes the evolution of clinical practice in the alcohol field. The increased availability of insurance coverage and of inpatient, partial-hospital, and outpatient services represents one of the most important developments of the past decade. This chapter on psychosocial approaches to treatment and rehabilitation serves to emphasize the wide range of necessary services required by the psychiatrically heterogeneous alcoholic patient population. The authors stress the importance of a partnership between psychiatrists and self-help programs, and they point out the importance of a rehabilitation model when working with alcoholic patients. This chapter will be of special clinical usefulness to many readers.

In Chapter 18, Kranzler and Orrok describe developments in the pharmacotherapy of alcoholism. Their chapter elaborates both the progress and the promise of this work. Research on alcohol's effects on the chloride ion channel portion of the benzodiazepine-GABA receptor complex, and the possible pharmacological modification of those effects, suggests the possibility of a true amethystic agent. While much about this work remains to be clarified, this chapter highlights the potential applicability of research in neurobiology to clinical practice. Research on locus coeruleus activity in alcohol withdrawal has led to studies of clonidine in alcohol withdrawal, while other research has highlighted the potential usefulness of beta blockers such as propranolol in the treatment of aspects of the withdrawal syndrome. As Kranzler and Orrok point out, none of this work has served to displace the central role of benzodiazepines in the treatment of alcohol withdrawal. Their chapter highlights the state of the art in the pharmacotherapy of the treatment of alcohol withdrawal. Finally, a number of studies suggest the promise and the complexity of pharmacotherapy in the treatment of alcoholism. After 50 years, disulfiram has now been subject to a large systematic clinical trial (Fuller et al, 1986), and the results are thoroughly described by Kranzler and Orrok. These authors also highlight the potential role of serotonin uptake inhibitors in future alcoholism treatment. Issues of psychiatric comorbidity must inevitably be considered in connection with pharmacotherapy.

As these chapters so clearly demonstrate, we are in the era of subspecialization within psychiatry. The vigorous growth of psychiatrists' interest in the addictions field has been reflected in the rapid rise of membership in the recently formed American Academy of Psychiatrists in Alcoholism and Addictions (AAPAA), which has grown to 800 members in its brief lifetime. Moreover, 24 universities now offer fellowships in the addictions and another thirty-three are planning to start such programs. The chapters in this section highlight the growing body of knowledge which serves the alcoholism field.

REFERENCES

American Psychiatric Association: The Diagnostic and Statistical Manual of Mental Disorders, Third Edition. Washington, DC, American Psychiatric Association, 1980

American Psychiatric Association: Diagnostic and Statistical Manual of Mental Disorders, Third Edition, Revised. Washington, DC, American Psychiatric Association, 1987

Babor TF, Cooney NL, Lauerman R: The drug dependence syndrome concept as a psychological theory of relapse behavior. An empirical evaluation. Br J Addict (in press a)

Babor TF, Kranzler HR, Kadden RM: Issues in the definition and diagnosis of alcoholism: Implication for a reformulation. Prog Neuropharmacol Biol Psychiatry (in press b)

Chick, J: Is there a unidimensional alcohol dependence syndrome? Br J Addict 1980; 75:265–280

Commission on Professional and Hospital Activities: International Classification of Diseases, Ninth Revision. Ann Arbor, MI, Commission on Professional and Hospital Activities, 1980

Dolinsky ZS, Morse DE, Kaplan RF, et al: Neuroendocrine, psychophysiological and subjective reactivity to an alcohol placebo in male alcoholic patients. Alcoholism: Clinical and Experimental Research 1987; 11:296–300

Edwards G, Gross MM: Alcohol dependence: provisional description of a clinical syndrome. Br Med J 1976; 1:1058–1061

Fuller RK, Branchey L, Brightwell DR, et al: Disulfiram treatment of alcoholism: a Veterans Administration cooperative study. JAMA 1986; 256:1449–1455

Goldstein DB: Ethanol-induced adaptation in biological membranes. Ann NY Acad Sci 1987; 492:103–111

Grinspoon L (Ed): Psychiatry Update: The American Psychiatric Association Annual Review, vol. 3. Washington, DC, American Psychiatric Press, Inc., 1984

Heather N, Rollnick S, Winton M: A comparison of objective and subjective measures of alcohol dependence as predictors of relapse following treatment. Br J Clin Psychol 1983; 22:11–17

Helzer JE, Robins LN, Taylor JR, et al: The extent of longterm moderate drinking among alcoholics discharged from medical and psychiatric treatment facilities. N Engl J Med 1985; 312:1678–1682

Hodgson R, Rankin H, Stockwell T: Alcohol dependence and the priming effect. Behav Res Ther 1979; 17:379–387

Jellinek EM: The Disease Concept of Alcoholism. New Brunswick, Hillhouse Press, 1960

Kaplan RF, Meyer RE, Stroebel CF: Alcohol dependence and responsivity to an ethanol stimulus as predictors of alcohol consumption. Br J Addict 1983; 78:259–267

Kaplan RF, Meyer RE, Virgilio LM: Physiological reactivity to alcohol cues and the awareness of an alcohol effect in a double-blind placebo design. Br J Addict 1984; 79:439–442

Kaplan RF, Cooney NL, Baker LH, et al: Reactivity to alcohol-related cues: physiological and subjective responses in alcoholics and non-problem drinkers. J Stud Alcohol 1985; 46:267–272

Laberg JC: Alcohol and expectancies: subjective, psychophysiological and behavioral responses to alcohol stimuli in severely, moderately and non-dependent drinkers. Br J Addict 1986; 81:797–808

Litman GK, Stapleton J, Oppenheim AN, et al: The relationship between coping behaviours, their effectiveness and alcoholism relapse and survival. Br J Addict 1984; 79:283–291

Morse DE, Dolinsky ZS, Kaplan RF, et al: Ethanol expectancy: effects on testosterone levels. Alcoholism: Clinical and Experimental Research 1985; 9:83 (abstract)

Murphy JM, Waller MB, Gatto WJ, et al: Monoamine uptake inhibitors attenuate ethanol intake in alcohol-preferring (P) rats. Alcohol 1985; 2:349–52

Murphy JM, McBride WJ, Lumeng L, et al: Contents of monoamines in forebrain regions of alcohol-preferring (P) and nonpreferring (NP) lines of rats. Pharmacol Biochem Behav 1987; 26:389–92

Oford J, Oppenheimer E, Edwards G: Abstinence of control: the outcome for excessive drinkers two years after consultation. Behav Res Ther 1976; 14:409–418

Polich AM, Armor DJ, Braiker HB: The course of alcoholism four years after treatment. Publication No. RAND Corp R-2433. Rockville, MD, National Institute on Alcohol Abuse and Alcoholism, 1980

Rush B: An Inquiry into the Effects of Spiritous Liquors on the Human Body. Boston, Thomas and Andrews, 1790

Skinner AJ, Allen BA: Alcohol dependence syndrome: measurement and validation. J Abnorm Psychol 1982; 91:199–209

Taraschi TF, Ellingson JS, Rubin E: Membrane structural alterations caused by chronic ethanol consumption: the molecular basis of membrane tolerance. Ann NY Acad Sci 1987; 492:171–180

Vaillant GE: The Natural History of Alcoholism: Causes, Patterns and Paths of Recovery. Cambridge, MA, Harvard University Press, 1983

Chapter 13

Explanatory Models of Alcoholism

by Roger E. Meyer, M.D., and Thomas F. Babor, Ph.D.

Alcoholism is a disorder for which the symptoms have been known since antiquity. While explanatory models, or theories of alcoholism, have had to await developments in the biological, behavioral, and social sciences, a rich tradition of theoretical speculation about the etiology of alcoholism has grown since the 1870s (Babor and Dolinsky, 1988). Alcoholism was either the first disease, or the second social problem (after homicide) mentioned in Genesis (Genesis 9:20–26), when Noah planted a grape orchard sometime after the flood and became intoxicated with wine. The conflict that ensued between Noah and his son Ham is the earliest known description of the problems that can develop for a child growing up in an alcoholic family. Alcoholism has affected the course of history: Alexander the Great, whose father was a heavy drinker and whose mother was a Dionysian, died at age 33 after a bout of heavy drinking. After the ancient Romans cleared large sections of the Italian landscape for the growing of grapes, alcoholism became a major problem for the upper classes and the early emperors (Nero, Caligula, Claudius). Following the introduction of Christianity, there was an apparent decline in the prevalence of problem drinking among the Roman nobility; but in the middle ages, when winemaking became an important occupation of the monasteries, alcoholism became a problem among the clergy.

With the development of distillation technologies, alcohol became more widely available in greater quantities to the poor of Europe. In 18th century England, alcoholism was rampant among the lower classes. In the United States, per capita alcohol consumption peaked in the early 19th century. It was at this time that Dr. Benjamin Rush described alcoholism as a *disease* for which the cure was total abstinence. In addition to his position as the founder of American psychiatry (and a signatory to the Declaration of Independence), Rush was regarded in the 19th century as the founder of the American temperance movement. Throughout the 19th century, American medicine (and psychiatry) viewed alcoholism as a disease (called dipsomania or inebriety), rather than a behavioral response to some other psychiatric condition. Nineteenth century physicians differentiated between chronic alcoholism and alcohol addiction. The former was defined on the basis of the physical and psychological consequences of prolonged alcohol use, while alcohol addiction was defined as an uncontrollable craving for alcohol (Lender, 1979). The symptoms of craving and loss of control were considered the necessary components of alcohol addiction.

In the 20th century, psychiatric perspectives on alcoholism have been influenced by a number of distinct events and trends. Prohibition converted alcohol use into a legal problem, with a consequent decline of the medical profession's interest in the disease of inebriety. During the 1930s, the influence of psychoanalysis on American psychiatry contributed to the view that alcoholic drinking

This work was supported by the National Institute on Alcohol Abuse and Alcoholism Grant #5 P50 AA03510.

behavior was symptomatic of underlying psychopathology. With the growth of the social sciences following World War II, social psychiatrists, anthropologists, and epidemiologists cited the pronounced ethnic and cultural differences in alcoholism rates as evidence that drinking problems had their origins in social behavior. By the 1970s, alcoholic drinking behavior could be explained on the basis of learning mechanisms, psychodynamic influences, family systems, and sociocultural factors, as well as the psychopharmacology of ethanol.

Explanatory models of alcoholism are designed to explain the etiology, natural history, and consequences of the disorder. Any given model needs to account for cultural heterogeneity, genetic as well as familial risk factors, biological vulnerability, premorbid personality characteristics, and the psychiatric and medical comorbidities found in alcoholic patients. A good model should be based upon empirical evidence and should have predictive validity. This chapter will review some explanatory models of alcoholism. It will serve as a summary of current theory and an introduction to the subsequent sections on recent developments in alcoholism research and clinical practice. Table 1 provides a summary of the major features and etiological foci of eleven representative explanatory models reviewed below.

THE DISEASE CONCEPT OF ALCOHOLISM

Dorland's *Illustrated Medical Dictionary* defines a disease as a "definite morbid process having a characteristic train of symptoms," affecting one or more organ systems, whose "etiology, pathology, and prognosis may be known or unknown." Historically, the validity and reliability of diagnoses have been more certain where organ-based pathology has been clearly described, etiology is clear-cut and uncomplicated, and at the end stages of illness where those who are clearly diseased may be differentiated from those who are clearly not diseased. In the case of alcoholism, the diagnosis is most certain in the presence of end-stage liver and brain pathology (including severe alcohol withdrawal). The diagnosis of alcoholism has seemed less clear when made on the basis of the quantity or pattern of alcohol consumption, or when diagnosticians have utilized criteria based on psychological or social disability. With regard to the latter, cross-cultural differences in the pattern of psychosocial consequences have raised questions about the usefulness of these criteria in the diagnosis of alcoholism. In general, substantial psychosocial disability is associated with alcoholism in cultures with a strong temperance tradition, such as Sweden, whereas such disabilities are less commonly associated with alcoholism in cultures that accept and even encourage heavy drinking, as in France. Moreover, comorbid psycho-pathology will also affect the nature and severity of psychosocial disability in alcoholics.

After the repeal of Prohibition, the strongest arguments for a disease-based model of alcoholism could be found in the tenets of Alcoholics Anonymous (AA), and in the writings of E.M. Jellinek, who was not a physician. Jellinek (1960) traced the roots of the disease model to nineteenth-century physicians and elaborated upon the cultural influences that shape different forms of the disorder in different countries. He postulated that there were five *species* of alcoholism: 1) purely psychological continual dependence, *alpha alcoholism*; 2) organ-based pathology in the absence of psychological dependence, *beta alco-*

holism; 3) acquired tissue tolerance, withdrawal symptoms, and craving associated with physical dependence, *gamma alcoholism*; 4) an inability to abstain without loss of control, *delta alcoholism*; and 5) episodic drinking bouts without dependence or organ damage, *epsilon alcoholism*. Jellinek reserved the notion of addictive disease for delta and gamma alcoholisms. Gamma alcoholism was the principal type observed in the United States, and delta alcoholism was the principal type in France. He described the disease as progressive, unless the individual was able to abstain. His pathophysiological model of "craving" in the alcoholic required the presence of physical dependence.

Jellinek's disease concept was modified slightly and adopted by AA as its basic definition of alcoholism. According to Pattison and colleagues (1977), the basic tenets of this *traditional* model of alcoholism can be summarized as follows: 1) alcoholism is a unitary phenomenon that can be considered a distinct entity; 2) alcoholics and those predisposed to become alcoholics react differently to alcohol than nonalcoholics; 3) alcoholism is a permanent and irreversible condition; 4) alcoholics experience an irresistible physical craving for alcohol, or a strong psychological compulsion to drink; 5) alcoholics gradually develop a process called *loss of control* over drinking, and possibly even an inability to stop drinking; 6) alcoholism is a progressive disease which follows an inexorable development through a distinct series of phases.

Beginning in the 1970s, the traditional disease concept of alcoholism was challenged by a succession of studies which seemed to question a number of Jellinek's major points. Davies' (1962) report on seven former alcohol addicts who had returned to "normal drinking" called into question the notion of a progressive disorder. Longitudinal surveys of drinking practices in the United States (Roizen et al, 1978), showing that drinking problems often go into remission, seemed to add additional evidence to Davies' observation that alcoholism was not progressive. In the mid-1970s, the Sobells reported on successful efforts to shape a moderate drinking outcome in alcohol-dependent patients (Sobell and Sobell, 1976). In the same year that their follow-up study was reported, the initial RAND Corporation report (Armor et al, 1978) suggested that relapse to dependent drinking was not inevitable in alcohol-dependent persons who resumed drinking after treatment. The notion of loss of control of drinking by alcoholics was called into question by alcohol self-administration studies which showed that drinking behavior, like any other operant, could be controlled by its consequences (Mello and Mendelson, 1971), Moreover, alcoholics did not appear to drink to avoid withdrawal symptoms (Mello and Mendelson, 1971).

Pattison and co-workers (1977) summarized the implications of these studies and proposed seven *emerging concepts* as a substitute for the traditional disease concept of alcoholism: 1) alcohol dependence summarizes a variety of syndromes defined by drinking patterns and the adverse physical, psychological, and social consequences of such drinking; 2) an individual's pattern of alcohol use lies on a continuum ranging from nonpathological to severely pathological; 3) any person who uses alcohol can develop a syndrome of alcohol dependence; 4) the development of alcohol problems follows variable patterns over time and does not necessarily proceed inexorably to severe fatal stages; 5) recovery from alcohol dependence bears no necessary relation to abstinence, although such a concurrence is frequently the case; 6) the consumption of a small amount of alcohol by an individual once labelled *alcoholic* does not initiate either physical depen-

Table 1. Major Propositions, Distinguishing Features, and Etiological Foci of Some Explanatory Models of Alcoholism

Models	Major Propositions, Distinguishing Features	Etiological Focus
Disease concept Jellinek (1960)	Gamma and delta alcoholisms are diseases characterized by tolerance, physical dependence, and impaired control over the frequency or amount of drinking	Mixed; biological, psychological, and sociocultural
Emerging concept Pattison et al. (1977)	There are multiple syndromes of alcoholism; alcoholism is not a unitary, discrete, progressive disorder	Psychological learning mechanisms
Biopsychosocial theory Kissin (1983)	Alcoholism results from the interaction among predispositional factors, heavy drinking, alcohol dependence, and the addictive cycle	Mixed; biological, psychological, and sociocultural "vulnerability" factors
Dependence syndrome concept Edwards and Gross (1976)	Alcohol dependence is a biobehavioral disorder distinct from alcohol-related disabilities	Social, personal antecedents
Conditioned abstinence Ludwig and Wikler (1974)	Conditioned withdrawal reactions maintain alcohol dependence and precipitate relapse	Classical conditioning processes
Social learning theory Abrams and Niaura (1987)	Individual differences, reinforcement history, and psychological expectations lead to alcohol dependence	Social learning processes
Personality theories	Antecedent personality and psychopathology influence the onset, course, and severity of alcoholism	Premorbid personality traits; psychiatric disorder
Tension-reduction theory	The tension-reducing effects of alcohol reinforce heavy drinking and maintain dependence	Anxiety/stress lead to alcoholism

Table 1. Major Propositions, Distinguishing Features, and Etiological Foci of Some Explanatory Models of Alcoholism (*continued*)

Models	Major Propositions, Distinguishing Features	Etiological Focus
Psychodynamic theory	Dependency needs, oral personality characteristics are satisfied by alcohol and maintain alcohol dependence	Various unconscious motives (e.g., latent homosexuality)
Psychosocial theory Kissin (1977)	Psychopathology is a more prominent feature of clinical picture in abstinence-oriented societies	Biological, psychological, social influences individually and combined
Addiction-experience model Peele (1985)	Society creates the need for addictive experiences by making it difficult to fulfill needs through effort and accomplishment	Stress, lack of opportunity, low self-esteem

dence or a physiological need for more alcohol by that individual; and 7) continued drinking of large doses of alcohol over an extended period of time is likely to initiate a process of physical dependence that will eventually be manifested as an alcohol withdrawal syndrome.

Although the first six items of this emerging concept are at variance with the traditional disease concept of alcoholism described by Jellinek, none, according to Kissin (1983), are inconsistent with the more recent disease formulations elaborated during the 1970s. This newer disease concept of alcoholism is best exemplified by Kissin's (1983) biopsychosocial theory, which postulates the following elements: 1) certain susceptible individuals are more likely to develop alcohol dependence because of biological (for example, genetic), psychological (depression), or social (peer influences) predispositional factors; 2) heavy drinking is intensified by precipitating factors such as stressful life events or psychological instigators (for example, anxiety, insomnia); 3) the susceptible individual finds alcohol rewarding, either because of the euphoria produced or the dysphoria assuaged; 4) primary psychological dependence is developed as a consequence, resulting in tolerance and increased drinking; 5) physical dependence follows, along with the need to drink to prevent withdrawal symptoms (secondary psychological dependence); 6) the addictive cycle is further intensified by the protracted abstinence syndrome with persistent physiological craving; and 7) physical dependence mechanisms tend to become reactivated by alcohol ingestion after a period of abstinence, with concomitant reinstatement of the addictive cycle.

At the core of this newer disease concept is an addictive cycle that results in a perpetuation of harmful drinking. The development of physical dependence marks a change in both the severity and the quality of the syndrome. Kissin's model differs from the emerging concept of alcohol dependence primarily in its emphasis on a broader view of etiology. Critics of the traditional disease concept tend to emphasize social influences in the development of alcoholism to the virtual exclusion of other factors, including the self-perpetuating nature of alcohol dependence.

Since the mid-1970s, the disease concept has enjoyed something of a rebirth. Edwards has recently reported on a long-term follow-up of the patients that Davies had described in 1962 (Edwards, 1985). Edwards' report not only calls Davies' original observations into question, it also indicates that only two of Davies' seven famous cases ever achieved the status of prolonged problem-free social drinking, and one of these had never been seriously dependent on alcohol. Pendery and colleagues (1982) followed up 20 patients 10 years after being exposed to controlled drinking therapy by the Sobells and argued against the feasibility of a long-term moderate drinking outcome in previously dependent alcoholics. The four-year follow-up by the RAND Corporation modified its earlier conclusions based on 18-month follow-up data. The second RAND report found that more severely dependent alcoholics who could maintain abstinence improved at follow-up (Polich et al, 1980). Less dependent alcoholics improved only if they were able to maintain a moderate drinking outcome over the first six-month period. Moderate drinking in this study was defined as six ounces of absolute ethanol per day, and it was not possible for more seriously alcohol-dependent individuals to achieve this.

At this writing, the newer disease concept of alcoholism is probably best expressed in the formulation of the alcohol dependence syndrome proposed by Edwards and Gross (1976), which was incorporated into the *International Classification of Diseases, Ninth Revision, Clinical Modification (ICD-9)*. This symptom complex includes a history of repeated withdrawal symptoms, increased tolerance, drinking to avoid withdrawal symptoms, and impaired control over alcohol intake. The latter is characterized by a strong desire to drink, increasingly stereotyped drinking with little day-to-day variability, a consistently high blood alcohol level, and a behavioral pattern that grants the highest priority to maintaining alcohol intake, despite negative social or medical consequences. This formulation presumes that the abstinent alcoholic who begins to drink again will quickly develop dependence symptoms and attain previously high levels of consumption because the syndrome has a tendency to redevelop more rapidly once acquired. Two other propositions of the dependence syndrome concept are: 1) dependence exists along a continuum of severity that ranges from social drinking to severe compulsive alcohol-seeking behavior; and 2) dependence symptoms are empirically and conceptually distinct from alcohol-related physical, mental, and social disabilities (Edwards et al, 1977). The dependence syndrome construct has been substantially incorporated into the *Diagnostic and Statistical Manual of Mental Disorders, Third Edition, Revised (DSM-III-R)* published in 1987 by the American Psychiatric Association (APA).

Twin and adoptee studies have helped to establish the case for a genetic vulnerability to alcoholism (see Chapter 14) and argue in favor of the disease concept. Studies of children of alcoholics have suggested that they differ from children of nonalcoholics in their biological response to ethanol (Schuckit, 1988) and in CNS function (Begleiter and Porjesz, 1988). Nevertheless, much remains to be done to define the disease of alcohol dependence beyond our present state of knowledge. For example, it is not clear how the biological markers observed in sons of alcoholics contribute to increased risk of alcoholism. Of critical importance, better understanding is needed of the biological substrate that accounts for the symptom complex of alcohol dependence described in DSM-III-R and ICD-9. In Chapter 15, Bloom describes the state of neurobiological research in the alcohol field. As a general rule, those effects of chronic ethanol administration that have been observed at the cellular and molecular level can be more clearly related to the development of tolerance than to other aspects of the alcohol dependence syndrome, such as impaired control over alcohol intake. This has also been true of studies of Pavlovian conditioning, which is described below.

As described above, Kissin (1983) postulated the existence of a protracted abstinence syndrome following acute alcohol withdrawal, which could contribute to risk of relapse (an essential tenet of the dependence syndrome construct). Porjesz and Begleiter (1983) reported electrophysiological evidence for the existence of protracted abstinence in detoxified alcoholics. These patients often complain of persistent insomnia and feelings of depression or anxiety. In studies using rat and monkey models of alcohol dependence, a challenge dose of alcohol elicited hyperexcitability in specific brain regions (mesencephalic reticular formation, hippocampus, frontal cortex, and posterior association cortex) in alcohol-dependent animals abstinent for 37 days, but not in control animals (Begleiter and Porjesz, 1977; Begleiter et al, 1980). These data suggest that alcohol consumption by an abstinent alcoholic may elicit withdrawal-like symptoms because of persistent latent CNS hyperexcitability. However, the latent hyperexcitability described in animal models has not been studied in human subjects. It is unclear whether this state persists beyond the period of time described by Begleiter and Porjesz. Suffice it to say, impaired control of drinking behavior—the hallmark of the dependence syndrome—is likely a function of CNS changes consequent to prolonged periods of heavy drinking. Genetically determined risk factors may influence the developmental course of dependence, and psychological and cultural factors also play a role as risk factors for heavy alcohol consumption. A comprehensive model of alcoholism must be based on a biobehavioral concept of alcohol dependence, a clear description of its biological substrate, and the genetic and psychosocial factors that contribute to risk.

CONDITIONING MODELS AND BEHAVIORAL THEORY

Pavlov originally suggested the importance of conditioning factors in addictive disorders in his classic text (Pavlov, 1927), but the seminal work in this area really began with Abraham Wikler. Based on studies of recovering narcotic addicts (Wikler, 1965), and in animal models (Wikler et al, 1963; Wikler and Pescor, 1967), he postulated that drug-free narcotic addicts reexperienced withdrawal symptoms in environments where they had previously experienced actual drug withdrawal. In this circumstance, addicts experienced craving and were likely to relapse to drug use. Interpreted within a classical Pavlovian conditioning paradigm, the withdrawal symptoms had been paired to environmental cues (conditioned abstinence) as a consequence of repeated episodes of pharmacological withdrawal. In later formulations of his theory, Wikler postulated that environmental cues could also elicit *counter adaptive* responses associated with the anticipation of intravenous drug administration. He proposed that these counter adaptive responses were mirror opposites of the morphine experience and predominantly dysphoric in tone. Ludwig and associates (Ludwig and Wikler, 1974; Ludwig, 1974; Ludwig et al, 1978) extended these observations to alcoholics. They found that alcoholics experienced physiological arousal and craving in association with alcohol-related cues. Following the Wikler paradigm, Ludwig and associates concluded that the physiological arousal was consistent with a conditioned withdrawal reaction.

Wikler's postulated conditioning of counter adaptive processes was further elaborated by Solomon and associates (Solomon, 1980; Solomon and Corbit, 1974) as the opponent process theory of acquired motivation. Solomon specifically linked opponent-process conditioning to addictive behaviors, including alcohol dependence. Siegel applied opponent process theory to studies of morphine tolerance (Siegel, 1975, 1977). Mansfield and Cunningham (1980) extended this model to alcohol tolerance in rats. Rats administered alcohol in distinctive environments demonstrate tolerance to the hypothermic effects of alcohol only in that environment. If given placebo injections in the distinct environment, these animals will demonstrate a hypothermic reaction, consistent with the conditioning of opponent processes.

Wikler's model and its derivatives have the advantage of experimental validation of conditioned abstinence (Wikler, 1974; O'Brien et al, 1977) and of conditioned tolerance (Siegel, 1975, 1977; Mansfield and Cunningham, 1980). But this model has been criticized when applied to opioid and cocaine addiction because of its reliance on a history of physical dependence to explain addictive behavior (Schuster and Villareal, 1968; Stewart et al, 1984). McAuliffe and Gordon (1974) have pointed out that most alcoholics and addicts do not experience craving in detoxification facilities, although they do experience craving in settings where drug consumption takes place. Recently, Ludwig (1985) has reported that abstinent alcoholics on the verge of relapse report that they can almost taste or smell a cold beer or experience the warm glow of a cocktail as they *imagine* themselves consuming these beverages, and this mental imagery induces a powerful urge to drink. These reports suggest that the subjective desire to drink prior to relapse is more compatible with conditioned alcohol effects than of conditioned alcohol withdrawal. It is consistent with the model of relapse to opioid and cocaine consumption proposed by Stewart et al (1984). These authors postulate that repeated episodes of drug reinforcement become paired with environmental stimuli, which in turn become conditioned stimuli for *incentive drug effects*. At this writing, it is fair to state that conditioning factors probably play some role in eliciting a desire to drink in abstinent alcoholics who relapse to drinking. Once drinking has resumed, other conditional and unconditional biological responses may come into play to contribute to the problem of diminished control over drinking behavior (Dolinsky et al, 1987).

Ludwig (1985) has noted that the experience of craving does not perforce mean inevitable relapse to heavy drinking. Social learning theory (Bandura, 1985) presumes individual differences related to self-regulatory and self-reflective abilities also contribute to relapse.

Within the framework of social-learning theory, Abrams and Niaura (1987) describe a sequence of events that leads individuals to dependent drinking patterns. They presume that there are individual differences in risk associated with pharmacogenetic and psychosocial factors; and a long-term reinforcement history associated with alcohol use sets up additional expectations for drinking. During periods of stress or impaired coping, individuals may turn to alcohol in increasing amounts. Tolerance and physical dependence will develop. Alcohol consumption will then be reinforced negatively by the avoidance of withdrawal symptoms associated with brief periods of abstinence from alcohol. Recovery, according to the social-learning model, depends upon the individual's ability to develop alternative coping strategies.

Abrams and Niaura (1987) specifically contrast a social-learning model of alcohol abuse with a medical model. Yet their description of the social-learning model is not unlike Ludwig's (1985) analysis of the processes that lead to relapse. Ludwig is identified with a disease model of alcoholism. Abrams and Niaura describe a developmental framework in which alcohol dependence can develop within a social-learning context; they see youthful drinking behaviors and expectancies concerning alcohol emerging from the combined influence of culture, family, and peers. Vaillant (1983) makes a similar point, albeit not from a social-learning framework.

Marlatt and Gordon (1985) have proposed a social-learning model of relapse for which they have developed a theoretically based treatment approach called relapse prevention therapy. They are especially concerned about the individual's response to a single drink, which may be associated with a sense of personal weakness and failure. This cognitive response to a drink is termed the *abstinence violation effect*. To counteract this, the relapse-prevention therapist attempts to re-cast the experience as a tool to improve performance the next time. The aim is to stop drinking early on, so that the behavior is seen as a *lapse* rather than a full-blown *relapse*.

Currently, social-learning theory is one of the most active areas of treatment research in the alcohol field. The aversion to a medical model among social-learning theorists seems more ideological than substantive. The traditional disease construct elaborated by Jellinek presumed that conditioned biological factors contributed to the risk of relapse and to the disease of alcoholism. Social-learning theory also incorporates findings on Pavlovian and opponent process conditioning. As more experience is gained with the relapse-prevention strategies developed by Marlatt and others, it should be possible to relate differential treatment efficacy to specific diagnostic, biological, and psychosocial characteristics of alcoholic patients.

PSYCHOLOGICAL THEORIES OF ALCOHOLISM

In a recent review article, six different possible relationships between addictive disorder (including alcoholism) and psychopathology have been described (Meyer, 1986). These can be summarized in relationship to alcoholism as follows:

1. *DSM-III-R* Axis 1 and Axis 2 psychopathological disorders can serve as risk factors for the development of alcoholism.
2. Comorbid psychiatric disorders can affect the course, symptom picture, and treatment response of alcoholic patients.

3. Chronic alcohol intoxication is marked by increased psychiatric symptoms including anxiety, panic symptoms, depression, and belligerence.
4. After withdrawal from alcohol, some patients continue to manifest symptoms of depression, personality change, and cognitive impairment for prolonged periods of time.
5. Meaningful significance can be attributed to an alcoholic's drinking behavior in the context of psychodynamic, personality, and family systems theory; mood states may also serve as conditional stimuli for craving for alcohol, based upon previous episodes of drinking behavior.
6. Some psychiatric disorders will occur in alcoholic patients with no greater frequency than in the general population (a chance occurrence).

Most psychological theories of alcoholism have been developed from observations of personality patterns of alcoholic patients in treatment. In this context, drinking behavior is thought to mediate some underlying motive(s) based upon the personality or affective state of the individual. With the introduction of *DSM-III*, a number of studies have identified the prevalence of comorbid Axis I and Axis II psychiatric disorders of alcoholics. For example, co-morbid psychopathology has been found to affect the symptom pattern, course, and treatment response of patients. Hesselbrock and associates (1985) found that male alcoholics with comorbid antisocial personality disorder manifested an earlier onset of alcohol problems, with a more rapid course from initial drinking to alcohol dependence. These patients also manifested more social disability and affective symptomatology than alcoholics without psychopathology. Cadoret and co-workers (1984) and Powell and colleagues (1982) have reported similar observations, which are consistent with Cloninger's (1987) type II alcoholics. Depressed alcoholics were more likely to manifest affective symptomatology associated with alcohol withdrawal (Hesselbrock et al, 1985). Depressed male alcoholics have a poorer prognosis than male patients with no other psychopathology; but, on some elements of treatment outcome, depressed female alcoholics do better than those with no other psychopathology (Rounsaville et al, 1987; Schuckit and Winokur, 1972).

Schuckit (1985) has emphasized the importance of primary versus secondary comorbid psychopathology in the prognosis of alcoholic patients. He finds that male alcoholics with primary drug abuse or primary antisocial personality have a poorer prognosis than *primary alcoholics*. McLellan and co-workers (1983) found that a global rating of psychopathology was a more useful predictor of treatment outcome than the specific comorbid *DSM-III* diagnosis. These findings, and those of Schuckit (1985), contrast with the results reported by Rounsaville and colleagues (1987). They found that the primary diagnosis—alcoholism versus depression—was of less importance than the specific *DSM-III* diagnoses. Comorbid *DSM-III* diagnosis, primary/secondary distinctions, and global measures of psychiatric disturbance may reflect different dimensions in the relationship between psychopathology and the course, symptom picture, and treatment response of alcoholic patients.

Psychological theories of alcoholism would appear to be most important in conceptualizing risk factors for the development of alcoholism, and devising therapeutic strategies for individual patients (see Chapter 16). In the context of the post-*DSM-III* literature, three disorders may serve as risk factors for the development of alcoholism: antisocial personality disorder and drug abuse in men, and major depressive disorder in women. These observations, however, are based on cross-sectional data on comorbidity: essential longitudinal studies are lacking.

Prior to *DSM-III*, risk factors for the development of alcoholism were seen in the psychopharmacology of ethanol and in psychodynamic and personality factors. The anxiolytic properties of ethanol were a major component of the tension reduction theory (Cappell, 1975). Studies employing conflict procedures provided support for the tension reduction hypothesis (Cappell, 1975). However, while alcohol is anxiolytic in nonalcoholic subjects, high doses of alcohol administered chronically have been found to be anxiogenic (Mello and Mendelson, 1971). In a recent study, Stockwell and colleagues (1984) found that while alcoholics in treatment attribute tension-reducing properties to alcohol, they also report that anxiety symptoms worsened as a consequence of heavy drinking. At this juncture, most theorists regard the tension-reduction hypothesis as excessively simplistic.

Psychodynamic theories of addiction have gone through a series of modifications since classical psychoanalysis first suggested that alcoholism was a regression to the oral stage of development (Khantzian, 1978). Fenichel (1945) described latent homosexual inclinations as another dimension underlying alcohol problems in men. McCord and McCord (1960) emphasized the dependent qualities of alcoholics, with heavy drinking and intoxication as evidence of a dependent personality orientation. David McClelland and colleagues (1972) believed that male alcoholics drank in order to feel powerful. Khantzian (1981) has described disturbances in self-regulation, self-care, and self-esteem in addicts and alcoholics. His formulations suggest therapeutic interventions designed to improve the patient's functioning in these areas. Khantzian's model is similar to the proposal for alcoholic rehabilitation developed by Alan Marlatt from a social-learning perspective. Indeed, Khantzian seems much closer to Marlatt than to his fellow psychoanalysts (Vaillant, 1983; Bean-Bayog, 1986; Zinberg, 1975), who have emphasized the disabling consequences to personality resulting *from* alcoholism.

The literature on personality, psychopathology, and alcoholism is vast—too vast to adequately summarize in a paper designed to contrast models of alcoholism. Unfortunately, the literature is heavily laden with the idiosyncratic theoretical terminology of the authors. In some cases, the constructs lack clearly defined objective criteria that could permit more systematic empirical research. It is easier for a writer to criticize the existing literature than to convince a wide audience about the veracity of his or her own propositions. Despite these drawbacks, one can discern a consistent pattern of theoretical and empirical observations. A substantial percentage of male alcoholics manifest personality characteristics that may be described as impulsive and novelty-seeking as indicated by their elevation on Scale 4 (psychopathic deviate) on the Minnesota Multiphasic Personality Inventory (MMPI). In addition to their primary elevation on Scale 4, alcoholics also show a characteristic elevation on Scale 2 (depression) and Scale 7 (psychasthenia). While Kammier and colleagues (1973) found that most of the MMPI differences in alcoholics appear to be a consequence of drinking, their longitudinal study also suggested that prealcoholics could be identified on the basis of their MMPI profiles as college freshmen.

One underlying assumption common to psychopathologically derived models of alcoholism is treatment relevance. In this regard, there has been interest in *treatment matching* strategies based on personality and other typologies, and psychotherapeutic interventions have been proposed based upon the perspectives of family and individual therapy. These models generally postulate one or more defects in function, including problems in affect regulation, anticipation of risks and consequences, difficult interpersonal and intrafamilial relations, and other dimensions of human behavior. Some of these deficits are undoubtedly antecedent to the development of alcoholism. More importantly, alcoholism can result in problems of self-care; and alcohol-related cognitive deficits in short-term memory, abstraction, and visuo-spatial relations will complicate a patient's response to psychotherapeutic intervention. The wise clinician will evaluate his or her patient thoroughly to assess *DSM-III-R* psychiatric comorbidity and severity of alcohol dependence, as well as other meaningful domains that will affect recovery. Such is the "real world" usefulness of psychopathological models of alcoholism.

SOCIOCULTURAL THEORIES OF ALCOHOLISM

The role of sociocultural factors in alcoholism was described extensively by Jellinek (1960), who argued that culture influences both the meaning and manifestations of alcohol problems. Jellinek suggested that the concept of alcoholism has different meanings throughout the world, primarily as a consequence of cultural differences in the way alcoholics drink, the symptoms they develop, the consequences they experience, and the attributed etiologies of their disorder. In England, Scandinavia, and North America, the terms alcoholic and alcoholism tend to be associated with what Jellinek (1960) referred to as the "steady symptomatic excessive drinker," that is, a drinker whose impaired control over drinking is a consequence of an underlying psychological problem. This view of alcoholism differs from medical concepts in the predominantly wine-drinking nations of southern Europe and South America. The French conception of alcoholism is considered to be typical of this alternative model. According to Jellinek (1962), the French literature on alcoholism makes frequent mention of *l'alcoolisme sans ivresse* (alcoholism without drunkenness); asserting that a drinker can become alcoholic without ever showing signs of intoxication. The absence of intoxication is not the only characteristic distinguishing this "inveterate" drinker. Whereas psychological disturbance is presumed to underlie symptomatic drinking in the Anglo-Saxon countries, social customs and economic incentives are seen as the major influences in French alcoholism. Termed *gamma* and *delta* alcoholics, respectively, these varieties of alcoholism are probably prevalent in every nation of drinkers. Because one variety or the other tends to predominate, the disease label brings with it a set of meanings consistent with the prevailing cultural view.

Jellinek's sociocultural typology of alcoholism has been reformulated by Kissin (1977) in terms of the *psychosocial principal*. This hypothesis states that the degree of psychopathology associated with the development of alcohol dependence is inversely related to the level of acceptance of alcohol abuse in that individual's subculture. A corollary of this hypothesis (Kissin, 1983, p. 104) is that "the degree of psychopathology necessary to develop alcoholism is inversely proportional to the strength of the biological and social influences tending in that direction." In this conceptualization, the etiological origins of alcoholism in a given individual may be biological, psychological, social, or a combination of each. The summation of these factors represents an index of predisposition. The more one factor is operative, the less others need to be present for the development of alcoholism. On the aggregate level, the rate and type of alcoholism will reflect the relative contributions of biological, psychological, and social influences. In France, where social encouragement is given to heavy drinking, psychopathology can be expected to play less of a role in the clinical profile of alcoholism than it does in countries such as the United States, where drinking is viewed as less a part of social custom and more as an escape from unpleasant feelings or circumstances. The history of drinking and alcohol problems in the United States has been influenced by cultural diversity, geographic mobility, the frontier style of drinking to intoxication, and the temperance movement. This may explain why the American drinking pattern is more erratic and socially disruptive than that observed in wine-producing countries like France.

One of the most provocative sociocultural theories of alcoholism is the addiction-experience model proposed by Peele (1985). This model combines cultural processes with individual and situational variables to argue that society creates the need for addictive experience by setting forth key values that are not realizable. People are susceptible to addictive experiences to the extent that they 1) occupy unsatisfying and stressful positions in society; 2) feel that social rewards are unobtainable; 3) relate to the world through dependencies; and 4) believe in the efficacy of external forces. Progressive involvement in substitute addictive experiences limits the alcoholic's ability to fulfill needs *naturalistically*, through effort and accomplishment. As a consequence, there is a drop in feelings of self-efficacy and social worth. This exacerbating cycle of experience achieves the extremes of addiction as drinking becomes a core part of the self-concept and the sole means of asserting control of the individual's emotional life. According to Peele (1985, p. 129), "no additional constructs are necessary to account for the fervor of pursuit of an addictive object (craving) and the anguish resulting from its abandonment (withdrawal)." This social-psychological model borrows from McClelland and associates' (1972) power theory to account for variations in addiction from one culture to another. That theory proposes that societies with high rates of alcoholism place a premium on individual power but at the same time make it difficult to achieve power. In these cultures, alcohol intoxication leads to fantasies of personal domination over other people and is associated with aggressive and disruptive social behavior.

INTEGRATIVE BIOPSYCHOSOCIAL MODELS AND TYPOLOGIES OF ALCOHOLISM

Beginning in the late nineteenth century, alcoholism theorists became uncomfortable with the ability of a unitary disease concept to account for the range of etiological phenomena and consequences manifested by persons with alcohol problems. To account for this diversity, a variety of typological theories were proposed that postulated different forms of alcoholism (Babor and Dolinsky, 1988). Initially, these theories tended to be one-dimensional, explaining the origins of different "alcoholisms" in terms of the presence or absence of single factors such as personality variables, genetic differences, or the presence or absence of antecedent psychopathology. More recently, typological theorists, taking their cues from the seminal work initiated by Jellinek (1960), have begun to incorporate multiple biopsychosocial influences and etiological processes into their theories. Jellinek's five species of alcoholism, described above, were explained on the basis of different combinations of biological, psychological, and social vulnerability that resulted in different patterns of drinking and alcoholism. Three typological models that can be considered in the Jellinek tradition are Morey and associates' (1984) hybrid model, Cloninger's (1987) neurobiological-learning model, and Zucker's (1987) general developmental model. The major features of these models are summarized in Table 2.

Zucker's developmental model is based on the assumption that there are at least four kinds of alcoholism, each having different developmental processes, natural histories, and presenting symptoms. Type I, *antisocial alcoholism*, is characterized by the early onset of both antisocial behavior and alcohol-related problems. A genetic diathesis is suggested by the high prevalence of parental alcoholism and antisocial behavior. More likely to occur in lower class males, this form of alcoholism is generally considered to have a poor prognosis.

Type II, *developmentally cumulative alcoholism*, is similar to what other theorists have called primary alcoholism—that is, the symptomatic drinking behavior is considered to have been established before the onset of any other psychiatric condition. The term developmentally cumulative implies that risk is tied to normal, culturally prescribed processes of drinking, rather than childhood antisocial antecedents. Over the life course, an addictive process has become sufficiently cumulative so that beyond a certain point, "it has a different trajectory than if it were simply regulated by normative developmental trends in the culture" (Zucker, 1987, p. 67).

Type III, *developmentally limited alcoholism*, is characterized primarily by frequent heavy drinking. An extension of adolescent problem drinking, it is often associated with separation from the family of origin in young adulthood. This form of problem drinking tends to dissipate in many individuals in the middle twenties, with successful assumption of adult career and family roles.

Type IV, *negative affect alcoholism*, tends to be more prevalent in women who use alcohol for affective regulation or to enhance social relationships. There may be a genetic diathesis associated with mood regulation in this type of alcoholism.

Cloninger (1987) has proposed a neurobiological-learning model of alcoholism that distinguishes two basic types, termed *milieu-limited* (type I) and *male-limited* (type II). Type I alcoholics tend to have a later onset of alcohol-related problems, develop psychological dependence, and have guilt feelings about their alcohol dependence. In contrast, type II alcoholics have an early onset of problems, exhibit spontaneous alcohol-seeking behavior (inability to abstain), and are socially disruptive when drinking. Three dimensions of personality, which in turn have their basis in different neural mechanisms and brain systems, are hypothesized to account for these different types of alcoholism. Thus, type I is associated with passive-dependent or anxious personality traits, while type II is characterized by traits associated with antisocial personality, such as high novelty seeking, low harm avoidance, and low reward dependence. Like Zucker's theory, Cloninger's model implicates developmental stages, learning mechanisms, personality variables, and genetic factors in its attempt to account for individual differences in the signs and symptoms of alcoholism.

Using a mathematical clustering procedure, Morey and co-workers (1984) identified three distinct types of drinkers within a large sample ($n = 725$) of individuals seeking help for alcohol-related problems. Type A (early-stage problem drinkers) represented a fairly heterogeneous group who showed evidence of drinking problems but who had not accrued major symptoms of alcohol dependence. Type B drinkers (affiliative alcoholics with moderate alcohol depen-

Table 2. Integrative Models and Typological Theories of Alcoholism

Model/Theorist	Major Subtypes	Subtype Features/ Characteristics
Zucker's (1980) developmental model	Antisocial	Early onset, genetic diathesis, poor prognosis
	Developmentally cumulative	Later onset, risk tied to participation in heavy drinking subcultures
	Developmentally limited	Frequent heavy drinking tends to mature out after adult roles are assumed
	Negative affect	More prevalent in women who drink to regulate mood states
Cloninger's (1987) neurobiological learning model	Milieu-limited	Later onset, psychological dependence, passive dependent personality
	Male-limited	Early onset, spontaneous alcohol-seeking, socially disruptive drinking, antisocial personality traits
Morey and associates' (1984) hybrid model	Early-stage problem drinkers	Heavy or intensive drinking associated with alcohol-related problems in the absence of serious dependence symptoms
	Affiliative	Daily drinkers with moderate alcohol dependence who drink primarily for social reasons
	Schizoid	Socially isolated binge drinkers with severe alcohol dependence

dence) were more socially oriented and tended to drink on a daily basis. Type C drinkers (schizoid alcoholics with severe alcohol dependence) were more socially isolative, tended to drink in binges, and reported the most severe symptoms of alcoholism. There were consistent differences in symptom severity among the three types of drinkers on measures of psychopathology, cognitive functioning, and social adjustment. A hybrid model was therefore proposed that superimposed the three types on an underlying continuum of alcohol dependence. Although speculative at this point, the model has heuristic value for stimulating further research on the etiology and differential treatment of alcohol abuse.

What is notable about these typological models is that, despite differences in theoretical focus and empirical support, there are some striking similarities in the subtypes they have identified. In particular, there is sufficient overlap in the characteristics of Zucker's antisocial alcoholic, Cloninger's male-limited type, and Morey and colleagues' schizoid drinker to suggest that each theorist is talking about a similar type of alcoholism. Another subtype identified by each theorist is the late onset, socially motivated habitual drinker, variously termed milieu-limited, developmentally cumulative, or affiliative alcoholics. As typology theories become more sophisticated, they are likely to invite more intensive efforts at empirical verification. Their appeal lies in their ability to account for heterogeneity and complexity among alcoholics. To the extent that they incorporate many of the premises of earlier theories, they hold promise as a means of building on the cumulative wisdom of the past.

CONCLUSIONS

A theory is a set of concepts related to each other by general principles or propositions. It is usually supported by considerable data and is proposed as an explanation for a set of phenomena. A model is a representational device designed to show how something works, especially by displaying the relationship between parts and the whole. Both theories and models have been used to describe, understand, and predict alcoholism, as indicated by the rich and often conflicting literature summarized in this chapter.

Models of alcoholism, like Wikler's conditioning model, have been most often conceptual, although there have been some attempts at more sophisticated mathematical modeling as well. Theories are more solidly supported by evidence than are models. Theories of alcoholism range from broad, multifaceted conceptions of the interactions among agent (alcohol), host (drinker), and environment, as in Cloninger's neurobiological learning model, to relatively narrowly focused statements about a limited set of alcohol-related phenomena, such as the relationship between anxiety, alcohol consumption, and tension-reduction (Cappell, 1975). More often theories of alcoholism tend to be in the middle range between minor working hypotheses, based on routine research, and all-inclusive speculations comprising a master conceptual scheme.

This chapter has reviewed representative models and theories of alcoholism to summarize some of the major issues that clinicians and research scientists have considered with respect to the nature of this disorder. Our approach has been more expository than critical, given that, within the scientific paradigm, behavioral, biological, and social scientists have often worked at different levels of analysis and have rarely even approximated the more formal deductive systems developed in the physical sciences. This is not to say that explanatory models should not be held accountable in some way. To bring a critical element to our review of models and theories, we need to approach them from the perspective of what constitutes a good and a useful contribution to the understanding of alcoholism.

A good theory serves as a guide to investigation, organization, and explanation. Not only does it stimulate inquiry and understanding, it also helps to predict the occurrence of new phenomena and influences the treatment or prevention of disease. A good model clarifies the relationships between concepts, suggesting hypotheses for further study or illustrating the possible ways in which alcoholism develops and manifests itself. Ideally, models and theories should have logical coherence, they should generate scientifically verifiable hypotheses, and they should be useful to researchers and clinicians.

By these standards, conditioning models and those based on social-learning theory have been useful to the extent that they have stimulated research and have inspired new approaches to treatment. Personality and sociocultural theories, on the other hand, have not easily been translated into systematic research or practical applications in prevention or therapy. With new advances in genetics, neurobiology, and multivariate statistics, there has been a revival of theory building in alcoholism research. These newer explanatory models (Cloninger, 1987; Zucker, 1987) integrate biological, psychological, and social levels of analysis and often postulate multiple etiological paths to account for different types of alcoholism. The usefulness and validity of these models must be examined in longitudinal research designs, and ultimately in the context of more effective programs of prevention and treatment.

REFERENCES

Abrams DB, Niaura RS: Social learning theory, in Psychological Theories of Drinking and Alcoholism. Edited by Blane HT, Leonard KE. New York, Guilford Press, 1987

American Psychiatric Association: Diagnostic and Statistical Manual of Mental Disorders, Third Edition, Revised. Washington, DC, American Psychiatric Association, 1987

Armor DJ, Polich JM, Stambul HB: Alcoholism and Treatment. New York, Wiley & Sons, 1978

Babor TF, Dolinsky ZS: Alcoholic typologies. Historical evolution and empirical evaluation of some common classification schemes, in Alcoholism: Origins and Etiology. Edited by Rose R, Barrett J. New York, Raven Press, 1988

Bandura A: Social Learning Theory: Social Foundations of Thought and Action. Englewood Cliffs, NJ, Prentice Hall, 1985

Bean-Bayog M: Psychopathology produced by alcoholism, in Psychopathology and Addictive Disorders. Edited by Meyer RE. New York, Guilford Press, 1986

Begleiter H, Porjesz B: Persistence of brain hyperexcitability following chronic alcohol exposure in rats. Adv Exp Med Biol 1977; 85B:209–222

Begleiter H, Porjesz B: Neurophysiological dysfunction in alcoholism, in Alcoholism: Origins and Outcome. Edited by Rose RM, Barrett JE. New York, Raven Press, 1988

Begleiter H, De Noble V, Porjesz B: Protracted brain dysfunction after alcohol withdrawal in monkeys, in Biological Effects of Alcohol. Edited by Begleiter H. New York, Plenum Press, 1980

Cadoret R, Troughtone E, Widmer R: Clinical differences between antisocial and primary alcoholics. Compr Psychiatry 1984; 25:1–8

Cappell H: An evaluation of tension models of alcohol consumption, in Research Advances in Alcohol and Drug Problems. Edited by Gibbins RJ, Israel Y, Kalant H, et al. New York, John Wiley & Sons, 1975

Cloninger CR: Neurogenetic adaptive mechanisms in alcoholism. Science 1987; 236:410–416

Commission on Professional and Hospital Activities: International Classification of Diseases, Ninth Revision, Clinical Modification. Ann Arbor, MI, Commission on Professional and Hospital Activities, 1980

Davies DL: Normal drinking in recovered alcohol addicts. Quarterly Journal for Studies on Alcohol 1962; 23:94–104

Dolinsky Z, Morse D, Kaplan R, et al: Neuroendocrine, psychophysiological and subjective reactivity to an alcohol placebo in male alcoholic patients. Alcoholism: Clinical and Experimental Research 1987; 11:296–300

Edwards G: A later follow-up of a classic case series: D.L. Davies's 1962 report and its significance for the present. J Stud Alcohol 1985; 46:181–190

Edwards G, Gross MM: Alcohol dependence: provisional description of a clinical syndrome. Br Med J 1976; 1:1058–1061

Edwards G, Gross MM, Keller M, et al: Alcohol-Related Disabilities. WHO Offset Publication No. 32. Geneva, World Health Organization, 1977

Fenichel O: The Psychoanalytic Theory of Neurosis. New York, W.W. Norton & Co., 1945

Hesselbrock M, Meyer RE, Keener JJ: Psychopathology in hospitalized alcoholics. Arch Gen Psychiatry 1985; 42:1050–1055

Jellinek EM: The Disease Concept of Alcoholism. New Haven, CT, College and University Press, 1960

Jellinek EM: Cultural differences in the meaning of alcoholism, in Society, Culture and Drinking Patterns. Edited by Pittman D, Snyder C. Carbondale, IL, Southern Illinois University Press, 1962

Kammier ML, Hoffman H, Loper RG: Personality characteristics of alcoholics as college freshmen and at time of treatment. Quarterly Journal for Studies on Alcohol 1973; 34:309–399

Khantzian EJ: The ego, the self and opiate addiction: theoretical and treatment considerations. Int Rev Psychoanal 1978; 5:189–198

Khantzian EJ: Some treatment implications of the ego and self disturbances in alcoholism, in Dynamic Approaches to the Understanding and Treatment of Alcoholism. Edited by Bean MH, Zinberg NE. New York, The Free Press, 1981

Kissin B: Theory and practice in the treatment of alcoholism, in Treatment and Rehabilitation of the Chronic Alcoholic. Edited by Kissin B, Begleiter H. New York, Plenum Press, 1977

Kissin B: The disease concept of alcoholism, in Research Advances in Alcohol and Drug Problems. Edited by Smart RG, Glaser FB, Israel Y, et al. New York, Plenum Press, 1983

Lender ME: Jellinek's typology of alcoholism: historical antecedents. J Stud Alcohol 1979; 40:361–375

Ludwig AM: Irresistible urge and the unquenchable thirst for alcohol, in Alcoholism: A Multilevel Problem. Edited by Chafetz ME. Proceedings of the Fourth Annual Alcoholism Conference of the National Institute on Alcohol Abuse and Alcoholism, Washington, DC, 1974

Ludwig AM: Cognitive processes associated with "spontaneous activity" from alcoholism. J Stud Alcohol 1985; 46:53–58

Ludwig AM, Wikler A: Craving and relapse to drink. Quarterly Journal for Studies on Alcohol 1974; 35:108–130

Ludwig AM, Bendfeld TF, Wikler A, et al: "Loss of control" in alcoholics. Arch Gen Psychiatry 1978; 35:370–373

Mansfield JG, Cunningham CL: Conditioning and extinction of tolerance to the hypothermic effect of ethanol in rats. J Comp Physiol Psychol 1980; 94:962–969

Marlatt GA, Gordon JR: Relapse Prevention: Maintenance Strategies in the Treatment of Addictive Behaviors. New York, Guilford Press, 1985

McAuliffe WE, Gordon RA: A test of Lindesmith's theory of addiction: the frequency of euphoria among long-term addicts. American Journal of Sociology 1974; 79:795–840

McClelland DC, Davis WM, Kalin R, et al: The Drinking Man: Alcohol and Human Motivation. New York, The Free Press, 1972

McCord W, McCord J: Origins of Alcoholism. Stanford, CA, Stanford University Press, 1960

McLellan AT, Luborsky L, Woody GE, et al: Predicting response to alcohol and drug abuse treatments: role of psychiatric severity. Arch Gen Psychiatry 1983; 40:620–625

Mello NK, Mendelson JH: Drinking patterns during work contingent and noncontingent alcohol acquisition, in Recent Advances in Alcoholism. Edited by Mello NK, Mendelson JH. Washington, DC, US Public Health Service, No. HSM 719045, 1971

Meyer RE: How to understand the relationship between psychopathology and addictive disorders: another example of the chicken and the egg, in Psychopathology and Addictive Disorders. Edited by Meyer RE. New York, Guilford Press, 1986

Morey LC, Skinner HA, Blashfield RK: A typology of alcohol abusers: correlates and implications. J Abnorm Psychol 1984; 93:408–417

O'Brien CP, Testa T, O'Brien TJ, et al: Conditioned narcotic abstinence in humans. Science 1977; 195:1000–1001

Pattison EM, Sobell MB, Sobell LC: Emerging Concepts of Alcohol Dependence. New York, Springer, 1977

Pavlov IP: Conditioned Reflexes: An Investigation of the Physiological Activity of the Cerebral Cortex (translated by G.V. Anrep). London, Oxford University Press, 1927

Peele S: The Meaning of Addiction. Lexington, MA, Lexington Books, 1985

Pendery ML, Maltzman IM, West LJ: Controlled drinking by alcoholics? New findings and a reevaluation of a major affirmative study. Science 1982; 217:169–175

Polich AM, Armor DJ, Braiker HB: The course of alcoholism four years after treatment. Publication No. RAND CR–2433. Santa Monica, CA, National Institute on Alcohol Abuse and Alcoholism, 1980

Porjesz B, Begleiter H: Brain dysfunction and alcohol, in Pathogenesis of Alcoholism: Biological Factors. Edited by Kissin B, Begleiter H. New York, Plenum Press, 1983

Powell BJ, Penick EC, Othmer E, et al: Prevalence of additional psychiatric syndromes among male alcoholics. J Clin Psychiatry 1982; 43:404–407

Roizen R, Cahalan D, Shanks P: Spontaneous remission among untreated problem drinkers, in Longitudinal Research on Drug Use. Edited by Kandel DB. New York, Wiley & Sons, 1978

Rounsaville B, Dolinsky ZS, Babor TF, et al: Psychopathology as a predictor of treatment outcome in alcoholics. Arch Gen Psychiatry 1987; 44:505–513

Schuckit MA: The clinical implications of primary diagnostic groups among alcoholics. Arch Gen Psychiatry 1985; 42:1042–1049

Schuckit MA: A search for biological markers in alcoholism: application to psychiatric research, in Alcoholism: Origins and Outcome. Edited by Rose RM, Barrett JE. New York, Raven Press, 1988

Schuckit MA, Winokur G: A short-term follow-up of women alcoholics. Diseases of the Nervous System 1972; 33:672–678

Schuster CR, Villareal: The experimental analysis of opioid dependence, in Psychopharmacology: A Review of Progress. Edited by Efron DH. Washington, DC, Public Health Service Publication No. 1836, 1968

Siegel S: Evidence from rats that morphine tolerance is a learned response. J Comp Physiol Psychol 1975; 89:498–506

Sobell MB, Sobell LC: Second year treatment outcome of alcoholics treated by individualized behavior therapy: results. Behav Res Ther 1976; 14:195–215

Solomon RL: The opponent-process theory of acquired motivation: the cost of pleasure and the benefits of pain. Am Psychol 1980; 35:691–712

Solomon RL, Corbit JD: An opponent process theory of motivation, I: temporal dynamics of affect. Psychol Rev 1974; 81:119–145

Vaillant GE: The Natural History of Alcoholism: Causes, Patterns and Paths of Recovery. Cambridge, MA, Harvard University Press, 1983

Wikler A: Conditioning factors in opiate addiction and relapse, in Narcotics. Edited by Wilmer DM, Kassebaum GG. New York, McGraw Hill, 1965

Wikler A: Dynamics of drug dependence: implications of a conditioning theory for research and treatment, in Opioid Addiction: Origins and Treatment. Edited by Fisher S, Freeman AM. Washington, DC, Winston, 1974

Wikler A, Martin WR, Pescor FT, et al: Factors regulating oral consumption of an opioid (Etonitazine) by morphine-addicted rats. Psychopharmacologia 1963; 5:55–76

Wikler A, Pescor FT: Classical conditioning of morphine abstinence, reinforcement of opioid-drinking behavior and relapse in morphine-addicted rats. Psychopharmacologia 1967; 10:255–284

Zinberg NE: Addiction and ego function. Psychoanal Study Child 1975; 30:567–588

Zucker RA: The four alcoholisms: a developmental account of the etiologic process, in Alcohol and Addictive Behavior. Edited by Rivers PC. Lincoln, NB, University of Nebraska Press, 1987

Chapter 14

Epidemiology and Genetics of Alcoholism

by C. Robert Cloninger, M.D., Stephen H. Dinwiddie, M.D., and Theodore Reich, M.D.

The prevalence of alcoholism in the general population and within families has increased exponentially, as have the average consumption rates in industrialized populations during the past generation (Cloninger et al, 1988b). The increased frequency of alcoholism has been associated with concomitant increases in depressive and anxiety disorders, which are often seen together in the same individual (Reich et al, 1988; Rose and Barrett, 1988; Helzer and Przybeck, 1988). Despite the repeated finding that alcoholism is strongly familial (Cotton, 1979), no simple genetic model has been shown to fit the pattern of inheritance, and the change in the prevalence of alcoholism and comorbid disorders has been so rapid that nongenetic factors, interacting in a complex fashion with constitutional elements, must be involved. Nevertheless, evidence from adoption and twin studies shows that genetic factors play a substantial role in the development of personality factors that may underlie differences between individuals in their susceptibility to alcoholism and related disorders (Cloninger, 1987a).

In this chapter, we will review recent progress in the genetic epidemiology of alcoholism. In particular, recent work has identified clinical subtypes of alcoholism with distinct genetic and epidemiological characteristics. Accordingly, we will review the classification of alcoholism, studies of its prevalence, potential markers for risk of developing alcoholism, and family adoption studies of alcoholic subtypes. Next, we will consider what is inherited and what influences the expression of heritable susceptibility factors. Finally, we will consider the implications of these findings for psychiatric practice and future research.

CLINICAL HETEROGENEITY

Alcoholics differ widely in their clinical features, which include different types of social and medical problems, varying ages of onset, and numerous associated personality traits (Park and Whitehead, 1973; Cloninger et al, 1988b). Recent clinical and treatment studies have emphasized these differences and highlighted the importance of distinguishing between individuals with and without severe dependency phenomena, such as loss of control and craving for alcohol. Although this distinction is of great importance in management and treatment, family and adoption studies indicate that it reflects the severity and duration of actual alcohol misuse, rather than the degree or type of susceptibility to alco-

This work was supported in part by Research Scientist Award MH-00048 and grants MH-31302 and MH-14677 from the National Institute of Mental Health, grant AA-03539 from the National Institute of Alcoholism and Alcohol Abuse, and a grant from the MacArthur Foundation Network on Risk and Protective Factors in Major Mental Disorders.

holism. Severity of alcohol misuse appears to be influenced largely by aspects of the nonheritable postnatal environment, such as the social status of the adoptive home or extent of postnatal hospital care prior to adoption (Cloninger et al, 1981). Accordingly, although the distinction between alcohol abuse and dependence may be important in treatment, it is doubtful that it is relevant to etiology.

Two clinical subgroups of alcoholics that differ in both their genetic and environmental backgrounds have been distinguished in family and adoption studies. Initially identified in the Stockholm Adoption Study of Alcoholism, these groups were characterized on the basis of differences in their pattern of inheritance of alcoholism (Cloninger et al, 1981). Type 1, *milieu-limited*, alcoholics were characterized by adult onset of either mild or severe alcohol abuse associated with little or no criminality; both their biological mothers and fathers often had a similar pattern of abuse. In contrast, type 2, *male-limited*, alcoholics were characterized by teenage onset of moderate alcohol abuse that was associated with frequent criminality; their biological fathers, but not their mothers, also had an early onset of alcohol abuse and criminality.

Later studies of type 1 and type 2 alcoholics revealed distinct alcohol-related symptoms and personality traits, as summarized in Table 1 (Cloninger, 1987a; Gilligan et al, 1987, 1988). Type 1 alcoholics have *anxious* or passive-dependent personality traits, including high harm avoidance (that is, anticipatory worrying, pessimism, fear of uncertainty, shyness, and fatigability), high reward dependence (sentimentality, warm social attachment, emotional dependence, and persistency), and low novelty seeking (rigid, stoical, reflective, slow-tempered). When they drink alcohol, they are positively reinforced by the reduction of anxiety they experience, so that they rapidly become tolerant and dependent (Cloninger, 1987a). In family studies, the type 1 alcoholics can be distinguished from other alcoholics by their greater frequency of onset after 25 years of age, loss of control, prolonged and repeated binges, guilt feelings about their drinking, and higher incidence of liver disorders from sustained high levels of alcohol intake (Gilligan et al, 1987, 1988).

Table 1.   Distinguishing Characteristics of Two Types of Alcoholism

Characteristic Features	Type of Alcoholism	
	type 1	type 2
Alcohol-related problems		
Usual age of onset (years)	after 25	before 25
Spontaneous alcohol-seeking (inability to abstain)	infrequent	frequent
Fighting and arrests when drinking	infrequent	frequent
Psychological dependence (loss of control)	frequent	infrequent
Guilt and fear about alcohol dependence	frequent	infrequent
Personality traits		
Novelty seeking	low	high
Harm avoidance	high	low
Reward dependence	high	low

Type 2 alcoholics have the opposite configuration of personality traits from type 1 alcoholics (Cloninger, 1987a,b; von Knorring et al, 1985, 1987). Type 2 alcoholics have antisocial personality traits, including high novelty seeking (that is, impulsiveness, curiosity, exploratory excitability, intuitiveness, quick-temperedness), low harm avoidance (risk-taking, optimism, self-confidence, outgoingness, vigor), and low reward dependence (practicality, social detachment, irresoluteness, and independence). When they drink alcohol, they are positively reinforced by feelings of pleasant activation or euphoria, so they often repeatedly seek out alcohol for euphoric stimulation (Cloninger, 1987a; Baer et al, 1988; Nordstrom and Berglund, 1987). In family studies, type 2 alcoholics are distinguished from others by their greater frequency of onset before age 25 years, inability to abstain entirely for prolonged periods, fighting when drinking, arrests for reckless driving when drinking, and treatment for alcohol abuse in programs other than Alcoholics Anonymous (Gilligan et al, 1987).

The distinction between these two groups of alcoholics is associated with many differences in epidemiology and genetics, as well as psychiatric diagnosis and treatment. For example, type 2 alcoholics are often impulsive and aggressive risk takers who abuse a variety of substances besides alcohol (Dinwiddie and Cloninger, in preparation). On the other hand, type 1 alcoholics are more cautious, but may develop prolonged and severe depressive responses to separation or loss of social attachments. Such differences have important implications in the practice of clinical psychiatry, as discussed later regarding treatment.

PREVALENCE IN THE GENERAL POPULATION

Recent surveys have revealed high lifetime rates of alcohol abuse in the general population. Averaged across the five sites of the Epidemiologic Catchment Area (ECA) study, lifetime incidence of alcohol abuse plus dependence was 13.5%, (Robins et al, 1988) with the risk being consistently higher for men than for women regardless of age. The finding that younger cohorts do not have markedly lower rates of alcoholism indicates that the prevalence may be increasing as shown in Table 2, which summarizes the cumulative lifetime prevalence of definite alcoholism in white men and women from the St. Louis portion of the ECA. Women born recently appear to have about the same risk of alcoholism as did men in their fathers' generation, as depicted in Figure 1. Age of onset is also earlier in more recently born individuals than in older individuals. These

Table 2. Population Prevalence of Definite Alcoholism in White Males and Females Based on the ECA (Feighner Criteria)

Age	Males		Females	
	N	% affected	N	% affected
18–24	45	11.1	45	4.4
25–44	289	21.8	331	5.1
45–64	141	19.9	169	0.6
65+	272	9.9	418	1.4

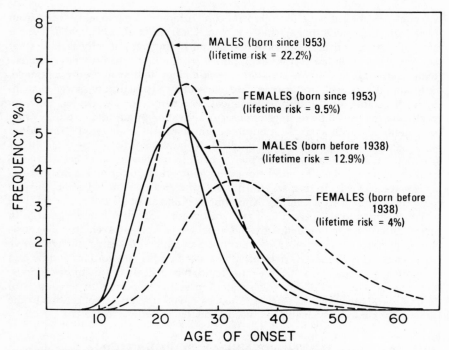

Figure 1. Risk of alcoholism among males and females of two generations.

secular changes are described in more detail elsewhere (Cloninger et al, 1988b; Reich et al, 1988).

Another survey has recently been completed to ascertain the lifetime risks of alcoholic subtypes in a national area probability sample of the United States, including an oversample of blacks. This was part of a reinterview study of the General Social Survey conducted in 1987, and will be reported in more detail elsewhere. The subtypes were identified by responses to questions that distinguished type 1 and type 2 alcoholics in family studies, as described in the prior section. Type 1 symptoms included loss of control, recurrent binges, guilt about drinking, liver disorders, and onset of alcohol problems after 25 years of age. Type 2 symptoms included inability to abstain, fights while drinking, reckless driving while drinking, and treatment for alcohol abuse in programs other than Alcoholics Anonymous. Probable cases had two of these symptoms, and definite cases had three or more. Preliminary estimates of lifetime risks are summarized in Table 3 by sex and race. These are preliminary because no adjustments have been made for biases in sampling according to sociodemographic variables. In any case, it is clear that women have fewer type 2 alcoholic symptoms than men, regardless of race.

STUDIES OF HIGH-RISK GROUPS

On both clinical and research grounds, discovery of a reliable, easily measured marker for vulnerability to developing alcoholism would be of great importance.

Table 3. Lifetime Risk of Alcoholic Subtypes by Sex and Race

Sex/Race	Total Number	Type 1, Definite	% Probable	Type 2, Definite	% Probable
White men	326	5.5	19.0	3.4	10.1
Black men	136	5.1	22.1	3.7	6.6
White women	350	2.6	13.1	0.6	1.7
Black women	207	2.9	8.2	0.5	3.9

However, because the expression of alcoholism appears to be dependent on numerous factors, both genetic and environmental, a trait marker for alcoholism could be a factor directly related in the pathogenesis of alcoholism, or it could be close to a locus closely linked to a genetic factor.

Earlier investigations concentrated on looking for behavioral antecedents to alcoholism or behavioral responses to alcohol challenges. For example, in a retrospective study, Goodwin and coworkers (1975) identified a population of 133 Danish male adoptees, and interviewed them during adulthood. Comparison of the 14 alcoholics in the sample with the 119 without alcoholism showed the alcoholic subgroup to have had elevated rates of problems with poor school performance, hyperactivity, truancy or antisocial behavior, disobedience, aggression, shyness, and insecurity. The authors went on to suggest that hyperactivity in childhood might predispose to later development of alcoholism.

Another approach has been to evaluate subjects at elevated risk for alcoholism for differences in subjective response to an alcohol challenge. Schuckit (1984) found that young men with family histories of alcoholism, who were therefore at higher risk for later development of alcoholism, had less intense subjective feelings of intoxication in response to standardized doses of ethanol, as compared with young men without a positive family history. This finding was later extended by showing that this population also demonstrated less body-sway after alcohol challenge (Schuckit, 1985).

Biochemical markers for susceptibility to alcoholism have also been investigated (Schuckit et al, 1987a, 1987b), showing that young men at higher risk for alcoholism demonstrated significantly lower blood levels of prolactin and cortisol following alcohol challenge than did controls. Such findings are of great interest, though their power in predicting later alcoholism has yet to be established.

Event-related potentials (ERPs) have also been used in an attempt to find trait markers. In particular, the P300 or P3 component, so named because it is a positive wave form with a latency of about 300 msec, has attracted considerable interest. This waveform may arise from the hippocampus and associated areas (Polich and Bloom, 1987) and has been related to sensory processing. In addition, it is highly similar between siblings, with even greater similarity between twins, indicating a high degree of genetic control (Steinhauer et al, 1987).

After finding a flattening of P3 amplitude in abstinent alcoholics, Begleiter and co-workers (1984), using a visual task, extended their investigation to preadolescent sons of alcoholics and again found consistent decreases in P3 amplitude, as compared to controls, a finding later replicated in young men aged 21 to 28

(O'Connor et al, 1986, 1987). However, other investigators, looking at both male and female subjects and using different stimulus modalities and methods of analysis, have not found group differences (Polich, Burns and Bloom, 1988).

In a later study, Begleiter et al (1987), again studying sons of alcoholic fathers, noted that the fathers of their subjects all had onset of alcohol abuse as teenagers, with a high incidence of antisocial behavior and repeated hospitalizations for alcoholism, and they could be characterized as type 2 alcoholics. In this study, their earlier finding of decreased P3 amplitude was confirmed. Interestingly, O'Connor et al (1986) had noted that, earlier than in their sample, a subset of high-risk subjects accounted for most of the group reduction in P3 amplitude. It may be that later studies, by categorizing subjects by alcoholism subtype, will resolve the discrepancies in this area. However, longitudinal studies will be necessary to establish the validity and reliability of these findings, and more work is needed to relate them to other evidence of risk for alcoholism.

Morbidity Risks in Family Members

The proportion of relatives of alcoholics who have similar problems depends on the degree of genetic relationship and sociodemographic variables, such as the sex, age, occupation, and birth cohort (year of birth) of the relative. The relevant sociodemographic variables are all associated with differences in the frequency and amount of alcohol consumed, thereby influencing exposure to the heavy drinking required to bring out susceptibility, if any, to alcoholism. For example, both consumption and complications have varied widely from one historical era to another and currently vary from country to country, between social classes, between persons of different occupation, and between men and women. Accordingly, the effect of degree of genetic relationship can be best assayed in observations about multiple classes of relationship in a single culture that is homogeneous and stable.

Fortunately, observations about multiple genetic classes of relatives have been made in Sweden, which is a relatively homogeneous population (Cloninger et al, 1988). The morbid risk of recurrent alcohol abuse in Sweden according to degree of genetic relationship is shown in Table 4. Recurrent alcohol abuse was defined as diagnosis and treatment for alcoholism or multiple registrations for

Table 4. Family Studies of Recurrent Alcohol Abuse in Swedish Men

Source	Relationship	Probandwise Concordance	
		N	%
Kaij (1960)	MZ twins	27	70
Kaij (1960)	DZ twins	60	33
Amark (1951)	singleton sib	349	31
	no alcoholic parent	252	17
	one alcoholic parent	97	33
Bohman (1978)	adopted-away sons	50	20
Kaij and Dock (1975)	grandsons	270	12
Census, 1968	general population		7

alcohol abuse by a social agency charged with maintaining sobriety in the community. The risk of recurrent alcohol abuse was seven percent in men in the general population and increased to 12 percent in individuals sharing one quarter of the same genes (grandsons), to 20 to 33 percent in individuals sharing half of the same genes (children or siblings), to 70 percent in genetically identical individuals (monozygotic twins). Compared to the general population, the relative risk of recurrent alcohol abuse is two in second-degree relatives, three or four in first-degree relatives, and ten in monozygotic twins. These risks provide an estimate of heritability for recurrent alcohol abuse of about 67 percent.

Family and adoption studies of alcoholism have been carried out that use explicit diagnostic criteria. Most of these have employed the criteria of Feighner et al (1972), which shows substantial concordance with *DSM-III* and *DSM-III-R* criteria. The lifetime risk of alcoholism in adult first-degree relatives of hospitalized alcoholics is summarized according to the sex of the alcoholic proband and the sex and severity of alcoholism in the relatives in Table 5. The data is based on the St. Louis Family Interview Study of Alcoholism, directed by Theodore Reich and Robert Cloninger (Cloninger et al, 1988a). Combining definite and probable cases, over 60 percent of the male relatives and 20 percent of the female relatives were alcoholic, regardless of the sex of the proband. Thus the sex of the relative, but not the proband, is associated with a large difference in the risk of alcoholism.

Coincident with increasing consumption of alcohol in the general population, the risk of alcoholism in relatives has also increased in more recently born individuals. This is depicted for men in the St. Louis Family Study in Figure 2. The cumulative risk of definite alcoholism by age 25 years increases progressively with the year of birth, from 26 percent of 61 men born before 1924, to 34 percent of the 56 born from 1925 to 1934, and increasing in each cohort to 67 percent of the 141 men born after 1954. The cumulative risks in the younger

Table 5. Alcoholism in Adult First-Degree Relatives of Hospitalized Alcoholics

Sex and Severity in Relatives	Male Probands (N = 132)		Female Probands (N = 52)	
	f/N	%	f/N	%
Father/Son				
definite alcoholism	24/67	35.8	13/32	40.6
probable alcoholism	7/67	10.4	6/32	18.8
Brother				
definite alcoholism	52/108	48.1	16/35	45.7
probable alcoholism	23/108	21.3	6/35	17.1
Mother/Daughter				
definite alcoholism	16/102	15.7	3/45	6.7
probable alcoholism	7/102	6.9	4/45	8.9
Sister				
definite alcoholism	17/113	15.0	10/46	21.7
probable alcoholism	7/113	6.2	2/46	4.3

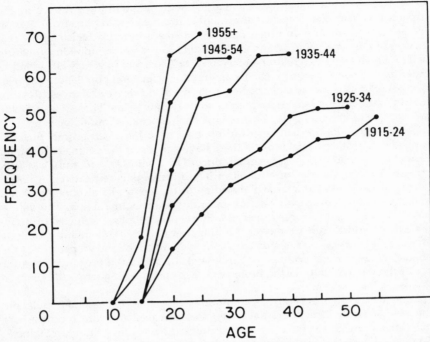

Figure 2. Effect of year of birth on frequency of alcoholism by age in first-degree male relatives of hospitalized alcoholics (Cloninger et al, 1988b).

cohorts are likely to increase further with age. For example, in the cohort born before 1924, the risk of alcoholism increases from 22 percent at age 25 to 28 percent by age 40. For those in the next cohort (born between 1925 and 1934), the risk increases from 36 percent to 48 percent, and in the cohort born between 1935 and 1944, it increases from 53 percent to 63 percent. A similar pattern has been described in women (Cloninger et al, 1988b; Reich et al, 1988).

Some studies have suggested that familial alcoholics can be distinguished from nonfamilial alcoholics because they show primary (that is, temporally antecedent to other diagnoses) and severe alcohol abuse, but these studies have not taken reliability of diagnosis into account (Cloninger, 1987c). Guze et al (1986) found in a six- to 12-year follow-up that diagnostic stability is higher in primary definite cases than in secondary probable cases, as summarized in Table 6. This suggests that many of the features that have been attributed to familial cases may actually define cases in which the diagnosis of alcoholism is most reliable. Furthermore, the increasing prevalence of alcoholism is not attributable to an increase in nonfamilial cases. Rather, increasing the prevalence of alcoholism in the general population has increased the proportion of familial cases and the proportion of alcoholic relatives in families. This suggests that familiarity alone is not an adequate way of subdividing alcoholics.

Nevertheless, type 2 alcoholics are more often familial than type 1 alcoholics (see Table 7) (Gilligan et al, 1987). Type 2 alcoholics also have early onset and

Table 6. Consistency of Alcoholism Diagnoses*

Initial Diagnosis of Alcoholism	Number of Cases	% Alcoholism Diagnosis at Follow-up
Primary definite	24	96%
Primary probable	4	100%
Secondary definite	27	89%
Secondary probable	15	53%

*From Guze SB, Cloninger CR, Martin R, et al: Alcoholism as a medical disorder. Compr Psychiatry 1986; 27:501–510.

more frequent treatment, so there is substantial overlap with other descriptions of familial or *process* alcoholics. However, the distinction based on personality and types of alcohol-related symptoms is more robust than that based on familiality alone. The greater robustness is based on evidence from adoption studies that familiality involves the interaction of genetic predisposition and postnatal environment in type 1 alcoholics.

Cross-Fostering Analysis in Adoptees

Adoption studies permit genetic and environmental influences on alcoholism and related psychopathology to be measured separately in terms of the characteristics of the biological parents and the postnatal milieu. In the Stockholm Adoption Study, all children who were born to single women in Stockholm from 1930 to 1949 and given up for adoption by nonrelatives at an early age were studied to identify background variables predictive of alcohol abuse in the adoptees. Alcohol abuse was identified using medical records and public registries that permit identification of about 70 percent of alcoholics without bias for any subtype (Cloninger et al, 1981; Bohman et al, 1981; Cloninger, 1987a). Alcohol abuse in the biological parents provided an index of genetic predisposition to alcoholism. A predisposition to type 1 alcohol abuse was identified by having biological parents who had adult onset of alcohol abuse with minimal criminality; in contrast, a predisposition to type 2 alcoholism was identified by having biological fathers, but not mothers, who had teenage onset of alcohol abuse associated with criminality.

Alcohol abuse in the adoptive parents was found not to increase the risk of alcohol abuse in the adopted children; in fact, the risk of alcohol abuse was slightly lower in children whose adoptive parents had problems with alcohol abuse. Thus alcohol abuse is clearly not the result of imitating parental alcohol abuse. However, low social status of the adoptive home and extent of hospital care in infancy provided an index of postnatal factors that were associated with increased environmental risk for heavy alcohol consumption and alcoholism.

Cross-fostering analyses revealed different patterns of inheritance for type 1 and type 2 alcoholic men. In men with a genetic predisposition to type 1 alcoholism, there was increased risk of alcoholism only if their adoptive home environment was associated with increased risk of heavy drinking (Table 8). In

Table 7. Characteristics of Alcoholic Women, Type 1 Men, and Type 2 Men*

Family History	Proband Type		
	type 2 men	type 1 men	women
Positive family history, %	68.8	16.7	39.2
Incidence of definite alcoholism, %			
male relatives[1]	51.9	30.0	43.3
female relatives	21.4	8.2	13.2
spouses	8.8	5.3	50.0
Age at onset of definite alcoholism, years (N)			
probands	22.1 (76)	25.0 (86)	30.5 (55)
mothers	26.0 (6)	41.8 (5)	—[2]
fathers	24.0 (8)	28.9 (5)	35.0 (8)
Incidence of antisocial personality, %			
probands	36.1	31.6	9.1
male relatives	15.1	7.1	9.0
female relatives	6.8	4.1	2.2
spouses	5.9	5.3	6.3

*From Gilligan SB, Reich T, Cloninger CR: Etiologic heterogeneity in alcoholism. Genet Epidemiol 1987; 7:395–414
[1]Relatives included all first-degree biological relatives: 243 male relatives (106 type 2 men, 70 type 1 men, and 67 female); 305 female relatives (117 type 2 men, 97 type 1 men, and 91 female)
[2]No mothers of female alcoholic probands received a diagnosis of definite alcoholism.

contrast, men with a genetic predisposition to type 2 alcoholism had an increased risk of alcoholism, regardless of their external circumstances (Table 9).

In order to evaluate whether the typological distinction was replicable regardless of the sex of the adoptee, the biological parent backgrounds of an independent group of female adoptees were classified by the same discriminant procedure derived for the men. Because the type 1, but not type 2, alcoholic men had an excess of alcoholic mothers, we predicted that the women with a genetic predisposition to type 1, but not type 2, alcoholism would have an excess of alcoholism compared to daughters of nonalcoholic (low risk) biological parents. These predictions were confirmed (Bohman et al, 1981; Cloninger et al, 1985). Specifically, type 1 daughters had a significant excess of alcoholism, but the type 2 daughters did not, as shown in Tables 10 and 11. In contrast, the type 2, but not type 1, daughters had an excess of somatization (that is, they were frequently disabled by complaints of headache, backache, and abdominal pain, as in DSM-III somatization disorder) (Cloninger et al, 1985, 1986; Bohman et al, 1984). The association between type 2 alcoholism and somatization was particularly interesting because antisocial personality traits are strongly associated with somatization, particularly in women in whom the overt antisocial behavior is less prominent.

Table 8. Cross-Fostering Analysis of Mild and Severe Type 1 Alcoholism

Is Genetic Background Type 1?	Is Environmental Background Mild or Severe?	Male Adoptees Observed total N	% with mild abuse	% with severe abuse
No	—	448	6.5	4.2
Yes	No	237	7.2	6.3
Yes	Mild	91	15.4*	7.7
Yes	Severe	86	4.7	11.6*

*Abuse is increased only given both genetic and postnatal predisposition (p<.05).

The genetic heterogeneity of type 1 and type 2 alcoholism has recently been confirmed in pedigree analysis of male and female alcoholics in the St. Louis Family Study (Gilligan et al, 1987). In treatment samples of alcoholics, about 80 percent of female and about 50 percent of male alcoholics are type 1 alcoholics.

What Is Inherited?

Individuals with both anxiety and somatization disorders were found to have an increased risk of alcoholism (Cloninger et al, 1986; Cloninger, 1987a). However, criminality in the biological parents was positively correlated with somatization and negatively correlated with anxiety disorders in the adopted-away children (Cloninger et al, 1986). Likewise, the numbers of type 1 and type 2 alcoholism symptoms were found to be negatively correlated when severity of illness is taken into account in general samples (Gilligan et al, 1988). This suggested that susceptibility to alcoholism was mediated by heritable personality traits, and that opposite configurations of personality traits predisposed to the two alcoholic subtypes (Cloninger, 1987a).

Personality can be defined in terms of individual differences in the adaptive brain systems involved in the reception, processing, and storing of information about the environment. Factor analytic studies consistently reveal that three higher-order dimensions of personality account for most variability between individuals, particularly those aspects that are heritable and stable across cultures and situations (Cloninger, 1987b). The heritability of such higher-order personality traits have consistently been found to be about 40 percent to 60 percent, so that genetic and environmental factors are roughly equally important in personality development. Elsewhere evidence has been presented that the underlying neurogenetic structure of personality reflects variation in three adaptive brain system processes for the activation, maintenance, and inhibition of behavioral responses to stimulation, including responses to alcohol and other drugs (Cloninger, 1987a, 1987b). Differences between individuals in the neuromodulation of these three brain systems are hypothesized to cause variation in the three personality dimensions of harm avoidance (behavioral inhibition), novelty seeking (behavioral activation), and reward dependence (behavioral maintenance).

Table 9. Cross-Fostering Analysis of Type 2 Alcohol Abuse in Men

Is Genetic Background Type 2?	Is Environmental Background Type 2?	Male Adoptees Observed	
		total N	% with type 2 abuse
No	No	567	1.9
No	Yes	196	4.1
Yes	No	71	16.9[a]
Yes	Yes	28	17.9[a]

[a]Risk is significantly increased in those with type 2 genetic background compared to others ($p < 0.01$).

Alcohol-seeking behavior is considered to be a special kind of exploratory appetitive behavior (Cloninger, 1987a). As seen in type 2 alcoholics, prominent alcohol seeking and inability to abstain is associated with rapid initiation of exploratory activity in response to novelty and rapid acquisition of rewarded behavior in response to cues to reward, as in individuals who are high in novelty seeking and low in dopaminergic turnover in the brain. Furthermore, prominent alcohol seeking is associated with low harm avoidance and low serotonergic turnover in the brain, so that their inclination to initiate activity is not readily inhibited by the potential risks. In fact, type 2 alcoholics have been found to have antisocial personality traits (von Knorring et al, 1985, 1987; Cloninger et al, 1988), to seek alcohol for pleasure and exhilaration (Nordstrom and Berglund, 1987), and to have low turnover of dopamine and serotonin in their cerebrospinal fluid (Cloninger, 1987a). In addition, abstinent type 2 alcoholics and their children have been found to be augmenters in their stimulus-intensity modulation (von Knorring et al, 1987; Cloninger, 1986) and to have low P3 amplitudes in evoked responses, suggesting deficient ability to allocate significance to targeted stimuli (Cloninger, 1987a; Begleiter et al, 1987).

On the other hand, psychological dependence and loss of control, as seen in type 1 alcoholics, is hypothesized to reflect rapid development of tolerance to the antianxiety effects of alcohol. The combination of high harm avoidance and high reward dependence is hypothesized to facilitate conditioned responses to relief of anxiety. Animal experiments documenting the essential roles of serotonergic and noradrenergic mechanisms in tolerance to sedative doses of alcohol have been reviewed elsewhere (See Cloninger, 1987a). In human alcoholics, those with type 1 features have low basal turnover of norepinephrine after prolonged abstinence, as predicted by the theory described here (Borg et al, 1986).

The critical test of the relationship between childhood personality and adult alcoholism is a prospective longitudinal study. Recently, childhood personality ratings at age 10 years were found to predict later alcohol abuse in 431 adoptees followed to age 28 years (Cloninger et al, 1988a). At age 28, most alcoholics had type 2 features and antisocial personality traits (namely high novelty seeking, low harm avoidance, and low reward dependence). However, the opposite traits were also associated with increased risk of alcoholism. Long-term follow-up is

Table 10. Psychopathology in the Adopted-out Daughters of Type 1 Biologic Parents and of Nonalcoholic Biologic Parents

	Classification of Daughters[a]		
Observed Psychopathology[b]	type 1 (N = 100) row %	low risk (N = 282) row %	significance level P
Alcohol abuse	7.3	2.5	<0.05[c]
Criminality only	0	1.4	NS
Somatization only	16.3	16.3	NS
Other disability	13.6	15.2	NS

[a]Classification of the biologic parents of the women was based on discriminant analysis of an independent sample of parents of adopted men.
[b]The classification system for adoptees was hierarchical, proceeding from alcohol abuse to other psychiatric disability. Thus criminality only indicates criminality and no alcohol abuse with or without somatization or other disability; somatization only indicates neither alcohol abuse nor criminality.
[c]Risk is increased compared with low-risk daughters.

planned to test the prediction that late onset cases will show type 1 features and anxious personality traits (namely, high harm avoidance, high reward dependence, and low novelty seeking).

DISCUSSION

Recent epidemiological work found an increasing prevalence of alcoholism in younger cohorts. Although this increase is too rapid to be accounted for solely by genetic factors, the rise in the proportion of familial cases indicates that the increase is largely to be found in those with constitutional vulnerabilities to the development of alcoholism. This susceptibility may be mediated by heritable personality traits.

Recent work on the genetic epidemiology of alcoholism has demonstrated two sets of interrelated findings. First, alcoholism is heterogeneous and different subtypes are associated with different kinds of psychiatric comorbidity. Type 1 alcoholism is associated with susceptibility to anxiety and resistance to antisocial behavior; it is associated with anxiety disorders and possibly neurotic depressive reactions to loss or separation. On the other hand, type 2 alcoholism is associated with antisocial personality traits; it is associated with criminality and somatoform disorders and abuse of stimulants and opiates. Type 2 alcoholics are overrepresented in psychiatric treatment settings, presumably because they are quicker to complain of discomfort and to require attention for acting-out behaviors, such as arrests and suicide attempts.

Secondly, these subtypes of alcoholism differ in age of onset and sex distributions. Type 2 alcoholics are more often men and develop problems earlier, usually before age 25 years. The motivation of these two groups for drinking is quite different: type 1 alcoholics seek relief of anxiety, and type 2 alcoholics seek

Table 11. Psychopathology in the Adopted-out Daughters of Type 2 Biologic Parents and of Nonalcoholic Biologic Parents

	Classification of Daughters[a]		
Observed Psychopathology[b]	type 2 (N = 105) row %	low risk (N = 282) row %	significance level P
Alcohol abuse	4.8	2.5	NS
Criminality only	2.9	1.4	NS
Somatization only	26.7	16.3	<0.05[c]
Other disability	13.3	15.2	NS

[a]Classification of the biologic parents of the women was based on discriminant analysis of an independent sample of parents of adopted men.
[b]The classification system for adoptees was hierachical, proceeding from alcohol abuse to other psychiatric disability. Thus criminality only indicates criminality and no alcohol abuse with or without somatization or other disability; somatization only indicates neither alcohol abuse nor criminality.
[c]Risk is increased compared with low-risk daughters.

stimulation and pleasure. Accordingly, the treatment of alcoholics needs to be individualized to the characteristics of the alcoholic.

The treatment of type 1 alcoholics with loss of control and prominent psychological dependence emphasizes the necessity of total, lifelong abstinence. In addition, these individuals need to find other ways to relax, relieve their anxiety, and maintain supportive social relationships. Nonsedating antidepressants that reduce postsynaptic sensitivity to serotonin (for example, fluoxetine) and norepinephrine (desipramine or maprotaline) may be considered if psychosocial approaches alone are unsuccessful.

On the other hand, the treatment of type 2 alcoholics should emphasize finding other ways to obtain stimulation and exhiliration, such as engaging in challenging activities and physical exercise. Noneuphoriant dopaminergic (for example, pemoline) or serotonergic (lithium with or without fluoxetine) drugs may be considered if psychosocial approaches alone are unsuccessful.

To date, no systematic controlled trials of alcoholism treatment based on this theoretical model have been conducted. Further studies of the personality, learning, neurophysiology, and neurochemical traits of alcoholics and their relatives are needed to test and extend the theoretical models described here. Along with these basic studies, there is clearly a need to begin trials of treatments guided by available knowledge about the basic mechanisms underlying the initial onset and later progression of alcoholism. Use of such an integrated approach, ideally targeting not only problematic behaviors but underlying personality traits as well, holds the promise of developing more specific and effective treatment modalities.

REFERENCES

Begleiter H, Porjesz B, Bihari B, et al: Event-related brain potentials in boys at risk for alcoholism. Science 1984; 225:1493–1496

Begleiter H, Projesz B, Rawlings R, et al: Auditory recovery function and P3 in boys at high risk for alcoholism. Alcohol 1987; 4:315–321

Bohman M, Sigvardsson S, Cloninger CR: Maternal inheritance of alcohol abuse: cross-fostering analysis of adopted women. Arch Gen Psychiatry 1981; 38:965–969

Bohman M, Cloninger CR, von Knorring AL, et al: An adoption study of somatoform disorders, III: cross-fostering analysis and genetic relationship to alcoholism and criminality. Arch Gen Psychiatry 1984; 41:872–878

Borg S, Liljeberg P, Mossberg D: Clinical studies on central noradrenergic activity in alcohol abusing patients. Acta Psychiatr Scand 1986; Suppl 327:43–60

Cloninger CR: Neurogenetic adaptive mechanisms in alcoholism. Science 1987a; 236:410–416

Cloninger CR: A systematic method for clinical description and classification of personality variants. Arch Gen Psychiatry 1987b; 44:573–588

Cloninger CR: Recent advances in family studies of alcoholism, in Genetics and Alcoholism. Edited by Goedde HW, Agarwal D. New York, Alan R. Liss. Progress Clinical Biological Research (series) 1987c; 241:47–60

Cloninger CR, Bohman M, Sigvardsson S: Inheritance of alcohol abuse: cross-fostering analysis of adopted men. Arch Gen Psychiatry 1981; 38:861–868

Cloninger CR, Bohman M, Sigvardsson S, et al: Psychopathology in adopted-out children of alcoholics. Recent Dev Alcohol 1985; 3:37–51

Cloninger CR, von Knorring AL, Sigvardsson S, et al: Symptom patterns and causes of somatization in men; II: genetic and environmental independence from somatization in women. Genet Epidemiol 1986; 3:171–185

Cloninger CR, Sigvardsson S, Bohman M: Childhood personality predicts alcohol abuse in young adults. Alcoholism: Clinical and Experimental Research 1988a; 12:494–505

Cloninger CR, Reich T, Sigvardsson S, et al: Effects of changes in alcohol use between generations on inheritance of alcohol abuse, in Alcoholism: Origins and Outcome. Edited by Rose RM, Barrett J. Raven Press, New York, 1988b

Cloninger CR, Sigvardsson S, Gilligan SB, et al: Genetic heterogeneity and the classification of alcoholism. Adv Alcohol Subst Abuse 1988c

Cotton NS: The familial incidence of alcoholism: a review. J Stud Alcohol 1979; 40:89–116

Feighner JP, Robins E, Guze SB, et al: Diagnostic criteria for use in psychiatric research. Arch Gen Psychiatry 1972; 26:57–63

Gilligan SB, Reich T, Cloninger CR: Etiologic heterogeneity in alcoholism. Genet Epidemiol 1987; 7:395–414

Gilligan SB, Reich T, Cloninger CR: Alcohol-related symptoms in heterogeneous families of hospitalized alcoholics. Alcoholism: Clinical and Experimental Research 1988

Goodwin DW, Schulsinger F, Hermansen L, et al: Alcoholism and the hyperactive child syndrome. J Nerv Ment Dis 1975; 160:349–53

Guze SB, Cloninger CR, Martin R, et al: Alcoholism as a medical disorder. Compr Psychiatry 1986; 27:501–510

Helzer JE, Pryzbeck TR: The co-occurrence of alcoholism with other psychiatric disorders in the general population and its impact on treatment. J Stud Alcohol 1988; 49:219–24

Nordstrom G, Berglund M: Different patterns of successful long-term adjustment in genetically defined subtypes of alcoholics. Alcohol Alcohol 1987; 1(Suppl):401–405

O'Connor S, Hesselbrock V, Tasman A: Correlates of increased risk for alcoholism in young men. Prog Neuropsychopharmacol Biol Psychiatry 1986; 10:211–218

O'Connor S, Hesselbrock V, Tasman A, et al: P3 amplitudes in two distinct tasks are decreased in young men with a history of paternal alcoholism. Alcohol 1987; 4:323–330

Park P, Whitehead PC: Developmental Sequence and Dimensions of Alcoholism. Quarterly Journal for the Study of Alcohol 1973; 34:887–904

Polich J, Bloom FE: P300 from normals and adult children of alcoholics. Alcohol 1987; 4:301-305

Polich J, Burns T, Bloom F: P300 and the risk for alcoholism: family history, task difficulty, and gender. Alcoholism: Clinical and Experimental Research 1988; 12:248–254

Reich T, Cloninger CR, Van Eerdewegh P, et al: Secular trends in the familial transmission of alcoholism. Alcoholism: Clinical and Experimental Research 1988

Robins LN, Helzer JE, Pryzbeck TR, et al: Alcohol disorders in the community: a report from the Epidemiologic Catchment Area, in Alcoholism: Origins and Outcome. Edited by Rose RM, Barrett J. New York, Raven Press, 1988

Rose RM, Barrett JE: Alcoholism: Origins and Outcome. New York, Raven Press, 1988

Schuckit MA: Subjective responses to alcohol in sons of alcoholics and control subjects. Arch Gen Psychiatry 1984; 41:879–884

Schuckit MA: Ethanol-induced changes in body sway in men at high alcoholism risk. Arch Gen Psychiatry 1985; 42:375–379

Schuckit MA, Gold E, Risch C: Serum prolactin levels in sons of alcoholics and control subjects. Am J Psychiatry 1987a; 144:854–859

Schuckit MA, Gold E, Risch C: Plasma cortisol levels following ethanol in sons of alcoholics and controls. Arch Gen Psychiatry 1987b; 144:942–945

Steinhauer SR, Hill SY, Zubin J: Event-related potentials in alcoholics and their first-degree relatives. Alcohol 1987; 4:307–314

von Knorring A-L, Bohman M, von Knorring L, et al: Platelet MAO activity as a biological marker in subgroups of alcoholism. Acta Psychiatr Scand 1985; 72:51–58

von Knorring L, von Knorring A-L, Smigan L, Lindberg U, Edholm M. Personality traits in subtypes of alcoholics. J Stud Alc 1987; 48:523–527

Chapter 15

Neurobiology of Alcohol Action and Alcoholism

by Floyd E. Bloom, M.D.

NEUROBIOLOGICAL APPROACHES TO ALCOHOL ACTION AND ALCOHOLISM

Historically, attempts to explain the actions of ethanol on the brain have focused on the ability of alcohol (ethanol) to perturb general membrane functions as measured *in vitro* (Goldstein, 1987; Taraschi et al, 1987, for review) through its chemical properties of a lipid permeant. In contrast, more recent *in vitro* biochemical assays, as well as cellular electrophysiologic studies supported by separate bodies of anatomic and neurochemical evidence, suggest the emergence of a more specific pharmacologic profile in which the membrane-mounted proteins of selected subsets of neurons are the main targets of the pharmacologically relevant actions of alcohol. This current view is based on data drawn from the full spectrum of levels of inquiry into the effects of ethanol on the brain.

Hierarchical Research Strategies in Central Nervous System (CNS) Alcohol Research

To understand modern methods of drug analysis in the CNS, it is useful to distinguish the levels of complexity of the brain and its composite elements. One approach is to distingush at least three related levels of complexity: molecular, cellular, and behavioral.

MOLECULAR STUDIES. At the molecular level, research strategies focus on the identification of new molecules involved in cellular structure and function. The past decade's research has emphasized those molecules that are critical for communication between neurons, such as the neurotransmitters, their receptors, and the complementary molecules associated with transmitter synthesis, storage, release, and response. In contrast to other major psychoactive drugs, no single known transmitter has yet been incriminated as the mediator of any specific action of alcohol. However, it is clear from the momentum of present work that not all transmitters have yet been identified.

More specifically, one can ask the general question, "How many kinds and types of neurotransmitters are there?" In current terms, the several different chemical classes of transmitters vary from the simple small molecules such as amino acids (for example, glutamate and gamma amino butyrate) and monoamines (serotonin, acetylcholine, and the catecholamines) on the one end, to the more complex forms such as neuropeptides, steroids, and lipid mediators

I thank Nancy Callahan for manuscript typing. This work was supported by USPHS grants from NIAAA (AA-06420, AA-07456), NIDA (DA-03665), and the Research Institute of Scripps Clinic BCR #5247.

of cell–cell messages. More than 100 examples of the neuropeptides have now been described, and new ones are being added continuously.

An additional important example of the growth at this level is that the actual amino acid sequences of neurotransmitter receptor molecules can now be specified, rather than being limited to a functional assay for the receptor. As a result, it is possible to discriminate between the varieties of receptors, to distinguish those that directly regulate ion channels from those that employ more complex mechanisms of signal transduction, and—critically—to define the sites at which the endogenous ligands activate the receptor. This capacity not only permits a rational basis for probing drug–receptor interactions, but also an intellectual platform to design agonist or antagonist drugs.

Despite the major advances that are incorporated in the findings that have generated these concepts, they in turn lead to a still more general and perhaps more profound index of our remaining ignorance of the brain: "How many genes (and gene products) are made by the brain?" Current research would place this number at well over half of the genome, and perhaps as many as 30,000 to 50,000 genes, of which much less than one percent can now be specified.

CELLULAR STUDIES. At the cellular level, research questions center on whether one or more sets of neurons can be viewed as the initial responders to alcohol, leading to either the effects of intoxication, the underlying rewarding or aversive effects of intoxication, or to the brain's adaptive responses to being intoxicated. Such questions are based upon the degree to which cell classes in the brain can be characterized by their shared and unique properties, and how these cell classes interact in circuits or ensembles of two more neurons to accomplish functions generally referred to as *information processing*. In this regard, one can consider the general question of "How many kinds of neurons are there?" Present estimates suggest that the human brain contains roughly 100 billion neurons.

Traditionally, neuroscientists have divided them up into specific classes of cells by their shape (pyramidal, mitral, stellate, etc.), their size (magnocellular, parvocellular), their location within the brain (cortical, spinal, thalamic) or in specific functional systems (motor, sensory), or their transmitter type (such as GABA-ergic, noradrenergic, cholinergic). Clearly, none of these features per se is an adequate index, since any given brain cell has multiple qualities on each of these lists.

Building on the new waves of specific genetic information, we anticipate that future categories will be based less on these qualitative phenotypic designations and more precisely on the molecular designations of their specific genetic categorizations. That information may also help determine why certain nerve cells are susceptible to the drug actions and their toxic long-term effects that other neurons are able to resist, and how some nerve cells within the brain are able to repair themselves after damage while others die.

The field of cell–cell communication, whether it be one of synaptic transmission between connected neurons or the poorly understood areas of neuron–glial interactions, has also benefitted from recent research efforts. Two major avenues of advance in the past decade have been 1) the ability to define neuronal circuitry experimentally by microscopic methods, and 2) the definition of the mechanisms of signal transduction for specific transmitters and receptors. In fact, the growth in factual information at the cellular level, largely from studies of the brains of small experimental animals, may be viewed as perhaps the leading edge of the neuroscientific information explosion. However, appreciation of the new advances remains fragmentary and is almost certainly not well integrated with the knowledge used by clinical neuroscientists to conjecture into the nature of a diagnostic behavioral entity, such as alcoholism, or to conceive of new mechanisms of pathogenesis, treatment, or prevention.

BEHAVIORAL STUDIES. Research at the behavioral (supracellular) level centers on the integrative phenomena that link populations of neurons, their supporting glia, and vasculature into ensembles specialized for performance of specifiable sensory, motor, or behavioral tasks. These global brain–body functions traditionally included the brain's abilities to monitor internal chemical signals and, thus, to provide regulatory responses over virtually all internal visceral systems, including specifically the endocrine system, the cardiovascular system, the gastrointestinal system, and the genitourinary system. More recently, because of the advances in neurotransmitter and receptor identification, and receptor the neuroscientific data avalanche has led to suggestions that neuronal events may also regulate the immune system and alter its abilities to respond to self and to foreign invaders, such as cancer-promoting viruses and other infectious agents.

Work at the behavioral level has perhaps the greatest apparent relevance to alcoholism because it seeks specifically to understand the basis for the behavioral functions of the brain. Such work extends from the complex but still poorly understood mechanisms of learning, reward, and reinforcement. To some experts, such work may only be properly pursued in human studies. The general field has gained importance in the recent past through development of noninvasive functional tests that permit identification of the sites in normal and patient samples that are altered in prolonged states of abnormal functional activities: vigilance, sleep, performing complex mental tasks, or exhibiting prolonged psychiatric phenomena such as hallucinations, delusional depression, or mania. The noninvasive imaging and assessment strategies have also pointed to specific sites at which alcohol may act.

INFERENCES FROM THE NEUROBIOLOGICAL STUDIES. Whole-animal behavioral investigations show clearcut selective drug interactions for ethanol that distinguish it from benzodiazepine actions, despite their shared ability to produce anxiolysis (see below). On the basis of single neuronal recordings, some brain systems, such as cerebellar neurons, seem to be relatively insensitive to ethanol at high concentrations, while other neuronal systems, such as the hippocampus, inferior olivary nucleus, and locus coeruleus, show much greater sensitivity.

Conceptually, one might prefer to derive from the host of diverse sensitivities and the range of types of changes observed in response to ethanol some common denominator as a mediating action that could explain all of the effects of ethanol on motor behavior, on emotion, and on arousal and attention. However, no such common mechanisms can now explain alcohol effects on either transmitter release generally (Hudspith et al, 1987) or the general membrane-mediated actions (Gordon et al, 1987); nor are there any solid clues as to the mechanisms by which chronic exposure to alcohol induces the cellular toxicity in chronic alcoholics or fetuses born to mothers who drink excessively.

While the effects of ethanol on the rodent and primate brains are no doubt widespread, there is emerging a specific pattern of ethanol-induced effects that would appear to begin to define the cellular basis for the complex behavioral state termed *intoxication*. Recognition of these cellular events and the mechanisms by which ethanol achieves them would in turn seem to be requisite starting points for understanding and perhaps preventing the deleterious dependence that can arise with chronic consumption.

CURRENT PROMISING DIRECTIONS

Having reviewed the general strategies of research within the domain of neurobiology generally, it should be clear that many opportunities exist for analyzing the effects of alcohol and by which to distinguish the sensitivity to alcohol between individuals. During the past decade, as a result of the infusion of research funds into the alcoholism and alcohol-abuse fields, many such studies have been initiated. Some of the more promising early results are reviewed below; more complete details are available in recent reviews (Bowen, 1987; Straus and Li, 1987).

Molecular Studies

MEMBRANES.   A perennial question in alcohol research is whether the effects of the drug are mediated through changes in the properties of plasma membrane lipids or membrane-mounted proteins. These data have recently been reviewed by Harris et al (1987), with particular regard to the possible actions of alcohol on the physical property of membrane *fluidity* or, more precisely, to the separable properties of viscosity of membrane lipid molecules and their relative ordered arrangements within the plane of the membrane. The conclusions reached were that, at concentrations up to lethal levels, ethanol does not alter the microviscosity of membrane lipids, nor can it be viewed as affecting membrane function during intoxication through alterations in membrane lipid order. While modest changes in lipid order can be observed after very large doses of alcohol, similar changes can also be produced without signs of intoxication by raising body temperature. On the other hand, after chronic exposure to alcohol, similar studies of membrane properties support the concept of a physicochemical adaptation that results in membranes able to resist the actions of alcohol. Harris et al (1987) noted that there was a correlation between sensitivity of membrane lipids, particularly the most external surface of the membrane and ethanol sensitivity of an individual animal, whether due to genetic differences or recent pharmacological exposure and tolerance; those correlations suggest, without conclusive proof, that the lipid changes, although minor, can influence membrane function (Goldstein, 1987).

PROTEINS.   Alcohol could influence neuronal function through membrane actions on the proteins within the membrane, such as the receptors for neurotransmitters or the macromolecular intermediates that allow the activated receptors to regulate ion movement through the membrane. Rabin and Molinoff (1983) established that very high doses of alcohol (far above levels attained during intoxication) can enhance basal activity of the enzyme adenylate cyclase, and that these same high doses enhance the ability of the transmitter dopamine to activate this second messenger response. Subsequently, Hoffman and colleagues (1987) reported similar effects for both norepinephrine and dopamine mediated activation of mouse brain adenylate cyclase. While the mechanisms of this effect remain unclear, the authors propose that ethanol is able to alter the affinity of the enzyme for the required binding of magnesium, so that both basal activity and transmitter activation are enhanced. The brain-specific protein IIIb has been identified as a substrate for cyclic adenosine monophosphate (cAMP) induced protein phosphorylation; this protein appears to be diminished in content in postmortem assays on abstinent alcoholics compared to alcoholics of comparable intensity who died while intoxicated (Perdahl et al, 1984; Browning et al, 1987).

At the cholinergic nicotinic receptor, in an *in vitro* purified model system, the effects of alcohol, like those of general anesthetics, have also been linked to effects on the protein itself, rather than on the surrounding lipids (Miller et al, 1987). No significant acute alterations in other receptor or ion channel functions have been reproducibly observed at pharmacologically relevant alcohol concentrations, although effects on tracer fluxes of both calcium and chloride channels have been reported. The reservations associated with these *in vitro* assessments of ion tracer movements are that comparable channels do not appear to be altered by phamacologically pertinent doses of ethanol, when assessed by electrophysiological measurements (Siggins et al, 1987a, 1987b).

TRANSMITTERS. Despite multiple studies, no consistent relationship has been established between the content, synthesis, or catabolism of any neurotransmitter and the doses of alcohol required to produce intoxication. Most such efforts have focused on the catecholamines (Weiner et al, 1987). More promising data on alterations in content but not reuptake of serotonin may underlie the neurochemical differences between alcohol-preferring rat lines relative to nonpreferring controls (Murphy et al, 1985, 1987). An alternative view that has been pursued unsuccessfully with near equal vigor is the concept that during exposure to ethanol the nervous system forms small amounts of monoamine catabolites that can form amine–aldehyde condensation products, whose pharmacologic actions produce the cellular effects of ethanol. The most popularized version of this hypothesis, the *tetrahydroisoquinoline (TIQ) hypothesis*, holds that reactive catabolites of dopamine may form complex metabolic byproducts whose pharmacologic profile accounts for reinforcing behavioral actions of alcohol (see Smith and Amit, 1987, for review). While the data on the behavioral effects of exogenously injected synthetic TIQs are quite contentious, no consistent evidence exists to support the detection of pharmacologically effective doses of any known TIQ after intoxicating amounts of ethanol (see Bloom et al, 1981, and below).

Cellular Level Studies

The past decade has witnessed a resurgence of interest in analysis of the intoxicating and dependence-forming actions of ethanol. Considerable attention has been directed, in animal brain studies, to the questions of how and where ethanol may act to produce the behavioral phenomena and neurological dysfunctions known colloquially as intoxication. The cellular effects of alcohol have been studied in the cerebellar cortex and within the hippocampal formation to develop model systems that may be readily assumed to represent sensitivity to ethanol. These studies have in turn suggested other fruitful neuronal populations to study.

CEREBELLAR ACTIONS. The actions of local (Siggins and French, 1979) and systemic (Rogers et al, 1980) ethanol on the discharge patterns of the cerebellar Purkinje neuron suggested that these cells were relatively resistant to locally applied ethanol even at very high doses (1–3 M) (also see Siggins et al, 1987a). Nevertheless, when rats were given systemic injections of ethanol, in doses that produce far lower local tissue concentrations (25–100 nM), significant acute actions of ethanol were observed on the typical distinctive firing pattern of the Purkinje neuron: an increased frequency of the climbing fiber bursts, with modest increases in modal intervals of single-spike firing (Rogers et al, 1980).

Climbing-fiber bursts reflect the activity of the neurons from which climbing fibers arise, namely neurons of the inferior olivary nucleus. Thus, the apparent activation of olivary neurons by systemic ethanol, as well as the evidence of resistance to direct effects of ethanol on Purkinje neurons, favors the interpretation that the known acute intoxicating effects of ethanol on cerebellar and vestibular function do not arise through actions at the synaptic level within the cerebellar cortex.

The extracellular electrical activity of single neurons of the inferior olivary nucleus, recorded by standard methods in alcohol-naive rats, confirmed that there were significant increases in olivary unit activity (70 percent to 80 percent over baseline), as inferred from recordings in cerebellum. Recovery occurred approximately 80 minutes or more after the ethanol injection (Rogers et al, 1986). Although the mechanism by which ethanol causes olivocerebellar activation remains unclear, several possibilities have been considered (Rogers et al, 1986). The indirect mediation of this effect by some metabolite of ethanol, such as a harmaline-like β-carboline (formed by condensation of acetaldehyde and serotonin) is a possibility that would explain the contrasting effects of systemically versus locally administered ethanol on several cells, including olivocerebellar neurons.

Indeed, it is well known that the rodent inferior olivary complex is heavily innervated with 5-hydroxytryptamine (5-HT)-containing fibers, ending in dense perineuronal networks on the large neurons of the olive (Steinbusch, 1984). We have confirmed these findings (Bloom, Battenberg, Madamba, and Siggins, unpublished), and have gone on to determine whether this innervation by 5-HT neurons is critical for the ability of ethanol to excite olivary cells. To investigate their role, the effects of ethanol in normal rats were compared with the effects of the same doses of ethanol (by the same route of administration and in the same acute experimental preparation) in rats that had been pretreated intracisternally or intracerebroventricularly with the 5-HT-specific toxin, 5,7-dihydroxytryptamine (Daly et al, 1974). This treatment greatly reduces the number of 5-HT immunoreactive terminals within the inferior olive, leaving a few grossly distorted preterminals. Animals given this pretreatment fail to exhibit the consistent and dramatic activation of olivary neuronal firing seen following alcohol dosing in the normals.

When rats were exposed for 10 to 14 days to intoxicating doses of ethanol, either by multiple daily gavages through an implanted intragastric cannula or more evenly by continuous exposure to atmospheric ethanolic vapors (Rogers et al, 1980), no statistically significant alteration of cerebellar Purkinje discharge patterns was seen. Because there had been significant effects on cerebellar unit firing after acute administration, the lack of effect after chronic continuous ethanol could only mean that a cellular tolerance had developed to the acute cellular responses.

Furthermore, after 12 to 32 hours of withdrawal from the chronic ethanol exposures, marked changes in Purkinje cell firing patterns were readily observed. Climbing-fiber bursts were now decreased in frequency, while spontaneous rates of discharge were depressed, and the modal interspike intervals as well as the proportion of long intervals were all significantly increased. These latter changes are quite reminiscent of the general qualitative changes in Purkinje discharge observed when norepinephrine (NE) is iontophoresed or when the locus ceruleus is stimulated (see Foote et al, 1983, for references). When these chronically ethanol-treated animals were again treated with ethanol, the firing abnormalities of the withdrawing rats returned to the normalized firing patterns of the chronically exposed (prewithdrawn) rats (Rogers et al, 1980). Thus, these simple spike effects of withdrawal from chronic ethanol exposure, as viewed through the discharge pattern abnormalities of the Purkinje neuron, would suggest that noradrenergic neuron function may be increased during early withdrawal. Such alterations would not be dissimilar to the changes proposed for the noradrenergic systems during opiate tolerance and withdrawal (Aghajanian, 1978).

LOCUS CERULEUS ACTIONS. These inferences are also testable directly on the neurons of the locus ceruleus (Aston-Jones et al, 1982), by measuring ethanol actions in terms of sensory response properties of these neurons in unanesthetized, freely behaving rats and squirrel monkeys (Foote et al, 1983). Ethanol had no significant effect on the mean spontaneous discharge rates of locus ceruleus (LC) neurons at any dose between 0.5 and 3.0 gm/kg, ip. Furthermore, ethanol had no effect on either latency or reliability of the response of LC neurons to antidromic stimulation. However, the LC was not insensitive to ethanol: When these same LC neurons were evaluated for their response to a standardized orthodromic sensory stimulus, there was a pronounced dose-dependent depression by ethanol ($p<0.0005$, $n=11$); this effect was detected at slightly lower ethanol levels in chloral hydrate than in halothane-anesthetized rats (Aston-Jones et al, 1982).

Significant effects of ethanol on LC neuronal properties were observed at even lower blood levels when the orthodromic sensory responses were evaluated for their fidelity of latency. Ethanol was observed to increase substantially the variations in trial-to-trial response latencies for single tests of sensory responsiveness. Several indices of the variations in afferent activation were evaluated statistically (Aston-Jones et al, 1982); of these, the greatest magnitude effect, as well as the lowest-dose ethanol effect, was related to the standard deviation of the response latencies (significantly increased at 0.5 gm/kg; maximal effect: 325% increase at 3.0 gm/kg). This increased variability of orthodromic sensory response latency may be associated with a second sensitive action of ethanol on LC neurons observed in our study, namely an increase in the inhibitory period that follows antidromic activation.

This effect of ethanol on the LC could be considered a major detriment to normative function. LC neurons have a highly divergent trajectory and produce potent and specific forms of conditional actions on their target neurons (Foote et al, 1983). Although LC or NE actions appear to be *inhibitory* when tested on the basal discharge properties of their cortical target neurons, LC and NE also enhance or *enable* those targets to respond more effectively when the targets are driven by other afferents (excitatory or inhibitory) that may be active simultaneously. Given the phasic discharge of the LC neurons in the awake, behaviorally responsive rat, we have suggested (Foote et al, 1983) that the LC system can bias its targets to favor phasic adaptation to unexpected external environmental stimuli. Significant alteration of the normally precise sensory responses of the LC would, under this view, significantly disrupt the ability of specific external sensory stimuli to elicit appropriate adaptive responses, as confirmed behaviorally (Robbins et al, 1985). Expressed more simply, ethanol-induced disruption of LC sensory responsiveness may be expected to alter cortical information processing and may thus be a basis for further investigation of how ethanol intoxication is produced.

More recently, Pineda and Foote (in preparation) examined squirrel monkeys, trained to sit in a chair and to respond to frequent or infrequent auditory cues, while an electroencephalogram (EEG) was recorded from chronically implanted screw electrodes. They observed (Pineda et al, 1987) that squirrel monkeys do generate a *late positive complex* wave, recorded from the lateral parietal cortical leads, when the infrequent attention-generating auditory cues were presented. The amplitude of this late positive complex was found to be inversely proportional to the frequency with which the eliciting cue was presented and to exhibit trial-to-trial sequential dependencies. Following bilateral electrolytic locus ceruleus lesions, in which the loss of ascending neocortical noradrenergic fibers was confirmed by immunohistochemistry of the synthetic enzyme dopamine-β-hydroxylase, there was a marked diminution of the amplitude of the late positive complex. The effects of LC lesions are thus similar in some respects to the effects of ethanol on LC firing.

HIPPOCAMPAL ACTIONS. The hippocampal pyramidal cell (HPC) has also provided much information on ethanol effects. Extracellular recordings *in vivo* indicate that systemically administered ethanol can alter hippocampal EEGs and multi- and single-unit firing rates, as well as field potential and single-unit responses evoked by stimulation of afferent inputs (Siggins et al, 1987a,b). Although most of these studies found depressant effects (usually at high supraintoxicating doses of ethanol), Newlin and associates (1981) noted that systemic ethanol also can facilitate both excitatory and inhibitory responses to certain afferent stimulation. Local application to HPCs of ethanol by microelectroosmosis or pressure can produce an early excitatory response, sometimes followed by a depression at higher doses, although depression alone is also seen (Siggins et al, 1987a).

To determine the transmitters involved in the enhancement by ethanol of the excitatory and inhibitory responses of pyramidal cells to stimulation of afferent pathways, Mancillas and colleagues (1986a) tested the effect of ethanol (blood levels of 80-150 mg%) on the responses of identified pyramidal cells to iontophoretically applied transmitters in the halothane anesthetized rat. Systemic ethanol markedly enhanced excitatory responses to iontophoresis of acetylcholine (ACh) in CA1 or CA3 pyramidal cells within 15 to 30 minutes, and recovered by about 60 minutes after injection. No comparable effect was observed on glutamate-induced excitation in cells tested alternatively with both transmitters. Similar enhancement of ACh effects have been seen in the *in vitro* hippocampal slice preparation (Siggins and Madamba, in preparation), suggesting that this effect is in no way attributable to anesthetic interactions.

Systemic ethanol also significantly increased the amplitude and duration of inhibitory responses to iontophoretically applied the neuropeptide somatostatin (somatostatin-14, SS-14). This enhancement was evident 10 to 15 minutes after ethanol injection and recovered at 60 to 80 minutes. Ethanol had no statistically significant effect on inhibitory responses to serotonin or norepinephrine. It is perhaps relevant that SS-14 potentiates of responses to ACh in the hippocampus (Mancillas et al, 1986b). Thus, it is possible that ethanol-induced enhancement of responses to ACh may be secondary to an enhancement of the effects of endogenously released somatostatin, which in turn enhances postsynaptic responses to iontophoretically applied ACh. The ethanol-induced alteration of ACh and SS-14 responses may underly the enhancement by ethanol of inhibitory and excitatory synaptic transmission previously described in hippocampus (Newlin et al, 1981).

GABA TRANSMISSION: LINKING CELLULAR AND BEHAVIORAL ALCOHOL ACTIONS. Because of reports that gamma aminobutyric acid (GABA) responses effects are enhanced by very low doses of ethanol (Nestoros 1980; Ticku et al, 1983; Ticku and Burch, 1980), we also examined GABA actions in some detail. Ethanol seemed to cause a small (average: 25%) but consistent potentiation of inhibitory responses to GABA, but most of these potentiations did not recover for up to three hours after ethanol administration, and, in control experiments, they occurred when neurons were tested with GABA repeatedly for comparable periods of observation without ethanol. These and other control experiments (Mancillas et al, 1986a) suggest that the apparent potentiation of GABA was an artifact of the repetitive iontophoretic application under these experimental conditions, rather than a true pharmacological interaction. In contrast, changes in responses to ACh and SS-14 were only observed after ethanol injections and all recovered within one to two hours.

Siggins and colleagues (1978a,b) have also examined the effects of ethanol superfusion on the responses of CA1 pyramidal cells to GABA as determined by intracellular recordings *in vitro*, to evaluate further whether ethanol potentiated GABAergic transmission and to determine the pre- or post-synaptic locus of action for their finding that ethanol reduces IPSP size (see above). GABA was applied locally by micropipette and uniform responses were obtained by repetitive testing. In all cells, GABA produced hyperpolarizations of 5 to 10 mV, accompanied by cessation of discharge. In four cells studied for the effects of ethanol on this GABA action, superfusion of 22 to 80 mM ethanol had little effect on the responses to GABA. These results, thus, do not support the conclusion that ethanol enhances GABAergic IPSPs. *In vitro* ethanol superfusion increased the size or duration of IPSPs in only 5 of 47 tests and had little effect on the hyperpolarizing, inhibitory responses to GABA applied locally to pyramidal neurons, in accord with our *in vivo* hippocampal studies (see above).

Results at the behavioral level (Ticku et al, 1983) and more recently at the *in vitro* biochemical level (Suzdak et al, 1986) have focused attention to ethanol-potentiating GABAergic synaptic transmission sites. Koob and his collaborators have found that ethanol and the benzodiazepines are synergistic in the anti-conflict test mode, and that both drug effects are antagonized by FG-7142, a carboline *inverse benzodiazepine agonist* (Koob et al, 1986), and by naloxone (Koob et al, 1980). However, ethanol probably does not release punished responses by acting on the benzodiazepine receptor at the benzodiazepine recognition site. Thus, the drug RO 15-1788, characterized as a benzodiazepine antagonist, does not, in fact, antagonize the effects of ethanol, although it completely reverses the effects of chlordiazepoxide (Koob et al, 1986). Nevertheless, as noted above, direct tests of GABA responsiveness (that is, iontophoretic dose response curves before and after ethanol) failed to confirm GABA potentiation in the cerebellum (Bloom et al, 1984) as have more recent tests in the hippocampus (Siggins et al, 1987a; Mancillas et al, 1986a).

Clearly, there is not yet sufficient agreement to conclude whether GABAergic mechanisms per se account for any, many, or all of the intoxicating effects of ethanol. It is possible that the behaviorally arousing effects of GABAergic antagonists overcoming ethanol intoxication could imply a nonspecific summation of more general analeptic actions. It is equally possible that the apparent mimicry of ethanol and GABA effects at both the behavioral and multicellular levels may derive from similar but distinct mechanisms. It is noteworthy that our recent intracellular records of CA1 and CA3 pyramidal neurons in the hippocampal slice showed no GABA-like effects (hyperpolarization) and that the GABAergic IPSPs evoked by pathway stimulation were most often reduced in size rather than potentiated.

FUTURE DIRECTIONS

Thus far, the effects of reasonable intoxicating doses of ethanol on neuronal properties have been examined in modest detail for only four regions of the rodent and primate brain: the cerebellum, the inferior olivary nucleus, the locus ceruleus, and the hippocampus. In all four regions, presentation of ethanol through the blood stream or by continuous superfusion *in vitro* does produce sensitive consistent and dose-dependent effects on some neurons, often at doses below those expected to produce intoxication in humans. Based on these data, the following sequence of cellular events may be critical for intoxication: low doses of ethanol first increase variability in responsiveness of locus ceruleus neurons to critical external sensory events; this leads to inattention and decreased arousal. In squirrel monkeys, lesions of the locus ceruleus result in surface potential recording alterations that are similar to those that have been reported in the children of alcoholics, namely reduced late (300 msec) event-related potentials (see Chapter 14).

Somewhat higher doses of ethanol activate neurons of the inferior olive, possibly indicating the endogenous formation of a serotonin-derived beta-carboline-like effect, that depends on the presence of an intact serotonin innervation of the inferior olive. Also, at modest doses of ethanol, responses of hippocampal pyramidal neurons to acetylcholine and to somatostatin are enhanced, and the effects of synaptic pathway activation are suppressed. With the exception of the enhanced responsiveness to somatostatin and to acetylcholine during ethanol administration in the hippocampus, no other specific transmitter (including other monoamines or GABA) responses have been observed. During longer-term administration of ethanol, healthy rats show no significant alteration in discharge properties, as long as intoxication is maintained, but they do show ethanol-reversible effects, suggestive of locus ceruleus hyperactivity, during withdrawal.

Thus each of the four regions show region specific effects of systemically or topically applied ethanol in doses throughout the range required to produce moderate intoxication in humans.

Proof that an ethanol action may be mediated through a specific chemical form of neurotransmission requires more than testing of exogenous transmitters. A unifying hypothesis of ethanol actions would require that a given system is both necessary and sufficient to explain all relevant actions of ethanol, from the most sensitive and earliest effects on neuronal synaptic transmission at discrete ion channel sites, to synaptic circuitry, through more global macroelectrode and behavioral actions. The ethanol actions should not only be simulated by the appropriate agonist or antagonist of the transmitter hypothesized as critical, but effects on that system must sooner or later be shown to produce similar shifts in the effectiveness of ethanol on membrane processes and behavioral states. For example, Aston-Jones and co-workers (1982) have demonstrated that the synaptic responsiveness of the locus ceruleus (but not its spontaneous activity) certainly ranks among the most sensitive and most rapid actions of ethanol at the whole-animal level. Others have hypothesized that the LC is critical to the changes seen during withdrawal from states of opioid addiction or the naloxone-antagonizable suppression of both benzodiazepine-induced and ethanol-induced increases in punished behavior (Aghajanian, 1978). The latter hypothesis has been directly tested (Koob et al, 1984). Those data indicate that neither naloxone-induced withdrawal symptoms in opiate dependent rats nor naloxone-sensitive anticonflict effects of ethanol or benzodiazepines requires an intact locus ceruleus forebrain projection, making this site an unlikely mediator of these ethanol actions.

At the present time however, the data on cellular actions of ethanol favors at least three cellular system mediators: First, the synchronous increased firing pattern of the inferior olive, perhaps due to formation of a carboline-like, 5-HT-derived condensation product, disrupts the cerebellar cortical operations to account for the incoordination of motor function that occurs with moderate to deep intoxication. Second, the disruption in the synchronous activation of the locus ceruleus by low doses of ethanol, resulting in a failure to synchronize brain attentional mechanisms with the external events that demand proper focused attention, may account for some of the attentional deficits associated with early intoxication. It is possible, although not described here, that the corticotropin releasing factor (CRF) system, known to produce proconflict behavioral effects that are sensitive to ethanol action (Thatcher-Britton et al, 1986) may underlie the disruption of the locus ceruleus neurons during intoxication, as this peptide activates the LC (Valentino and Foote, 1987) but does not facilitate its sensitivity to sensory stimuli. Furthermore, endocrine studies suggest that in rodents at least, acute ethanol intoxication does release CRF (Rivier et al, 1986). Third, the effects of ethanol on hippocampal function, possibly reflective of the effects of the drug through the memory systems, may in part underlie the ability of ethanol to modify emotional activity. A critical aspect for future investigation is the issue of which of these or other ethanol-sensitive systems underlies the tolerance and dependence that develops in both human alcoholics and rats bred for their willingness to drink intoxicating amounts of alcohol (Gatto et al, 1987a, 1987b).

As neuroscientific research proliferates, novel new mechanisms, potentially capable of acting as intermediaries of ethanol perturbations, will naturally continue to appear. One such recent unexpected intermediate is the evidence suggesting that brain-produced steroids may be selectively and rapidly depleted by low doses of ethanol (Corpechot et al, 1983). It is further interesting in this regard that the steroids produced by the rodent brain are quite similar to synthetic steroids shown to be powerful general anesthetics that operate through GABA-like actions (Harrison et al, 1987). While the brain-produced steroids that have been detected thus far do not appear to share in these actions, it is possible that under the influence of intoxicating doses of ethanol, changes in brain oxidation-reduction reactions (Anderssen et al, 1986) suppress brain steroid synthesis and result in the production of abnormal metabolites of these steroids. Such metabolites could, for example, produce some or all of the intoxicating actions of ethanol. Given the present momentum in the field, the likelihood is high that these or far better paths not now visible will provide further unroads into the puzzling cellular neuropharmacology of alcohol.

REFERENCES

Aghajanian G: Tolerance of locus coeruleus neurones to morphine and suppression of withdrawal response by clonidine. Nature 1978; 276:186–188

Anderssen S, Cronholm T, Sjovall J: Redox effects of ethanol on steroid metabolism. Alcoholism: Clinical and Experimental Research 1986; 10:55S–63S

Aston-Jones G, Foote SL, Bloom FE: Low doses of ethanol disrupt sensory responses of brain noradrenergic neurones. Nature 1982; 296:857–860

Bloom F, Barchas J, Sandler M, et al: Beta-carbolines and Tetrahydroisoquinolines. New York, Alan R. Liss, Inc., 1981

Bloom FE, Siggins GR, Foote SL, et al: Noradrenergic involvement in the cellular actions of ethanol, in Catecholamines, Neuropharmacology and the Central Nervous System. Edited by Usdin E. New York, Alan R. Liss, Inc., 1984

Bowen OR: Alcohol and Health. Washington, DC, Government Printing Office, 1987, pp 1–147

Browning MD, Huang CK, Greengard P: Similarities between protein IIIa and protein IIIb, two prominent synaptic vesicle-associated phosphoproteins. J Neurosci 1987; 7:847–53

Corpechot C, Shoemaker WJ, Bloom FE, et al: Endogenous brain steroids: effect of acute ethanol ingestion. Soc Neurosci Abstr 1983; 13:1237

Daly J, Fuxe K, Jonsson G: 5,7-dihydroxytryptamine as a tool for the morphological and functional analysis of central 5-hydroxytryptamine neurons. Res Comm Chem Patholo Pharmacol 1974; 7:175–187

Foote SL, Bloom FE, Aston-Jones G: Nucleus locus ceruleus: New evidence of anatomical and physiological specificity. Physiol Rev 1983; 63:844–914

Gatto GJ, Murphy JM, Waller MB, et al: Chronic ethanol tolerance through free-choice drinking in the P line of alcohol-preferring rats. Pharmacol Biochem Behav 1987a; 28:105–110

Gatto GJ, Murphy JM, Waller MB, et al: Persistence of tolerance to a single dose of ethanol in the selectively-bred alcohol-preferring P rat. Pharmacol Biochem Behav 1987b; 28:111–115

Goldstein DB: Ethanol-induced adaptation in biological membranes. Ann NY Acad Sci 1987; 492:103–111

Gordon AS, Wrubel B, Collier K, et al: Adaptation to ethanol in cultured neural cells and human lymphocytes. Ann NY Acad Sci 1987; 492:367–374

Harris RA, Burnett R, McQuilkin S, et al: Effects of ethanol on membrane order: fluorescence studies. Ann NY Acad Sci 1987; 125–132

Harrison NL, Vicini S, Barker JL: A steroid anesthetic prolongs inhibitory post-synaptic currents in cultured rat hippocampal neurons. J Neurosci 1987; 7:604–609

Hemmings HC Jr, Nairn AC, Greengard P: Protein kinases and phosphoproteins in the nervous system. Res Publ Assoc Res Nerv Ment Dis 1986; 64:47–69

Hoffman PL, Saito T, Tabakoff B: Selective effects of ethanol on neurotransmitter receptor-effector coupling systems in different brain areas. Ann NY Acad Sci 1987; 492:396–397

Hudspith MJ, Brennan CH, Charles S, et al: Dihydropyridine-sensitive Ca^{2+} channels and inositol phospholipid metabolism in ethanol physical dependence. Ann NY Acad Sci 1987; 492:156–170

Koob GF, Strecker RE, Bloom FE: Effects of naloxone on the anticonflict properties of alcohol and chlordiazepoxide. Substance and Alcohol Actions/Misuse 1980; 1:447–457

Koob GF, Thatcher-Britton K, Britton DR, et al: Destruction of the locus coeruleus or the dorsal NE bundle does not alter the release of punished responding by ethanol and chlordiazepoxide. Physiol Behav 1984; 33:479–485

Koob GF, Braestrup C, Thatcher-Britton K: The effects of FG 7142 and RO 15-1788 on the release of punished responding produced by chlordiazepoxide and ethanol in the rat. Psychopharmacology 1986; 90:173–178

Mancillas J, Siggins GR, Bloom FE: Systemic ethanol: selective enhancement of responses to acetylcholine and somatostatin in the rat hippocampus. Science 1986a; 231:161–163

Mancillas J, Siggins GR, Bloom FE: Somatostatin selectively enhances acetylcholine-induced excitations in rat hippocampus and cortex. Proc Natl Acad Sci USA 1986b; 83:7518–7521

Miller KW, Firestone LL, Forman SA: General anesthetic and specific effects of ethanol on acetylcholine receptors. Ann NY Acad Sci 1987; 492:71–85

Murphy JM, Waller MB, Gatto WJ, et al: Monoamine uptake inhibitors attenuate ethanol intake in alcohol-preferring (P) rats. Alcohol 1985; 2:349–352

Murphy JM, McBride WJ, Lumeng L, et al: Contents of monoamines in forebrain regions of alcohol-preferring (P) and -nonpreferring (NP) lines of rats. Pharmacol Biochem Behav 1987; 26:389–392

Nestoros JN: Ethanol specifically potentiates GABA-mediated neurotransmission in feline cerebral cortex. Science 1980; 209:708–710

Newlin SA, Mancillas-Trevino J, Bloom FE: Ethanol causes increase in excitation and inhibition in area CA3 of the dorsal hippocampus. Brain Res 1981; 209:113–128

Perdahl E, Wu WC, Browning MD, et al: Protein III, a neuron-specific phosphoprotein: variant forms found in human brain. Neurobehav Toxicol Teratol 1984; 6:425–431

Pineda J, Foote SL, Neville H: Effects of noradrenergic locus coeruleus lesions on squirrel monkey event-related potentials. Electroenceph Clin Neurophysiol 1987; 67:77–90

Rabin RA, Molinoff PB: Multiple sites of action of ethanol on adenylate cyclase. J Pharmacol and Experimental Therapeutics 1983; 227:551

Rivier C, Rivier J, Vale W: Stress-induced inhibition of reproductive functions: role of endogenous corticotropin-releasing factor. Science 1986; 231:607–609

Robbins TW, Everitt BJ, Cole BJ: Functional hypotheses of the coeruleocortical noradrenergic projection: A review of recent experimentation and theory. Physiol Psychol 1985; 13:127–150

Rogers J, Siggins JR, Schulman JR, et al: Physiological correlates of ethanol intoxication, tolerance, and dependence in rat cerebellar Purkinje cells. Brain Res 1980; 196:183–198

Rogers J, Madamba SG, Staunton DA, et al: Ethanol increases single unit activity in the inferior olivary nucleus. Brain Res 1986; 385:253–262

Siggins GR, French E: Central neurons are depressed by iontophoretic and micro-pressure applications of ethanol and tetrahydropapaveroline. Drug Alcohol Depend 1979; 4:239–243

Siggins GR, Gruol, DL: Synaptic mechanisms in the vertebrate central nervous system, in Handbook of Physiology, Volume on Intrinsic Regulatory Systems of the Brain. Edited by Bloom FE. Maryland, The American Physiological Society, pp 1–114, 1986

Siggins GR, Bloom FE, French ED, et al: Electrophysiology of ethanol on central neurons. Ann NY Acad Sci 1987a; 492:350–366

Siggins GR, Pittman QJ, French ED: Effects of ethanol on CA1 and CA3 pyramidal cells in the hippocampal slice preparation: an intracellular study. Brain Res 1987b; 414:22–34

Sinclair JG, Lo GF: The effects of ethanol on cerebellar Purkinje cell discharge pattern and inhibition evoked by local surface stimulation. Brain Res 1981; 204:465–471

Sinclair JG, Lo GF, Tiem AF: The effects of ethanol on cerebellar Purkinje cells in naive and alcohol-dependent rats. Can J Physiol Pharmacol 1980; 58:429–432

Smith BR, Amit Z: False neurotransmitters and the effects of ethanol on the brain. Ann NY Acad Sci 1987; 492:384–389

Steinbusch HWM: Serotonin-immunoreactive neurons and their projections in the CNS, in Handbook of Chemical Neuroanatomy, volume three: Classical Transmitters and Transmitter Receptors in the CNS, Part II. Edited by Bjorklund A, Hokfelt T, Kuhar MJ. Amsterdam, Elsevier Science Publishers, 1984, pp 68–125

Straus F, Li TK (eds): Causes and Consequences of Alcohol Problems: an Agenda for Research. Report of a Study by a Committee of the Institute of Medicine. Washington, DC, National Academy Press, 1987, pp 1–218

Suzdak PD, Glowa JR, Crawley JN, et al: A benzodiazepine that antagonizes alcohol actions selectively. Science 1986; 234:1243–1247

Taraschi TF, Ellingson JS, Rubin E: Membrane structural alterations caused by chronic ethanol consumption: the molecular basis of membrane tolerance. Ann NY Acad Sci 1987; 492:171–180

Thatcher-Britton K, Koob GF: Alcohol reverses the proconflict effect of corticotropin-releasing factor. Regulatory Peptides 1986; 16:315–320

Thatcher-Britton KT, Ehlers CL, Koob GF: Is ethanol antagonist RO 15-4513 selective for ethanol? Science 1988; 239:648–649

Thatcher-Britton K, Ehlers CL, Koob GF: Ethanol antagonist RO 15-4513 is not selective for ethanol. Science (in press)

Ticku MK, Burch T: Alterations in GABA receptor sensitivity following acute and chronic ethanol treatments. J Neurochem 1980; 34:417–423

Ticku MK, Burch TP, Davis WC: The interactions of ethanol with the benzodiazepine GABA receptor ionophore complex. Pharmacol Biochem Behav 1983; 18:Suppl 15–18

Valentino RJ, Foote SL: Corticotropin-releasing factor disrupts sensory responses of brain noradrenergic neurons. Neuroendocrinology 1987; 45:28–36

Volicer L, Gold BI: Effect of ethanol on cyclic AMP levels in rat brain. Life Sci 1973; 13:269–280

Weiner N, Disbrow JK, French TA, et al: The influence of catecholamine systems and thyroid function on the actions of ethanol in long sleep (LS) and short sleep (SS) mice. Ann NY Acad Sci 1987; 375–384

Chapter 16

The *DSM-III-R* Diagnosis of Alcoholism

by *Bruce J. Rounsaville, M.D., and Henry R. Kranzler, M.D.*

Diagnosis is a crucial first step in the treatment of alcoholism. Its fundamental purpose is to distinguish clinically significant patterns and consequences of alcohol use from those that are clinically insignificant. Beyond this, diagnosis should impart information that reflects current knowledge about underlying processes of alcoholism and that can guide treatment decisions.

The most recent version of the *Diagnostic Statistical Manual of Mental Disorders, Third Edition, Revised* (*DSM-III-R*) of the American Psychiatric Association (APA) (American Psychiatric Association, 1987) includes a number of changes in criteria for the diagnosis of alcohol abuse and dependence that reflect the evolution in knowledge of the clinically relevant features of compulsive alcohol use. In addition, *DSM-III-R* shares with previous editions a set of guidelines encouraging assignment of multiple diagnoses when patients meet criteria for more than one disorder. The purpose of this chapter is to 1) describe the *DSM-III-R* changes in alcohol use disorders along with the rationale and guidelines for use of the new criteria, and 2) suggest guidelines for the diagnosis of coexistent psychiatric disorders in alcoholics.

CHANGES IN *DSM-III-R* ALCOHOL USE DISORDERS

Features of DSM-III *Alcohol Abuse and Dependence*

To help the reader understand the changes described below, we will briefly describe the *Diagnostic and Statistical Manual of Mental Disorders, Third Edition* (*DSM-III*) (American Psychiatric Association, 1980) alcohol use disorders. In *DSM-III*, substance use disorders were conceived of as conceptually independent of one another, with comparatively little effort made to identify the nomothetic principles that underlie them. Alcohol use disorders were divided into two major types: *abuse and dependence*. Alcohol abuse was defined by a pattern of pathological use for at least one month that causes impairment in social or occupational functioning. Indications of a pathological pattern of use include perceived need for daily use, inability to cut down or stop drinking, repeated efforts to control or reduce excess drinking, binges, occasional consumption of a fifth of spirits or more, blackouts, continuation of drinking despite a serious physical disorder that the individual knows is exacerbated by alcohol use, or drinking of nonbeverage alcohol. Alcohol dependence was defined by a combination of a patho-

This study was supported by Public Health Service grant 5P50–AA03510 from the National Institute of Alcohol Abuse and Alcoholism, and by Research Scientist Award K05DA00089 (to BJR) and grants P50DA04060 and R01 DA04753 from the National Institute on Drug Abuse.

logical pattern of use or social or occupational impairment *and* tolerance or withdrawal. The pattern of use or course of alcohol abuse or dependence was coded in the fifth digit as continuous, episodic, or in remission.

Revisions in DSM-III-R

In contrast to the idiographic approach to substance use disorders in *DSM-III*, the revised edition reflects a growing recognition that dependence is a biobehavioral construct that can be used to characterize compulsive use of a variety of substances. The principal change in *DSM-III-R* alcohol use disorders was to broaden the meaning of alcohol dependence to not only include tolerance and withdrawal but also denote a range of behavioral indices of diminished control over alcohol use (Rounsaville et al, 1986). Alcohol dependence can now be diagnosed if an individual meets three of the nine criteria listed in Table 1, even if tolerance or withdrawal have never been present. While the diagnosis of alcohol abuse is still available and is defined by hazardous use of alcohol or alcoholic-related impairment, it is intended to be a residual category. It is to be used in comparatively rare instances in which alcohol-related impairment is present without two additional dependence symptoms.

For alcohol dependence, severity can be designated as *mild, moderate,* or *severe.* Current course can be designated as being *in partial remission* if there has been some alcohol use in the past six months without meeting three dependence criteria and *in full remission* if there has either been no alcohol use in the past six months or no dependence criteria have been met.

Rationale and Implications of DSM-III-R *Changes*

The revisions included in the *DSM-III-R* criteria are not anticipated to change markedly the overall rates of alcohol use disorders. The results of field trials suggest that the practical effect of the revisions will be to redesignate as *dependent* all individuals who meet *DSM-III* criteria for either dependence or abuse (Rounsaville et al, 1987b). However, the new criteria have a number of implications reflecting evolving concepts of alcoholism: 1) use of criteria that are consistent with the alcohol dependence syndrome, first proposed in 1976 by Edwards and Gross (1976); 2) removal of primary emphasis on the physical aspects of dependence, exemplified by tolerance and withdrawal; 3) shifting of the criteria away from emphasis on social consequences of alcohol use; 4) greater emphasis on the idea that alcohol dependence may be seen at different levels of severity; and 5) recognition that reduction of drinking associated with avoidance of recurrent dependence symptoms may justify a current designation that the disorder is in partial or full remission. Each implication will be discussed below.

Relationship of DSM-III-R *to the Alcohol Dependence Syndrome*

A factor guiding the choice of *DSM-III-R* alcohol dependence criteria was the body of theoretical and empirical work on the alcohol dependence syndrome (Edwards, 1986; Edwards et al, 1981). According to this formulation, alcohol syndromes develop in accordance with behavioral principles via a system of reinforcement that initiates and perpetuates substance taking and dependence. The positive and negative reinforcement contingencies involved in heavy alcohol use lead to the development of a core set of symptoms designated as the *depen-*

dence syndrome; it is seen as multidimensional with *biologic, social, and behavioral components*. The cardinal feature of this syndrome is impaired control over alcohol use. The syndrome elements, most of which are incorporated in *DSM-III-R* criteria, are as follows: 1) narrowing of the substance use repertoire such that substance use becomes stereotyped around a regular schedule of almost continuous or daily consumption; 2) salience of substance-taking behavior such that,

Table 1. *DSM-III-R* Diagnostic Criteria for Psychoactive Substance Dependence and Abuse

I. Dependence

A. At least three of the following:
  1. Substance often taken in larger amounts or over a longer period than the person intended
  2. Persistent desire or one or more unsuccessful efforts to cut down or control substance use
  3. A great deal of time spent in activities necessary to get the substance, take the substance, or recover from its effects
  4. Frequent intoxication or withdrawal symptoms when expected to fulfill major role obligations at work, school, or home, or when substance use is physically hazardous
  5. Important social, occupational, or recreational activities given up or reduced because of substance use
  6. Continued substance use despite knowledge of having a persistent or recurrent social, psychological, or physical problem that is caused or exacerbated by the use of the substance
  7. Marked tolerance: need for markedly increased amounts of the substance (at least a 50 percent increase) to achieve intoxication or desired effect, or markedly diminished effect with continued use of the same amount
  8. Characteristic withdrawal symptoms
  9. Substance often taken to relieve or avoid withdrawal symptoms

B. Some symptoms of the disturbance have persisted for at least one month or have occurred repeatedly over a longer period of time

II. Abuse

A. A maladaptive pattern of psychoactive substance use indicated by at least one of the following:
  1. Continued use despite knowledge of persistent or recurrent social, occupational, psychological, or physical problems that are caused or exacerbated by use of the psychoactive substance
  2. Recurrent use in situations when use is physically hazardous

B. Some symptoms of the disturbance have persisted for at least one month or have occurred repeatedly over a longer period of time

C. Never met the criteria for psychoactive substance dependence for this substance

despite negative consequences, substance use is given higher priority than are other activities that previously had been important; 3) increased tolerance; 4) withdrawal symptoms; 5) substance use to avoid withdrawal; 6) subjectively experienced compulsion to use the substance; and 7) readdiction liability.

Regarding the alcohol dependence syndrome, Edwards (1986, p. 1058) asserts the following essential postulates:

1. The syndrome may be recognized by the clustering of certain elements. Not all elements need always be present or present in the same degree, but with mounting intensity the syndrome is likely to show increasing coherence.
2. The syndrome is not all-or-none, but occurs with graded intensity.
3. Its presentation will be shaped by the pathoplastic influence of personality and culture.
4. A bi-axial concept is introduced, with the dependence syndrome constituting one axis and alcohol-related problems the other.

Two of these postulates, syndrome coherence and the biaxial concept suggesting an orthogonal relationship between syndrome elements and alcohol-related problems, are empirically testable. In fact, a major strength of the alcohol dependence construct is the large amount of empirical research that it has inspired, most of which has supported its propositions.

A number of instruments have been devised to assess alcohol dependence syndrome elements (Hodgson et al, 1978; Skinner, 1981; Chick, 1980; Stockwell et al, 1979; Hesselbrock et al, 1983), a development that has facilitated work in this area. Regarding syndrome coherence, all available research suggests that the syndrome elements are highly intercorrelated. Regarding the biaxial concept, evidence is more mixed and dependent on the type of population studied (Edwards, 1986). However, from a clinical standpoint, the most important findings are those related to the prognostic implications of severity of alcohol dependence. Research in both experimental and clinical settings suggests that the severity of alcohol dependence predicts attendance at a treatment clinic (Skinner and Allen, 1982), craving for alcohol after a "priming" drink (Hodgson et al, 1979; Kaplan et al, 1983), relapse to uncontrolled drinking following an initial "slip" (Hesselbrock et al, 1983; Polich and Armour, 1981; Hodgson, 1980; Orford et al, 1976; Foy et al, 1984), and poorer post treatment outcome along a range of dimensions (Rounsaville et al, 1987a). Moreover, severity of dependence shows promise as a dimension on which to match patients to treatments, with relatively low severity patients requiring only ambulatory, nonintensive interventions and high severity patients receiving inpatient or intensive outpatient treatment (Hodgson, 1980). The goals of treatment may also be based on the severity of dependence, such that controlled drinking may be an option for low severity alcoholics while abstinence is the optimal goal for more dependent alcoholics (Hodgson, 1980; Orford et al, 1976; Foy et al, 1984). While further research is called for, and two studies have failed to support the predictive validity of dependence (Heather et al, 1983; Litman et al, 1984), it appears that the dependence syndrome construct has considerable promise for diagnosis, early detection, and treatment planning.

Deemphasis of Tolerance and Withdrawal

In the *DSM-III* system, tolerance and withdrawal were the cardinal elements of alcohol dependence, and one of these two symptoms was required to make the diagnosis. While these symptoms have been retained in the *DSM-III-R* dependence criteria, they are no longer of pivotal importance, as it is possible to have three of the nine broadened dependence symptoms and meet criteria for dependence without having either tolerance or withdrawal. The deemphasis of these physiological indices of dependence is in keeping with clinical knowledge about the salient features of alcoholism. The behavioral dependence elements that emphasize diminished control over drinking appear to be more at the center of this syndrome, the principle clinical feature of which is its chronic, relapsing nature. If the syndrome of dependence were confined to tolerance or withdrawal symptoms, then brief detoxification programs would suffice as treatment. Instead, effective treatments of substance use disorders must extend far beyond the point at which the individual remains vulnerable to withdrawal symptoms and must emphasize preventing relapse over an extended time period (Marlatt and Gordon, 1985).

In addition to the above, there are several practical and conceptual difficulties in placing tolerance in a key position for the diagnosis of dependence. While an essential criterion for dependence in *DSM-III* is a marked change in the amount of substance necessary to achieve the desired effect, there are large individual differences in the amount of substance necessary to cause intoxication. These individual variations make it difficult to translate a history of amounts of alcohol consumed into a decision regarding the presence or absence of tolerance.

Tolerance is a complex phenomenon and may develop through diverse mechanisms. For example, *pharmacodynamic tolerance* is present when, after exposure to a drug, higher levels of the drug are required at its site of action to produce a given response. *Metabolic tolerance* is the increased capacity to metabolize a drug: it can be induced by the substance itself or by some other agent (Edwards et al, 1981). Related to the diversity of underlying mechanisms, tolerance may develop to some aspects of a drug's effects and not to others, as in the case of barbiturates, in which continued use may lead to a decreased euphoriant effect but an unchanged respiratory depressant effect (Jaffe, 1980). The fact that different patterns and amounts of tolerance can develop across different categories of drugs (for example, marked tolerance to opiates, minimal tolerance to alcohol) limits the utility of this criterion for many drug categories. These complexities of tolerance limit both the degree to which it can be rated reliably and its theoretical meaningfulness for different categories of substances.

The criterion of tolerance may not be stringent enough to exclude individuals whose substance use is not excessive. Although some *marked* changes in *desired effects* of alcohol are required by *DSM-III*, these changes may be manifested by the subject's using much more of the substance or using the same amount but getting less of an effect from it. Getting much less of an effect may be more related to factors such as loss of novelty or the learning of social rituals for drinking than to physiological adaptation to the substance. As noted by Segal (1981) for many individuals with chronic alcoholism and abuse of other substances, reverse tolerance is displayed, with less drug required to achieve the desired effect.

A primary problem with placing heavy emphasis on withdrawal symptoms as evidence for alcohol dependence is the often nonspecific nature of symptoms associated with abstinence from most classes of psychoactive substances. For example, diagnostic symptoms of alcohol withdrawal include nausea, malaise, and irritability, a syndrome that can be equivalent to a "hangover," following even a single episode of heavy use. Other criteria, such as coarse tremor or seizures, may be more specific to the withdrawal syndrome but are inadequately sensitive. A second difficulty with placing heavy diagnostic emphasis on withdrawal symptoms is that many individuals use large amounts of a substance with either a sufficient supply or an adequately long substance half-life to prevent their ever experiencing or recognizing withdrawal symptoms; this pattern is noted in French alcoholics, who may be mildly but continuously intoxicated every day (Babor et al, 1985).

The Shift Away from Social Consequences as Criteria

While social and occupational impairment caused by alcohol use were essential criteria for the *DSM-III* diagnosis of either alcohol abuse or alcohol dependence, they are no longer required criteria for either diagnosis in *DSM-III-R*. Elements of this alcohol-related impairment are implicated in both the dependence and abuse criteria, but the emphasis is now on the drug-using behaviors linked with the impairment—continuing to use alcohol despite negative consequences—rather than with the impairment itself. This change was partly based on the theoretical concepts and empirical findings concerning the alcohol dependence syndrome that suggest the comparative independence of the syndrome from consequences (Edwards, 1986). However, it was also based on a number of additional conceptual and practical difficulties in making the consequences of a disorder part of the criteria for its initial diagnosis.

A crucial difficulty with the requirement that social or occupational impairment be shown to make the diagnosis of substance use disorders is the wide variability in acceptable uses of psychoactive substances. The *DSM-III* system was vulnerable to powerful, swiftly changing social forces such as the tightening of laws restricting alcohol use while driving. Thus, for example, actions of a legislature in a particular state can determine the number of residents who meet *DSM-III* criteria for a mental disorder such as alcohol abuse.

Evaluating the social consequences of substance use can be difficult in practice because of an often unclear temporal relationship between the onset of heavy substance use and the onset of social impairment. Requiring social impairment may miss many individuals in whom pathological compulsive substance use is present but in whom social impairment has not yet been detected. An example would be an alcohol abusing housewife who has so far been able to hide her dependence.

Determining the diagnosis of a substance use disorder on the basis of its social consequences may place insufficient emphasis on defining and detecting the essential process of the disorder. As noted earlier, the process of substance abuse may be well under way before consequences emerge, just as the process of essential hypertension may have a long course before symptoms are evident. Although social consequences are frequently a motivation to seek treatment, the use of social consequences as a diagnostic criterion unnecessarily blurs the distinction between the disorder itself and its consequences.

Explicit Recognition of Syndrome Severity

Although the *DSM-III-R* system is categorical, with diagnoses given as either present or absent, the criteria for alcohol dependence presented may be conceptualized as arrayed along an underlying continuum of increasing severity, in a manner analogous to hypertension or fever in general medicine. A concept of severity of alcoholism is at variance with a unitary disease model of this disorder, which suggests that it is a lifelong disease that one either has or doesn't have and that it has an inevitably progressive course. One argument that can be made in support of a unitary concept of alcoholism is that mild cases are simply those that have not had a long enough time to progress. However, data regarding antisocial and nonantisocial subgroups of alcoholics suggest that some of the more severe alcoholics are those whose disorder has an early age of onset and a very rapid progression, while less severely dependent alcoholics are frequently those whose disorder has developed more slowly over a number of years (Cloninger, 1987; Hesselbrock et al, 1985). As noted above, recognition of severity of alcoholism may have treatment and prognostic implications, as less severely dependent alcoholics may require less intensive treatment interventions and may be able to formulate treatment goals of controlled drinking (Hodgson, 1980; Orford et al, 1976; Foy et al, 1984). More empirical work in this area is clearly needed.

Designating Dependence as in Remission

Because *DSM-III-R* is meant to allow diagnosis of all psychiatric disorders that an individual may have had during his or her lifetime, it is important to include the designation that a disorder is not currently symptomatic. This is preferable to simply omitting diagnoses that are not current. For alcoholism, including the diagnosis of alcoholism even when the individual is currently abstinent or not symptomatic, this is important because of the chronic, recurrent nature of the disorder. The designation *in remission* is not equivalent to being *cured* or *absent*, as a similar designation may apply to serious, life-threatening, recurrent diseases in other branches of medicine. Still, it is important to be able to designate an individual as currently asymptomatic, as many individuals with alcohol abuse or dependence appear able to maintain abstinence indefinitely or to avoid problem drinking with or without treatment. Evidence for this can be found in epidemiological surveys that indicate that alcohol use disorders and alcohol-related problems are most commonly seen in young adults (Robins et al, 1984; Meyers et al, 1984) and rates drop off sharply in older adults. This age-related variability in rates is not simply cross-sectional, as it has been observed in many different surveys conducted at different times. It appears that many young adults with alcohol use disorders are able to change their drinking behavior as they age and thereby no longer meet criteria for these diagnoses. For these individuals, it is inappropriate to give a current diagnosis.

DIAGNOSING COEXISTENT PSYCHIATRIC DISORDERS IN ALCOHOLICS

DSM-III-R, like *DSM-III*, encourages the use of multiple diagnoses when an individual meets criteria for more than one disorder. This is true of dependence or abuse of multiple substances, except when there is a time period in which no single substance predominates or the individual does not clearly know the range of substances being taken. It is also true of psychiatric disorders other than substance use disorders. Hence, if an individual meets diagnostic criteria for an alcohol use disorder, a mood disorder, and a personality disorder, all should be listed. Moreover, there are no diagnostic heirarchies in *DSM-III-R* regarding alcoholism, so that any other category of diagnosis can be made in alcoholic patients. Finally, while some authors have recommended making a primary/secondary distinction based on the temporal sequence in which an individual met criteria for alcoholism and another disorder (Schuckit, 1985; Schuckit, 1986), this has not been included in the formal diagnostic system and no code numbers are available for making this distinction. In this section, we will briefly review both the rationale and the methods for making dual diagnoses in alcoholics.

Rationale for Diagnosing Psychiatric Disorders in Alcoholics

While the major problem that alcoholics present with is excessive drinking, it is seldom the only problem. Impairment is frequently seen in multiple domains, including problems in social, medical, psychological, legal, and occupational areas (McLellan et al, 1980; McLellan et al, 1981). While it has been long known that alcoholics seeking treatment commonly present with symptoms of anxiety, depression, and irritability, the recent development of specified diagnostic criteria and structured diagnostic interviews has facilitated recognition of potentially treatable disorders in this group. As reviewed below, recently gathered evidence suggests that psychiatric disorders are common in alcoholics and that they confer a poorer prognosis in treatment and are likely to have implications for the choice of treatment.

RATES OF DISORDERS AND PROGNOSTIC SIGNIFICANCE. A number of studies have now been completed that document rates of psychiatric disorders diagnosed according to *DSM-III* criteria in alcoholics seeking treatment (Hesselbrock et al, 1985; Powell et al, 1982; Schuckit, 1985; Ross et al, in press). These studies are consistent in that the diagnoses must commonly seen are major depression, anxiety disorders, antisocial personality, and drug abuse/dependence. They are also in agreement that alcoholics seeking treatment appear not to have excessive rates of mania or schizophrenic disorders, in comparison to nonalcoholic community samples. We will briefly review findings regarding prevalence rates and the prognostic significance of the more frequently diagnosed disorders.

Major depression has been reported in lifetime rates ranging from 18–25 percent (Powell et al, 1982; Hesselbrock et al, 1985; Weissman et al, 1980; Schuckit, 1985) of alcoholics and in current rates of 9–38 percent (Ross et al, in press; Dorus et al, 1987; Keeler et al, 1979). These rates are many times those of rates reported for community samples in the Epidemiology Catchment Area (ECA) Study (4–7 percent for lifetime and 2–4 percent for current diagnoses) (Robins et al, 1984; Myers et al, 1984). The prognostic significance of depression in treated alcoholics has been less frequently studied. Few differences between depressed and nondepressed alcoholics at one-year posttreatment follow-up were reported by two studies (Schuckit, 1985; Penick et al, 1984), but the number of depressives was very small. In a third study, male depressives had a poorer treatment outcome compared to males with no other psychiatric disorder, but female depressives had a better outcome (Rounsaville et al, 1987a).

Anxiety disorders, especially panic disorder and phobic disorders, have been found to be highly prevalent in alcoholics. Panic disorder has been estimated at 8–16 percent lifetime and is currently at less than 1–9 percent (Hesselbrock et al, 1985; Powell et al, 1982; Ross et al, in press; Bowen et al, 1984). Phobias have been reported at 3–55 percent lifetime and 15–29 percent current (Schuckit, 1985; Hesselbrock et al, 1985; Powell et al, 1982; Ross et al, in press; Mullaney and Trippet, 1979; Bowen et al, 1984; Smail et al, 1984). Low prevalence rates tend to be from single reports, while the preponderance of results suggest higher prevalence rates. These rates are also many times those of community rates from the ECA study, which are 1–2 percent lifetime for panic disorder and 8–23 percent lifetime for phobias (Robins et al, 1984). No data on the prognostic significance of anxiety disorders in alcoholics are available, although one unpublished analysis showed no difference in the course of anxiety disordered patients and those without additional diagnoses (Rounsaville et al, unpublished).

Antisocial personality rates have been reported as ranging from 20–79 percent of treated alcoholics (Hesselbrock et al, 1985; Powell et al, 1982; Schuckit, 1985; Ross et al, in press; Grande et al, 1984). Two follow-up studies have shown antisocial alcoholics to have a poorer treatment prognosis than primary alcoholics or those without psychiatric comorbidity (Schuckit, 1985; Rounsaville et al, 1987a). Community rates of antisocial personality are around one percent (Robins et al, 1984). Schubert and associates (in press) showed a significant association between alcoholism and antisocial personality in seven of the eight studies that they reviewed.

Drug abuse/dependence has been reported in 12–25 percent of alcoholics (Hesselbrock et al, 1985; Schuckit, 1985; Powell et al, 1982; Ross et al, in press) and has been shown in two studies to be associated with poorer one-year treatment outcome (Schuckit, 1985; Rounsaville et al, 1987a). These prevalence rates are compared to rates in the community of around 6 percent (Robins et al, 1984).

To highlight the prognostic significance of coexistent psychopathology in alcoholics, several studies have shown that a global rating of overall severity of psychiatric symptoms is among the most powerful predictors of treatment outcome in substance abusers (Woody et al, 1984; McLellan et al, 1983). Given the limitations in long-term diagnostic reliability for psychiatric disorders in substance abusers, it can be argued that simply rating global severity of psychiatric problems may be preferable to the more time-consuming procedure of determining whether an individual meets criteria for particular diagnostic groups. However, one study has shown that specific diagnostic categories, particularly depression, has prognostic significance that remains even after controlling for a global rating of psychopathology (Rounsaville et al, 1987a). Furthermore, categorical diagnoses have the advantage of suggesting specific treatments (for example, lithium for bipolar illness, specific psychotherapies and medications for depression) while ratings of global psychopathology do not point the clinician to a specific psychotherapeutic or pharmacologic strategy.

Treatment Implications for Patients with Dual Diagnoses

If dual diagnoses in alcoholics are common and confer a poorer prognosis, what are the treatment implications? To begin with, many disorders, notably depression and panic and phobic disorders, have been shown to respond well to psychotherapeutic and pharmacologic treatments in nonalcohol abusing populations. Attention to coexistent psychiatric disorders may improve treatment efficacy through three mechanisms. First, reducing painful psychological symptoms, like depression and panic anxiety, may be useful in relieving suffering, even if it has no impact on alcoholics' patterns of problem drinking. Second, treating coexistent depression or anxiety disorders may also have an impact on drinking behaviors. Marlatt and Gordon (1985) have shown that the most commonly endorsed category of relapse precipitants is dysphoric moods, and two other studies have shown that coexistent psychopathology confers a poorer prognosis regarding drinking outcomes in alcoholics (Schuckit, 1985; Rounsaville et al, 1987a). Third, even if no particular treatment has been shown to be successful in treating an alcoholic's coexistent psychiatric disorder (for example, antisocial personality), making the diagnosis may have important implications for matching patients to programs. For example, it is likely that antisocial alcoholics may respond better to group settings, because they have a more externally based locus of control, and to treatments which emphasize structure and limit setting. Preliminary results from a study of group alcoholism aftercare treatment (Ronald Kadden, Ph.D., personal communication, January 1988) have suggested that a more structured, skills-training format was more efficacious with antisocial alcoholics than a more open-ended, exploratory approach.

While the mechanisms described above suggest a plausible rationale for detecting and treating psychopathology in alcoholics, the empirical research on targeted treatments is sparse. Regarding psychotherapeutic approaches, there have been no clinical trials aimed at specific psychotherapies for dually diagnosed alcoholics. Studies of opioid addicts suggest that those with major depression are particularly likely to respond to professional psychotherapy even if the patient also met criteria for antisocial personality. Regarding pharmacological approaches, the most commonly studied treatment has been with tricyclic antidepressants (TCAs) for depressed alcoholics. Ciraulo and Jaffe (1981) reviewed nine placebo-controlled studies of this approach and found that none showed tricyclics to be superior to placebo in drinking outcomes. Some studies did show decreased depression and anxiety in medicated patients, but these differences tended to disappear after the first several weeks of treatment. All of the studies were considered to have major methodological shortcomings, the most important of which was inadequate dosages of the tricyclic medications, a problem that is underscored by evidence that TCA-treated alcoholics have consistently lower plasma levels of drug than nonalcoholics. These authors concluded that new studies with improved designs are needed. However, none have appeared in the literature since this review was published in 1981. A new class of antidepressants, the serotonin-uptake inhibitors, represented in the United States by fluoxetine, has shown promise with depressed alcoholics, as it reduced depression in nonalcoholics and, in laboratory and clinical settings, this class of drugs also reduced drinking behavior (Naranjo et al, 1986; Naranjo et al, 1984; Amit et al, 1985; Naranjo et al, in press). However, no studies of serotonin-uptake inhibitors with depressed alcoholics have been conducted to date.

Treatment of depression with monoamine oxidase inhibitors may be complicated by serious side effects in this population, and alcoholics' ability to comply with dietary and pharmacological prohibitions may be limited (Schottenfeld et al, in preparation). As reviewed by Kranzler and Liebowitz (in press), other pharmacotherapies have been evaluated in only a few studies, most of them not double-blind or placebo-controlled. Lithium has been evaluated with mixed results regarding mood and alcohol use. Treatment of phobic and panic patients with TCAs has been supported by open trials (Quitkin et al, 1972). Other pharmacological treatments of anxiety symptoms are complicated by the addictive potential of most minor tranquilizers, especially the benzodiazepines. Meyer (1986) has suggested that anxious alcoholics may be treated with buspirone, a new, nonbenzodiazepine anxiolytic with limited euphorigenic and withdrawal effects. A recent open trial by Kranzler (1987) also provides pilot data suggesting that buspirone reduces craving and anxiety in anxious alcoholics.

To conclude this section, the categories of coexistent psychiatric disorders seen in alcoholics are clinically significant and likely to be treatable with psychotherapeutic approaches and a number of standard and new pharmacologic agents. However, strong empirical evidence supporting the efficacy for particular treatments of dually diagnosed alcoholics is not available at this time. Given the high rates of dual diagnosis in alcoholics described above, this is an area that requires more attention. For the clinician, it is advisable to make treatment decisions on a case-by-case basis, weighing the severity and duration of psychiatric symptoms along with likelihood of patient compliance and presence of medical contraindications for pharmacologic agents.

How Should Assessments of Dual Diagnosis Be Made?

In devising an assessment system, the clinician can choose from a variety of techniques: self-reports versus clinician interviews, structured interviews versus unstructured interviews, paraprofessional interviewers versus professional interviewers, and screening versus diagnostic evaluations.

SELF-REPORTS. When patients are literate, use of self-reported assessments saves considerable staff time and can frequently be accomplished during the time the patient is waiting for an appointment. Although self-report instructions can yield inadequate information because patients misunderstand the forms or omit items, these drawbacks can be avoided if the clinical evaluator reviews the answers with the patient after the forms have been completed. Self-report forms are most acceptable if they are brief and simple. These properties are most common in measures that are conceived as screening tests, such as the Beck Depression Inventory, which is a useful screen for depression (Beck and Beck, 1979), or the Drug Abuse Screening Test, which can detect unsuspected drug abuse in an alcoholic patient group (Skinner, 1982).

STRUCTURED VERSUS UNSTRUCTURED INTERVIEWS. While structured interviews have the disadvantage of allowing less time for spontaneous exploration of a patient's problems, this is far outweighed by the advantages of increased reliability, avoidance of significant omissions, and efficiency. Several structured, reliable methods for making psychiatric diagnoses in alcoholics are now available (Robins et al, 1981a; Robins et al, 1981b; Spitzer and Endicott, 1979; Endicott and Spitzer, 1978; Spitzer and Williams, 1985; Othmer et al, 1981; Mathisen et al, in press). These include clinician interviews, lay interviews, and even computer-administered questionnaires. Although a full diagnostic interview may be lengthy (30 to 90 minutes), the assessment of selected disorders that alcoholics are likely to have can be done using portions of existing interview guides.

SCREENING AND DIAGNOSTIC INTERVIEWS. Because professional time is usually a scarce resource in most substance abuse treatment programs, it is desirable to develop an assessment system that can be conducted largely by staff with varying degrees of formal training. This is facilitated by the use of structured-interview scales that ensure uniformity in the areas assessed and the ways that questions are phrased. When counseling staff are trained to use structured assessments, the results can be superior to those yielded by professionals using unstructured interviews (Rounsaville et al, 1980). The use of a paraprofessional assessment staff is particularly justified when evaluations are a two-stage process, with the first stage consisting of screening and the second composed of more definitive diagnosis.

The screening phase is meant to provide a highly sensitive, if less specific, assessment of areas in which the alcoholic is likely to have clinically significant problems. For example, initial screening with the Beck Depression Inventory is highly sensitive to the presence of depression (Rounsaville et al, 1979). In the diagnostic phase, a more thorough, professional evaluation can be done only with those patients who have high enough screening scores to determine whether the screening results were indicative of a clinically significant problem, such as a current diagnosis of major depression. Use of diagnostic interview guides, such as the Diagnostic Interview Schedule (Robins et al, 1981a) or the Structured Clinical Interview for DSM-III (Spitzer and Williams, 1985) may facilitate a more definitive diagnosis.

To facilitate a multidimensional, structured evaluation system that can be conducted by counselors in substance abuse treatment programs, McLellan and associates (1980) have developed the Addiction Severity Index (ASI), a clinician-administered instrument that elicits information in six areas: substance use and medical, psychological, legal, social, and occupational problems. The ASI can be administered in 30 to 45 minutes and provides reliable ratings that agree well with longer assessments of the six problem areas; the ratings are also highly correlated with treatment outcome (McLellan et al, 1983). Moreover, it is useful as a method for assessing a patient's progress in treatment by comparing reevaluations of the six problem areas with those made on entrance into the program. Given its clinical utility, this instrument has gained progressively widespread acceptance. In the several areas, including psychopathology, it is useful as a screening tool, with more extensive psychiatric evaluation reserved for those whose ASI ratings of psychological problems are high.

When Should Dual Diagnoses Be Made in Alcoholics?

Acute alcohol intoxication, chronic heavy alcohol use, and recent withdrawal from heavy alcohol use can have profound effects on a patient's mental status, especially in the areas of cognitive functioning (memory, concentration) (Goldman, 1986; Tarter and Edwards, 1986; Wilkison and Sanchez-Craig, 1981) and mood (depression, anxiety) (Mendelson and Mello, 1966; Nathan and O'Brien, 1971). Because of these major alcohol-induced mental states, diagnosis of psychiatric disorders in alcoholics is complicated by the questions of when assessment procedures should be conducted and when reports of psychiatric symptoms should be judged as meeting criteria for coexistent psychiatric diagnoses.

TIMING OF ASSESSMENTS. The psychiatric assessment would ideally be held off until the patient has been abstinent from alcohol for at least four weeks. This time period is recommended on the basis of neuropsychological studies suggesting that significant improvement of presenting levels of impairment takes place during the first few weeks of abstinence (Goldman, 1986). Similarly, levels of depressive and anxiety symptoms improve considerably in abstinent alcoholics over the course of a four-week inpatient stay (Dorus et al, 1987). Time to improve neuropsychological status is important, because impairment can reduce the patient's ability to remember major events related to psychiatric diagnoses (for example, episodes of disorder, periods of treatment, disorder-related consequences) or age at onset of disorders in relation to onset of alcoholism, a sequence issue fundamental for the primary/secondary diagnostic decision. High levels of dysphoric symptoms that are completely substance-induced may result in overreporting of symptoms and selective remembering of dysphoric events (Beck, 1967).

In many treatment settings, it is not feasible to assess patients during a protracted period of abstinence. In outpatient settings, many patients are unable to achieve lengthy periods of abstinence, and those with dual diagnoses are less likely to remain abstinent (Rounsaville et al, 1987a). In 28-day inpatient settings, it is possible to hold off evaluation until the final week, but this procedure does not permit diagnosis among early dropouts and does not leave any time during an inpatient stay to provide treatment for psychiatric disorders that may be diagnosed. As a compromise, it is reasonable to attempt psychiatric diagnosis of alcoholics after a brief period of abstinence, such as 3 to 10 days, if one can be sure that the patient is not either acutely intoxicated or experiencing severe withdrawal symptoms at the time of the interview. In addition, a brief mental status examination to assess memory and concentration can screen out patients whose neuropsychological status is so impaired that valid assessment cannot take place.

ALCOHOL-INDUCED SYMPTOMS OR PSYCHIATRIC DISORDERS? Laboratory studies with humans have shown that prolonged consumption of alcohol and alcohol withdrawal can both induce symptoms of anxiety and depression that are indistinguishable from those characteristic of major depression and panic disorder (Mendelson and Mello, 1966; Nathan and O'Brien, 1971). Moreover, depressive symptoms have been shown to improve during the initial weeks following abstinence, without the institution of specific antidepressant treatments (Dorus et al, 1987). These observations suggest the need for guidelines that determine whether the depressive and anxiety symptoms seen in treatment-seeking alcoholics are part of clinically significant syndromes or are likely to resolve, untreated, with prolonged abstinence. When determining whether to treat alcoholics' depressive and anxiety symptoms, both overaggressive treatment of symptoms that may resolve spontaneously with abstinence and inadequate treatment of painful, debilitating syndromes should be avoided.

A conservative approach to diagnosing depressive and anxiety syndromes in alcoholics has been advocated by Schuckit (1986). Diagnoses of current depressive or anxiety disorders should be made only if the disorders 1) preceded the initial onset of alcoholism; 2) persisted during past alcohol-free periods; and/or 3) continued during the present episode after four weeks of abstinence from alcohol. For a diagnosis of major depression, this approach would preclude a positive diagnosis in 80 percent to 90 percent of those who would otherwise meet diagnostic criteria, as most depression in alcoholics has its first onset after the onset of alcoholism, especially men (Hesselbrock et al, 1985). The advantage of this approach lies in saving trivially depressed alcoholics from being treated with antidepressant medications that have significant side effects and overdose potentials, especially if used in combination with large quantities of alcohol.

There are, however, several drawbacks to a conservative approach. First, selectively attending to primary depression or primary anxiety disorders excludes the majority of alcoholics who have significant symptoms of these disorders. These symptoms have been shown to confer a poorer prognosis in treatment, whether or not they were primary or secondary to the alcoholic diagnosis (Rounsaville et al, 1987a). Moreover, continued presence of dysphoric symptoms may have a negative impact on the patient's ability to maintain abstinence, as Marlatt and Gordon (1985) have shown that one of the most common precipitants for relapse was dysphoria.

Excluding all but primary depression of anxiety disorders in alcoholics has the paradoxical effect of "protecting" alcoholics from these diagnoses, because these disorders are not suspected as long as the patient is drinking heavily. The paradox is more apparent if the alcoholism occurs over a period of many years and the age of onset antedates typical ages of onset of depressive and anxiety disorders.

A second set of problems arises from the conservative approach because it depends on the patient's ability to remember a sequence of events—onset of significant depression versus onset of heavy drinking from the relatively distant past. In general, the types of past events that are best remembered are discrete, major changes (for example, moves, hospitalizations, imprisonments), while onset of psychiatric symptoms can be subtle and not well demarcated. Memory confusion is compounded in alcoholics by the relatively common incidence of neuropsychological impairment.

The conservative approach can lead to a third set of problems pertaining to the requirement that alcoholics remain abstinent for four weeks or more before persistent depressive or anxiety symptoms are deemed clinically relevant. In an outpatient setting, it is difficult to verify prolonged abstinence, and patients with clinically significant psychiatric symptoms are least likely to achieve sobriety (Rounsaville et al, 1987a). Hence, diagnosis and treatment of psychiatric disorders are withheld from those who are likely to need them most. In an inpatient setting, waiting four weeks to diagnose disorders may delay pharmacotherapy until after discharge from a 28-day program, thereby reducing the advantages of intensive monitoring of medication compliance, side effects, and efficacy that can take place while the patient is hospitalized.

A more aggressive approach to the diagnosis and treatment of depressive or anxiety disorders in alcoholics can be taken by positively diagnosing these conditions if symptoms do not occur only when the patient is making large changes in the amount of alcohol consumed. This excludes depressive and anxiety symptoms that occur only when the patient discontinues or reduces alcohol use or when he or she increases the average amount being consumed. With this approach, institution of antidepressant or antianxiety treatment might be started for those remaining symptomatic after one to two weeks of abstinence.

An advantage of this approach is the relatively rapid institution of treatment for serious psychiatric disorders and the potential reduction of dropout rates; furthermore, treatment decisions are based on the recent clinical picture, rather than poorly remembered past symptom sequences. Precautions are also clearly needed to avoid giving potentially toxic medications to outpatients who present a significant suicide risk or whose drinking is clearly out of control; but, such patients are likely to be the minority of those whose dual diagnoses persist after one to two weeks of abstinence.

Placebo-controlled trials of pharmacologic agents in dual-diagnosis patients will provide measurements of the clinical usefulness of an aggressive approach, but care must be taken to ensure an adequate medication dose (Ciraulo and Jaffe, 1981). Newer antidepressants, such as the serotonin-uptake inhibitor fluoxetine, may provide better treatment for this population than tricyclics or "second generation" antidepressants (Naranjo et al, 1986).

SUMMARY AND CONCLUSIONS

In this chapter we have described the *DSM-III-R* changes in alcohol use disorders and suggested guidelines for the diagnosis of coexistent psychiatric disorders in alcoholics. The principal change in *DSM-III-R* alcohol use disorders was to broaden the meaning of alcohol dependence to not only include tolerance and withdrawal but also denote a range of behavioral indices of diminished control over alcohol use. While the diagnosis of alcohol abuse is still available and is defined by hazardous use of alcohol or alcohol-related impairment, it is intended to be a residual category. Some major intended results of *DSM-III-R* changes are to base diagnostic criteria on the theoretically important and clinically relevant alcohol dependence syndrome first proposed by Edwards and Gross (1976), to deemphasize the importance of tolerance and withdrawal in the dependence diagnosis, to shift the diagnostic criteria away from heavy emphasis on social consequences, to recognize dependence as a syndrome with varying grades of severity, and to allow an *in-remission* designation of the disorder.

Regarding diagnosis of coexistent psychiatric disorders in treatment seeking alcoholics, this chapter reviews the growing evidence that this clinical population has high rates of depression, anxiety disorders, antisocial personality, and other substance use disorders and that dual diagnosis is associated with a generally poorer prognosis in treatment. While it makes clinical sense to detect and treat coexistent psychiatric disorders, empirical studies of the efficacy of psychotherapies or pharmacotherapies for dually diagnosed alcoholics have been infrequently performed and should be replicated with more adequate research methodology. Although more research on treatment of this group is needed, we recommend that clinicians be alert to dual diagnostic procedures to detect coexistent psychiatric disorders.

REFERENCES

American Psychiatric Association: Diagnostic and Statistical Manual of Mental Disorders, Third Edition. Washington DC, American Psychiatric Association, 1980

American Psychiatric Association: Diagnostic and Statistical Manual of Mental Disorders, Third Edition, Revised. Washington DC, American Psychiatric Association, 1987

Amit Z, Brown Z, Sutherland A, et al: Reduction in alcohol intake in humans as a function of treatment with zimelidine: implications for treatment, in Research Advances in New Psychopharmacologial Treatments for Alcoholism. Edited by Naranjo CA, Sellers EM. Amsterdam, Elsevier Science Publishers, 1985

Babor TF, Lauerman RJ, Cooney NL: In search of the alcohol dependence syndrome: a cross-national study of its structure and validity. Paper presented at the Conference on Cross-Cultural Studies on Alcohol, Finnish Foundation of Alcohol Studies, Helsinki, September 1985

Beck AT: Depression: Clinical, Experimental and Therapeutic Aspects. New York, Harper & Row, 1967

Beck AT, Beck RW: Screening depressed patients on family practices: a rapid technique. Postgrad Med 1972; 52:1191–1195

Bowen RC, Cipywnyk D, D'Arcy C, et al: Alcoholism, anxiety disorders, and agoraphobia. Alcoholism: Clinical and Experimental Research 1984; 8:48–50

Chick J: Alcohol dependence: methodological issues in its measurement: reliability of the criteria. Br J Addict 1980; 75:175–186

Ciraulo DA, Jaffe JH: Tricyclic antidepressants in the treatment of depression associated with alcoholism. J Clin Psychopharmacol 1981; 1:146–150

Cloninger CR: Neurogenic adaptive mechanisms in alcoholism. Science 1987; 236:410–416

Dorus W, Kennedy J, Gibbons RD, et al: Symptoms and diagnosis of depression in alcholics. Alcoholism: Clinical and Experimental Research 1987; 11:150–154

Edwards G: The alcohol dependence syndrome: a concept as stimulus to enquiry. Br J Addict 1986; 81:171–183

Edwards G, Gross MM: Alcohol dependence: provisional description of a clinical syndrome. Br Med J 1976; 1:1058–1061

Edwards G, Arif A, Hodgson R: Nomenclature and classification of drug and alcohol related problems. Bull WHO 1981; 59:225–242

Endicott J, Spitzer RL: A diagnostic interview: the Schedule for Affective Disorders and Schizophrenia. Arch Gen Psychiatry 1978; 35:837–844

Foy DW, Nunn LB, Rychtarik RG: Broad-spectrum behavioral treatment for chronic alcoholics: effects of training controlled drinking skills. J Consult Clin Psychol 1984; 52:218–230

Goldman MS: Neuropsychological recovery in alcoholics' endogenous and exogenous processes. Alcoholism: Clinical and Experimental Research 1986; 10:136–144

Grande TP, Wolf AW, Schubert DSP, et al: Associations among alcoholism, drug abuse and antisocial personality: a review of literature. Psychol Rep 1984; 55:455–474

Heather N, Rollnick S, Winton M: A comparison of objective and subjective measures of alcohol dependence as predictors of relapse following treatment. Br J Clin Psychol 1983; 22:11–17

Hesselbrock M, Babor TF, Hesselbrock V, et al: Never believe an alcoholic? On the validity of self-report measures of alcohol dependence and related constructs. Int J Addict 1983; 18:593–609

Hesselbrock MN, Meyer RE, Keener JJ: Psychopathology in hospitalized alcoholics. Arch Gen Psychiatry 1985; 42:1050–1055

Hodgson RJ: Treatment strategies for the early problem drinker, in Alcoholism Treatment in Transition. Edited by Edwards G, Grant M. Baltimore, University Park Press, 1980

Hodgson R, Stockwell T, Rankin H, et al: Alcohol dependence: the concept, its utility and measurement. Br J Addict 1978; 73:339–342

Hodgson RJ, Rankin JJ, Stockwell TR: Alcohol dependence and the priming effect. Behav Res Ther 1979; 17:379–387

Jaffe JH: Drug addiction and drug abuse, in The Pharmacological Basics of Therapeutics, sixth edition. Edited by Goodman LS, Gilman L. New York, Macmillan, 1980

Kaplan RF, Meyer RE, Stroebel CF: Alcohol dependence and responsivity to an ethanol stimulus as predictors of alcohol consumption. Br J Addict 1983; 78:259–267

Keeler MH, Taylor CI, Miller CW: Are all recently detoxified alcoholics depressed? Am J Psychiatry 1979; 136:586–588

Kranzler HR: Preliminary studies on the effects of buspirone on craving in alcoholics. Presented at the Annual Meeting of the American College of Neuropsychopharmacology, 1987

Kranzler HR, Liebowitz N: Depression and anxiety in substance abuse: clinical implications, in Depression and Anxiety. Edited by Frazier S. Med Clin North Am (in press)

Litman GK, Stapleton J, Oppenheim AN, et al: Relationship between coping behaviors, their effectiveness and alcoholism relapse and survival. Br J Addict 1984; 79:283–291

Marlatt GA, Gordon JR (Eds): Relapse Prevention. New York, Guilford Press, 1985

Mathisen KS, Evans FJ, Meyers K, et al: Interactive computerized DIS (DSM-III) diagnosis (in press)

McLellan AT, Luborsky L, Woody GE, et al: An improved diagnostic evaluation instrument for substance abuse patients: the Addiction Severity Index. J Nerv Ment Dis 1980; 168:26–33

McLellan AT, Luborsky L, Woody GE, et al: Are the "addiction related" problems of substance abusers really related? J Nerv Ment Dis 1981; 169:232–239

McLellan AT, Luborsky L, Woody GE, et al: Predicting response to alcohol and drug abuse treatments: role of psychiatric severity. Arch Gen Psychiatry 1983; 40:620–625

Mendelson JH, Mello NK: Experimental analysis of drinking behavior in chronic alcoholics. Ann NY Acad Sci 1966; 133:828–845

Meyer RE: Anxiolytics and the alcoholic patient. J Stud Alcohol 1986; 47:269–273

Myers JK, Weissman MM, Tischler GL, et al: Six-month prevalence of psychiatric disorders in three communities. Arch Gen Psychiatry 1984; 41:959–967

Mullaney JA, Trippet CJ: Alcohol dependence and phobias: clinical description and relevance. Br J Psychiatry 1979; 135:565–573

Naranjo CA, Sellers EM, Roach CA, et al: Zimelidine-induced variations in alcohol intake by nondepressed heavy drinkers. Clin Pharmacol Ther 1984; 35:374–381

Naranjo CA, Sellers EM, Lawrin MO: Modulation of ethanol by serotonin uptake inhibitors. J Clin Psychiatry 1986; 47:16–22

Naranjo CA, Sellers EM, Sullivan JD, et al: Serotonin uptake inhibitors (SUI) consistently moderate ethanol intake (EI) in humans: citalopram (c) effects. Clin Pharmacol Ther (in press)

Nathan PE, O'Brien JS: An experimental analysis of the behaviour of alcoholics and nonalcoholics during prolonged experimental drinking: a necessary precursor of behaviour therapy? Behav Ther 1971; 2:455–476

Orford J, Oppenheimer E, Edwards G: Abstinence or control: the outcome for excessive drinkers two years after consultation. Behav Res Ther 1976; 14:409–418

Othmer E, Penick EC, Powell BJ: Psychiatric Diagnostic Interview (PDI) (manual). Los Angeles, Western Psychological Services, 1981

Penick EC, Powell BJ, Othmer E, et al: Subtyping alcoholics by co-existing psychiatric syndromes: course, family history, outcome, in Longitudinal Research in Alcoholism. Edited by Goodwin DW, Van Dusen RT, Mendick SA. Hingham, MA, Kluwer-Nijhoff Publishing Co., 1984

Polich JM, Armour DJ: The Course of Alcoholism: Four Years After Treatment. New York, John Wiley & Sons, 1981

Powell BJ, Penick EC, Othmer E, et al: Prevalence of additional psychiatric syndromes among male alcoholics. J Clin Psychiatry 1982; 43:404–407

Quitkin FM, Rifkin A, Kaplan J, et al: Phobic anxiety syndrome complicated by drug dependence and addiction: a treatable form of drug abuse. Arch Gen Psychiatry 1972; 27:159

Robins LN, Helzer JE, Croughan J, et al: NIMH Diagnostic Interview Schedule, Version III. St. Louis, Washington University School of Medicine, 1981a.

Robins LN, Helzer JE, Croughan J, et al: National Institute of Mental Health Diagnostic

Interview Schedule: its history, characteristics, and validity. Arch Gen Psychiatry 1981b; 38:381–389

Robins LN, Helzer JE, Weissman MM, et al: Prevalence of specific psychiatric disorders in three sites. Arch Gen Psychiatry 1984; 41:949–958

Ross HE, Glaser FB, Germanson T: The prevalence of psychiatric disorders in patients with alcohol and drug problems. Arch Gen Psychiatry (in press)

Rounsaville BJ, Weissman MM, Rosenberger PH, et al: Detecting depressive disorders in drug abusers: a comparison of screening instruments. J Affective Disord 1979; 1:255–267

Rounsaville BJ, Rosenberger P, Wilbur CH, et al: A comparison of the SADS/RDC and the DSM-III: diagnosing drug abusers. J Nerv Ment Dis 1980; 168:90–97

Rounsaville BJ, Spitzer RL, Williams JB: Proposed changes in DSM-III substance use disorders: description and rationale. Am J Psychiatry 1986; 143:463–468

Rounsaville BJ, Dolinsky ZS, Babor TF, et al: Psychopathology as a predictor of treatment outcome in alcoholics. Arch Gen Psychiatry 1987a; 44:505–513

Rounsaville BJ, Kosten TR, Williams JBW, et al: A field trial of DSM-III-R substance dependence disorders. Am J Psychiatry 1987b; 144:351–355

Schubert DSP, Wolf AW, Patterson MP, et al: A statistical evaluation of the literature regarding the associations among alcoholism, drug abuse and antisocial personality. Int J Addict (in press)

Schuckit MA: The clinical implications of primary diagnostic groups among alcoholics. Arch Gen Psychiatry 1985; 42:1081–1086

Schuckit MA: Genetic and clinical implications of alcoholism and affective disorder. Am J Psychiatry 1986; 143:140–147

Selzer ML: The Michigan Alcoholism Screening Test: the quest for a new diagnostic instrument. Am J Psychiatry 1971; 127:1653–1658

Segal BM: Alcohol disorders and DSM-III (letter). J Clin Psychiatry 1981; 42:448

Skinner HA: Primary syndromes of alcohol abuse: their management and correlates. Br J Addict 1981; 76:63–76

Skinner HA: The Drug Abuse Screening Test. Addict Behav 1982; 7:363–371

Skinner HA, Allen BA: Alcohol dependence syndrome: measurement and validation. J Abnorm Psychol 1982; 91:199–209

Smail P, Stockwell T, Canter S, et al: Alcohol dependence and phobic anxiety states: a prevalence study. Br J Psychiatry 1984; 144:53–57

Spitzer RL, Endicott J: Schedule for Affective Disorders and Schizophrenia (SADS), Third Edition. New York, New York State Psychiatric Institute, January 1978-October 1979

Spitzer RL, Williams JBW: Structured Clinical Interview for DSM-III—Patient Version (SCID-P). New York, New York State Psychiatric Institute, 1985

Stockwell T, Hodgson R, Edwards G, et al: The development of a questionnaire to measure severity of alcohol dependence. Br J Addict 1979; 74:79–87

Tartar RE, Edwards KL: Multifactorial etiology of neuropsychological impairment in alcoholics. Alcoholism: Clinical and Experimental Research 1986; 10:128–135

Weissman MM, Meyers JK, Harding PS: Prevalence and psychiatric heterogeneity of alcoholism in a United States urban community. J Stud Alcohol 1980; 41:672–681

Wilkison DA, Sanchez-Craig M: Relevance of brain dysfunction to treatment objectives: should alcohol-related cognitive deficits influence the way we think about treatment? Addict Behav 1981; 6:253–260

Woody GE, McLellan AT, Luborsky L, et al: Psychiatric severity as a predictor of benefits from psychotherapy: the Penn-VA study. Am J Psychiatry 1984; 141:1172–1177

Chapter 17

Psychosocial Approaches to Treatment and Rehabilitation

by Richard J. Frances, M.D., Marc Galanter, M.D., and Sheldon I. Miller, M.D.

WIDENING THE SCOPE OF TREATMENT

The development of inpatient rehabilitation programs in general hospitals, free-standing residential programs, and dual-diagnosis alcoholism facilities in psychiatric hospitals has been a major growth industry. Over 1.2 million patients with alcoholism were seen in inpatient, outpatient, and halfway houses in 1985 and approximately three-quarters of these were in nonhospital treatment units (State Alcohol and Drug Abuse Profile [SADAP] Data for States, unpublished report, 1986). In a six-year period the American Hospital Association (1984) reports a 78 percent rise in the number of alcoholism and drug treatment units and a 62 percent rise in the number of inpatient beds. Many states have mandated third-party reimbursement for outpatient alcoholism treatment, and there has been growth in organized day and evening treatment programs and halfway houses. Comprehensive alcoholism treatment facilities provide a variety of settings and continuity of care for patients with alcoholism. In addition to professionally organized treatment, it is estimated that there are 70,000 Alcoholics Anonymous (AA) self-help groups and between 1 and 1.5 million AA members. Alanon, which provides self-help for the friends and relatives of alcoholics, has approximately 13,000 groups in the United States.

In an era of subspecialization, clinical knowledge about addictions is growing: Tailored approaches to individual, group, and family treatment have been developed; and the use of many treatment modalities, such as behavioral therapy, insight-oriented treatment, cognitive and psychoeducational approaches, vocational therapy, counselling, and others has increased. In addition, vigorous growth of interest in addictions by psychiatrists has been reflected in the rapid rise in membership of the recently formed American Academy of Psychiatrists in Alcoholism and Addictions (AAPAA), which currently has approximately 800 members. A recent AAPAA survey found that 24 universities offered fellowships in the addictions field and another 33 were planning to start fellowship programs (Galanter and Frances, 1988).

The revision of the *Diagnostic and Statistical Manual, Third Edition (DSM-III)*, published by the American Psychiatric Association in 1980, led to major changes in the diagnosis of alcoholism, including expansion of the concept of dependency to include psychosocial problems, as well as tolerance and withdrawal. This change, along with identification of risk factors for alcoholism and a narrowed concept of alcohol abuse, should ultimately lead to earlier diagnosis and treatment (American Psychiatric Association, 1987; Rounsaville et al, 1987). Advances in multiaxial diagnosis have led to increased recognition of the dual-diagnosis patient and greater attention to questions concerning the interaction of several disorders in one patient (Meyer, 1985; Frances, 1986).

When diagnosing alcoholism and associated pathologies, the clinician must differentiate between the effects of overdose, states of intoxication and withdrawal, and the consequences of chronic alcohol use, and must identify whether the alcoholism is primary, secondary, or concomitant to another disorder (Schuckit, 1983). Multiple substance use, drug interactions or adverse effects, or withdrawal might also account for alcoholic symptomatology (Meyer, 1985; Bean-Bayog, 1987). Frequently, the psychiatrist is part of a treatment team that utilizes modalities such as family and group therapy, education, and 12-step programs, such as Alcoholics Anonymous. A broadly based biopsychosocial model must take into account genetic factors, perinatal issues, and child development, and the value of good, old-fashioned, careful history taking cannot be overstated. This should include an evaluation of mental status and close attention to the signs and symptoms of substance disorders, as they interact with other psychiatric disorders (Frances, 1987). Suicide potential should be assessed, as well as the level of functioning of object relations, reality testing, defenses, and superego. Khantzian and Mack (1983) also emphasize the importance of assessing the role of substance abuse in affect regulation, self-governance, and self-care.

The medical and social complications of alcoholism must be considered in an appropriate treatment plan. Specific needs and cultural sensitivities should be taken into account in planning treatment for special populations such as women, minorities, adolescents, geriatric patients, homosexuals, children of alcoholics, victims of abuse, veterans, the handicapped, the homeless, and AIDS patients (Caetano, 1984).

This chapter will review the literature, including the treatment outcome literature and the implications of new research for treatment, on psychosocial approaches to treatment of patients with alcoholism. The importance of early diagnosis, the differential therapeutics of alcohol treatment, selection of settings for inpatient and outpatient rehabilitation, modalities of treatment, and the tailoring of therapists' characteristics to the special needs of specific populations will be discussed. The value of self-help groups is now widely appreciated, and this approach is becoming an important research focus (Miller and Frances, 1986).

REVIEW OF ALCOHOLISM TREATMENT OUTCOME RESEARCH LITERATURE

Emrick and Hansen (1983) discussed the following factors that can affect research on the treatment outcome of alcoholism: 1) patient characteristics; 2) sample selection and attrition; 3) patient experiences outside of and after treatment; 4) duration of follow-up; 5) type of outcome variables examined; 6) analysis and interpretation of data; and 7) a host of methodological problems related to the conduct of outcome research. Because of the numbers of problems and their interactions, it is not surprising that, although most studies indicate positive results for alcoholism treatment, it has been hard to differentiate treatment outcome on the basis of modality of treatment, setting, or therapist characteristics. While most studies have shown that treatment is effective, it is difficult to differentiate which treatments are best for which patients. Treatment outcome studies using different modalities or lengths of treatment often report tie scores and have not yielded clear answers (Edwards et al, 1977).

In a well-controlled study, Edwards and colleagues (1977) compared treatment outcome in patients who were receiving only advice to patients getting intensive outpatient treatments. Low intensity of treatment generally led to poor results for both treatment groups, although this result may be related in part to a lack of therapeutic zeal on the part of the researchers. In uncontrolled studies, highly motivated clinicians report favorable results when using their preferred modes of treatment.

Patient characteristics, such as good socioeconomic stability, a lack of psychiatric and medical problems, low sociopathy, and a family history negative for alcoholism, seem to be positive prognostic features in many studies (Baekeland, 1977; McLellan, 1983; Gibbs and Flanagan, 1977). Work history, marriage or cohabitation, high-status occupations, a history of AA contact prior to treatment, higher social class, fewer arrests, and employment were all factors in a positive outcome. Moreover, programs that tend to select clients with these characteristics and that do not do controlled studies, such as the Hazelden Treatment Center in Minnesota, report success rates as high as 62 percent after 18 months of follow-up, with a follow-up response rate of 75 percent (Patton, 1979). On the other hand, programs that serve inner city populations with high unemployment rates report abstinence rates of only 32 percent after one year (Gordis et al, 1981).

Most studies of treatment settings have not yielded differences in outcome between patients treated in inpatient versus outpatient settings or partial hospitalization versus day clinic settings. However, there may be problems with patient selection for comparison groups, as patients often are not randomly assigned to an inpatient setting. Sicker patients are more often referred for hospitalization and are more likely to stay for a complete course of treatment. Though most studies have demonstrated no advantages to increasing the length of the hospital stay, Welte and associates (1981) found that patients who stayed in inpatient treatment longer were more likely to be abstaining or drinking less at follow-up. Bromet and Moos (1977) also found that increasing the length of stay reduced the relapse rate in three out of the five alcoholism treatment facilities studied.

McLellan and co-workers (1983) found that severity of psychiatric disturbance in general was a factor useful in predicting outcome of treatment for alcoholism and that it might also help predict which kind of treatment setting might be needed for psychiatrically ill patients. Improvement was measured by decrements in drinking and family problems, reduction of severity of psychiatric problems, and increases in income. Patients with less severe psychiatric problems did well in both inpatient and outpatient programs, while patients with more severe psychiatric problems had poorer prognoses, regardless of treatment modality. Patients with psychiatric problems in the middle range of severity who also had employment or family problems were less successfully treated with outpatient treatment relative to inpatient care. Moreover, patients who had legal problems did poorly in both inpatient and outpatient programs. McLellan's work demonstrated that alcohol treatment is effective overall and that effectiveness of treatment is improved when patients are matched to the most appropriate treatment setting. When the patient's severity of illness was matched to an appropriate treatment setting, they had a 19 percent better outcome than unmatched patients. A well-controlled study by Woody and colleagues (1984) also showed that appropriate treatment of psychiatric diagnoses concomitant with substance use disorders improves the outcome for patients who otherwise have a poor prognosis.

In general, alcoholism treatment has been shown to be cost-effective and to result in reduction of inpatient and outpatient medical costs. Research in relapse prevention is still needed, however. Vaillant (1983) found that, eight years after treatment, 29 percent of a sample of 100 inpatients had achieved stable abstinence of at least three years' duration, 24 percent had intermittent alcoholism, and 47 percent had continuing serious alcohol problems. High AA attendance and premorbid social stability, along with sustained abstinence, were indicators of good psychosocial outcome at eight years.

Helzer and co-workers (1985b) studied a five-to-seven-year outcome for 1289 patients; of 83 percent of the sample, only 1.6 percent were found to be drinking moderately (up to six drinks per day) at follow-up. It was concluded that stable moderate drinking is likely to be a rare outcome among treated alcoholics. Pettinati and associates (1982) followed 61 hospitalized alcoholics in a four-year study. Similarly, they found a low (three percent) nonproblem rate of drinking in the follow-up period. They also found a return to normal Minnesota Multiphasic Personality Index (MMPI) profiles in subjects who maintained long-term abstinence, with a general improvement in psychological function and no rehospitalization for those who achieved complete abstinence. These outcome studies have lent support to the widely accepted view that abstinence is the best goal for alcoholic patients and that there is no way of predicting which patients are likely to be the rare ones returning to nonproblem drinking in a follow-up period.

Treatment Implications of Research Advances

Current and future increases in scientific knowledge will affect the identification of high-risk populations and the prevention and treatment of addictions, and this trend is likely to continue. Such knowledge will include increased understanding of 1) fetal alcohol syndrome; 2) electrophysiological studies, such as evoked potentials (Begleiter et al, 1984); 3) molecular genetics and linkage studies; 4) biological markers; 5) animal models; 6) imaging technologies (Chao and Foudin, 1986); 7) neurotransmitter and receptor studies; 8) studies of endogenous opioids and other ligands; 9) newer generations of useful medications; 10) treatment of AIDS (Flavin and Frances, 1987); and 11) epidemiological studies (Myers et al, 1984). New scientific findings support and are compatible with the AA notion of alcoholism as an illness with an etiology, pathophysiology, course of treatment, epidemiological pattern, and means of prevention, and these results have led to greater cooperation among addictions therapists, researchers, and the AA community. Further, the discovery of endorphins has led to greater optimism about understanding opioid addiction in a broader biological, psychological, and social context.

Increased knowledge of epidemiology through the Epidemiological Catchment Area (ECA) study, which used standardized techniques, has led to the development of important data bases that clarify the extent of addictive problems

(Helzer et al, 1985a). The development of clear operational criteria and a broadened concept of dependency in the *Diagnostic and Statistical Manual of Mental Disorders, Third Edition, Revised (DMS-III-R)*, published by the American Psychiatric Association (1987), which includes psychosocial problems, has aided in earlier diagnosis, treatment, and prevention.

Importance of Early Diagnosis

Psychiatrists have a role in prevention, early intervention, and treatment along a continuum of problem severity. Early diagnosis can prevent progression of the illness in patients identified as being at high risk because they have a positive family history of alcoholism, harmful or hazardous patterns of use, or are already abusing or mildly dependent on alcohol. Long before severe alcoholism major medical complications develop and family, work, and legal difficulties appear, early signs of problems are likely to emerge. Alcohol can be used to change mood or to get to sleep, and it can disrupt communication in families and affect the ability to carry out social roles. Confrontation of denial may be needed to get the patient to accept help early, which is important for outcome. Late in the course of alcoholism, it may be very easy to identify the alcoholism but much harder to treat the problem. Early in its course, the converse is often true: The disease may be much easier to treat but harder to identify.

DIFFERENTIAL THERAPEUTICS

Choice of Setting

Patients who are not able to maintain abstinence as outpatients or who relapse repeatedly require inpatient treatment, but wherever possible, an outpatient trial is indicated first. Outpatient treatment is an alternative to hospitalization and is always a part of the long-term management of patients with alcoholism. Outpatient treatment is preferred by most patients because it is less disruptive in terms of work and family life, and it costs less than inpatient treatment (see Table 1).

Table 1. Indications for Inpatient Treatment*

---

1. Presence of a serious medical condition, including severe withdrawal, such as DT's and other medical complications of alcoholism
2. Presence of major psychiatric problems in addition to alcoholism, including psychosis, depression, suicidal behavior, panic disorders, anorexia
3. Failed attempt at outpatient treatment
4. Lack of social support from family or friends who might provide encouragement for abstinence
5. Multiple addiction to substances in addition to alcohol which would require inpatient management

---

*Reprinted from Frances RJ, Franklin JE: Alcohol-induced organic mental disorders, in Textbook of Neuropsychiatry. Edited by Hales RE, Yudofsky SL. Washington, DC, American Psychiatric Press, 1987

The Psychosocial Inpatient Rehabilitation Model of Addiction and Recovery

There has been an increasing emphasis in psychiatry on use of a rehabilitation treatment model for a variety of categories of psychiatric illness. The model was pioneered in alcohol and drug abuse and includes combinations of self-help, counselling, psychoeducation to patients and families, group treatment, use of a warm supportive environment, and an emphasis on a medical model aimed at reduction of stigma and blame. Alcohol and drug programs generally provide high degrees of structure, insist on abstinence as a goal, and emphasize cognitive and psychoeducational approaches that include lectures, films, and discussion groups. They often serve as a means of induction into self-help programs and professionally led after-care. An awareness of the needs of patients with dual diagnoses or medical complications, as well as the problems of special populations, has led to programs that better tailor treatment to specific patient needs and give greater attention to differential therapeutics in treatment planning. Integration of treatments—such as cognitive and behaviorial therapy that includes relapse prevention strategies, interpersonal therapy, family therapy, group treatment, psychoanalytically oriented psychotherapy, brief psychodynamically oriented psychotherapy, social network approaches to treatment, counselling, and psychoeducation—leads to the need for a highly skilled professional staff and the ready availability of consultation.

Most inpatient programs include five to seven days for detoxification and approximately three to six weeks for rehabilitation; longer stays tend to be necessary for patients with dual diagnosis, adolescents, and patients with severe medical problems (Frances and Allen, 1982). Many patients can begin an outpatient rehabilitation program as an alternative to hospitalization or after a brief detoxification.

A careful psychiatric evaluation is needed in every case, because the interactions between alcoholism, depression, and characterologic problems are quite complex (Weissman et al, 1980). An abstinence-oriented approach during treatment is valuable for both diagnostic and therapeutic reasons. Patients with substance use disorders often have combinations of denial, dissimulation, and memory problems, related to organicity, that make obtaining a clear history difficult. After years of social isolation, or when intoxicated or overdosed, the patient may have no family or friends who can be interviewed and may not be able to answer questions coherently. The patient who is coerced into seeking help by family, employer, the court, or family physician may initially be uncooperative and ambivalent.

Because alcoholic patients are frequently children of alcoholics, they may have little trust in authority and a lack of insight into their own high dependency needs (Frances and Allen, 1986). This may have led to bad past experiences with physicians who did not understand patients with addictions. Unless the reasons are carefully and thoroughly explained, it may be harder to achieve compliance with prescribed psychotropic medications because the need for medication may not be well accepted, given the distrust recovering patients can feel towards any chemical treatment of emotional problems.

The rehabilitation model takes into account that alcoholic patients have been socially isolated for a long time and have had few opportunities to practice social skills. They are likely to have regressed in superego function and ability to control impulses, and may use primitive defenses such as denial, splitting, and projection. In a rehabilitation program, patients get a chance to practice their social skills in group and self-help settings. The highly structured nature of such a program provides an auxiliary superego with clear limits and aids in self-control and self-examination of values, including self-honesty.

Many patients with substance abuse will appear to be sociopathic because they have had a regression, resulting from their addiction, in superego function; but, in recovery, they are found not to have a personality disorder (Frances, 1986). Rehabilitation programs foster movement from primitive levels of defense to use of higher levels of defense, such as intellectualization, isolation of affect, and reaction formation. The patient moves from saying "I'm not an alcoholic" to being able to identify with other patients with an alcohol problem and becoming a "grateful alcoholic" for the opportunity to be in the program. Instead of feeling isolated from others with the same problem, a patient may, over time, begin to feel helpful to other people with similar problems. Instead of self-loathing, there can be a development of pride in recovery. Issues of self-care, self-control, and self-governance have been emphasized by Khantzian and Mack 1983) as important parts of rehabilitation.

Outpatient Treatment: Office Practice and Organized Programs

Most experts feel that outpatient treatment requires complete abstinence from alcohol and all other psychoactive substances, except in the treatment of opioid addiction, in which methadone maintenance plays a major role (Miller et al, in press; Peachey and Naranjo, 1984). Although almost all patients seek to achieve controlled drinking, and some researchers have set this goal for patients as well, most experts feel that a total abstinence approach yields best results and is an essential goal for relapse prevention (Vaillant, 1983). Mandatory urine testing may be a useful adjunct to ensure an abstinence approach, especially for patients with multiple substance dependence. The need for urine testing obviously becomes critical, depending upon the addictive drugs of choice; it is especially important when treating the cocaine-addicted individual.

Outpatient treatment may involve a variety of modalities of treatment provided either by a solo practitioner, an organized outpatient alcohol program, or in conjunction with a halfway house program (McLachlan and Stein, 1982). Organized outpatient alcohol programs may provide anywhere from several hours of individual, family, group, and psychoeducational treatment per week to a full-service day or evening hospital program. Though generally cost-effective, the cost of community-based day and evening hospitals plus halfway houses may approach or exceed the cost of residential treatment or inpatient facilities (McCrady et al, 1986a). However, they are less restrictive and provide an alternative to hospitalization, as well as being a useful part of after-care programs.

Discharge from an inpatient facility without planned after-care can hardly be considered a complete treatment plan. Similarly, however, a single group meeting per week for a severely addicted individual will only on rare occasions be considered a comprehensive treatment approach. Few providers would fail to refer an addict to AA, Narcotics Anonymous, or another program, as part of their outpatient therapeutic approach. While, for some patients, these and other self-help groups are effective only when complementary to other therapeutic interventions, self-help programs may be sufficient for others when attended faithfully. Long-lasting recovery may be effected without further intervention from a professional or from an organized therapeutic program (Vaillant, 1983). It is hard to study the effectiveness of 12-step programs, such as AA (see Miller and Hester, 1986), because of the anonymity of these fellowships and the accompanying difficulty in following a given individual or a sample of randomly assigned individuals.

Perhaps the most intensive outpatient approach is the addiction day-treatment program (Bast, 1984). This type of care utilizes many of the same techniques in inpatient treatment programs. It can be hospital-based or freestanding; it is typically staffed by an interdisciplinary team made up of both professionals from traditional mental health backgrounds and drug addiction treatment staff. Patients are evaluated carefully by members of the team, which then forms an individualized treatment plan. Often, but not frequently enough, psychiatric evaluations are included in the process. The inclusion of the psychiatric evaluation may well indicate how thoroughly the team has considered the critical issues and complications in the drug- or alcohol-dependent individual. Careful attention should always be given to the possibility that a second psychiatric diagnosis that can complicate the treatment process may be present.

Interventions are typically offered as part of a program that requires attendance for several hours each day at least five days per week and that includes individual, group, family, and cognitive approaches. For those patients whose illness has not yet resulted in loss of employment, such programs meet in the evenings; others occur during the day. The programs run for several weeks and are followed by a longer period of decreasing treatment intensity. Generally speaking, attendance at self-help groups is strongly encouraged throughout the total period of treatment and for many years beyond. During the phasing-down of the organized program, individual psychotherapeutic efforts may continue, if indicated for secondary illnesses. The approaches and the duration of long-term intervention are best decided by continually evaluating both patient and family.

The above approach is generally used regardless of the addictive drug of choice. Obviously, in some situations, adding special features will be necessary, depending on the drug involved. For example, the treatment of cocaine withdrawal may include the use of tricyclic antidepressants (Kleber and Gawin, 1987).

Other less intensive outpatient approaches may be employed according to patient need. For example, a session of group therapy each week coupled with weekly individual therapy may be sufficient for some patients, especially when there is also attendance at a self-help group such as AA. Other combinations are offered, depending on individual situations, but it should be pointed out that for most addicted patients, individual psychotherapy once a week is probably not enough to produce and maintain sobriety, the ultimate goal for all addicted patients regardless of the drug he or she is using or the setting in which therapy is offered.

It is becoming obvious that the majority of alcoholics can be safely detoxified as outpatients (Naranjo et al, 1983), although it needs to be done with the full understanding of the strength of the addictive drive and, hence, in the context of an organized program, not an isolated treatment. It is best done as a part of the same program that will eventually become the outpatient rehabilitation program. Establishing continuity of care will help to decrease patient drop-out once relief from the discomfort associated with detoxification is achieved.

In summary, the treatment of addictive disorders in an outpatient setting is gaining in popularity as concern about the cost of health care grows and increasing data suggest an effectiveness for some patients equal to the more costly and time-consuming inpatient care. However, careful evaluation of each individual is crucial. Finally, just as is true for the inpatient setting, successful treatment in the outpatient setting is often dependent on an interdisciplinary team approach, as well as a multimodality treatment plan.

Choice of Modality or Combination of Modalities

Choice of modality or a combination of treatments will depend on factors listed in Table 2. The differential therapeutics of depression, anxiety disorders, attention deficit disorder, and so on will affect the choice of treatment for patients with these additional problems (McLellan et al, 1980; Hesselbrock et al, 1985). Most often, a patient is coerced into treatment by the employer, family, physician, probation officer, or teacher. An empathic therapist can anticipate and work through typical resistances of patients who feel frightened, hostile, and trapped and is best able to form a therapeutic alliance with them. Most inpatient alcohol treatment services offer combinations of modalities including psycho-education, 12-step programs, individual, group, and family counselling, and chemical aversive conditioning (described below). Unless a clear diagnosis of another psychiatric disorder has been made previously, drug-free periods of approximately two to four weeks with medication trials may also be indicated.

Chemical aversive conditioning (CAC), which consists of pairing a drinking stimulus with emetine to initiate nausea and vomiting, is widely used in the Soviet Union and has been used by several American hospital chains. Due to the risks of CAC, which include cardiac toxicity and risk for Malory Weiss syndrome, other equally efficacious but less risky forms of treatment should be tried first. On the other hand, disulfiram is a form of chemical conditioning that is widely used as an adjunct to other treatments (Azrin et al, 1982).

Table 2. Factors Influencing Choice of Treatment Modality or Combination

1. Individual patient characteristics
2. Illness severity
3. Cultural issues
4. Availability of treatment modality
5. Finances
6. Differential therapeutics of co-existing disorders

MODALITIES OF TREATMENT

Individual Therapy

Alcoholics can be effectively treated with individual therapy, but it is best combined with additional modalities, such as Alcoholics Anonymous, disulfiram administration, and family support (McClellan et al, 1983b; Zimberg et al, 1985, Frances and Allen 1986, Bean-Bayog, 1987). A strong and active relationship with the therapist is encouraged, and abstinence is considered the only acceptable treatment goal. Occasionally patients who are only abusers not dependent on alcohol, particularly those who are secondary alcoholics, may achieve controlled drinking with psychotherapy (Orford et al, 1984). However, there are no reliable ways to predict which patients can do this. For practical purposes, alcohol-dependent patients in the United States are encouraged to consider abstinence as their only option.

Psychoanalytic psychotherapy alone has been found to have little impact on alcohol dependence during the early phases of treatment. It is also generally agreed that psychoanalytic therapy cannot be conducted with an alcoholic who is actively drinking. Once abstinence has been established, however, insight-oriented therapy can be prescribed, for a selected subgroup, to facilitate the resolution of problems in mood or interpersonal function. Problems in identity, separation and individuation, affect regulation, self-governance, and self-care may be addressed in individual insight-oriented treatment (Khantzian and Mack, 1983). Indications for psychodynamically oriented therapy include psychological mindedness; capacities for honesty, intimacy, and identification with the therapist; average or superior intelligence; economic stability; high motivation; and a willingness to discuss conflict. Expressive psychotherapy may lead to deepening the capacity to tolerate depression and anxiety without using substances. However, when patients are not abstinent, exploratory treatment may do more harm than good, as the reactivation of painful conflicts can contribute to further drinking and regression.

Individual treatments may range from psychoanalytically informed supportive and expressive therapy to cognitive and behaviorally oriented treatments, and they are sometimes used alone when a patient refuses to become involved in Alcoholics Anonymous, group, or family treatments. Though possibly over-prescribed, individual treatment plays an important role, especially for patients who are facing bereavement, loss, and social disruption and who may have targeted problems, such as anxiety or panic disorders. Patients with anxiety disorders may especially benefit from a cognitively or behaviorally oriented treatment.

In the preliminary stages, the therapist should concentrate on how the patient can achieve and maintain abstinence by relying on specified sources of social support, resorting to the directive psychotherapy process itself, attending AA, and consistently following a disulfiram regimen (Zimberg, 1982; Galanter, 1984). In addition, limits must be set regarding the continuation of treatment in the face of repeated relapses. Appropriate referrals to more intensive treatment programs should be made, in the event the patient cannot achieve abstinence by these means. Terminating individual treatment should not be considered until abstinence has been long established, usually following as many as two years of treatment (Zimberg, 1982). Additional supportive strategies are described in Table 3.

Group Therapy

In many programs, therapeutic groups and group therapy are the principle treatment modalities for alcoholism, and a large variety of group-therapy formats have been employed by ambulatory, residential, hospital, and community programs (Brandsma and Pattison, 1984). Groups provide an opportunity for resocialization, practicing object-relatedness skills and impulse control, and accepting the identity of a recovering person. Groups that provide acceptance and support for an ego ideal of sober living foster the patient's development of self-esteem and reality testing. Despite their popularity, however, many group approaches can provide neither adequate descriptions of their design nor substantive evidence to document their superiority over other treatment approaches (Galanter, 1987). At present, some documentation of the positive effects in the treatment of alcoholism is available for the following: marital couples groups (Arieti, 1981); assertiveness-training groups (Hirsch et al, 1978) and groups for self-control (Miller et al, 1981), for ego strength, for self-concept, and for mood problems such as anxiety and depression. These groups generate a sense of mutual commitment and provide a cognitive basis for recognizing conditioned drinking-cues that can lead to relapse. Further, they provide consensual vali-

Table 3. Supportive Strategies

1. Exercise
    Provides outlet for aggression
    Enhances self-image
    May increase endorphins
    Reduces mild depression

2. Changes in Life Style
    Develops network of nonusing friends
    Removes alcohol from house
    Reduces exposure to availability
    Reduces high-risk situations

3. Relapse Preventions
    Stress reduction
    Refusal training—rehearse "no"
    Reaching out to others
    Life skills training
    Learning to live with craving
    Maintaining progress after lapses

4. Contingency Contracting
    Agreement that negative consequences will occur with relapse

From Marlatt GA, Gordon JR: Relapse Prevention. New York, Guilford Press, 1985

dation for the concept of abstinence, thereby combating the denial typical of alcoholism.

Traditional therapy groups are generally composed of six to ten members. They provide the alcoholic with the opportunity to learn about alcoholism, socialize with other alcoholics in different stages of sobriety, and benefit from focused interventions for specific behavioral problems. Importantly, it appears that the clinical outcome for these patients is greatly improved if the group is conducted in the context of a multi-modality program, irrespective of the philosophical orientation of the group leader. Psychotherapy groups serve mainly to prevent relapses by identifying and addressing psychological and interpersonal problems. The orientations and structures of these groups can be psychoanalytical, confrontational and problem-solving, couples/marital therapy, psychodrama, or interactional (Greenbaum, 1954; Rathod et al, 1966).

Among other types of groups frequently employed by alcoholism treatment programs are orientation and didactic groups; these help to engage the patient in the initial stages of treatment and improve retention and attendance in longer-term rehabilitation. Diagnostic groups are helpful during the psychosocial evaluation of new patients. Ward and milieu groups provide an opportunity to enforce more adaptive behavioral patterns by focusing on the patient's interactions with the ward therapeutic environment (Westfield, 1972); after discharge, they may lead to after-care groups and clubs that afford their members a continuous opportunity for socialization and reinforcement of accepted norms.

Successful outcomes have been studied in outpatient groups that lasted from one to two years (Rathod et al, 1966; Westfield, 1972), and from briefer courses of group therapy. Positive results have been reported with couples groups and behaviorally oriented and psychoanalytically oriented groups (Edwards et al, 1977; Miller et al, 1981).

Family and Social Network Therapy

A good diagnostic evaluation of the families of alcoholic patients is crucial in every case. Family treatment is frequently indicated and may be especially helpful to prevent problems in the children of alcoholics. The family system frequently has been altered to accommodate a patient's drinking and may in some cases reinforce it (McCrady et al, 1986b). In many cases, it is a family crisis that first brings the patient to treatment, and engaging the family may be crucial in both providing support for the patient and in helping him or her remain in treatment. One such approach is based on the concept of the *alcoholic system*. The focus of treatment is on the correction of dysfunctional patterns of interactional behavior within the family, and therapeutic success is measured not only by the degree of abstinence achieved, but also by improvement in the level of functioning of the family unit. Some of the techniques employed in the family therapy systems approach are conjoint family therapy (Usher et al, 1982); marital group therapy (Gallant et al, 1970); and conjoint hospitalization for marital couples (Steinglass et al, 1977).

Family and network modalities can also be used as an adjunct to individual management in office treatment. This is particularly useful because it is important that the clinician have access to effective supports in rehabilitation of these patients, as traditional office psychotherapeutic approaches alone have limited impact on addictive illness. In this approach (Galanter, 1984), a network of family or friends is forged into a working group to provide necessary support for the patient between the initial sessions. Membership ranges from one to several persons close to the patient. Contacts between network members initially include telephone calls (usually at the patient's initiative), dinner arrangements, and social encounters, and they should be planned, to a fair extent, during each early joint session. These encounters are usually planned for a time when alcohol or drug use is likely to occur.

In planning encounters, however, the psychiatrist should make clear to network members that relatively little unusual effort will be required for the long term, and that, after the patient is stabilized, their participation will come to little more than attendance at scheduled meetings with the patient and therapist. This is reassuring to those network members who may be unable to make a major time commitment to the patient, as well as to those patients who do not want to be placed in a dependent position.

Establishing a social network is a task that requires the active collaboration of patient and therapist. These two, sometimes aided by those parties who initially join the network, must search for the right balance of members. The process is not without problems, and the therapist must think in a strategic fashion to assure a balanced group. Also, the administration of disulfiram under observation is a treatment option easily adapted to work with social networks (Azrin et al, 1982). A patient who takes disulfiram cannot drink; a patient who agrees to be observed by a family member while taking disulfiram will not miss a dose without the observer knowing.

At the outset of therapy, it is important to see the patient within the network on a weekly basis for at least the first month, and unstable circumstances demand more frequent contacts with the network. Sessions can be tapered off to biweekly and then monthly intervals after a time, but to sustain the continuing commitment of the group, network sessions should be held every three months for the duration of the individual therapy. Once the patient has stabilized, reflections on the patient's progress and goals or on relationships between network members can be discussed.

Unlike family members involved in system-oriented family therapy, network members are not led to expect personal symptom relief or self-realization. This helps avoid the development of competing goals for the network's meetings. It also assures the members protection from having their own motives scrutinized and thereby supports their continuing involvement without threat of an assault on their psychological defenses.

Alcoholics Anonymous

AA is a voluntary, self-supporting fellowship, regarded by most alcoholism treatment institutions as a vital adjunct to the management of alcoholics. It is generally considered the ideal setting for long-term maintenance of sobriety. It was established in 1935 in response to the lack of available medical treatment for alcoholics, and it has since grown into an international movement with over one million members. While not formally affiliated with any professional organization or institution, AA now represents a major referral resource for alcoholic patients, and, according to one AA report (unpublished, 1984), 31 percent of AA members credit a rehabilitation center or some form of professional counseling with responsibility for their joining AA.

Although AA operates independently of the referring physician, there are certain steps that a psychiatrist can take to enhance the likelihood of the patient having a constructive experience with that fellowship. The patient should be made to appreciate that the psychiatrist is actively involved in the referral, and expects it to succeed. To underline this, the referring psychiatrist can call AA, while the patient is in the office, and help select a convenient meeting to attend. (Most cities have an Alcoholics Anonymous information bureau listed in the phone book.) The clinician can then arrange to meet the patient after the first AA meeting to continue to discuss the treatment plan. After the patient has attended the initial Alcoholics Anonymous meeting, the clinician should query the patient's impressions and help to dispel concerns or negative responses felt after the first encounter with the group. Patients are often unaware of the purpose of many of the AA rituals. Over the course of treatment, too, the clinician should make an effort to stay informed about the nature of the patient's involvement with AA and should be sensitive to the patient manifesting negative feelings toward the group, as these may be an expression of ambivalence about the abstinence regimen.

The clinician should encourage the patient to work with an AA sponsor and should promote the development of a good working relationship between patient and sponsor. At the same time, however, the patient's growing commitment to AA should be respected as an independent entity, and the psychiatrist should not intrude on the patient's strong feelings of affiliation. The patient's acceptance of AA and the resultant dependent feelings on the group should be taken at face value and not interpreted.

Professionally Led Self-Help

Most ambulatory problems for alcoholism treatment are modeled after ones used in general psychiatric clinics; they rely primarily on professionally conducted individual and small-group therapy. On the other hand, by incorporating self-help techniques, an alternative approach to alcoholism treatment, designed to allow for decreased staffing, can be effected (Galanter, 1987). This treatment format draws on the principles of large-group psychology observed in free-standing self-help approaches to addictive illness, such as Alcoholics Anonymous and the drug-free therapeutic communities, as well as certain other zealous self-help movements. These group formats have effected changes in addictive behavior by means qualitatively different from the usual hospital-based therapy.

Within this institutionally based format, therapy groups are led by patients who have established sobriety and have demonstrated a measure of social stability over several months. These senior patients monitor the progress of patients in orientation and ongoing therapy groups and are supervised by the primary therapists, who participate in a limited fashion only. New patients are encouraged to seek out peers and senior patients who will be available to assist them through the program. Senior patients are supervised when assisting with crises, if that is judged clinically appropriate by the primary therapist. Patients are thereby made aware that the primary source of support in the clinic is derived from the peer group.

CHOICE OF THERAPIST

When selecting a therapist, patients may wish to seek out therapists who can provide the modalities of treatment they need, who have expertise in the areas of addictions and concomitant psychiatric disorders, who can provide treatment at a cost the patient can bear, and who are comfortable referring the patient for additional consultation if needed (Perry et al, 1985). Patients should seek out second opinions and change approach or therapist when treatment is not effective. Patients may also be interested in the training background, experience, and associations to which the therapist belongs. Patients may have been advised to see a psychiatrist when issues of alcohol and drug-induced organicity—including intoxication effects, withdrawal effects, and chronic organic effects on mood, memory, or personality—and concurrent medical complications (including AIDS) interact and complicate differential diagnosis. Psychiatrists are also seem when psychotropic medications are indicated. A psychiatrist well trained in the addictions is best able to bring together basic science, medical, psychological, social, and cultural perspectives, and address each particular problem at its most appropriate level of understanding.

CONCLUSION

Improved understanding of the biological basis of alcoholism and other addictions and their interaction with environmental issues affects the way patients, families, and the public view addictions and the development of rational treatment approaches. The medical model has begun to replace a moral model in mass media presentations of alcoholism, and a wider public acceptance of the disease model affects the way patients and their families view addictions. There has been increased hope, reduced stigma, and reductions in guilt, self-blame, and blame projection within the family. There is also a heightened respect for professionals that accompanies any maturing field with an increased knowledge base.

REFERENCES

American Hospital Association, Hospital Statistics, 1984 Edition: Data from the American Hospital Association 1983. Clinical Service Chicago; American Hospital Association, 1984

American Psychiatric Association: Diagnostic and Statistical Manual of Mental Disorders, Third Edition. Washington, DC, American Psychiatric Association, 1980

American Psychiatric Association: Diagnostic and Statistical Manual of Mental Disorders, Third Edition, Revised. Washington, DC, American Psychiatric Association, 1987

Arieti A: A multicouple group therapy of alcoholics. Int J Addict 1981; 16:733–782

Azrin NH, Sisson RW, Meyers R, et al: Alcoholism treatment by disulfiram and community reinforcement therapy. J Behav Ther Exp Psychiatry 1982; 13:105–112

Baekeland F: Evaluation of treatment methods in chronic alcoholism, in The Biology of Alcoholism, Volume 5: Treatment and Rehabilitation of the Chronic Alcoholic. Edited by Kissin B, Begleiter H. New York, Plenum Press, 1981

Bast RJ: Classification of Alcoholism Treatment Settings. Rockville, MD, National Institute on Alcohol Abuse and Alcoholism, 1984

Bean-Bayog M: Inpatient treatment of the psychiatric patient with alcoholism. Gen Hosp Psychiatry 1987; 9:203–209

Begleiter H, Porjesz B, Bihari B, et al: Event-related potentials in boys at risk for alcoholism. Science 1984; 225:1493–1496

Brandsma JM, Pattison EM: Group treatment methods with alcoholics, in Advances in the Psychosocial Treatment of Alcoholism. Edited by Galanter M, Pattison EM. Washington, DC, American Psychiatric Press, Inc., 1984

Bromet E, Moos RH: Environmental resources and the posttreatment functioning of alcoholic patients. J Health Soc Behav 1977; 18:326–338

Caetano R: Ethnicity and drinking in northern California: A comparison among whites, blacks, and Hispanics. Alcohol Alcohol 1984; 19:31–44

Chao HM, Foudin L: Symposium on imaging research. Alcoholism: Clinical and Experimental Research 1986; 10:223–258

Edwards G, Orford J, Egert S: Alcoholism: a controlled trial of "treatment" and "advice." J Stud Alcohol 1977; 38:1004–1031

Emrick CD, Hansen J: Assertions regarding effectiveness of treatment for alcoholism: fact or fantasy? Am Psychologist 1983; 1078–1088

Flavin DK, Frances RJ: Risk-taking behavior, substance abuse disorders, and the acquired immune deficiency syndrome. Adv Alcohol Subst Abuse 1987; 6:223–233

Frances RJ: Signs and symptoms of alcoholism and substance abuse, in Textbook of Diagnostic Medicine: Psychiatric Problems. Edited by Samiy A, Gordon RD, Barondes J. Philadelphia, Lee and Feibiger, 1987

Frances RJ, Allen M: The interaction of substance-use disorders with nonpsychotic psychiatric disorders, in Psychiatry. Edited by Michels R. Philadelphia, J.B. Lippincott Co, 1986

Frances FJ, Franklin JE: Alcohol-induced organic mental disorders, in Textbook of Neuropsychiatry. Edited by Hales RE, Yudofsky SC. Washington, DC, American Psychiatric Press, Inc., 1987

Galanter M: The use of social networks in office management of the substance abuser, in Advances in the Psychosocial Treatment of Alcoholism. Edited by Galanter M, Pattison EM. Washington, DC, American Psychiatric Press, Inc., 1984

Galanter M: Institutional self-help therapy for alcoholism: clinical outcome. Alcoholism: Clinical and Experimental Research 1987; 11:424–429

Galanter M, Frances R: American Academy of Psychiatrists in Alcoholism and Addictions newsletter, Spring, 1988

Gallant DM, Rich A, Bey E, et al: Group psychotherapy with married couples: a successful technique in New Orleans alcoholism clinic patients. Journal of the Luisilan Medical Society 1970; 122:41–44

Gibbs L, Flanagan J: Prognostic indicators of alcoholism treatment outcome. Int J Addict 1977; 12:1097–1141

Gordis E, Dorph D, Sepe V, et al: Outcome of alcoholism treatment among 5,578 patients in an urban comprehensive hospital-based program: application of a computerized data system. Alcohol Clin Exp Res 1981; 5:509–522

Greenbaum H: Group psychotherapy with alcoholism in conjunction with antabuse treatment. Int J Group Psychother 1954; 4:30–45

Helzer JE, Robins LN, McEvoy LT, et al: A comparison of clinical and Diagnostic Interview Schedule diagnoses. Arch Gen Psychiatry 1985a; 42:657–666

Helzer JE, Robins LN, Taylor JR, et al: The extent of long-term moderate drinking among alcoholics discharged from medical and psychiatric treatment facilities. N Engl J Med 1985b; 313:1678–1682

Hesselbrock M, Meyer RE, Keener JJ: Psychopathology in hospitalized alcoholics. Arch Gen Psychiatry 1985; 42:1050–1055

Hirsch SM, Rosenberg RV, Phelam C, et al: Effectiveness of assertiveness training with alcoholics. J Stud Alcohol 1978; 39:89–97

Khantzian EJ, Mack JE: Self-preservation and the care of the self, in Ego Instincts Reconsidered. Psychoanal Study Child 1983; 38:39–232

Kleber HD, Gawin FH: Pharmacological treatments of cocaine abuse, in Cocaine: A Clinician's Handbook. Edited by Washton AW, Gold MS. New York, Guilford Press, 1987

Marlatt GA, Gordon JR: Relapse Prevention. New York, Guilford Press, 1985

McCrady BS, Longabagh R, Fink EB, et al: Cost-effectiveness of alcohol treatment in partial hospital versus inpatient settings after brief inpatient treatment: 12-month outcomes. J Consult Clin Psychol 1986a; 54:708–713

McCrady BS, Noel NE, Abrams DB, et al: Comparative effectiveness of three types of spouse involvement in outpatient behavioral alcoholism treatment. J Stud Alcohol 1986b; 47:459–467

McGinnis CA: The effect of group therapy on the ego-strength scale scores of alcoholic patients. J Clin Pschol 1963; 19:346–347

McLachlan JFC, Stein RL: Evaluation of a day clinic for alcoholics. J Stud Alcohol 1982; 43:261–272

McLellan AT: Predicting outcome from methadone maintenance: role of patient factors, in A Review of Methadone Maintenance. Edited by Cooper J, Scholl S. National Institute on Drug Abuse Research Monograph. Washington, DC, U.S. Government Printing Office, 1983

McLellan AT, O'Brien CP, Kron R: Matching substance abuse patients to appropriate treatments: a conceptual and methodological approach. Drug Alcohol Depend 1980; 5:189–195

McLellan AT, Woody GE, Luborsky L, et al: Is treatment for substance abuse effective? JAMA 1982; 247:1423–1427

McLellan AT, Luborsky L, Woody GE, et al: Predicting response to alcohol and drug abuse treatments: role of psychiatric severity. Arch Gen Psychiatry 1983a; 40:620–625

McLellan AT, Woody GE, Luborsky L, et al: Increased effectiveness of substance abuse treatment: a prospective study of patient-treatment "matching." J Nerv Men Dis 1983b; 171:597–605

Meyer R (Ed): Psychopathology of Addiction. New York, Guilford Press, 1985

Myers JK, Weissman MM, Tischler G, et al: Six-month prevalence of psychiatric disorders in three communities. Arch Gen Psychiatry 1984; 41:959–967

Miller SI, Frances RJ: Psychiatrists and the treatment of addictions: perceptions and practices. American Journal of Alcohol and Drug Abuse 1986; 12:187–197

Miller SI, Frances RJ, Holmes DJ: Alcoholism and psychotropic medications, in Comprehensive Handbook of Alcoholism Treatment Approaches. Edited by Hester RK, Miller WR. New York, Pergamon Press (in press)

Miller WR, Hester RK: The effectiveness of alcoholism treatment: what research reveals, in Treating Addictive Behavior: Processes of Change. Edited by Miller WR, Heather N. New York, Plenum Press, 1986

Miller WR, Pechocek TF, Hamburg S: Group behavior therapy for problem drinkers. Int J Addic 1981; 16:829–839

Naranjo EA, Sellers EM, Chatter K, et al: Nonpharmacologic intervention in acute alcohol withdrawal. Clin Pharmacol Ther 1983; 34:214–219

Orford J, Oppenheimer E, Edwards G: Abstinence and control. Behav Res Ther 14:409–418, 1984

Patton M: Validity and reliability of Hazelden treatment follow-up data. City Center, MN, Hazelden Educational Services, 1979

Peachey JE, Naranjo CA: The role of drugs in the treatment of alcoholism. Drugs 1984; 27:171–182

Perry S, Frances A, Clarkin J, et al: A DSM-III Casebook of Differential Therapeutics. New York, Brunner-Mazel, 1985

Pettinati HM, Sugerman AA, DiDonato N, et al: The natural history of alcoholism over four years after treatment. J Stud Alcohol 1982; 43:201–215

Rathod NH, Gregory E, Blows P, et al: A two-year follow-up study of alcoholic patients. Br J Pschiatry 1966; 72:683–692

Rounsaville BJ, Kosten TR, Williams JBW, et al: A field trial of DSM-III-R psychoactive substance dependence disorders. Am J Psychiatry 1987; 144:351–354

Schuckit MA: Alcoholism and other psychiatric disorders. Hosp Community Psychiatry 1983; 34:1022–1027

Steinglass P, Davis DI, Berenson D: Observations of conjointly hospitalized "alcoholic couples" during sobriety and intoxication: implications for theory and therapy. Fam Process 1977; 16:1–6

Swinner P: Treatment approaches, in Alcoholism in Perspective. Edited by Grant M, Swinner P. Baltimore, Baltimore University Park Press, 1979

United States Department of Health and Human Services: Sixth Special Report to the U.S. Congress on Alcohol and Health. Rockville, MD, Public Health Service, 1987

Usher ML, Jay J, Glass DR: Family therapy as a treatment modality for alcoholism. J Stud Alcohol 1982; 43:927–938

Vaillant GE: The Natural History of Alcoholism. Cambridge, MA, Harvard University Press, 1983

Weissman MM, Meyers JK, Harding PS: Prevalence and psychiatric heterogeneity of alcoholism in a United States urban community. J Stud Alcohol 1980; 41:672

Welte J, Hynes G, Sokolow L, et al: Effect of length of stay in inpatient alcoholism treatment on outcome. J Stud Alcohol 1981; 42:483–491

Westfield, DR: Two years experience of group methods in the treatment of male alcoholics in a Scottish mental hospital. Int J Addict 1972; 67:267–276

Woody GE, McLellan AT, Luborsky L, et al: Psychiatric severity as a predictor of benefits from psychotherapy. Am I Psychiatry 1984; 141:1171–1177

Zimberg S: The Clinical Management of Alcoholism. New York, Brunner/Mazel, 1982

Zimberg S, Wallace J, Blume S (eds): Practical Approaches to Alcoholism Psychotherapy. New York, Plenum Press, 1985

Chapter 18
The Pharmacotherapy of Alcoholism
by Henry R. Kranzler, M.D., and Barbara Orrok, M.D.

Although there is little evidence that current pharmacotherapies are widely effective in alcoholism treatment, other than for the treatment of acute withdrawal, a number of drugs are widely used by physicians treating alcoholics (Jones and Helrich, 1972). Recent research suggests that pharmacotherapy may increase the efficacy of alcoholism treatment by serving as an adjunct to the modalities currently available, including psychological therapies such as relapse prevention (Marlatt, 1985) and self-help groups, such as Alcoholics Anonymous.

This chapter begins with a discussion of drugs that affect the intoxicating capacity of ethanol. This is followed by a review and update on the treatment of alcohol withdrawal, including commonly observed complications. Subsequent sections are devoted to the treatment of recurrent or chronic alcohol dependence and focus on aversive drugs, drugs that may indirectly decrease alcohol consumption by affecting concomitant psychopathology, and drugs that appear to act directly on the reinforcing effects of alcohol.

THE TREATMENT OF ALCOHOL INTOXICATION

A variety of attempts have been made to find a safe, effective amethystic (sobering) agent. However, with the exception of hemodialysis (Koppanyi et al, 1961), no method has been shown to reverse completely the central depressant effects of ethanol in humans (Noble, 1984). Recent developments (Suzdak et al, 1986a), however, hold considerable promise of drugs with clinical utility in reversing the intoxicating effects of alcohol.

Since blood alcohol concentration (BAC) represents a balance between absorption and metabolism, pharmacokinetic antagonism of ethanol's effects may result from inhibition of absorption or by enhancement of metabolism. An increase in gastric emptying time or decreased gastrointestinal circulation, as with the ingestion of food or the administration of sympathomimetic or anticholinergic drugs (Kalant, 1971), will decrease absorption. Enhanced metabolism (as great as twofold compared to a control) has been demonstrated to occur with the administration of fructose, but this effect is inconsistent and there is a potential for serious adverse effects. Consequently, the small pharmacokinetic antagonism (compared with the ten-fold enhancement of metabolism needed to produce sobriety in an intoxicated individual) makes fructose of only limited value as an amethystic agent (Noble, 1984).

Based upon clinical evidence that naloxone reversed alcohol-induced coma, Jeffcoate and co-workers (1979) evaluated the effects of alcohol administration

This work was supported by grants P50-AA03510 and T32-AA07290 from the National Institute on Alcohol Abuse and Alcoholism. The authors wish to thank Jerome Jaffe, M.D., and Louis Gottlieb, M.D., for their helpful comments.

in normal volunteers pretreated with the drug; they found that naloxone prevented the impairment in psychomotor performance induced by low BACs. Based on these findings, the authors raised the possibility that the intoxicating effects of ethanol are mediated by endogenous opioids. However, five other controlled studies have failed to replicate these findings (Dole et al, 1982). While apparently ineffective at counteracting the effects of low BACs, there is considerable evidence that naloxone has specific effects on shock and cerebral ischemia, both of which may be important in intoxicated, comatose patients (Dole et al, 1982).

Pharmacodynamic antagonism may be feasible via effects on at least two neurotransmitter systems, including central catecholamines, the activity of which is inversely related to ethanol effects. Agents that increase catecholamine function (either directly or via effects on cyclic adenosine monophosphate, cAMP) appear to reverse some of ethanol's depressant effects. Inhibitors of phosphodiesterase, such as caffeine, produce an increase in cAMP (among other effects), which may explain the enhanced cognitive function observed upon its coadministration with ethanol (Noble, 1984). The effects of caffeine, however, are inconsistent and dependent on its concentration (Forney and Hughes, 1965). Similar findings have been reported for amphetamine (Hughes and Forney, 1964). The antagonism of a limited number of ethanol's effects has also been found to result from treatment with aminophylline and ephedrine, singly or in combination (Alkana et al, 1977).

A more promising line of inquiry relates to gammaaminobutyric acid (GABA), the most abundant of the neurotransmitters. Its inhibitory activity is mediated via effects on neuronal chloride ion flux (Allan and Harris, 1987), which appears to be the basis for many of the effects of both benzodiazepines (BZs) and barbiturates. Since these drugs are cross-tolerant with ethanol (hence their utility in the treatment of alcohol withdrawal), it is not surprising that some of ethanol's effects may occur via a similar mechanism (Suzdak et al, 1986b).

Recent work using Ro15-4513, an imidazobenzodiazepine that acts at GABA-BZ receptors, indicates that a specific antagonism of ethanol is possible at pharmacologically relevant concentrations and may ultimately be of clinical relevance. Using rat synaptoneurosomes, Suzdak and colleagues (1986a) demonstrated that the drug potently antagonizes ethanol-induced changes in chloride flux, but it had no such effect on changes induced by other agents that stimulate chloride uptake, including barbiturates. Similarly, Ro15-4513 antagonized the behavioral effects, including substantial degrees of intoxication, of ethanol in rats. The drug did not produce changes in BAC, which suggests that the observed behavioral changes were pharmacodynamic effects. Another group of investigators (Britton et al, 1988) has, however, adduced evidence that Ro15-4513 nonselectively antagonizes the behavioral effects of ethanol, pentobarbital, and chlordiazepoxide. These conflicting data make evident the need for further investigation of this partial inverse benzodiazepine agonist.

The availability of a specific antagonist of ethanol's effects would contradict the assertion by Sellers and Kalant (1976) that no such antagonism is possible. These authors based their conclusion on evidence that ethanol exerts it effects on the lipid bulk phase of neuronal membranes. While there is no evidence for a direct effect of ethanol on GABA receptors, the data on Ro15-4513 support the notion that "nonspecific membrane effects of alcohol may result in specific alterations in membrane function, including changes in the conformation of membrane-bound receptors such as those coupled to adenylate cyclase and ion channels" (Suzdak et al, 1986a, p. 1243).

However, Ro15-4513 does not prevent the lethal effect of very high doses of ethanol (Kolata, 1986). Perhaps the conformational changes in the receptor that permit specific antagonism at low to moderate BACs are not operative at high BACs, where bulk effects on the membrane may assume relatively greater importance. It is unclear whether Ro15-4513 will itself be of clinical use, as it is at high BACs that antagonism is most desirable, when reversing ethanol-induced coma, for example. Furthermore, it has both anxiogenic and proconvulsant properties (Britton et al, 1988).

Thyrotropin releasing hormone (TRH) has been shown to be an antagonist of pentobarbital-induced sedation and of both the sedative and hypothermic effects of ethanol (Erickson, 1983). The antagonism appears to be pharmacodynamic, consistent across species, and independent of the pituitary-thyroid axis. The actions of TRH do not appear to be mediated by effects on a single neurotransmitter system.

In summary, a variety of agents demonstrate amethystic effects. None, however, has consistently demonstrated efficacy and is sufficiently free of significant toxicity to permit widespread clinical application. Furthermore, the relatively limited effects of alcohol that particular agents antagonize may, paradoxically, have adverse consequences. This can result from partial antagonism of, for example, behavioral effects, such that people taking the drug may continue to drink beyond the level at which they ordinarily would stop, producing metabolic and respiratory effects that are potentially lethal (Kolata, 1986).

THE TREATMENT OF ALCOHOL WITHDRAWAL

Theories concerning the role of alcohol withdrawal and its treatment in the long-term outcome of alcohol-dependent patients have been based on unsystematic, anecdotal data (Gorelick and Wilkins, 1986), but carefully controlled studies are necessary to clarify these issues (Moskowitz et al, 1983). The best approach to the treatment of alcohol withdrawal remains in dispute, and two major areas of controversy have developed: the modality of treatment (sedative medication versus social detoxification) and the setting for treatment (inpatient versus outpatient).

The objectives in treating alcohol withdrawal are the relief of discomfort, prevention or treatment of complications, and preparation for rehabilitation. A corollary of these objectives is the need to minimize adverse consequences of therapy, including drug dependence or toxicity (Naranjo and Sellers, 1986). Social detoxification, which involves the nonpharmacologic treatment of withdrawal reactions, has been shown in both uncontrolled (Whitfield et al, 1978) and controlled (Naranjo et al, 1983; Sellers et al, 1983) trials to be an effective treatment strategy. It consists of frequent reassurance, reality orientation, monitoring of vital signs, personal attention, and general nursing care (Naranjo and Sellers, 1986).

Social detoxification is most appropriate for patients in mild to moderate withdrawal and has been shown to be useful in outpatient (Whitfield et al, 1978), inpatient (Sellers et al, 1983) and emergency room (Naranjo et al, 1983) settings. Based on clinical impressions, proponents of this approach suggest that it is a more rapid, cost effective approach than pharmacotherapy (Whitfield et al, 1978). Furthermore, it may avoid the sedation and cognitive impairment that are associated with drug therapy and that may adversely affect early efforts at rehabilitation (McGovern, 1983). However, the data on the relative merits of social and medical detoxification are equivocal (Gorelick and Wilkins, 1986).

Careful screening for concurrent medical problems and medical backup when needed are essential ingredients of social detoxification (Naranjo and Sellers, 1986). As with medical detoxification, administration of thiamine (50 to 100 mg, po or im) and multivitamin preparations is a low-cost, low-risk intervention with important potential utility in the prophylaxis and treatment of neurologic disturbance. Decisions regarding repletion of fluid volume and electrolytes must be based on careful clinical assessment. The need for good supportive care and treatment of concurrent illness should be stressed (Naranjo and Sellers, 1986).

The decision as to whether treatment of withdrawal requires a hospital admission depends on a number of factors, although detoxification is increasingly being done on an ambulatory basis. Concurrent serious medical or surgical illness requires inpatient treatment, which is also indicated for those individuals with a past history of serious withdrawal reactions or those with current evidence of more serious withdrawal, including changes in mental status or extreme autonomic lability (Feldman et al, 1975). The health problems of alcoholics are often multiple and are particularly relevant during withdrawal, when they may substantially complicate therapy. Adverse effects of chronic ethanol consumption include gastrointestinal, neurologic, cardiovascular, hematologic, and endocrine disorders (Eckardt et al, 1981). The psychiatric complications are discussed elsewhere in this volume (see Chapter 16). Comorbidity is an important consideration in the treatment of alcoholism, and coexistent medical and/or psychiatric disorders can add to the utility of pharmacotherapy or limit it, due to increased potential for adverse effects.

A wide variety of medications have been used for the treatment of alcohol withdrawal, including antihistamines, antipsychotics, barbiturates, benzodiazepines, and other sedative/hypnotics (for example, chlormethiazole, chloral hydrate, paraldehyde). Despite the established efficacy of many of these agents, in North America the use of benzodiazepines, due to their more favorable side effect profile, has largely supplanted that of other sedative/hypnotics (Naranjo and Sellers, 1986). There is no evidence that any one benzodiazepine is superior to another for this purpose, but different pharmacokinetic profiles make some more useful under certain circumstances (Gessner, 1979). Table 1 provides information on a number of currently available benzodiazepines.

Since both diazepam and chlordiazepoxide are metabolized to long-acting compounds, which in effect are self-tapering, these are the most widely used of the benzodiazepines for treatment of withdrawal. However, because metabolism is dependent upon liver function, hepatitis or cirrhosis can complicate their use. Both have the related disadvantage of accumulating over a period of days if the dosage is not reduced adequately, producing intoxication, particularly among the elderly. Furthermore, when given intramuscularly, these drugs are absorbed erratically, requiring that their administration be limited to the oral or intravenous routes. Since oxazepam, lorazepam, and temazepam are not oxidized to long-acting metabolites, there is less risk of accumulation. Lorazepam is also suitable for intramuscular administration (Harvey, 1985).

Table 1. Benzodiazepines and Their Use in the Therapy of Moderate to Severe Alcohol Withdrawal

Generic Name	Trade Name	Initial Biotransformation Pathway	Range of Elimination Half-Life (Includes Active Metabolites)	Total Daily Dosage (in Divided Doses, q4–6h)
Alprazolam	Xanax	oxidation	8–15 h	2.0–8.0 mg
Chlordiazepoxide	Librium	oxidation	36–96 h	100–400 mg
Clorazepate	Tranxene	oxidation	36–96 h	30–120 mg
Diazepam	Valium	oxidation	36–96 h	20–80 mg
Lorazepam	Ativan	conjugation	10–20 h	4–16 mg
Oxazepam	Serax	conjugation	5–15 h	60–240 mg
Prazepam	Centrax	oxidation	36–96 h	40–160 mg

In uncomplicated cases of withdrawal, two approaches to the use of long-acting benzodiazepines are recommended. The first employs chlordiazepoxide in gradually decreasing dosage over four days. Depending on the severity of the withdrawal reaction, on the first day up to 400 mg may be given in divided doses (that is, every 4-6 hours). Toxicity is avoided by the gradual reduction of dosage and limited duration of therapy (Sellers and Kalant, 1976). Alternatively, diazepam may be given in 20 mg doses every two hours until signs and symptoms are completely suppressed. This provides a loading dose, the activity of which gradually diminishes. Further dosing is unnecessary due to diazepam's long-acting metabolites (Sellers et al, 1983). Regardless of which approach is employed, careful monitoring of the patient's mental status and vital signs is necessary.

Of the other sedative-hypnotics employed for treatment of alcohol withdrawal, chlormethiazole is among the most widely used, particularly in Europe and Great Britain; it is not approved for use in the United States. While chemically related to thiamine, it is an effective sedative-hypnotic that possesses anticonvulsant activity. Cases of abuse and overdosage have been reported (Jaffe and Ciraulo, 1985).

Antipsychotics are not indicated for the treatment of withdrawal except when hallucinations or severe agitation are present, in which case they should be added to a benzodiazepine. Under those circumstances, haloperidol (0.5–2.0 mg im every two hours) until control of symptoms is achieved or five doses have been given is a suitable treatment (Sellers and Kalant, 1976). In addition to their potential to produce extrapyramidal side effects, antipsychotics lower seizure threshold. There is little advantage to the use of antihistamines in the treatment of withdrawal, and they have the potential for problematic side effects. Their use in this setting is not recommended (Sellers and Kalant, 1976).

The utility of anticonvulsants is a more complicated issue. The seizures associated with withdrawal occur generally between 21 and 48 hours after the last drink (Sellers and Kalant, 1976). Since phenytoin does not appear to be useful in suppressing withdrawal seizures (Gessner, 1979), it should be used, along with a benzodiazepine, only in those patients with a history of underlying seizure disorder. Valproic acid is effective in suppressing alcohol withdrawal seizures in animals and has been used with success in humans in Europe and Australia (Gessner, 1979), and carbamazepine also appears to be useful as a primary treatment of withdrawal (Poutanen, 1979). However, the liver dysfunction common in alcoholics may affect the metabolism of anticonvulsants, which makes careful blood level monitoring necessary.

Given the increased adrenergic activity associated with alcohol withdrawal (Carlsson and Haggendal, 1967), efforts have been made to assess the clinical utility of sympathetic-blocking drugs. Two alpha-adrenergic blockers, clonidine and lofexidine, and two beta-blockers, propranolol and atenolol, have been shown to reduce withdrawal symptoms. In a placebo-controlled trial, patients treated with clonidine showed more rapid improvement in withdrawal symptoms, particularly those of an autonomic or psychiatric nature (Bjorkqvist, 1975). No significant adverse effects were observed, but concomitant treatment of all patients with a sedative/hypnotic was provided, confounding evaluation of the effects of the adrenergic drug. In a Swedish study (Manhem et al, 1985), patients treated with carbamazepine were randomly assigned to receive clonidine or chlormethiazole concomitantly. The addition of clonidine was more effective in the reduction of plasma catecholamines, blood pressure, and pulse than was the addition of chlormethiazole. In a placebo-controlled trial, lofexidine was shown to be of significant utility in the treatment of withdrawal symptoms (Cushman et al, 1985). Hypotension was the most prominent side effect of lofexidine therapy, but one of the patients treated with the drug suffered hallucinations.

Sellers and associates (1977) found that propranolol alone was more effective in alleviating symptoms of alcohol withdrawal than were chlordiazepoxide alone or both drugs in combination. However, propranolol was given in a much lower dose (10 mg) in combination with the benzodiazepine than the dose (40 mg) given alone. A number of psychotic reactions have been reported to occur with propranolol treatment in alcohol withdrawal (Jacob et al, 1983). Kraus and co-workers (1985) found that, in combination with oxazepam, atenolol was significantly more effective than placebo. Atenolol-treated patients spent less time in hospital, required a lower dosage of benzodiazepine, and had a more rapid return to normal in their vital signs and abnormal behavioral and clinical features than did placebo-treated patients. Adverse effects in both groups were comparable, and none were serious. Similar results have been obtained by these investigators in a study of alcoholics in outpatient detoxification with oxazepam and either atenolol or placebo. There was evidence in this trial that atenolol also decreased desire for alcohol and kept more patients in treatment than did placebo (Horwitz et al, 1987). Combined treatment involving a benzodiazepine and a sympathetic-blocking drug appears to hold promise as a means of enhancing the effects of the standard benzodiazepine therapy of alcohol withdrawal (Lerner and Fallon, 1985).

Table 2 provides a summary of adjunctive therapies for alcohol withdrawal. In general, the treatment of alcohol withdrawal can be accomplished on an ambulatory basis, given the absence of serious medical or surgical illness or past history of severe withdrawal reactions and the presence of adequate social support, such as family members to oversee the patient's progress. Administration of thiamine (50 to 100 mg po or im) and daily multivitamins is highly recommended. Among patients with elevated vital signs, the most conservative approach is to administer benzodiazepine either as a loading dose or as a tapering dose, as described above. For moderate to severe withdrawal, the addition of atenolol may be considered, although further investigation of adjunctive treatment with beta-blockers is required. In patients with a preexisting seizure disorder, treatment with phenytoin is recommended. For hallucinations or severely agitated behavior, an antipsychotic is warranted, with the recognition that seizure threshold may be reduced.

PHARMACOTHERAPY IN ALCOHOLISM REHABILITATION

Despite the lack of convincing evidence concerning their safety and efficacy, as recently as 1972 greater than 90 percent of physicians in private practice reported the use of drugs to treat alcoholism (Jones and Helrich, 1972). Perhaps in an effort to temper what they saw as unjustified optimism concerning their use, Sellers and colleagues (1981) predicted that drugs were unlikely ever to play a

Table 2. Drug Therapy of Problems That Commonly Arise During Alcohol Withdrawal

Clinical Problem	Drug	Route	Dose	Interval	Comment
Withdrawal moderate to severe	diazepam chlordiazepoxide oxazepam	po po po	5–20 mg 25–100 mg 15–60 mg	every 4–6 hr	Dose and interval determined by vital and other signs. Oxazepam is preferred in the presence of serious liver disease
Hallucinations, extreme agitation	haloperidol	im	0.5–5.0 mg	every 2 hr	Until controlled or to maximum of five doses; appropriate doses of diazepam should be used concurrently
Seizure history of seizure disorder or previous withdrawal seizures	phenytoin	po	Diphenylhydantoin detected in blood, maintenance dose: 100 mg; No diphenylhydantoin detected in blood, loading dose: 200–300 mg, maintenance dose: 100 mg	every 8 hr	Repeated seizures may require phenytoin or diazepam i.v.

Note. Adapted from Naranjo CA, Sellers EM: Clinical assessment and pharmacotherapy of the alcohol withdrawal syndrome, in Recent Developments in Alcoholism, vol. 4. Edited by Galanter M. New York, Plenum Press, 1986

primary role in the rehabilitation of alcoholics. They anticipated that when drugs with demonstrated efficacy become available, they would serve only as adjuncts to behavioral and social therapies. Due to the multidimensional nature of alcoholism, no single approach is likely to be useful for all patients. However, a drug that reduces the risk of relapse would permit the patient to participate more effectively in psychosocial treatment, in much the same way that antidepressants are used with other therapies in the treatment of depression.

Aversive Drugs

Drugs that cause an unpleasant reaction when combined with alcohol have considerable intuitive appeal for use in alcoholism treatment. This may explain the widespread popularity of disulfiram in the rehabilitation of alcoholic patients (Favazza and Martin, 1974). However, there have been few methodologically sound evaluations of the efficacy of aversive drugs (Liskow and Goodwin, 1987). Studies undertaken prior to this decade have not included measures of compliance, have not provided adequate controls, or have used small samples or ill-defined outcome measures (Fuller et al, 1986).

A variety of agents (including the trichomonacides, oral hypoglycemic agents, and monoamine oxidase-inhibiting antidepressants) may produce unpleasant effects when combined with ethanol. A comparatively minor aversive reaction and the potential for other toxic reactions have made these drugs unsuitable for widespread use in alcoholism treatment. The bulk of research has focused on disulfiram and calcium carbimide which, along with the newest agent nitrefazole, will be discussed here.

THE ACETALDEHYDE SYNDROME.   All aversive drugs in current use block hepatic oxidation of acetaldehyde by aldehyde dehydrogenase. The resulting five- to ten-fold increase in blood acetaldehyde accounts for most of the unpleasant effects of the alcohol–drug reaction. Shortly after alcohol is consumed by an individual taking an aversive drug, vasodilation results. This leads to facial flushing, often with progression to throbbing headache, nausea and vomiting, sweating, thirst, chest pain, palpitations, increased pulse rate, orthostatic syncope, marked uneasiness, weakness, vertigo, blurry vision, and confusion. As the symptoms remit, the exhausted individual may fall asleep. Severe reactions may include respiratory depression, arrhythmias, myocardial infarction, acute congestive heart failure, seizures, cardiovascular collapse, and death. An elevated acetaldehyde level is probably the principle mechanism involved in the reaction; however, particularly in severe reactions, many aspects remain to be explained (Ritchie, 1985).

In combination with the usual dosage of an aversive drug, mild reactions can occur with ingestion of as little as 7 ml of alcohol, which gives rise to a BAC of 5–10 mg per dl. Full symptoms result from a BAC of 50–100 mg per dl. Symptoms can result from ethanol consumption as long as aldehyde dehydrogenase is inactivated. Once precipitated, the reaction may last from 30 minutes to several hours, and treatment is limited to supportive measures. It may be possible to provide rapid relief from a severe reaction with the administration of 4-methylpyrazole, which decreases the conversion of alcohol to acetaldehyde (Lindros et al, 1981). There are reports of mild reactions that result from ingestion of alcohol from hidden sources (for example, cough syrups, added flavoring) and from topical application (Ritchie, 1985).

DISULFIRAM. Disulfiram is the most extensively researched aversive medication and the only one approved for use in the United States. It is given in a single daily dose of 125–500 mg. Within about 12 hours of administration, it binds irreversibly to aldehyde dehydrogenase, with permanent inactivation of the enzyme. This inhibition lasts for up to two weeks, until new enzyme is synthesized (Ritchie, 1985). Consequently, disulfiram will not produce an aversive reaction immediately after therapy is begun, but may produce discomfort when alcohol is taken for up to two weeks following the last dose.

In addition to its effects on acetaldehyde dehydrogenase, disulfiram inhibits the enzyme dopamine beta-hydroxylase, resulting in elevated levels of the neurotransmitter dopamine (Ritchie, 1985). This may be the basis for the observation that, in susceptible individuals, disulfiram therapy may elicit psychotic symptoms (Nasrallah, 1979). Disulfiram has also been shown to inhibit the metabolism of serotonin (Fukumori et al, 1980). Uncommon adverse effects of disulfiram include an immune-mediated hepatitis, peripheral neuropathy, and cardiac conduction abnormalities (Ritchie, 1985).

There are anecdotal reports that alcoholics can become intoxicated from the combination of disulfiram and small amounts of alcohol. In a double-blind, controlled study of 23 nonalcoholic subjects, Brown and associates (1983) reported that disulfiram (and calcium carbimide, see below) can enhance intoxication and euphoria when combined with small doses of ethanol. The effect is apparently mediated by a limited (three- to four-fold) increase in serum acetaldehyde, rather than a direct effect of BAC (Brown et al, 1983). In addition, reports that some people can "drink through" or overcome their acetaldehyde reactions may have validity (Peachey et al, 1983).

As mentioned above, the efficacy of disulfiram in the maintenance of abstinence in alcoholics, while widely assumed, has undergone comparatively little systematic assessment. A large, multicenter study was recently completed in the Veterans Administration (Fuller et al, 1986), and the investigators were careful to control for a variety of potentially confounding variables, including the rate of compliance, validity of self-reported consumption, concurrent treatment, and placebo effects. More than 600 male alcoholics were randomly assigned to treatment with 250 mg per day of disulfiram, 1 mg per day of disulfiram (to control for the threat of a disulfiram-ethanol reaction), or placebo. Patients who were given either dosage of disulfiram were told that they were receiving the drug, and neither they nor the treatment or research staff knew the actual dosage. Patients in the third group (which served as a control for the counselling that all patients received) were given 50 mg of riboflavin, of which they were informed.

There were several significant findings: The first was a direct relationship between compliance with drug therapy (in any of the three treatments, including disulfiram 250 mg, disulfiram 1 mg, or riboflavin) and complete abstinence. The second was that, among the patients who drank, those on the therapeutic dosage of disulfiram had significantly fewer drinking days than did the other groups. There was also a suggestion that this smaller number of drinking days represented a real difference from pretreatment patterns, but this could not be measured accurately. There was no significant difference among the three groups in number of men totally abstinent, length of time to first drink, unemployment, or social stability. The authors concluded that disulfiram may be helpful in reducing the frequency of drinking in men who cannot remain abstinent (Fuller et al, 1986). An important limitation in the study was the fact that only 10 percent of patients screened were eligible and willing to participate. More than three-quarters of the 6,000 patients screened were ineligible, and, of those who were eligible, more than 60 percent refused to participate. Consequently, generalization of the results of the study to the larger population of alcoholics is limited.

Efforts to enhance the effectiveness of disulfiram by improving patient compliance have proceeded in two directions. Surgical implantation of depot pellets (in doses of from 500-1500 mg) in abdominal or inguinal areas provides a continued source of the drug for up to several years. While this technique appears not to result in significant elevations in blood acetaldehyde levels acutely in response to an alcohol challenge (Johnsen et al, 1987), there is clinical evidence that implants increase abstinence in alcoholics (Wilson et al, 1984). Because of the unpredictability of this route of administration, disulfiram implantation appears to have the greatest potential for use only in patients for whom little else holds promise, and disulfiram implantation is not approved for general use in the United States. A second approach to improving compliance is behavioral (Azrin et al, 1982). A trial program that involved five sessions of stimulus control training, role playing, and communication skills training was effective in promoting abstinence in married patients. When more intensive behavioral training and recreational and vocational counselling were added, single patients benefitted as well. Taken together, the evidence on disulfiram suggests that the patient's willingness to use the drug may reflect a motivation to modify behavior and that only with substantial efforts (either surgical or behavioral) can compliance be enhanced. Use of the drug outside of the context of a well-organized treatment program appears unwarranted.

CALCIUM CARBIMIDE. Calcium carbimide is in use in Europe and Canada, but it is not yet available for use in the United States; the usual dosage is 50 mg twice a day. In contrast to disulfiram, calcium carbimide binds rapidly and reversibly to aldehyde dehydrogenase. The result is a more rapid onset of action and a more rapid recovery of the capacity to metabolize acetaldehyde than with disulfiram. These characteristics may make the drug useful on an intermittent basis, rather than for long-term daily use (Liskow and Goodwin, 1987), which could reduce the potential for adverse effects associated with chronic administration. Although the acetaldehyde syndrome appears to be similar with both disulfiram and calcium carbimide, fewer serious side effects have been reported with the latter, which may reflect the fact that disulfiram has been in use longer and more widely than calcium carbimide. However, hepatitis has been reported with calcium carbimide and may be more severe than that associated with disulfiram (Vasquez et al, 1983).

Evaluation of the efficacy of calcium carbimide in the treatment of alcoholism is more limited than with disulfiram. A double-blind, placebo-controlled study in 24 nonalcoholics showed that while the initial acetaldehyde reaction was more severe in subjects pretreated with calcium carbimide, it was more easily overcome by continued drinking than in subjects receiving disulfiram (Peachey et al, 1983). There has not yet been a study of calcium carbimide comparable in size and scope to the recent multicenter trial of disulfiram (Fuller et al, 1986). As with disulfiram, calcium carbimide, combined with small doses of alcohol, may produce euphoria (Brown et al, 1983).

NITREFAZOLE. Originally developed as a trichomonacide, nitrefazole is available for use in Europe (Stockwell et al, 1984). There is, as yet, little experience with the drug as therapy for alcoholism, and it has not been approved for use in the United States. In combination with ethanol, nitrefazole produces a reaction (within one to four hours of a single oral dose of 800 mg) that may persist for up to six days, and these features may enhance compliance. However, there have been reports of serious side effects (including cardiovascular collapse) from the drug (Suokas et al, 1985), which if confirmed would limit its utility.

The Treatment of Psychiatric Co-Morbidity in Alcoholics

A variety of psychiatric disorders have been shown to co-exist with alcohol dependence (Meyer, 1986a). Because these comorbid disorders may predispose to the development or maintenance of heavy drinking, one approach to treating alcoholism has been to treat the concomitant psychopathology. Drug treatment has played an important part in this effort; and use of antidepressants, lithium, antipsychotics, and benzodiazepines has been most notable, given their use in the treatment of disorders characterized by negative emotional states. These states, including frustration, anger, anxiety, depression, and boredom, have been shown to contribute to relapse in a substantial proportion of alcoholics (Marlatt, 1985).

TRICYCLIC ANTIDEPRESSANTS. In general, placebo-controlled trials of tricyclic antidepressants (TCAs) in depressed alcoholics have not shown them to be useful beyond the first two weeks of abstinence. Research in this area is characterized by substantial methodologic problems, including a failure to distinguish primary from secondary depression, symptoms related to withdrawal from enduring disorders, and family-history-positive from family-history-negative cases. It may be that subgroups of depressives respond differently to antidepressant medication (Ciraulo and Jaffe, 1981).

Although depressive symptoms are common early in alcohol withdrawal, they frequently remit spontaneously with time (Dorus et al, 1987). For depression that persists well past the period of acute withdrawal, a TCA is the usual first-line drug. There is no evidence for greater efficacy of any particular TCA for treating depression in alcoholics (Sellers et al, 1981), and dosage may be a more important variable. Depressed alcoholics have been shown to clear imipramine more rapidly and to have lower blood levels on the same dosage than nonalcoholic depressives. The result was a greater improvement in depressive symptomatology among the nonalcoholics (Ciraulo et al, 1982). It is likely that the pharmacokinetics of other TCAs are similarly affected. To date, there have been no studies reported of the efficacy of TCAs for the treatment of depression in alcoholics in which adequate blood levels have been demonstrated.

MONOAMINE OXIDASE INHIBITORS (MAOIs). The similarities between atypical depression and the depression associated with alcoholism (including dysphoria and anxiety without typical neurovegetative signs) suggest that MAOIs may be of particular use in depressed alcoholics. MAOIs may also be helpful in alcoholics with panic disorder and mixed anxiety and depressive disorders. While the pharmacokinetics of MAOIs in alcoholics have not been studied, the potential for serious side effects (including hypertensive crisis precipitated by relapse) appears to limit the usefulness of these drugs in alcoholics.

LITHIUM CARBONATE. Evaluation of the usefulness of lithium carbonate in the treatment of alcoholism has focused on the relief of affective symptoms, as well as the effects on drinking behavior. A chart review based on data from one year prior to and one year subsequent to starting lithium showed some improvement in affective symptoms, but little change in drinking behavior in a group of manic alcoholics (Young et al, 1981). Three controlled trials of lithium in alcoholics have focused on depressive symptoms (Kline et al, 1974; Merry et al, 1976; Pond et al, 1981). All were plagued by high dropout rates, which make evaluation of the findings difficult. Lithium generally did not decrease depressive symptoms, but in two studies it appeared to result in a decrease in total incapacity due to drinking (Kline et al, 1974, Merry et al, 1976). In the third study (Pond et al, 1981), there was no difference between lithium and placebo.

In a study of alcoholics who were not selected for coexistent depression, Fawcett and colleagues (1987) found that compliance, with either lithium or placebo, was associated with abstinence. Compliant patients who were on active medication and who had therapeutic serum levels (0.4 meq/l or greater) were abstinent more often than compliant subjects with subtherapeutic lithium levels. Beyond the first six months, even the subjects who were compliant early on tended to stop their medication. Nevertheless, the association between early compliance and sobriety persisted, suggesting that the beneficial effects of lithium are most crucial in the early months after detoxification. Lithium was not found to affect mood in those patients who were depressed, indicating that the beneficial effect was not mediated by an antidepressant effect.

Lithium may produce its clinical effects in alcoholics via increased serotonergic tone (Zucker and Branchey, 1985). The role of serotonin (5-HT) will be discussed in a subsequent section of this chapter. Judd and Huey (1984) showed that, among inpatient alcoholics, lithium antagonized the intoxicating effects of ethanol and decreased the desire to continue drinking, compared with placebo. There was no significant difference in the effect of the drug on patients with coexistent affective disorders.

A multicenter, double-blind trial comparing lithium with placebo in depressed and nondepressed alcoholic veterans has recently been completed. The study may clarify the effect of lithium on both depressive symptoms and drinking behavior in alcoholics, but it will not shed light on other potentially lithium-responsive disorders that may be prevalent in alcoholics, such as attention deficit, anxiety, or antisocial personality disorders (Liskow and Goodwin, 1987). Results of this trial were not available at the time of this writing.

In general, there is empirical support for the use of lithium in the treatment of alcoholism. However, the results of a number of studies argue against an effect on mood as an explanation for the observed decreases in alcohol consumption. An advantage to the use of lithium is the ability to measure serum levels for routine assessment of compliance. However, because of the potential for a variety of unpleasant side effects, including serious toxicity, a role for lithium in the treatment of alcoholism remains to be defined.

BENZODIAZEPINES. Kissin (1975) reviewed a number of studies that showed chlordiazepoxide to be effective in the maintenance of alcoholics in long-term outpatient treatment. Other investigators, using double-blind, placebo-controlled trials, have shown a similar advantage to chlordiazepoxide (Ditman, 1961; Rosenberg, 1974). However, the potential for additive central nervous system depression produced by the concurrent use of alcohol and benzodiazepines is well recognized. Furthermore, the use of a benzodiazepine may itself result in tolerance and dependence, particularly in alcoholics (Schuster and Humphries, 1981). This concern, however, may be exaggerated (Bliding, 1978), and all benzodiazepines may not be equal in their capacity to produce dependence in alcoholics (Jaffe et al, 1983). Finally, for some alcoholics it may be preferable to substitute benzodiazepine dependence for alcohol dependence, in that the former may be less toxic (Jaffe and Ciraulo, 1985). Generally speaking, however, the use of benzodiazepines in alcoholics is best limited to the period of detoxification (Meyer, 1986b).

BUSPIRONE. Buspirone (Taylor et al, 1985) is a selective nonbenzodiazepine anxiolytic that has a site of action independent of the benzodiazepine-GABA complex. It appears to exert its effects largely via its activity at serotonergic receptors, where it is a potent agonist. In outpatients with moderate to severe anxiety, buspirone consistently relieved anxiety and associated depression. Buspirone was equal in efficacy to diazepam; however, the newer compound offers several advantages: 1) it is less sedating than diazepam or clorazepate; 2) it does not interact with alcohol to impair psychomotor skills; and 3) it does not appear to have abuse liability. A double-blind trial of buspirone in patients with mild to moderate alcohol abuse (Bruno and Casten, 1987) showed an advantage over placebo in terms of retention in treatment and on measures of anxiety and depression. There was no significant difference in alcohol consumption between the two treatment groups after eight weeks of treatment. An open trial by Kranzler (1987) showed that buspirone treatment in alcohol-dependent patients following detoxification reduced both anxiety and desire to drink in those with generalized anxiety.

BETA-BLOCKERS. As with buspirone, beta-blockers appear not to have potential for abuse or dependence. Several trials in alcoholics have shown that propranolol is superior to diazepam or placebo in reducing tension (Rada and Keller, 1979, Carlsson and Fasth, 1976), although these studies have not included data on the effects of the drug on drinking behavior. Data showing that atenolol increases retention in treatment and decreases anxiety and desire to drink (Horwitz et al, 1987) suggest that, in addition to being useful during alcohol withdrawal, beta-blockers may play a role in the rehabilitation of alcoholics.

ANTIPSYCHOTICS. Currently, antipsychotics are indicated only in alcoholics with a coexistent psychotic disorder or for the treatment of alcoholic hallucinosis (Naranjo and Sellers, 1986). Because of their capacity to lower seizure threshold, they should be used with caution in this population. Several placebo-controlled studies have found no advantage to the use of phenothiazines for treatment of anxiety, tension, and depression following detoxification (Jaffe and Ciraulo, 1985). In one study, phenothiazine treatment resulted in a decrease in tension and insomnia but also produced less improvement in measures of work and activity than did treatment with placebo (Hague et al, 1976).

Tiapride, a selective dopaminergic receptor blocker, has recently been used in Europe with favorable results in anxious and depressed alcoholics. It appears to reduce tremor, agitation, gastrointestinal disturbance, appetite disturbance, anxiety, depression, and craving for alcohol, without risk of dependence and without the sedative or parkinsonian side effects associated with typical antipsychotics. A recent double-blind, randomized trial of the drug in depressed and anxious alcoholics showed an advantage over placebo, in that the tiapride-treated subjects drank less; had longer periods of abstinence; showed decreased neuroticism, anxiety, and depression; expressed greater satisfaction with their social situations and physical health; and had fewer physical complications of alcoholism (Shaw et al, 1987). The study's findings, however, are limited by a high dropout rate. Given the equivocal results of trials of antipsychotics in alcoholics and the potential for adverse effects such as tardive dyskinesia, long-term use of these medications in alcoholics without coexistent psychotic disorder is unwarranted.

Drugs That May Directly Reduce Alcohol Consumption

Three major central neurotransmitter systems have been implicated in the reinforcing effects of ethanol: endogenous opioids (Martin et al, 1983), catecholamines (Amit et al, 1977), and serotonin (5-HT) (Myers and Melchior 1977, Naranjo et al, 1986). Although these systems may function interactively in their effects on drinking behavior, each will be discussed separately here.

There is experimental evidence that ethanol in high concentrations and the condensation products of ethanol metabolites and catecholamines interact with opiate receptors (Hiller et al, 1981, Lucchi et al, 1981). Despite the high face-validity of this mechanism for the reinforcing effects of ethanol, the bulk of available evidence argues against a role for condensation products such as tetrahydroisoquinolones (Amit et al, 1982). Other opiate-mediated mechanisms may be involved (Volpicelli et al, 1986), however, and these may explain the observation that naltrexone, an opiate antagonist, decreases ethanol consumption in experimental animals (Myers et al, 1986). Furthermore, a recent, double-blind, placebo-controlled trial in detoxified alcoholics suggests that the drug may have an important role in relapse prevention (Volpicelli et al, in preparation).

The evidence that catecholamines act to reinforce ethanol consumption is contradictory, but experimental evidence has implicated norepinephrine as a reinforcer of ethanol consumption in animals (Amit et al, 1977). The use of beta-blockers and alpha-agonists in the treatment of alcohol withdrawal has been discussed earlier in this chapter. In one series of outpatient alcoholics given atenolol in combination with oxazepam for alcohol withdrawal, the beta-blocker resulted in decreased desire to drink when compared with placebo (Horwitz et al, 1987). This has resulted in a one-year follow-up study to assess the effects of ongoing treatment with atenolol on relapse to drinking (L. Gottlieb, personal communication, March 22, 1988).

Mention has already been made of the effects of disulfiram on the enzyme dopamine-beta-hydroxylase, inhibition of which results in increased levels of dopamine (Ritchie, 1985). This increase may explain the euphoria-enhancing effects of the drug in combination with ethanol (Brown et al, 1983). A role for dopamine in the reinforcing effects of ethanol has also been proposed by Borg (1983), on the basis of a placebo-controlled trial of bromocriptine in chronic alcoholics. Patients treated with this dopamine agonist had a significantly better outcome at six months, as measured by desire to drink and psychosocial functioning. Drinking measures were also substantially better at outcome for the active drug group, but the lack of careful measurement made statistical evaluation impossible. Data indicating that both agonists and antagonists of catecholamines produce similar behavioral effects indicate the need for more experimental work to clarify what may be a complex interaction.

Of the neurochemical systems implicated in alcohol's reinforcing effects, the role of 5-HT has been best documented. Myers and Melchior (1977) and Naranjo and associates (1986) have reviewed the extensive experimental literature that links 5-HT to alcohol consummatory behavior. A variety of studies in animals and humans have linked 5-HT with violent and suicidal behavior and with alcoholism (Roy et al, 1987). In rodents, 5-HT agonists, particularly serotonin uptake inhibitors (SUIs), consistently decrease ethanol consumption (Naranjo et al, 1986). SUIs produce a decrease in intracranial self-stimulation, a paradigm usually considered analogous to drug self-administration (Naranjo et al, 1984). In humans the data are much more limited, but the results are similar. Zimelidine, an SUI that has been removed from clinical trials due to toxicity, was shown to attenuate ethanol consumption with both acute (Amit et al, 1985) and chronic administration (Naranjo et al, 1984). Other SUIs that have been tested for their effects on alcohol consumption in humans include fluoxetine (Gorelick, 1987) and citalopram (Naranjo et al, 1987). Although a variety of settings and methodologies have been employed, there is consistent evidence to suggest that SUIs may have an important role to play in alcoholism rehabilitation. Although their use has not yet been paired with a program of after-care involving skills training in relapse prevention (Marlatt, 1985), the results obtained by Naranjo and colleagues (1984, 1987) argues strongly in favor of such combined treatment.

SUMMARY AND CONCLUSIONS

We have selectively reviewed the literature on the drug treatment of alcoholism. In general, the use of pharmacologic agents that are currently available has added little to alcoholism treatment, with the exception of the central role that benzodiazepines play in the treatment of withdrawal. Recent developments, however, suggest that the adjunctive use of drugs with specific effects on identifiable neurotransmitter systems may eventually improve the treatment of acute intoxication and chronic alcoholism.

The identification of a benzodiazepine derivative (Ro15-4513) that interacts with the GABA-benzodiazepine receptor complex to reverse the pharmacologic and behavioral effects of ethanol (Suzdak et al, 1986a) has relevance for understanding the mechanism of action of the alcohols. Though not effective in reversing the effects of high ethanol concentrations, Ro15-4513 may be the first of a series of progressively more effective antagonists.

Benzodiazepines have supplanted most other sedative drugs in the treatment of alcohol withdrawal (Naranjo and Sellers, 1986). However, recent evidence suggests that the addition of a beta-blocker to standard benzodiazepine therapy may enhance both acute treatment and longer-term rehabilitative efforts. The careful combination of drugs, vitamin and mineral supplements to replete deficiencies, and good supportive care appears to provide a firm foundation upon which rehabilitative efforts may proceed.

Attention to psychiatric comorbidity is increasingly being recognized as essential to effective rehabilitation. While the relationship between substance use and psychiatric symptomatology is complex (Meyer, 1986b), new pharmacologic agents effective in treating the latter may provide important benefits for relapse prevention. Anxiolytics without evidence of abuse potential, such as buspirone (Bruno and Casten, 1987; Kranzler, 1987), and antidepressants with specific effects on neurotransmitter systems implicated in ethanol's reinforcing effects, such as the SUIs (Naranjo et al, 1986), warrant careful evaluation in the treatment of anxious and depressed alcoholics.

Finally, drugs that directly affect the desire to drink may have utility as adjuncts to either treatments oriented to relapse prevention (Marlatt, 1985) or treatment based on involvement with self-help groups, such as Alcoholics Anonymous. This is particularly true during the first months following detoxification, which may correspond to a period of protracted abstinence (Gorelick and Wilkins, 1986). Both SUIs and lithium have potential utility here. Multicenter trials, such as those conducted in the Veterans Administration system with disulfiram and lithium, appear to be an efficient approach to evaluation that may have far-reaching effects comparable to those of earlier Veterans Administration-based studies of antihypertensive drugs.

REFERENCES

Alkana RL, Parker ES, Cohen HB, et al: Reversal of ethanol intoxication in humans: an assessment of the efficacy of L-dopa, aminophylline, and ephedrine. Psychopharmacology 1977; 55:203–212

Allan AM, Harris RA: Involvement of neuronal chloride channels in ethanol intoxication, tolerance and dependence, in Recent Developments in Alcoholism, Volume 5. Edited by Galanter M. New York, Plenum Press, 1987

Amit Z, Levitan DE, Brown ZE, et al: Catecholaminergic involvement in alcohol's rewarding properties: implications for a treatment model for alcoholics. Adv Exp Med Biol 1977; 85A: 486–494

Amit Z, Smith BR, Brown ZW, et al: An examination of the role of TIQ alkaloids in alcohol intake: reinforcers, satiety agents or artifacts, in Beta-Carbolines and Tetrahydroisoquinolines. Edited by Bloom F, Barchas J, Sandler M, et al. New York, Alan R. Liss, Inc., 1982

Amit Z, Brown Z, Sutherland A, et al: Reduction in alcohol intake in humans as a function of treatment with zimelidine: implications for treatment, in Research Advances in New Psychopharmacological Treatments for Alcoholism. Edited by Naranjo CA, Sellers EM. Amsterdam, Elsevier, 1985

Azrin NH, Sisson RW, Meyers R, et al: Alcoholism treatment by disulfiram and community reinforcement therapy. J Behav Ther Exp Psychiatry 1982; 13:105–112

Bjorkqvist SE: Clonidine in alcohol withdrawal. Acta Psychiatr Scand 1975; 52:256–263

Bliding A: The abuse potential of benzodiazepines with special reference to oxazepam. Acta Psychiatr Scand 1978; 24(Suppl):111–116

Borg V: Bromocriptine in the prevention of alcohol abuse. Acta Psychiatr Scand 1983; 68:100–110

Britton KT, Ehlers CL, Koob GF: Is ethanol antagonist Ro15-4513 selective for ethanol? Science 1988; 239:648–650

Brown ZW, Amit Z, Smith BR, et al: Alcohol induced euphoria enhanced by disulfiram and calcium carbimide. Alcoholism: Clinical and Experimental Research 1983; 7:276–278

Bruno F, Casten G: Buspirone in the treatment of alcoholic patients. Presented at the 39th Institute on Hospital and Community Psychiatry, Boston, MA, October, 25–29, 1987

Carlsson C, Haggendal J: Arterial noradrenaline levels after ethanol withdrawal. Lancet 1967; 2:889

Carlsson C, Fasth BG: A comparison of the effects of propranolol and diazepam in alcoholics. Br J Addict 1976; 71:321–326

Ciraulo DA, Jaffe JH: Tricyclic antidepressants in the treatment of depression associated with alcoholism. J Clin Psychopharmacol 1981; 1:146–150

Ciraulo DA, Alderson LM, Chapron DJ, et al: Imipramine disposition in alcoholics. J Clin Psychopharmacol 1982; 2:2–7

Cushman P, Forbes R, Lerner W, et al: Alcohol withdrawal syndrome: clinical management with lofexidine. Alcoholism: Clinical and Experimental Research 1985; 9:103–108

Ditman KS: Evaluation of drugs in the treatment of alcoholics. Quarterly Journal of Studies on Alcohol 1961; 1(Suppl): 107–116

Dorus W, Kennedy J, Gibbons RD, et al: Symptoms and diagnosis of depression in alcoholics. Alcoholism: Clinical and Experimental Research 1987; 11:150–154

Dole VP, Fishman J, Goldfrank L, et al: Arousal of ethanol-intoxicated comatose patients with naloxone. Alcoholism: Clinical and Experimental Research 1982; 6:275–279

Eckardt MJ, Harford TC, Kaelber CT, et al: Health hazards associated with alcohol consumption. JAMA 1981; 246:648–666

Erickson CK: Amethystic agents in the treatment of alcohol intoxication, in The Pathogenesis of Alcoholism, Volume 7. Edited by Kissin B, Begleiter H. New York, Plenum Press, 1983

Favazza AR, Martin P: Chemotherapy of delirium tremens: a survey of physicians' preferences. Am J Psychiatry 1974; 131:1031–1033

Fawcett J, Clark DC, Aagesen CA, et al: A double-blind, placebo-controlled trial of lithium carbonate therapy for alcoholism. Arch Gen Psychiatry 1987; 44:248–256

Feldman DJ, Pattison EM, Sobel LC, et al: Outpatient alcohol detoxification: initial findings on 564 patients. Am J Psychiatry 1975; 132:407–412

Forney R, Hughes F: Effect of caffeine and alcohol on performance under stress of audio-feedback. Quarterly Journal of Studies on Alcohol 1965; 26:206–212

Fukumori R, Minegishi A, Satoh T, et al: Changes in the serotonin and 5-hydroxyindoleacetic acid contents in rat brain after ethanol and disulfiram treatments. Eur J Pharmacol 1980; 61:199–202

Fuller RK, Branchey L, Brightwell DR, et al: Disulfiram treatment of alcoholism: a Veteran's Administration cooperative study. JAMA 1986; 256:1449–1455

Gessner PK: Drug therapy of the alcohol withdrawal syndrome, in Biochemistry and Pharmacology of Ethanol, Volume 2. Edited by Majchrowicz E, Noble E. New York, Plenum Press, 1979

Gorelick DA: Effect of fluoxetine on alcohol consumption in male alcoholics. Alcoholism: Clinical and Experimental Research 1986; 10:13

Gorelick DA, Wilkins JN: Special aspects of human alcohol withdrawal, in Recent Developments in Alcoholism, Volume 4. Edited by Galanter M. New York, Plenum Press, 1986

Hague WH, Wilson LG, Dudley DL, et al: Post-detoxification drug treatment of anxiety and depression in alcoholic addicts. J Nerv Ment Dis 1976; 162:354–359

Harvey SC: Hypnotics and sedatives, in The Pharmacological Basis of Therapeutics, Seventh Edition. Edited by Gilman AG, Goodman LS, Rall TW, et al. New York, MacMillan Publishing Co, 1985

Hiller JM, Angel LM, Simon EJ: Multiple opiate receptors: alcohol selectively inhibits binding to delta receptors. Science 1981; 214:468–469

Horwitz RI, Kraus ML, Gottlieb LD: The efficacy of atenolol and the mediating effects of craving in the outpatient management of alcohol withdrawal. Clin Res 1987; 35:348A

Hughes FW, Forney RB: Dextro-amphetamine, ethanol and dextro-amphetamine-ethanol combinations on performance of human subjects stressed with delayed auditory feedback. Psychopharmacologia 1964; 6:234–238

Jacob MS, Zilm DH, MacLeod SM, et al: Propranol-associated confused states during alcohol withdrawal. J Clin Psychopharmacol 1983; 3:185–187

Jaffe JH, Ciraulo DA, Nies A, et al: Abuse potential of halazepam and diazepam in patients recently treated for acute alcohol withdrawal. Clin Pharmacol Ther 1983; 34:623–630

Jaffe JH, Ciraulo DA: Drugs used in the treatment of alcoholism, in The Diagnosis and Treatment of Alcoholism, Second Edition. Edited by Mendelson JH, Mello NK. New York, McGraw-Hill, 1985

Jeffcoate WJ, Cullen MH, Herbert M, et al: Prevention of effects of alcohol intoxication by naloxone. Lancet 1979; 2:1157–1159

Johnsen J, Stowell A, Bache-Wiig JE, et al: A double blind placebo controlled study of male alcoholics given subcutaneous disulfiram implantation. Br J Addict 1987; 82:607–613

Jones RW, Helrich AR: Treatment of alcoholism by physicians in private practice: a national survey. Quarterly Journal for Studies on Alcohol 1972; 33:117–131

Judd LL, Huey LY: Lithium antagonizes ethanol intoxication in alcoholics. Am J Psychiatry 1984; 141:1517–1521

Kalant H: Absorption, diffusion, distribution and elimination of ethanol: Effects on biological membranes, in Biology of Alcoholism, Volume 1. Edited by Kissin B, Begleiter H. New York, Plenum Press, 1971

Kissin B: The use of psychoactive drugs in the long-term treatment of chronic alcoholics. Ann NY Acad Sci 1975; 252:385–395

Kline NS, Wren JC, Cooper TB, et al: Evaluation of lithium therapy in chronic and periodic alcoholism. Am J Med Sci 1974; 268:15–22

Kolata G: New drug counters alcohol intoxication. Science 1986; 234:1198–1199

Koppanyi T, Canary JJ, Maengwyn-Davies GD: Problems in acute alcohol poisoning. Q J Stud Alcohol 1961; 1(Suppl):24–36

Kranzler HR: Preliminary studies on the effects of buspirone on craving in alcoholics. Presented at the Annual Meeting of the American College of Neuropsychopharmacology. San Juan, Puerto Rico, December 7–11, 1987

Kraus ML, Gottlieb LD, Horwitz RI, et al: Randomized clinical trial of atenolol in patients with alcohol withdrawal. N Engl J Med 1985; 313:905–909

Lerner WD, Fallon JH: The alcohol withdrawal syndrome. N Engl J Med 1985; 313:951–952

Lindros KO, Stowell A, Pikkarainen, et al: The disulfiram (Antabuse) reaction in male alcoholics: its efficient management by 4-methylpyrazole. Alcoholism: Clinical and Experimental Research 1981; 5:528–530

Liskow BI, Goodwin DW: Pharmacological treatment of alcohol intoxication, withdrawal and dependence: a critical review. J Stud Alcohol 1987; 48:356–370

Lucchi L, Bosio A, Spano PF, et al: Action of alcohol and salsolinol on opiate receptor function. Brain Res 1981; 232:506–510

Manhem P, Nilsson LH, Moberg A-L, et al: Alcohol withdrawal: effects of clonidine treatment on sympathetic activity, the renin-aldosterone system, and clinical symptoms. Alcoholism: Clinical and Experimental Research 1985; 9:238–243

Marlatt GA: Relapse prevention: theoretical rationale and overview of the model, in Relapse Prevention. Edited by Marlatt GA, Gordon JR. New York, Guilford Press, 1985

Martin A, Pilotto R, Singer G, et al: The suppression of ethanol self-injection by buprenorphine. Pharmacol Biochem Behav 1983; 19:985–986

McGovern MP: Comparative evaluation of medical vs. social treatment of alcohol withdrawal syndrome. J Clin Psychol 1983; 39:791–803

Merry J, Reynolds CM, Bailey J, et al: Prophylactic treatment of alcoholism by lithium carbonate. Lancet 1976; 2:481–482

Meyer RE: How to understand the relationship between psychopathology and addictive disorders: another example of the chicken and the egg, in Psychopathology and Addictive Disorders. Edited by Meyer RE. New York, Guilford Press, 1986a

Meyer RE: Anxiolytics and the alcoholic patient. J Stud Alcohol 1986b; 47:269–273

Moskowitz G, Chalmers TC, Sacks HS, et al: Deficiencies of clinical trials of alcohol withdrawal. Alcoholism: Clinical and Experimental Research 1983; 7:42–46

Myers RD, Melchior CL: Alcohol and alcoholism: role of serotonin, in Serotonin in Health and Disease, Volume II. Edited by Essman WB. New York, Spectrum Publications, Inc., 1977

Myers RD, Borg S, Mossberg R: Antagonism by naltrexone of voluntary alcohol selection in the chronically drinking macaque monkey. Alcohol 1986; 3:383–388

Naranjo CA, Sellers EM: Clinical assessment and pharmacotherapy of the alcohol withdrawal syndrome, in Recent Developments in Alcoholism, Volume 4. Edited by Galanter M. New York, Plenum Press, 1986

Naranjo CA, Sellers EM, Chater K, et al: Non-pharmacological interventions in acute alcohol withdrawal. Clin Pharmacol Ther 1983; 34:214–219

Naranjo CA, Sellers EM, Roach CA, et al: Zimelidine-induced variations in alcohol intake by nondepressed heavy drinkers. Clin Pharmacol Ther 1984; 35:374–381

Naranjo CA, Sellers EM, Lawrin MO: Modulation of ethanol intake by serotonin uptake inhibitors. J Clin Psychiatry 1986; 47(Suppl):16–22

Naranjo CA, Sellers EM, Sullivan JT, et al: The serotonin uptake inhibitor citalopram attenuates ethanol intake. Clin Pharmacol Ther 1987; 41:266–274

Nasrallah HA: Vulnerability to disulfiram psychosis. West J Med 1979; 130:575–577

Noble EP: Pharmacotherapy in the detoxification and treatment of alcoholism, in Psychiatry Update, Vol. 3. Edited by Grinspoon L. Washington, DC, American Psychiatric Press, Inc., 1984

Peachey E, Zilm DH, Robinson GM, et al: A placebo-controlled double-blind comparative clinical study of the disulfiram and calcium carbimide-acetaldehyde mediated ethanol reactions in social drinkers. Alcoholism: Clinical and Experimental Research 1983; 7:180–187

Pond SM, Becker CE, Vandervoort R, et al: An evaluation of the effects of lithium in the treatment of chronic alcoholism. I. Clinical results. Alcoholism: Clinical and Experimental Research 1981; 5:247–251

Poutanen P: Experience with carbamazepine in the treatment of withdrawal symptoms in alcohol abusers. Br J Addict 1979; 74:201–204

Rada RR, Kellner R: Drug treatment in alcoholism, in Psychopharmacology Update: New and Neglected Areas. Edited by Davis JM, Greenblatt D. New York, Grune & Stratton, 1979

Ritchie JM: The aliphatic alcohols, in The Pharmacological Basis of Therapeutics, Seventh Edition. Edited by Gilman AG, Goodman LS, Rall TW, et al. New York, MacMillan Publishing Co., 1985

Rosenberg CM: Drug maintenance in the outpatient treatment of chronic alcoholism. Arch Gen Psychiatry 1974; 30:373–377

Roy A, Linnoila M, Virkkunen M: Serotonin and alcoholism. Substance Abuse 1987; 8:21–27

Schuster CL, Humphries RH: Benzodiazepine dependence in alcoholics. Conn Med 1981; 45:11–13

Sellers EM, Kalant H: Alcohol intoxication and withdrawal. N Engl J Med 1976; 294:757–762

Sellers EM, Zilm DH, Degani NC: Comparative efficacy of propanolol and chlordiazepoxide in alcohol withdrawal. J Stud Alcohol 1977; 38:2096–2108

Sellers EM, Naranjo CA, Peachey JE: Drugs to decrease alcohol consumption. N Engl J Med 1981; 305:1255–1262

Sellers EM, Naranjo CA, Harrison M, et al: Diazepam loading: simplified treatment of alcohol withdrawal. Clin Pharmacol Ther 1983; 34:822–826

Shaw GK, Majumdar SK, Waller S, et al: Tiapride in the long-term management of alcoholics of anxious or depressive temperament. Br J Psychiatry 1987; 150:164–168

Stockwell T, Sutherland G, Edwards G: The impact of a new alcohol sensitizing agent (nitrefazole) on craving in severely dependent alcoholics. Br J Addict 1984; 79:403–409

Suokas A, Kupari M, Petterson J, et al: The nitrefazole-ethanol interaction in man. Cardiovascular responses and the accumulation of acetaldehyde and catecholamines. Alcoholism: Clinical and Experimental Research 1986; 9:221–227

Suzdak PDH, Glowa JR, Crawley JN, et al: A selective imidazobenzodiazepine antagonist of ethanol in the rat. Science 1986a; 234:1243–1247

Suzdak PD, Schwartz RD, Skolnick P, et al: Ethanol stimulates gamma-aminobutyric acid receptor-mediated chloride transport in rat brain synaptoneurosomes. Proc Natl Acad Sci 1986b; 83:4071–4075

Taylor DP, Eison M, Riblet LA, et al: Pharmacological and clinical effects of buspirone. Pharmacol Biochem Behav 1985; 23:687–694

Vasquez JJ, Diaz de Otazu R, Guillen FJ, et al: Hepatitis induced by drugs used as alcohol aversion therapy. Diagnostic Histopathology 1983; 6:29–37

Volpicelli JR, Davis MA, Olgin JE: Naltrexone blocks the post-shock increase of ethanol consumption. Life Sciences 1986; 38:841–847

Whitfield EL, Thompson G, Lamb A, et al: Detoxification of 1,024 alcoholic patients without psychoactive drugs. JAMA 1978; 293:1409–1410

Wilson A, Blanchard R, Davidson W, et al: Disulfiram implantation: a dose response trial. J Clin Psychiatry 1984; 45:242–247

Young LD, Patel M, Keeler MH: The effect of lithium carbonate on alcoholism in 20 male patients with concurrent major affective disorder, in Currents in Alcoholism, Volume Eight. Edited by Galanter M. New York, Grune & Stratton, 1981

Zucker DK, Branchey L: Lithium, CNS serotonergic tone, and intoxication. Am J Psychiatry 1985; 142:886–887

Afterword

by Roger E. Meyer, M.D.

Where is the alcoholism field going? The preceding chapters highlight some likely directions for the next five years. In Chapter 13, "Models of Alcoholism," Meyer and Babor describe the historical aspects of this disorder, the evolution of the disease model, and the current status of genetically based models which may account for the psychopathological heterogeneity of the disorder. Future research on the disease concept must come from neurobiological research. In Chapter 14, Cloninger, Dinwiddie, and Reich describe the status of research in human genetics in the alcohol field which now seems ripe for molecular genetic studies in extended family pedigrees. The availability of possible phenotypic markers of risk in sons of alcoholics, and the definition of distinct heritable subtypes of the disorder, makes alcoholism a very promising area for genetics research. In Chapter 15, "Neurobiology of Alcoholic Action and Alcoholism," Bloom describes the challenge: More than 50 percent of the human genome is devoted to the brain; much less than one percent can now be specified. Despite the limitations in our knowledge, a number of leads begin to suggest mechanisms of alcohol intoxication. In his clear and concise manner, Bloom describes the status of this research. The absence of a specific alcohol *receptor* increases the complexity of the task, but the hierarchial strategy described by Bloom represents a workable approach to an understanding of the neurobiological basis of alcohol intoxication, reinforcement, tolerance, withdrawal symptoms, and dependence. The findings in neurobiology and in human genetics find a meeting point in the field of molecular genetics. In Chapter 16, by Rounsaville and Kranzler, Chapter 17, by Frances, Galanter, and Miller, and Chapter 18, by Kranzler and Orrok, the status of clinical research and clinical practice in the alcohol field are described. Issues of psychiatric comorbidity are also discussed in each of these chapters. This psychiatric heterogeneity must be considered in the contexts of pharmacotherapy and the extant psychosocial approaches to treatment and rehabilitation. In all of this, psychiatry must play a critical role.

To a very strong degree, the chapters in this section cohere nicely with each other. Basic research in neurobiology and genetics will increasingly augment clinical practice, while the nature of alcohol dependence described by the new *DSM-III-R* criteria (and the psychiatric heterogeneity of patient populations) will continue to affect basic and clinical investigations. It will be the challenge of the next decade to integrate research findings into clinical practice, as research moves beyond its present frontier.

This work was supported by the National Institute on Alcohol Abuse and Alcoholism grant 5 P50 AA03510.

IV

Psychiatry and the Law

Contents

Section IV

Psychiatry and the Law

Foreword

by Paul S. Appelbaum, M.D., Section Editor

Seven years ago, in the first volume of this Annual Review series (then entitled *Psychiatry 1982: The American Psychiatric Association Annual Review*) Alan Stone edited a section entitled "Law and Psychiatry" (Stone, 1982). Developments in the intervening years persuaded the editors of the series that a new section on the subject was needed. A reading of the chapters that follow will, I believe, confirm the correctness of their judgment.

I was a contributor to that first section on law and psychiatry. Being asked to edit its successor has afforded me the opportunity to reflect on the changes in psychiatry's relationship with the law that have transpired in the interim. To a large extent, these differences are a function of new actors setting the mental health law agenda and advocating new goals and new methods of achieving them. The initial section on law and psychiatry summarized the results of the first wave of mental health law reform in the 1970s; the chapters in this section reveal the effects of a second, less radical but no less important, period of change.

Our predecessors in these pages described the impact of laws and court decisions resulting from concerted efforts by a relatively young mental health bar to transform the nature of psychiatric care systems. Steeped in the civil libertarian ethos of the early 1970s, encouraged by judges willing to order massive changes in mental health systems when constitutional violations were found, and determined to eliminate the worst abuses in public facilities, these energetic advocates undertook litigation that changed the historic patterns of regulation of psychiatric care.

Their earliest successes came in court decisions and statutory changes that altered the traditional standard for involuntary commitment—based on patients' needs for care and treatment—in favor of a dangerousness-based approach (Stromberg, 1982). Bowing to the arguments of the mental health bar, courts and legislatures agreed that the older standards were distressingly, even unconstitutionally, vague. Further, the existing statutes swept into the mental health system a group of people who could not be said to be endangering themselves or others, but who required psychiatric treatment for their own benefit. To civil libertarians, this exercise of paternalism in the absence of threatened harm was anathema. Beginning in California with the Lanterman-Petris-Short Act, in 1969, and stimulated by subsequent court decisions, nearly every state in the nation altered its commitment criteria to embody a more circumscribed approach to involuntary hospitalization. Commitment was limited to those (in a variety of formulations) thought likely to be harmful to themselves or others. Simultaneously, procedures for commitment were tightened and made more analogous to those found in the criminal justice system.

As Chapter 21 by Hoge, Appelbaum, and Geller demonstrates, this was not the end of the story. Within a few years of their adoption, the dangerousness-oriented standards had provoked considerable dissatisfaction. From a societal point of view, they were seen as a major component of a policy of deinstitutionalization that bordered on deliberate neglect of the severely mentally ill. Although it is unclear to what extent statutory change, as opposed to progressive restriction of available inpatient beds and a crippled system of community-based care, is responsible for the spectre of homeless mentally ill people in our urban areas, the new statutes have taken a large share of the blame. Few clinicians are unable to offer anecdotes of people, desperately in need of care, who have been allowed to return to a miserable, psychotic existence in a shelter or on the streets because they did not qualify for commitment under the operative dangerousness criteria. From a professional point of view, the new standards were equally distressing, asking psychiatrists to become prognosticators of violence—an extraordinarily difficult, many would say impossible, task—rather than assessors of patients' need for treatment.

There appeared to be little question in most people's minds that the commitment system had swung too far from its paternalistic roots. The last decade, particularly the last five years, has been dominated by efforts of a new coalition of advocates, including family members of the mentally ill and mental health professionals, to broaden criteria for commitment, while leaving procedural protections for mentally ill individuals predominantly intact. Hoge and colleagues review the status of what promises to be the next important step in this direction: the development of systems of involuntary outpatient care. Although problematic from a legal perspective and beyond the capacity of many community-based systems to implement at this time, outpatient commitment can be seen as yet another response to the highly restrictive commitment policies of the 1970s.

Along with frontal attacks on the constitutional legitimacy of commitment statutes, civil liberties-oriented litigators of the 1970s argued that, under our Constitution, state interference with an individual's liberty had to be limited to the least restrictive alternative necessary to achieve the government's ends (Klein, 1982). Since they believed that community-based care often would be possible for patients who would otherwise be committed, advocates of mental health law reform saw the least restrictive alternative doctrine as a means of compelling the states to create community-based systems of care. The controversy over the least restrictive alternative—once fighting words in mental health law debates—has cooled, as the doctrine has seen its theoretical successes unmatched by practical impact. So much of a commonplace has this idea become that the least restrictive alternative is now a component of many state mental health codes. On the other hand, its presence is often a formality, as, in the absence of good community-based care, involuntary hospitalization is frequently the only alternative. The failure of the least restrictive alternative rationale to achieve the original goal of forcing creation of community-based mental-health systems is closely related to the fate of another of the major mental health law initiatives of the 1970s.

If the attack on civil commitment can be seen as the first prong of the civil libertarian agenda for mental health law, the second, equally important, prong was the desire to create a constitutionally grounded right to treatment (Mills,

1982). This effort was predicated on the unfairness of a system that involuntarily hospitalized mentally ill persons, but provided them with inadequate or even no meaningful treatment. There is still debate over the motives of legal advocates for a right to treatment. A skeptical view holds that they never believed the states would provide adequate care, and thus sought the establishment of a right to treatment to provoke the courts to order wholesale closure of mental hospitals, on the basis that "if you can't treat them, you can't keep them." Other observers are more generous in granting the advocates a real desire to improve state hospital conditions and a belief that they possessed a tool that could do so. As usual, the truth probably lies somewhere in between, with the major participants having different or mixed agendas.

Just months after the forerunner of this section appeared in 1982, the U.S. Supreme Court addressed the question of a constitutional right to treatment in *Youngberg v. Romeo*. It recognized only a circumscribed right: Patients might be entitled to freedom from assault and unnecessary restraint, but not to the array of treatment programs for which advocates of the right had argued. It seemed to most observers as though a broadly conceived right to treatment—which, alone among the major items in the mental health law agenda, had united lawyers and psychiatrists—was dead. Legally that conclusion was premature. Courts so inclined have found creative ways around the Supreme Court's restrictions. The Civil Rights of Institutionalized Persons Act (CRIPA) has given the U.S. Justice Department a mechanism for asking the courts to intervene in institutions where patients' rights are being abused, and ways have been found to apply state laws to the same end. The right to treatment still lives, but its partisans function more as a guerilla force, striking here and there in the night, than as an army capable of sweeping through the nation's inadequate state hospitals (Appelbaum, 1987).

But the libertarian agenda of the 1970s, targeted towards reducing governmental power over the mentally ill, has not disappeared altogether. The effort to sever the link between the state's power to commit patients and to treat those patients with medication has achieved a marked measure of success in the courts. Where two major cases dominated discussion of the right to refuse treatment in the early 1980s (Gutheil, 1982), Hoge and colleagues note that today a slew of courts have found such a right exists on a variety of legal grounds. Although the extent of the federal constitutional right is uncertain, given the U.S. Supreme Court's failure to resolve the issue to date, state courts are increasingly basing a right to refuse treatment on state common law, statutory, and constitutional grounds.

The orientation of the first generation of mental health law advocacy toward constitutional argument aimed at dismemberment of public mental health systems no longer characterizes the cutting edge of mental-health law. President Reagan's impact on the courts has resulted in a judiciary unwilling to order radical change, on constitutional grounds, of the sort usually considered a legislative prerogative. Although the old issues still retain some vitality, the interest of many advocates has shifted to a second generation of issues that might be considered more "needs-oriented" than "rights-oriented." In-hospital advocacy, supported by federal funding, more often focuses on the adequacy of care provided individual patients, than on class actions designed to reorient systems. Along the same lines, many legal advocates now engage in extensive lobbying and litigation to protect and expand funding for entitlement and service programs for the mentally ill, such as Social Security Disability. While significant differences in perspective on many issues remain between clinicians and the mental health bar, this new emphasis tends to accentuate the commonalities of their concerns (Rubinstein, 1986).

No better example of these changes can be found than that discussed in Schwartz and Roth's chapter (Chapter 20) on informed consent. The struggle over the right to refuse treatment—essentially an effort to extend the doctrine of informed consent to patients involuntarily committed—has held psychiatry's attention, while much more significant, though less noticed, progress has been made applying informed consent to the vastly larger group of voluntary patients. As Schwartz and Roth explain, psychiatry is no longer exempt from the premise that patients have the right to determine what medical interventions should be performed for their benefit. Efforts to apply informed consent in psychiatry have not proceeded from a desire to destroy institutional care, but out of a belief that substantial improvement in the therapeutic relationship and the quality of care will result. Whatever the reality of that conviction, it reflects motives very different from those behind the attempts in the 1970s to impede the ability of psychiatrists to treat patients in need.

Yet, like the earlier issues, informed consent comes with its share of dilemmas for psychiatrists. How can a doctrine premised on rational discourse between physician and patient be applied in settings where the absence of rationality is the very precipitant of treatment? Already, nearly a decade ago, the significance of patients' impaired competence to consent was recognized (Roth, 1982). Today it achieves even greater importance. Can institutionalized patients meet the other prerequisite of informed consent, the ability to decide without undue coercion? To what extent can information disclosure be limited, modified, or delayed in acute settings, particularly when dealing with conditions that may soon resolve with treatment, rendering patients then more capable of dealing with the implications of prolonged therapy? Although psychiatry is not alone in coping with the difficulties raised by informed consent, its peculiar problems, as Schwartz and Roth demonstrate, require the most careful consideration.

A second example of the new mental-health law agenda can be found in the attention being given to psychiatric malpractice. In the early 1980s, psychiatrists enjoyed relative immunity from suits by patients alleging professional negligence. Malpractice as an independent topic was not even addressed in the predecessor to this section. The one chapter on psychiatrists' obligations to their patients dealt with confidentiality—then, as now, an important issue—but noted that the weakness of legal remedies for breach of confidentiality rendered the duty to respect patients' confidences more of an ethical than legal concern (Appelbaum, 1982). That is certainly no longer the case. Although psychiatry is still a low-risk specialty, data presented by Wettstein in Chapter 19 on malpractice indicate that today approximately four percent of psychiatrists will be sued by their patients each year. Malpractice law has replaced constitutionally based mental health law as the primary stimulus for change in psychiatric practices, and, though problematic in some respects, the focus here is again on improving, rather than deconstructing, both institutional and noninstitutional psychiatry.

One of the most important areas of psychiatric malpractice concern that has developed in the last several years is the duty to protect potential victims of their patients' violent acts. This obligation, first enunciated with regard to outpatients in the mid-1970s in *Tarasoff v. Regents of the University of California (1974, 1976)*, had been adopted in only a handful of states by the early 1980s. Today the obligation has been recognized by approximately a score of courts and, at this writing, 20 percent of our state legislatures. In states where no law exists on the subject, clinicians are uniformly advised to act as if some version of a duty to protect were in place. Like informed consent, it has become a cornerstone of daily practice.

Other issues that were relatively hidden not long ago are now also serving as a frequent basis for litigation. Adverse effects of psychopharmacologic agents, as Dr. Wettstein notes, including the development of tardive dyskinesia, are increasingly the focus of malpractice allegations. Another major basis for litigation highlighted in Chapter 19—sexual contact with patients—is a disturbing feature of contemporary psychiatric care. Despite threats of malpractice suits, real risk of loss of licensure, and a consensus that erotic involvement with patients is unethical, psychiatrists continue to succumb to the temptations evoked by their intense involvements with their patients. Is it overly optimistic to hope that this problem will fade in prominence over the next decade?

Thus far we have considered the impact of law on psychiatric practice in the context of a changing set of goals and concerns, but the relationship between law and psychiatry has always been a two-way street. Although there was no lack of practical and ethical dilemmas for psychiatrists who lent their expertise to the courts in the early part of this decade (Halleck, 1982), Showalter and Fitch demonstrate in Chapter 24 that the situation has become still more complex. The debate over the trial of John Hinckley and the role of psychiatrists in his acquittal on the basis of insanity focused public and professional attention on what psychiatrists do in court. Their ethical standards, indeed the possibility even of formulating ethical standards, have been called into question. Simultaneously, the demand for forensic psychiatric services has increased, as the courts look for help in resolving morally loaded issues that often involve imposition of the death penalty. Psychiatrists' clinical skills in performing the requisite evaluations answer only half the need; they must be equally adept at dealing with the ethical problems that arise.

To whom does the psychiatrist in court owe allegiance, and how should that affect his or her evaluation and testimony? Can the effects of being hired by, and therefore aligned with, one side of a case ever be mitigated? What is the basis for our participation in courtroom proceedings, particularly in the criminal arena? Is such behavior consonant with our ethical responsibilities as physicians? If so, in general, do *any* ethical limits exist on the functions that we can perform at the request of the courts or other components of the criminal justice system?

Halleck's chapter in this section highlights one function of psychiatrists in court that has always evoked more attention and concern than any other: our participation in trials where a defendant's criminal responsibility is at issue. Controversy pervades the entire subject, from the philosophical rationale for responsibility and nonresponsibility, to the extent to which psychiatrists should address the ultimate issue of legal insanity in their testimony, to the mechanisms by which those found to lack responsibility should be supervised and treated. We appear to be making progress with the last issue, as exemplified by the

Oregon model of caring for offenders found not responsible by reason of insanity, now adopted in several other states, but the more basic questions remain.

Indeed, the problems grow more complex. New diagnostic categories carry implications for individuals' abilities to control or recognize the implications of their behavior. Post-traumatic stress disorder, pathological gambling, premenstrual syndrome, and syndromes associated with a variety of victimization experiences have all attained prominence recently, as purported exculpatory factors in criminal violence. In fact, so concerned have we become with the implications our diagnoses hold for the courts' determinations of criminal responsibility, that new formal diagnostic categories are now opposed because of their presumed impact in the courts—witness the fate of coercive paraphilic rapism. The reciprocal impact of the courts on psychiatry demonstrates Halleck's thesis of the centrality of questions concerning the impact of illness on individual responsibility to both psychiatry and law.

Finally, Chapter 23 by Schetky, on child psychiatry and the law, reviews and contributes to a literature that barely existed when the first section on law and psychiatry in this series appeared. For many years, child psychiatrists interacted with the legal system only in the context of juvenile-delinquency proceedings and disputes over child custody. While there is no gainsaying the continuing importance of these areas, in the last decade we have seen the rapid evolution of numerous other issues. Many child psychiatrists now frequently evaluate sexual abuse and other forms of abuse and neglect. They are called upon to assess children's capacity to testify in court, often in abuse cases, and their competence to consent to medical procedures independently of their parents. Waiver of juveniles to adult courts is another nascent issue that almost always calls for psychiatric input.

As the contributions of child psychiatrists have been sought increasingly by the courts, many have felt pushed to the limits of their expertise while addressing the new questions that have arisen. Is it possible to determine whether the best interests of a child lie in continuing to have contact with a biological parent after placement with a foster family or in adoption and severance of the parental relationship? Can we say whether children born by surrogate mothers should remain in contact with them, even though raised by a different set of parents? What is the impact likely to be of a young child testifying in court against a sexually abusive parent? Do new technologies aimed at protecting children who testify—e.g., testifying via closed-circuit video—truly detoxify the experience? Like the adult forensic realm, child forensic psychiatry struggles with exceedingly complex dilemmas, many crying out for empirical investigation.

Society's concerns about the manner in which psychiatric care is delivered, and the simultaneous desire for psychiatric participation in adjudications of a diverse nature, have combined to create continued ferment in that hybrid field called law and psychiatry. The issues are as challenging as any in psychiatry, and their resolutions call for the keenest clinical and analytical skills. The contributors to this section, for whom law and psychiatry is both a subspecialty and a passion, hope that the following chapters will convey the fascination we feel for this ever-evolving field. More importantly, we trust that the information and perspectives offered will assist the clinical psychiatrist who is dealing with the constant challenge presented by the legal system in the practice of psychiatry.

REFERENCES

Appelbaum PS: Confidentiality in psychiatric treatment, in Psychiatry 1982: The American Psychiatric Association Annual Review. Edited by Grinspoon L. Washington, DC, American Psychiatric Association, 1982

Appelbaum PS: Resurrecting the right to treatment. Hosp Community Psychiatry 1987; 38:703–704, 721

Gutheil TG: The right to refuse treatment, in Psychiatry 1982: The American Psychiatric Association Annual Review. Edited by Grinspoon L. Washington, DC, American Psychiatric Association, 1982

Halleck SL: The role of the psychiatrist in the criminal justice system, in Psychiatry 1982: The American Psychiatric Association Annual Review. Edited by Grinspoon L. Washington, DC, American Psychiatric Association, 1982

Klein JI: The least restrictive alternative: more about less, in Psychiatry 1982: The American Psychiatric Association Annual Review. Edited by Grinspoon L. Washington, DC, American Psychiatric Association, 1982.

Mills MJ: The right to treatment: little law but much impact, in Psychiatry 1982: The American Psychiatric Association Annual Review. Edited by Grinspoon L. Washington, DC, American Psychiatric Association, 1982

Roth LH: Competency to consent to or refuse treatment, in Psychiatry 1982: The American Psychiatric Association Annual Review. Edited by Grinspoon L. Washington, DC, American Psychiatric Association, 1982

Rubenstein L: Treatment of the mentally ill: legal advocacy enters the second generation. Am J Psychiatry 1986; 143:1264–1269

Stone AA (Ed): Law and psychiatry, in Psychiatry 1982: The American Psychiatric Association Annual Review. Edited by Grinspoon L. Washington, DC, American Psychiatric Association, 1982

Stromberg CD: Developments concerning the legal criteria for civil commitment: who are we looking for? in Psychiatry 1982: The American Psychiatric Association Annual Review. Edited by Grinspoon L. Washington, DC, American Psychiatric Association, 1982

Tarasoff v. Regents of the University of California, 529 P.2d 553 (Cal. 1974), 551 P.2d 334 (Cal. 1976)

Youngberg v. Romeo, 457 U.S. 308 (1982)

Chapter 19

Psychiatric Malpractice

by Robert M. Wettstein, M.D.

Much of contemporary medical and psychiatric practice is guided with an eye to the possibility of an adverse clinical outcome, with its attendant legal consequences. Today, a lawsuit against the physician for professional liability, even if unsuccessful, can result in disruption and harm to one's private practice, an increase in the cost of liability insurance, social and professional stigma, and considerable emotional distress and dysfunction. If successful, a suit can be the initial step in revocation of professional license, ejection from membership in professional societies, loss of hospital privileges, or personal financial loss, even bankruptcy.

This chapter will review some of the important elements in psychiatric malpractice, discuss several of the most significant areas of litigation for the psychiatrist, and highlight several principles of professional liability prevention.

OVERVIEW OF THE PROBLEM

Frequency and Severity of Psychiatric Malpractice Claims

Several medical malpractice "crises" have been declared in the last two decades. It is, however, more accurate to refer to these as crises in medical malpractice insurance rather than in iatrogenic injury. In the 1970s, many insurance companies withdrew from the medical professional liability market, leaving physicians to select from fewer, if any, insurers. Many state medical associations then initiated their own insurance companies, which provided coverage when none was previously available. Joint insurance underwriting associations and reinsurance exchanges were also established (Posner, 1986). In the 1980s, the malpractice crisis has been experienced in escalating costs insurance coverage for physicians, approaching $200,000 a year for some high risk specialists (New York Times, 1988). In response to this, access to certain specialists has been reduced in some areas. In addition, the cost to society of medical professional liability has been of increasing concern; direct and indirect liability costs accounted for one-half of the increase in society's expenditures on physicians' services from 1983 to 1984 (Reynolds et al, 1987). This includes higher liability insurance premiums, changes in clinical practice designed to reduce liability risk, and other unreimbursed costs incurred by physicians in managing liability claims. The costs of litigating medical malpractice claims in the courts (for example, fees for attorneys, courtrooms, and courtroom personnel) are an additional, though sometimes inconspicuous, burden to society.

The recent changes in medical professional liability should be viewed in the context of injury litigation in the United States in general. Broader legal standards of responsibility, as well as an increased readiness by injured individuals to seek legal redress, have increased the liability of professional service providers, such as physicians, attorneys, accountants, and real estate agents, among many others. Product manufacturers and municipalities have been similarly confronted by increased litigation for the use of their products and facilities. Litigation for such agents as environmental pollutants (*toxic torts*), asbestos, contraceptives, and vaccines have been particularly affected. Yet some areas of insurance, such as automobile liability, life, and property, have remained relatively stable (Huber, 1987).

There seems little doubt that medical malpractice claims have increased in incidence and severity (amount per paid claim) in the last two decades, yet the magnitude of these increases remains in dispute. Data about medical professional liability is compiled from a variety of sources, including surveys of physicians and insurers and court records from various jurisdictions (Zuckerman et al, 1986; Danzon, 1986). Some statistics include malpractice claims with other types of civil lawsuits, such as personal injury claims (automobile accidents) and product liability claims, making it difficult to assess the frequency of malpractice suits alone. Severity data can be presented with regard to claims, settlements, jury awards, or actual award (jury awards are sometimes subsequently reduced by a court). Severity of claims data are sometimes presented as the mean award rather than the median award. The increase in million and multimillion dollar claims, still relatively few in number compared to the total volume of litigation, skews the mean data but not the median data (Localio, 1985).

According to recent American Medical Association (AMA) data, the average annual incidence of professional liability claims per 100 physicians increased from 3.2 prior to 1981 to 10.1 in 1985 (AMA, 1987). Between 1981 and 1985, 25.4 percent of physicians were sued once; by 1985, 36.5 percent of physicians had been sued at least once in their careers (AMA, 1987). Between 1982 and 1985, physicians' insurance premiums increased by 21.9 percent annually, a total of 81.0 percent over the three years (AMA Board of Trustees, 1987).

Lawsuits against psychiatrists are relatively infrequent compared to those against nonpsychiatric physicians. Prior to 1981, the average incidence of professional liability claims per 100 psychiatrists was 0.6; this increased to 2.4 in 1985 (AMA, 1987). In 1982, more than 4 percent of psychiatrists insured through the American Psychiatric Association (APA) program filed a claim for insurance coverage (Slawson, 1984). Between 1981 and 1985, 10.3 percent of psychiatrists were sued at least once; by 1985, 15.8 percent of psychiatrists had been sued at least once in their careers (AMA, 1987).

This relatively lower liability for psychiatric physicians has been ascribed to a variety of factors: 1) the imprecise nature, definition, and taxonomy of psychiatric disorders; 2) difficulty establishing the origin of psychiatric injuries, given our limited knowledge about etiology; 3) problems in establishing definitive clinical standards, given the diversity of clinical techniques and strategies; 4) reluctance of psychiatric patients to publicize their psychiatric conditions in the courtroom; 5) reluctance of psychiatric patients to bring suit against their psychiatrists; 6) the clinical ability of the psychiatrist to dispel the patient's negative therapeutic reaction or transference; 7) the problems of evidentiary proof in the psychiatrist–patient interaction, given the absence of witnesses; and 8) the relatively low risk of psychiatric diagnostic and therapeutic procedures (Fishalow, 1975).

Tort Law

Tort law is the law governing civil damages that arise from breach of a legal duty, other than that which is defined by contract. Medical professional liability, like other tort actions, provides compensation for a person injured by a negligent defendant (the *tortfeasor*). As well, medical tort liability attempts to deter the physician and hospital from similar negligent behavior in the future. Many observers, however, have questioned how effectively the law deters medical negligence or provides fair compensation to the injured party (Schwartz and Komesar, 1978).

Malpractice is an action in negligence, though there may be other bases for liability, such as intentional torts, violation of civil rights, and criminal liability. Negligence has been described as "conduct which falls below the standard established by law for the protection of others against unreasonable risk of harm" (Restatement, 1965). Thus, *medical malpractice*, with regard to professional negligence causes of action, is largely predicated on the *fault* of the defendant, though unintentional. To recover for medical liability, the plaintiff-patient has the burden of proving that: 1) the physician-defendant owed a legal duty to the patient; 2) the physician breached that duty in the care rendered to the patient; 3) the patient suffered an injury or damages, whether physical or emotional; and 4) the damages resulted from the physician's negligence (proximate causation). Each element bears elaboration.

1. Establishing the psychiatrist's legal duty to the patient requires proof of the existence of a physician–patient relationship, as well as proof of the applicable standard of care. The existence of the physician–patient relationship can be established when the physician accepts the person as a patient or begins an examination (King, 1986). The standard of care required of the defendant is established through medical expert witness testimony, as judged by a reasonable and prudent practitioner practicing in the same or similar circumstances. The legal standard of care is usually based upon, if not identical with, customary medical practice, which tends to promote normative rather than innovative clinical care (Bovbjerg, 1975). The legal standard is sometimes additionally established by the use of authoritative psychiatric literature, professional association guidelines, hospital and clinic policy, accreditation policy, and relevant statutes or regulations. As a specialist, the psychiatrist is held to a higher standard of care than a general medical practitioner.

2. The plaintiff must also prove that the defendant deviated from the standard of care. Such a deviation may be due to the psychiatrist's error of omission (*nonfeasance*) or error of commission (*misfeasance*). On occasion, such negligence can be established solely through proof that the defendant violated a state law or regulation (*negligence per se*). A psychiatrist is required to possess and use the knowledge and skill of a reasonably well-qualified psychiatrist. Psychiatrists are typically judged according to objective, national standards of psychiatric practice, rather than exclusively those of their local community; they are not expected to provide the highest possible level of knowledge and skill. As well, it is not a defense that the psychiatrist provided his or her best possible care to the patient. The psychiatrist is not, however, held responsible for an error in judgment about the patient, so long as the clinical care conforms

to the standard of care.

Proof that the defendant failed to provide care in conformity with the legal standard is offered through expert witness testimony. Here, it is not enough for the plaintiff's expert to merely testify that he or she would have managed the patient differently. As well, the expert will judge the defendant's conduct with regard to the standard of care at the time of the allegedly wrongful treatment, rather than at a later time when clinical advances may have occurred.

3. Damages to the patient compensate the patient for injuries or are punitive to the practitioner, as a civil fine. Proof of the patient's injuries can be established by testimony from the patient, other lay persons familiar with the patient, and clinicians who have subsequently treated the plaintiff. Economic damages can be established by subsequent medical and rehabilitation expenses and loss of income.

4. Finally, using expert witness testimony, the plaintiff must establish that the injury resulted from the psychiatrist's negligent care. The psychiatrist is not a guarantor of a good result for the patient, and an adverse clinical outcome does not presume malpractice; an adverse outcome may, of course, result from the disorder itself, as well as from the treatment (Lakshmanan et al, 1986). Similarly, negligent conduct that does not result in injury to the patient is not actionable. Depending on the applicable law, the plaintiff must establish that the defendant's negligence was necessary to, or a substantial factor in, the clinical outcome.

Problems of Proof in Psychiatric Malpractice

In medicine, but particularly in psychiatry, there are several accepted methods of diagnosis and treatment (Franklin et al, 1980). A multitude of effective clinical strategies may be used, alone or in combination, to deal with a particular problem. Given different and competing "schools of thought," there may be a lack of universal consensus about the usefulness of a particular treatment modality. Thus, there may be legitimate differences in expert opinions about the use of hospitalization, psychotherapy, pharmacotherapy, or electroconvulsive therapy for a patient with a disorder such as major depression (Malcolm, 1986). In such cases, courts have indicated that a clinician is not negligent if, exercising reasonable and prudent judgment, he or she selects one of the accepted treatment modalities, even if it later turns out to be without benefit or is harmful. Further, the clinician may select a treatment modality that is recognized and accepted by a respectable minority of practitioners, rather than be confined to a modality used by the majority. Sometimes, however, clinical standards in psychiatric care are vague or ill defined.

The plaintiff may also have difficulty establishing the patient's damages. As individuals who present to psychiatrists seek care for emotional injuries, those who are negligently injured are likely to continue to complain of similar injuries. Yet there are obvious problems in identifying, defining, proving, quantifying, and valuing emotional injuries. There may be no objective method or verification, and the possibility of malingered or exaggerated injuries is everpresent. Society has historically been reluctant to compensate psychic injuries in the absence of physical injuries, though this has been liberalized in recent years.

Causation is a final problem for the plaintiff. Given psychiatry's limited ability to determine the etiology of psychiatric complaints and disorders, as well as the likelihood that such complaints and disorders are in fact multiply determined, it is difficult to determine when an injury is a product of the underlying illness, an expected outcome of treatment, the psychiatrist's or other defendants' negligence, or some combination of these, as well as the proportion for each. Variation in the response to psychiatric treatment modalities between patients also complicates the determination of causation.

Tort Reform

All parties involved in medical professional liability have, in recent times, been alleged to be responsible for the current liability situation. These include plaintiff's attorneys, physicians, hospitals and medical societies that fail to discipline incompetent physicians, plaintiff-oriented courts and legislatures, insurance companies, and patients with unrealistic expectations (Barsky, 1988). The current system is said to result in awards that are delayed, random, inequitable, fail to approximate the true economic costs of iatrogenic injury, and grossly exceed compensation for identical injuries not involving physicians (for example, industrial or auto accidents). Even though there appears to be a variety of contributing causes to the recent series of medical professional liability crises, more than one-third of states have recently enacted tort reforms in this area (Perkins and Stoll, 1987). The reforms have been directed to many of the involved parties, yet there are few studies that assess how any of these reforms have affected insurance premiums and availability (Zuckerman et al, 1986). Many of the reforms are of recent origin, most have been enacted as a package, and many vary from state to state (Danzon and Lillard, 1983; Sloan, 1985). Many have been enacted but later withdrawn by the legislature or ruled unconstitutional by state courts. Some of the provisions either proposed or enacted include the following:

1. *Limitations on liability.* These take the form of a limit on certain damages such as noneconomic ("pain and suffering"), or on total liability. Both types have been challenged as to their constitutionality.
2. *Modification of the collateral source rule.* This rule of evidence prohibits the jury from learning that the plaintiff's medical expenses have already been paid by another source, such as first-party health insurance or worker's compensation. Modification or elimination of this rule thus prohibits "double-recovery" for these expenses.
3. *Shortened statutes of limitation.* A reduced tail of vulnerability for the physician-defendant will, in theory, reduce the number of claims filed and help the insurer predict awards. This is of particular concern in the case of minors, whose statute may not begin to run until the age of majority.
4. *Attorney fee regulation.* Some states have begun to limit attorney's fees to a fixed percentage of the award, to a sliding scale that is reduced as the award increases, or to a set hourly charge.
5. *Abolition of joint and several liability.* Such liability permits recovery in full from any negligent defendant regardless of his or her contribution to the injury. Thus, a codefendant with 10 percent liability could be made to pay the entire award, if the codefendant with 90 percent liability were insolvent. Abolition of this rule results in liability for damages which is apportioned to the defendant's relative fault.

6. *Periodic payments.* This provision permits awards to be paid over time in a structured manner, rather than in a lump sum after the trial. Such a provision in effect reduces the total amount of the award and protects the award from being squandered.
7. *Pretrial screening panels.* A panel composed of physicians, attorneys, and laypersons reviews each liability claim prior to trial. The review may be voluntary or mandatory, and the panel's findings can be introduced as evidence at trial. Such panels were originally adopted in more than half the states, but some states have subsequently withdrawn them.
8. *Binding arbitration.* Patients and physicians may voluntarily agree to submit any present or future liability claim to binding arbitration, rather than litigation. Some statutes provide that the patient may later revoke the arbitration agreement, either following the execution of the contract or after the provision of the services.
9. *Standards for expert witnesses.* Some states have limited expert-witness testimony to those physicians who practice within the plaintiff's community or to those physicians who actively practice medicine within the specialty of the defendant (*Sutphin v. Platt, 1986*).
10. *Mandatory reporting.* A federal law, the Health Care Quality Improvement Act of 1986, requires that insurance carriers and self-insurers report any payments for a judgment, settlement, or claim of medical malpractice to a central clearinghouse; the name of the physician, the amount of the payment, and a description of the acts or omissions must be provided, under threat of fine up to $10,000 for each payment (Iglehart, 1987). In addition, each state medical licensing board and hospital must report to the clearinghouse disciplinary actions against a physician for reasons related to medical competence. Many states also require that insurance companies or state insurance officials report all medical liability settlements or awards to the state medical licensing board for review.
11. *No-fault-based resolution.* Finally, several major reforms of the current fault-based adversarial system for resolving medical professional liability claims have been proposed but not enacted. These may rely on private contracts between health care providers and patients and restrict or eliminate the role of tort law in compensating iatrogenic injuries (Epstein, 1976). The plans may be compulsory or elective, depending upon the parties involved, the nature of the medical care (prepaid or fee-for-service), as well as the nature and severity of the injury. Such reforms include a no-fault, social insurance system used in Sweden (Brahams, 1988); elective no-fault insurance; a workers' compensation approach; and medical adversity insurance (Havighurst and Tancredi, 1973). In these plans, compensation for covered injuries may be paid according to a predetermined schedule, without regard to the physician's negligence, and payment is more promptly and efficiently made, in comparison with the delays and litigation costs inherent in the current system (General Accounting Office, 1986; Havighurst, 1986). Such proposals have, however, sometimes given rise to fears of large increases in compensated claims that would offset any cost savings obtained (Danzon, 1985).

PSYCHIATRIC MALPRACTICE ISSUES

Overview

A variety of claims are brought against psychiatrists under the general rubric of malpractice, yet there is no standard nosology for such claims. A claim for suicide, for example, might be reported as a failure to diagnose, failure to supervise, improper treatment, or negligent psychopharmacology. Litigation against psychiatrists can be brought on grounds of negligence (malpractice), as discussed above, as well as other causes of action, such as battery, defamation, breach of contract guaranteeing a specific therapeutic result, intentional infliction of emotional distress, fraud, intentional misrepresentation, civil rights violations, and criminal behavior.

In a nationwide survey of 217 closed claims against psychiatrists from 1974 to 1978, 58 percent were closed with payment to the plaintiff; the payment was limited to $30,000 in 79 percent of paid claims (Slawson and Guggenheim, 1984). The distribution of closed claims against psychiatrists from 1980 to 1985 included: suicide, 21 percent; medication (overdose and addiction), 20 percent; miscellaneous (including failure to diagnose a medical condition), 18 percent; failure to treat psychosis, 14 percent; psychotherapy, 14 percent; sexual contact, 6 percent; and restraints (including ECT), 7 percent (Psychiatric News, April 3, 1987, p.12). Just 17 cases were brought against psychiatrists insured by the American Psychiatric Association insurance program from 1972 to 1983, all for ECT; indemnity was made in seven of these (Slawson, 1985).

Suicide and Parasuicide

Issues. Professional liability claims against psychiatrists for suicide and parasuicide are among the most common claims in psychiatric practice. Suicides and parasuicides occur during the course of outpatient treatment, in the hospital, or after release from the hospital or emergency room; there is corresponding litigation for self-inflicted injuries by patients in all contexts. Apart from the clinic or hospital where the patient is treated, psychiatrists bear individual liability for their patients' self-inflicted injuries when they are not employed by that facility.

An ironic aspect of malpractice litigation against psychiatrists for suicide and parasuicide is that the psychiatrist is asked to bear the responsibility for an intentional action of the patient. Tensions and conflicts arise between the psychiatrist's responsibility and that of the patient for the patient's own injury, and the patient's role in causing his or her own injury in other forms of psychiatric malpractice is much less prominent. In suicide litigation, the courts have tended to see the patient as child-like or unable to control self-destructive impulses, while simultaneously viewing psychiatrists as able to predict and prevent intentionally self-destructive behavior. The issues are such that juries and judges alternately identify with both psychiatrist and patient. Nevertheless, given the availability of insurance coverage for psychiatrists and hospitals, as well as an inclination to compensate a bereaved family, there is a tendency to hold the psychiatrist liable for a patient's self-injury despite the absence of negligence by the physician.

Similar tensions are created in the hospital setting, between protecting the patient's safety through continued confinement and releasing the patient to a less restrictive environment, which increases the risk of self-injury. In their use of contemporary standards of care for hospitalized patients, courts sometimes acknowledge the potentially antitherapeutic effects of prolonged or restrictive hospitalization, as well as the therapeutic importance of exposing the patient to the community.

The clinical dilemmas presented by suicidal patients are well known and can have significant legal impact: imprecision in assessing and predicting suicide; assessing acute suicide risk in chronically suicidal patients or those with significant character pathology; deciding whether there is adequate evidence of self-destructiveness to justify civil commitment; managing the patient who is unable to assess the risks and benefits of increasing hospital privileges with the psychiatrist; dealing with the patient who withholds information from staff about suicide; and managing the patient who consciously or unconsciously manipulates staff resulting in accidental self-injury (Bursztajn et al, 1983; Gutheil, 1985).
Litigation.   Professional liability for a patient's suicide or parasuicide is predicated upon the psychiatrist's deviation from the requisite standard of clinical care, as well as legal causation. A necessary component of causation with regard to suicide is the foreseeability of the patient's injury, judged from the perspective of the defendant at the time of the treatment, rather than with the benefit of hindsight.

Particular legal grounds for suicide include failure to diagnose a suicidal condition (including failure to take a history and perform an examination), failure to predict suicide, failure to treat a condition associated with suicidal behavior, failure to protect a suicidal patient once the diagnosis and prediction have been made, and abetting a suicidal patient to suicide. Most suits allege a negligent omission by the psychiatrist to evaluate, predict, or prevent a patient's self-inflicted injury, but it is conceivable that a psychiatrist could be held to have precipitated a patient's suicide through an error of commission. As noted earlier, an error of clinical judgment in assessing or managing a suicidal patient is not, by itself, actionable for negligence.

It may be difficult to establish legal causation between the psychiatrist's negligence and the patient's injury. It may be unclear whether responsibility lies with the patient's underlying illness or disorder, volitional behavior unrelated to the patient's illness, or the clinician's negligence. Suicides that occur in the outpatient setting cannot easily be attributed to the negligence of the psychiatrist, given the reduced ability to control the patient in that environment. Further, the longer the time interval between discharge from the hospital or last psychiatric contact and the suicide, the less likely liability will attach to the psychiatrist for negligence during the course of the treatment.

While there is much published suicide litigation, mention of a few cases is sufficient to illustrate the issues. In *Pisel v. Stamford (1980)*, a hospitalized patient with command hallucinations to hurt herself wedged her head between her mattress and the siderail of the bed while in seclusion. There was evidence that she had been inadequately monitored and treated. She survived in a semicomatose state and was awarded $3.6 million.

In another hospital case, the appellate court overturned a jury verdict against the psychiatrist for the widow of a patient who committed suicide by hanging

(Topel v. Long Island, 1981). Contrary to the plaintiff's contention, the court indicated that it was a matter of professional judgment whether to maintain observation of a suicidal patient on either a continuous basis or at 15-minute intervals. According to the court, it was proper for the physician to consider the patient's reaction to constant surveillance and the expected benefit of less restrictive treatment.

Claiming negligent release, a man who attempted suicide by dousing himself with gasoline and setting himself on fire one week after his discharge from a psychiatric hospital recovered damages against the hospital (*Bell v. New York City, 1982*). The treating psychiatrist had allegedly failed to inquire about the patient's delusions and hallucinations during the hospital stay; the jury verdict was upheld on appeal because of the absence of a careful examination. By contrast, in another case a court rejected a widow's claim that the psychiatrist had negligently released her husband from the hospital. The court ruled that "modern psychiatric practice does not require a patient to be isolated from normal human activities until every possible danger has passed" (*Johnson v. United States, 1981*, p. 1293).

Suicide litigation in the outpatient setting sometimes involves patients who take overdoses of prescribed medication. In *Speer v. United States (1981)*, the widow of a patient who overdosed with amitriptyline and perphenazine unsuccessfully brought suit alleging that the prescribing psychiatrist was negligent and that this breach of the standard of care was the cause of the patient's death. The court ruled that the psychiatrist had not breached the standard of care in prescribing a month's dosage or in monitoring the patient. The opposite result was obtained in a death involving the accidental or voluntary overdose of controlled medications (*Argus v. Scheppegrell, 1986*).

Psychopharmacology

Issues. Litigation in psychopharmacology may be brought against drug manufacturers, prescribing physicians, hospitals, pharmacists, and nurses. Malpractice claims against psychiatrists in this area are primarily brought on grounds of negligence, but some are brought by alleging failure to obtain informed consent from patients, sometimes considered a separate tort.

In prescribing medication, psychiatrists may be liable on any of several grounds of negligence. These include:

1. failure to obtain a relevant history prior to prescription
2. failure to conduct an examination or evaluation prior to treatment
3. prescription of the wrong medication
4. prescription of improper dosage
5. prescription for inappropriate duration
6. improper administration
7. failure to monitor the patient during the course of treatment
8. failure to recognize or treat side effects and toxicity
9. failure to anticipate drug–drug or food–drug interactions
10. failure to refer or consult with the appropriate experts
11. improper recordkeeping (Wettstein, 1983).

Informed consent claims in psychopharmacology have been brought against psychiatrists, usually for failure to warn of the side effects of medication that later eventuate. According to current law, the prescribing physician functions as a *learned intermediary* between the manufacturer and the patient. With few exceptions, manufacturers have a legal duty to provide the physician, rather than the patient, with information about medication side effects and toxicity. Patients may bring claims against a manufacturer for failure to warn their prescribing physicians of the necessary information and may also bring claims against their physicians for failure to obtain informed consent to treatment (see Chapter 20).

Litigation. As in much of medical practice, clinical standards in the prescription and administration of psychotropic medication are not rigidly defined. There is often considerable variation in what might be clinically appropriate treatment with regard to selection of medication, dosage, duration, and monitoring, yet much litigation occurs in this area.

Case law in psychopharmacology is best illustrated in the area of neuroleptic-induced movement disorders, principally tardive dyskinesia and tardive dystonia. Litigation here is modest in frequency but increasingly severe in outcome, and several multimillion dollar judgments have resulted. Much litigation has been settled out of court, without trial or appeal, leaving the details unknown. Litigation is brought on grounds of inappropriate prescription, failure to monitor the patient for side effects, failure to diagnose side effects, and failure to reveal the risks of treatment (Wettstein, 1985).

In *Clites v. Iowa (1982)*, a mentally retarded patient at a state hospital was treated for five years with antipsychotic medication to manage aggressive behavior before tardive dyskinesia of the face and extremities developed. There was evidence of negligent failure in prescribing, without proper indication, antipsychotic medication for this duration; failure to monitor the patient for side effects; and failure to diagnose tardive dyskinesia. The parents also alleged that they had never been informed of the risk of prolonged treatment, nor had they authorized consent to treatment. Damages of $760,165 were awarded and upheld on appeal.

In *Hedin v. U.S. (1985)*, after a two-month psychiatric hospitalization for treatment of alcohol abuse, the plaintiff was treated with thioridazine and then chlorpromazine as an outpatient. He continued to take 600 mg chlorpromazine daily for nearly four years, before his physicians noted his movement disorder and discontinued the medication. The patient had been aware of the movements, which involved the face, mouth, trunk, and extremities, but testified that he was unaware they were due to the medication. The government admitted that it had been negligent in prescribing excessive amounts of medication, over a prolonged period of time, without proper supervision. Damages of nearly $2.2 million were awarded to the plaintiff, who had become functionally disabled because of the tardive dyskinesia.

A sample of other litigation against physicians involving antipsychotic medication includes alleged overdosage resulting in accidental death (*Moon v. U.S., 1981*); overdosage resulting in quadriplegia (*Tucker v. Hutto, 1979*); cardiorespiratory death allegedly from haloperidol and chlorpromazine (*Allen v. Kaiser, 1985*); failure to diagnose chlorpromazine-induced jaundice (*Brown v. City of New York, 1978*); inadequate treatment resulting in serious physical injury (*Jansen v.*

University Hospital, 1982); and excessive dosage of thioridazine resulting in visual loss (*Chasse v. Banas, 1979*).

A vast array of other litigation over psychopharmacologic issues has been brought against physicians. Of benzodiazepines, plaintiffs have claimed, with various success, that these medications have resulted in delirium and accidental death (*Fleming v. Prince George's County, 1976*), or cerebral damage (*Crooks v. Greene, 1987*). Litigation for the improper use of antidepressants has included undertreatment of depression resulting in a suicide attempt (*Gowan v. U.S., 1985*), as well as overdosage resulting in suicide, described above (*Moon*). In at least one case, a patient recovered damages for the defendant's failure to monitor lithium carbonate (*Wright v. Louisiana, 1986*).

Accidental injuries to third parties inflicted by patients driving automobiles under the influence of prescribed psychotropics have also been the subject of suit against the prescribing physician. Legal grounds for suit here, with or without success, include negligent prescription, failure to warn the driver, and failure to warn the passenger. The medications at issue have included metha-qualone (*Gooden v. Tips, 1983*), diazepam (*Watkins v. U.S., 1979*), and fluphen-azine and chlorpromazine (*Kirk v. Michael Reese Hospital, 1987*).

Duty to Protect Third Parties

Issues. For many years, psychiatrists and hospitals have been found liable for the injuries their patients inflicted on others after release or escape from the hospital. In these cases, liability was predicated on the hospital's negligence in permitting escape or release. In the 1970s, this duty to a potentially injured third party, rather than to the patient alone, was extended to the outpatient-treatment setting, through the analogy of the physician's obligation to inform others who are placed at risk because of the patient's contagious disease. This legal duty to protect a third party is ultimately derived from the "special relationship" that the therapist has with the patient. In a landmark decision, the California Supreme Court formulated the rule that, "when a therapist determines, or pursuant to the standards of his profession should determine, that his patient presents a serious danger of violence to another, he incurs an obligation to use reasonable care to protect the intended victim" (*Tarasoff v. Regents, 1976*, p. 340).

The major problem in implementing any duty to protect a third party is the difficulty of assessing and predicting the behavior of the patient. The generally low prevalence of violence, particularly in the outpatient setting, is likely to result in significant overpredictions of violence by mental health professionals. As well, except in the case of civil commitment, therapists enjoy relatively little control over their outpatients, even if a risk of violence has been identified.

These cases also create a conflict between the third party duty and the clinician's ethical, and perhaps legal, duty to maintain the confidentiality of the treatment. Nevertheless, the potential harm to the treatment through the third party disclosure, if such is necessary, can be minimized by communicating with third parties in the presence of the patient, with the consent of the patient, or even with the assistance of the patient (Roth and Meisel, 1977). At times, the need to contact others can be turned to therapeutic advantage (Wexler, 1979).

In the vast majority of cases, therapists should be able to discharge their legal duty to a third party exclusively through a clinical intervention, without resorting to third party contact (Appelbaum, 1985).

Surveys of mental health professionals conducted subsequent to the *Tarasoff* ruling have indicated increased anxiety in the management of potentially dangerous patients (Wise, 1978). Therapists appear to have become more conservative in this regard, as seen by a lower risk of patient danger before intervention, but most clinicians misunderstand the legal requirement as a duty to warn rather than protect the victim (Givelber et al, 1984).

Litigation. There have been many lawsuits against psychiatrists and hospitals for the violent acts of their patients after release from the hospital. Plaintiffs in these cases have claimed that the decision to release the patient was negligent. In some cases, the patient has not become violent for several months following release (*Leverett v. Ohio, 1978*).

Subsequent to the *Tarasoff* holding, many suits alleging failure to protect a third party in the outpatient setting have occurred. These allege that the therapist failed to recognize the risk of violence to another, or, having done so, nevertheless failed to adequately protect the other from the patient. Courts in many states have considered the *Tarasoff* doctrine in a particular case, and some have upheld it (*McIntosh v. Milano, 1979*). Still others have appeared to accept the doctrine in principle, but not in a particular case (*Leedy v. Hartnett, 1981*).

Litigation against therapists has also involved a patient's violence directed to the general public, rather than to specific individuals. Though one court ruled that the therapist's duty to protect extended to the general public (*Lipari v. Sears, Roebuck, 1980*), other courts have refused to hold professionals to this standard (*Thompson v. Alameda, 1980*).

The question of whether a patient's threat to damage another person's property gives rise to a clinician's legal duty was raised in a Vermont case (*Peck v. Counseling Service, 1985*). In a therapy session, an outpatient threatened to set fire to his parents' barn and later did so. Ruling on his parents' claim for damages, the Vermont Supreme Court held that the therapist breached her duty to the parents, notwithstanding the fact that property rather than person was damaged. The court saw arson as a "violent act [that] represents a lethal threat to human beings who may be in the vicinity" (*Peck v. Counseling Service, 1985*, p. 424).

In response to the uncertainties regarding liability in this area, several states have enacted statutory immunity provisions for mental health professionals. In some cases, these statutes delineate the clinician's legal duty to protect third parties. Generally, however, they provide clinicians with immunity against third party liability for the failure to protect when the patient has threatened an identifiable victim or has acted in a threatening manner to that person, and the therapist has taken reasonable steps to prevent the violence by committing the patient, notifying the victim, and/or contacting the police. Some statutes also immunize the therapist from charges of breach of confidentiality in the course of a good-faith effort to discharge this duty. It remains to be determined, however, whether such statutes will reduce outpatient violence or only reduce the likelihood of a plaintiff verdict. Also, excessive reliance upon such statutes in marginal situations may unnecessarily disrupt treatment in the service of defensive practice.

Erotic Contact with Patients

Issues. Erotic contact of all types between psychiatrists and their patients appears to be prevalent. A recent survey of psychiatrists, with a 26 percent return rate, revealed that 7 percent of the male and 3 percent of the female respondents admitted to "sexual contact" with their patients (Gartrell et al, 1986). Though the majority of cases involved male psychiatrists and female patients, there were no gender boundaries to this behavior.

Erotic contact with patients is no longer, if it ever was, considered to be appropriate psychiatric care. Taking psychiatrists' attitudes as evidence of the legal standard of care, surveys reveal that 98 percent of psychiatrists believe that sexual contact between the psychiatrist and a current patient is always inappropriate (Herman et al, 1987). Similarly, the annotated *Principles of Medical Ethics of the American Psychiatric Association* indicates that such behavior is unethical (APA, 1985).

An issue which is perhaps less settled from clinical, legal, and ethical viewpoints is the appropriateness of erotic contact between the psychiatrist and a former patient. Nearly 30 percent of responding psychiatrists thought that such behavior could be acceptable under some circumstances (Herman et al, 1987). Any proscription of erotic conduct with patients raises questions about what can be considered appropriate, nonerotic contact (Pope et al, 1987).

Litigation. This area of psychiatric liability is perhaps more likely to result in adverse consequence to the defendant than elsewhere. Issues include negligence, intentional torts, criminal charges, ethical sanction, and revocation of professional license. Recent state laws have criminalized such behavior in some jurisdictions, even if the erotic contact occurs with the patient's consent. In some cases, the patient's spouse has a cause of action for alienation of affection. Many professional liability insurance policies provide coverage for the defense costs of these claims, but not for an adverse judgment or settlement, which then becomes the personal responsibility of the defendant. Further, employers and their insurers will not be held vicariously liable for the psychiatrist's erotic behavior, if it occurs outside the scope of the psychiatrist's employment (for example, away from the office, outside of office hours).

While the defendant may attempt to prove that there was patient consent, that the contact was intended to be therapeutic, or, on the contrary, that the contact occurred outside the parameters of treatment and thus did not constitute a breach of the legal duty to the plaintiff, negligence is usually not easily disputed in these cases. Litigation may also surround the questions of whether the erotic contact in fact occurred, the extent of the patient's damages, and causation. The potential damages include emotional distress, injury to reputation, deprivation of the necessary treatment for the patient's psychiatric disorder, aggravation of the patient's disorder, dissolution of the patient's marriage or relationship, and need for subsequent treatment.

Liability for damages may be mitigated in the eyes of the fact finder if the patient appears to have granted fully competent consent to, or even encouraged, the sexual activity, and when the contact occurs outside of the treatment milieu. Mitigation is less likely if the patient's psychiatric disorder is more severe and when there is a significant disparity in ages between the parties. Specific illustrations of these cases may be found elsewhere (Smith, 1987).

PREVENTION

While there is no substitute for excellent clinical care of patients, the psychiatrist must pay heed to the ever-present liability risks of psychiatric practice. This does not require a defensive practice, which essentially serves the interests of the physician rather than the patient. Rather, both patients and clinicians can benefit from a risk management approach to the high-risk situations reviewed above. The most important general clinical strategies here include: 1) attention to the therapeutic alliance; 2) consultation with other physicians and specialists; and 3) documentation of significant information and decisions in the patient's medical record. While no clinical strategy can in fact prevent a lawsuit, such efforts can help to successfully defend one.

The practice of psychiatry, as in the practice of medicine in general, requires attention to interpersonal relationships. Though litigation against the psychiatrist can be triggered by a variety of events, lawsuits often reflect problems in the physician–patient relationship, whether past or present. Patients usually do not sue their psychiatrist solely because of an adverse outcome to treatment; the physician's attitude or approach to the patient, for example, may facilitate the patient's decision to sue. While psychiatrists are, by training and experience, more capable than most physicians of dealing with surprised, disappointed, neglected, angry, or grieving patients and families, psychiatrists must nevertheless anticipate, recognize, and contend with such reactions in their patients. A disparity of expectations for treatment between the patient and psychiatrist or a misunderstanding of the roles of the patient and the psychiatrist must also be addressed by the clinician. Lack of rapport and communication with the patient will not only lead to limitations in the progress of the patient's treatment, but also create the potential for a lawsuit against the clinician. Attention to these factors will allow the patient and family to deal with unanticipated results or complications of treatment that might otherwise prompt litigation.

Consultation with other psychiatrists can improve the patient's care, as well as help to defend against subsequent charges of inadequate or inappropriate care, yet many psychiatrists are reluctant to obtain consultation. Such consultations may be formal or informal, single or ongoing; consultation with subspecialists within psychiatry, such as psychopharmacologists, may be particularly valuable when dealing with severely mentally ill patients. From a litigation potential viewpoint, such consultation provides evidence that the psychiatrist is providing consensually derived clinical care, as required by the legal standard, as well as good-faith efforts to treat the patient appropriately. The attending and consulting psychiatrists must, however, be careful to avoid a misunderstanding of their respective roles and responsibilities with regard to the patient and each other. It is also often useful to contact psychiatrists or attorneys who are experienced in the legal aspects of psychiatric care, particularly when the clinician is unfamiliar with the relevant law or clinical–legal issue.

The importance of appropriate documentation of clinical care cannot be overstated. Inadequate recordkeeping can not only make a lawsuit difficult to defend, it can trigger a lawsuit once a plaintiff's attorney and plaintiff's expert review the records. Indeed, recordkeeping is required by the standard of psychiatric care; it is not simply a clerical chore to be dismissed or delegated to nonmedical personnel. Clinicans typically fail to appreciate the importance of recording relevant clinical data, which should include past psychiatric history, pertinent positive and negative signs and symptoms, telephone contacts with patients and third parties, medication changes and refills, and, above all, treatment planning and clinical decision-making. Recording the risk-benefit rationale for any significant clinical decision, such as hospital admission, hospital privileges, hospital discharge, or change in medication, by "thinking aloud on paper" will provide valuable evidence that the psychiatrist approached the patient's care in a responsible manner. In the absence of this information, the trier of fact is left to speculate about the bases for the clinical decisions which were made. This is compounded by the operating principle in litigation that if something is not documented, then it did not in fact occur (Gutheil and Appelbaum, 1982). In general, documentation in the medical record need not be voluminous, but it must be directed to the particular problems for which the patient has sought treatment.

As in any risk-taking situation, psychiatrists should be familiar with the terms and coverage of their liability insurance policies in advance of any claim. This is particularly important for psychiatrists who change their place of employment, as insurance coverage for the earlier care may not follow them (claims-made coverage). Should a lawsuit ensue, claims should be reported immediately to the carrier, which will appoint a defense attorney for the case. Failure to report may jeopardize insurance coverage for the incident. Psychiatrist-defendants can additionally retain their own attorneys, at personal expense, to guide them through the litigation, and the defendant should avoid contact with the plaintiff's attorney except through the defendant's attorney. Review of some of the literature in this area will assist psychiatrists to effectively prepare and participate in their own defense (Fish et al, 1985; Fish and Ehrhardt, 1987).

REFERENCES

Allen v. Kaiser, 707 P.2d 1289 (Or. 1985)

American Medical Association: Professional liability. Citation 1987; 54:90

American Medical Association Board of Trustees: Report of the special task force on professional liability and insurance and the advisory panel on professional liability. JAMA 1987; 257:810–812

American Psychiatric Association: The Principles of Medical Ethics With Annotations Especially Applicable to Psychiatry. Washington, DC, American Psychiatric Association, 1985

Appelbaum PS: Tarasoff and the clinician: problems in fulfilling the duty to protect. Am J Psychiatry 1985; 142:425–429

Argus v. Scheppegrell, 489 So.2d 392 (La. 1986)

Barsky AJ: The paradox of health. N Engl J Med 1988; 318:414–418

Bell v. New York City Health and Hospitals Corporation, 456 N.Y.S.2d 787 (N.Y. 1982)

Bovbjerg R: The medical malpractice standard of care: HMOs and customary practice. Duke Law Journal 1975; 1975:1375–1414

Brahams D: The Swedish medical insurance schemes. Lancet 1988; 1:43–47

Brown v. City of New York, 405 N.Y.S. 2d 253 (1978)

Bursztajn H, Gutheil TG, Hamm RM, et al: Subjective data and suicide assessment in the light of recent developments, part II. International Journal of Law and Psychiatry 1983; 6:331–350

Chasse v. Banas, 399 A.2d 608 (N.H. 1979)

Clites v. Iowa, 322 N.W. 2d 917 (Iowa 1982)

Crooks v. Greene, 736 P.2d 78 (Kan. 1987)

Danzon PM: Medical Malpractice: Theory, Evidence and Public Policy. Harvard University Press, Cambridge, MA, 1985

Danzon PM: The frequency and severity of medical malpractice claims: new evidence. Law and Contemporary Problems 1986; 49:57–84.

Danzon PM, Lillard LA: Settlement out of court: the disposition of medical malpractice claims. Journal of Legal Studies 1983; 12:345–377

Epstein RA: Medical malpractice: the case for contract. American Bar Foundation Research Journal 1976; 1976:87–149

Fish RM, Ehrhardt ME, Fish B: Malpractice: Managing Your Defense. Oradell, NJ, Medical Economics Books, 1985

Fish RM, Ehrhardt ME: Malpractice Depositions: Avoiding the Traps. Oradell, NJ, Medical Economics Books, 1987

Fishalow SE: The tort liability of the psychiatrist. Bull Am Acad Psychiatry Law 1975; 3:191–230

Fleming v. Prince George's County, 358 A.2d 892 (Md. 1976)

Franklin SS, Hunt MT, Vogt T, et al: Hypertension and cerebral hemorrhage: a malpractice controversy. West J Med 1980; 133:124–140

Gartrell N, Herman J, Olarte S, et al: Psychiatrist-patient sexual contact: results of a national survey, I: Prevalence. Am J Psychiatry 1986; 143:1126–1131

General Accounting Office: Medical malpractice: no agreement on the problems or solutions. GAO/HRD–86–50, Washington, DC 1986

Givelber DJ, Bowers WJ, Blitch CL: *Tarasoff*, myth and reality: an empirical study of private law in action. Wisconsin Law Review 1984; 1984:443–497

Gooden v. Tips, 651 S.W.2d 364 (Texas 1982)

Gowan v. United States, 601 F.Supp. 1297 (Or. 1985)

Gutheil TG: Medicolegal pitfalls in the treatment of borderline patients. Am J Psychiatry 1985; 142:9–14

Gutheil TG, Appelbaum PS: Clinical Handbook of Psychiatry and the Law. New York, McGraw-Hill, 1982

Havighurst CC: Private reform of tort-law dogma: market opportunities and legal obstacles. Law and Contemporary Problems 1986; 49:143–172

Havighurst CC, Tancredi LR: Medical adversity insurance—a no-fault approach to medical malpractice and quality assurance. Milbank Memorial Fund Quarterly 1973; 51:125–168

Hedin v. U.S., Civil Docket No. 5–83–3, District Court, Fifth Division (Minn. 1985)

Herman JL, Gartrell N, Olarte S, et al: Psychiatrist–patient sexual contact: results of a national survey, II: psychiatrists' attitudes. Am J Psychiatry 1987; 144:164–169

Huber P: Injury litigation and liability insurance dynamics. Science 1987; 128:31–36

Iglehart JK: Congress moves to bolster peer review: The Health Care Quality Improvement Act of 1986. N Engl J Med 1987; 316:960–964

Jansen v. University Hospital, King County Superior Court, No. 81–2–06914–2 (Wash. 1982)

Johnson v. United States, 409 F.Supp. 1283 (M.D. Fla. 1976)

King J: The Law of Medical Malpractice, second edition. St. Paul, MN, West Publishing Co., 1986

Kirk v. Michael Reese Hospital, 513 N.E.2d 387 (Ill. 1987)

Lakshmanan MC, Hershey CO, Breslau D: Hospital admissions caused by iatrogenic disease. Arch Intern Med 1986; 146:1931–1934

Leedy v. Hartnett, 510 F.Supp. 1125 (Pa. 1981)

Leverett v. Ohio, 399 N.E.2d 106 (Ohio 1978)

Lipari v. Sears, Roebuck & Co., 497 F.Supp. 185 (D.Neb. 1980)

Localio AR: Variations on $962,258: The misuse of data on medical malpractice. Law, Medicine and Health Care 1985; 13:126–127

Malcolm JG: Treatment choices and informed consent in psychiatry: implications of the Osheroff case for the profession. Journal of Psychiatry and Law 1986; 14:9–107

Malpractice claims for suicides top list. Psychiatric News, April 3, 1987, p. 12

McIntosh v. Milano, 403 A.2d 50C (N.J. 1979)

Moon v. United States, 512 F.Supp. 140 (Nev. 1981)

New York Times: Florida to weigh crisis over doctors' malpractice insurance. New York Times, page 11Y, February 2, 1988

Peck v. Counseling Service of Addison County, 499 A.2d 422 (Vt. 1985)

Perkins J, Stoll K: Medical malpractice: a "crisis" for poor women. Clearinghouse Review 1987; 20:1277–1286

Pisel v. Stamford Hospital et al, 430 A.2d 1 (Conn. 1980)

Pope KS, Tabachnick BG, Keith-Spiegel P: Ethics of practice: the beliefs and behaviors of psychologists as therapists. Am Psychol 1987; 42:993–1006

Posner JR: Trends in medical malpractice insurance 1970–1985. Law and Contemporary Problems 1986; 49:37–56

Restatement (Second) of Torts, section 282, 1965

Reynolds RA, Rizzo JA, Gonzalez ML: The cost of medical professional liability. JAMA 1987, 257: 2776–2781

Roth LH, Meisel A: Dangerousness, confidentiality, and the duty to warn. Am J Psychiatry 1977; 134:508–511

Schwartz WB, Komesar NK: Doctors, damages and deterrence. N Engl J Med 1978; 298:1282–1289

Slawson PF: The clinical dimension of psychiatric malpractice. Psychiatric Annals 1984; 14:358–364

Slawson PF: Psychiatric malpractice: the electroconvulsive therapy experience. Convulsive Therapy 1985; 1:195–203

Slawson PF, Guggenheim FG: Psychiatric malpractice: a review of the national loss experience. Am J Psychiatry 1984; 141:979–981

Sloan FA: State responses to the malpractice insurance "crisis" of the 1970s: an empirical assessment. Journal of Health Politics, Policy and Law 1985; 9:629–646

Smith JT: Medical Malpractice: Psychiatric care. Colorado Springs, Colorado, McGraw-Hill, 1987

Speer v. United States, 512 F.Supp 670 (N.D. Texas 1981)

Sutphin v. Platt, 720 S.W.2d 455 (Tenn. 1986)

Tarasoff v. Regents of the University of California, 551 P.2d 334 (Ca. 1976)

Thompson v. Alameda, 614 P.2d 728 (Cal. 1980)

Topel v. Long Island, 431 N.E. 2d 293 (N.Y. 1981)

Tucker v. Hutto, No. 78-0161-R, U.S. District Court (E.D. Vir. 1979)

Watkins v. United States, 589 F.2d 214 (5 Cir. 1979)

Wettstein R: Tardive dyskinesia and malpractice. Behavioral Sciences and the Law 1983; 1:85–107

Wettstein R: Legal aspects of neuroleptic-induced movement disorders, in Legal Medicine 1985. Edited by Wecht CH. New York, Praeger, 1985

Wexler DB: Patients, therapists, and third parties: the victimological virtues of *Tarasoff*. Int J Law Psychiatry 1979; 2:1–28

Wise TP: Where the public peril begins: a survey of psychotherapists to determine the effects of *Tarasoff*. Stanford Law Review 1978; 31:165–190

Wright v. Louisiana, Docket Number 83–5035, Civil District Court New Orleans (La. 1986)

Zuckerman S, Koller CF, Bovbjerg R: Information on malpractice: a review of empirical research on major policy issues. Law and Contemporary Problems 1986; 49:85–112

Chapter 20

Informed Consent and Competency in Psychiatric Practice

by Harold I. Schwartz, M.D., and Loren H. Roth, M.D., M.P.H.

BACKGROUND

Informed consent is a doctrine intended to transform the very essence of the doctor-patient relationship (Stone, 1979) by shifting the balance of power from the physician to the patient. Since introduction of the term in 1957 in the *Salgo* case, the informed-consent doctrine has been shaped by the ethical mandate and a growing body of the law (Appelbaum et al, 1987; Meisel and Kabnick, 1980; Roth, 1985). Informed consent requires that physicians reconsider their use of authority and reorder their priorities so as to promote individual autonomy, possibly, though not necessarily, at the expense of more traditional medical values. That controversy and resistance continue to accompany informed consent should come as no surprise. In psychiatric practice, legal notions of autonomy often seem poorly matched to the clinical reality of mental illness. In one recent study, fewer than 10 percent of responding physicians reported that informed consent had something to do with a patient making a choice or stating a preference about treatment (Harris et al, 1982).

Though informed consent requires that patients be given sufficient information to make intelligent, free, and competent treatment decisions, a host of unanswered questions remains about the implementation of these requirements (Pernick, 1982): How much information is enough? By what criteria shall a patient's competency be assessed? Who shall decide for the incompetent patient? These are but a few of the important questions whose answers are in evolution in clinical practice, legal theory, and the courts.

Controversy continues to surround informed consent because the doctrine touches on an age old conflict of values, the strain between individual autonomy versus the benefits of medical paternalism (Pernick, 1982). Western medical tradition has long been ambivalent about the role of the patient in decision-making. Hippocrates, championing the authority of the physician, advised: "Perform [these duties] calmly and adroitly, concealing most things from the patient while you are attending to him" (President's Commission, 1982). The locus of control of decision-making has, however, shifted back and forth in response to social pressures and schools of thought. Eighteenth and nineteenth century physicians—for example, Benjamin Rush—were impressed with the relationship between health and the individual's moral, social, and psychic environment; they therefore viewed patient autonomy in decision-making in a more favorable light. But control shifted back to the professional in the late nineteenth and twentieth century, as discoveries in microbial science externalized the cause of disease, leading to technologies that were highly reliant on professional expertise (Pernick, 1982). Regardless of shifts in medical philosophy, the position of the common law has been to create a clear and consistent requirement that the patient must consent to medical treatment (Meisel et al, 1977). This view was crystalized in 1914 by Judge Benjamin Cardoza, who wrote in *Schloendorff v. Society of New York Hospital (1914)* that "every human being of adult years and sound mind has a right to determine what shall be done with his own body."

Ethical Background

Authoritarian models of physician-patient decision-making run contrary to a number of fundamental principles in Western social and political thought, especially the value of individual autonomy (Faden and Beauchamp, 1986). Two primary schools of ethical thought, deontological and utilitarian, are often used to justify the use of informed consent to promote autonomy. The ethical background of the informed consent doctrine is reviewed by Appelbaum and colleagues (1987). Deontological ethics posit a set of transcendant values which can be translated into duties that are binding in all situations. Immanuel Kant, prizing rationality as an end in itself, represents this school (Appelbaum et al, 1987).

Utilitarian ethics require an examination of the outcome of any action. In the absence of transcendant values the outcome or "utility" of an action must be the measure of its value. Utilitarian ethicists such as John Stuart Mill and Jeremy Bentham made major contributions to the notion of individual liberty in Western democracies. Mill argued that individual freedom should be constrained only when the rights of others are contravened. He believed that utility would be maximized when individuals knew what enhanced their personal happiness and were allowed to act on this knowledge (Mill, 1955). Both ethical schools have contributed to the doctrine of informed consent with their emphasis on rational decision-making and freedom from coercion.

Other Influences

A number of trends have come together in the mid-twentieth century to promote the growth of informed consent. Revelations of the horrific experimentation performed by Nazi doctors on concentration camp victims culminated in consent requirements for human research contained in the Nuremberg Code (Benson and Roth, in press). Though consent requirements for research are not wholly analogous to those for medical treatment, a number of concepts in the Nuremberg Code were ultimately reflected in informed consent requirements for medical treatment. The post-World War II era was marked by mushrooming medical technology and a rapid growth in subspecialization. The fragmentation of medical care contributed to the demystification of the physician's persona and led to requests for increased accountability and patient autonomy. The consumer and civil rights movements, beginning in the 1950s, empowered ordinary citizens in their relations with institutions and contributed to a shift from patients' passive acceptance of their status to active medical consumerism. A growing body of federal legislation, including the Truth in Lending Act and the Freedom of Information Act, promoted the value of informed consumerism in various aspects of public and private life (Schwartz and Rachlin, 1985). Increasing malpractice litigation and a growing patient advocacy bar were additional important influences.

Legal Background

To understand informed consent, it is necessary to briefly review its legal development. The requirement for patient consent to medical treatment is a common law principle; failure to obtain consent can leave the physician vulnerable to the charge of battery, an unlawful touching. In the eighteenth-century British case of *Slater v. Baker and Stapleton (1767)*, two clinicians were found guilty of disuniting a fracture on a patient from whom they had not obtained consent. The court noted that obtaining consent was a customary practice of surgeons and that informing patients about what is to be done to them could improve outcome by allowing the patient to "take courage."

The legal requirements for consent went essentially unchanged until the 1950s, when the notion that consent must, to some degree, be fully informed first emerged. In *Salgo v. Leland Stanford Jr. University Board of Trustees (1957)* a California court first used the phrase *informed consent*. In *Salgo*, a patient who had suffered spinal injury due to translumbar aortography alleged that he had not been adequately informed of the risks beforehand. The court ruled that "a physician violates his duty to his patients and subjects himself to liability if he withholds any facts which are necessary to form the basis of an intelligent consent by the patient to the proposed treatment." Yet the court also expressed its concern that disclosing every risk "no matter how remote" could be harmful: ". . . the patient's mental and emotional condition is important and in certain cases may be crucial, and . . . in discussing the element of risk a certain amount of discretion must be employed consistent with the full disclosure of facts necessary for an informed consent."

In 1960 a Kansas court made the next significant contribution in the case of *Natanson v. Kline (1960)*. A patient, burned by cobalt irradiation following a mastectomy, alleged that she had been inadequately informed of the risks of treatment. The *Natanson* court outlined the elements of disclosure, which have subsequently become standard: "the nature of the ailment, the nature of the proposed treatment, the probability of success or of alternatives, and perhaps the risks of unfortunate results . . ." The court significantly qualified its disclosure rule by limiting "the duty of the physician . . . to those disclosures which a reasonable medical practitioner would make under the same or similar circumstances. How the physician may best discharge his obligation to the patient in this difficult situation involves primarily a question of medical judgment . . ." (*Natanson v. Kline*, 1960, p. 1106).

The *reasonable medical practitioner* standard was adopted by other courts and went largely unchallenged for more than ten years (Meisel, 1977). This standard assumes professional consensus on recognizable and uniform standards of disclosure that also meet patients' needs. This assumption was challenged in the landmark case of *Canterbury v. Spence (1972)*. In *Canterbury*, the court rejected the professional standard, proposing in its place that clinicians be required to disclose what a *reasonable person* would want to know in making a treatment decision. This *lay* standard requires the physician to disclose information that is *material* to a patient's decision. However, the *Canterbury* standard (see also *Cobbs v. Grant, 1972*) does not require that disclosure be tailored to the individual needs of a particular patient but instead to the needs of a hypothetical reasonable person. Though the reasonable person standard was rapidly adopted by many courts, about half of the states continue to hold to the reasonable medical practitioner standard by case law or statute (President's Commission, 1982).

As this brief review suggests, the law provides only a bare outline of the minimal requirements for informed consent. To discuss informed consent from a legalistic point of view is to focus attention on what the physician must do to avoid liability. This misses the point. In the next section, we will review the components of informed consent, not with an eye cast over our shoulder for the malpractice lawyer, but looking forward to what the physician-patient relationship can become when these principles are valued for their own sake. At the same time, we take note that the tendency to approach informed consent legalistically reflects the degree to which many physicians resent the doctrine. The authors believe that many such objections are based on conscious and unconscious biases; others may reflect legitimate practical concerns that arise in the application of the doctrine.

THE COMPONENTS OF INFORMED CONSENT

Information (Disclosure)

Information is the foundation of the informed-consent dialogue. Initially, a patient must be informed of his current medical status to be able to assess the value of any strategies to alter the course of illness. He must be informed of the nature of the treatment being suggested, of the risks attached to the treatment, and of the benefits that might reasonably be expected from it. To weigh these risks and benefits, the patient must be informed of possible alternative treatments and of the risks and benefits attached to these, as well as the likely consequences of no treatment at all (Meisel et al, 1977).

The informed-consent doctrine has been challenged at its foundation by assertions that patients do not want to be informed or that they are uniformly frightened, to their detriment, by disclosure (Lankton et al, 1977). A small body of literature on patient attitudes toward disclosure argues otherwise (Strull et al, 1984). In a broad survey of patients and physicians performed by Louis Harris and Associates (Harris et al, 1982), most patients felt adequately informed of the common risks of treatment but wanted more information about less common risks than doctors reported providing.

Why do doctors make the assumption that patients do not want information? One answer may be that when disclosure is made contingent upon the patient's request, few patients ask for disclosure of the risks (Alfidi, 1975). Though patients may display passivity with regard to acquiring information, it is a mistake to equate passivity with lack of interest. It is equally likely that such passivity is reflective of the relative disadvantage at which patients often feel in a rushed encounter with an authoritative physician.

Another concern that may underlie physicians' reluctance to disclose is that detailed information about side effects will discourage compliance with treatment regimens. The reluctance to divulge detailed information about the risks of tardive dyskinesia is based on this clinical intuition but is not supported by empirical research. Munetz and Roth (1985) reported, in a study comparing written and oral approaches to informed consent for neuroleptic treatment, that providing detailed information about the risk of tardive dyskinesia to their study sample did not decrease compliance measured at a one-year follow-up. Though the belief that patients will be harmed by disclosure commonly appears to underlie physicians' reluctance to provide information, there are few studies that systematically examine what the nature of this harm might be and what kinds of disclosure might induce it (Meisel and Roth, 1981). In individual cases, when the clinician is convinced that a specific disclosure will cause serious mental or physical harm to a patient, he may withhold it, invoking therapeutic privilege (therapeutic privilege will be discussed below). In a review of physician behaviors in the issuance of do-not-resuscitate (DNR) orders, Schwartz (1987) reported that many physicians routinely fail to include their patients in the decision to write a DNR order, not because of evidence that such discussion will harm their patient, but rather as a product of their own psychological difficulties in conceding control, particularly when confronting a death. The reluctance to disclose detailed information to patients is often grounded in the psychology of the clinician. Likewise, the mistaken belief that patients cannot be adequately informed without providing them a medical education reflects a legalistic resistance to the doctrine rather than a legitimate objection (*Cobbs v. Grant, 1972*).

Voluntariness

Voluntariness, the second building block of informed consent, requires that a patient's consent be given free from coercion. Of course, when treatment is forced, as in the administration of involuntary medication, the application of restraints, or civil commitment, the patient's consent is not required. Society has a long history of approval of forced medical intervention in the form of mandatory vaccinations, quarantine, fluoridation, and so forth.

In other cases, however, the requirement that consent be given free of coercion stands. This may raise problems in practice because of difficulties in drawing clear lines between coercion and persuasion. An extreme interpretation of the informed consent doctrine would have the physician merely reporting the facts, much like a weather report (Lidz, 1980), to a medical-consumer who weighs all the evidence before rationally choosing a course of action. This model, which has the physician abandoning even persuasion or advice-giving for the sake of absolute patient autonomy, reduces the physician–patient relationship to absurdity and is of value only for dramatizing one end of a theoretical voluntariness spectrum.

At the other end of the voluntariness spectrum lies coercion, the threat of force or the application of influences so great as to rob the patient of free choice. Some elements of coercion may be inherent in institutionalization or other systemic components of medical care. In the case of *Kaimowitz v. Michigan Department of Mental Health* (1973), the court ruled that a patient, committed to a state hospital for seventeen years under a criminal sexual psycopath law and with no reasonable hope for discharge in the foreseeable future, could not voluntarily consent to an experimental psychosurgery procedure. The decision stated:

It is impossible for an involuntarily detained mental patient to be free of ulterior forms of restraint or coercion when his very release from the institution may depend upon his cooperating with the institutional authorities and giving consent to experimental surgery. . . . Involuntarily confined mental patients live in an inherently coercive institutional environment. Indirect and subtle psychological coercion has profound effect upon the patient population.

While experimental psychosurgery is an admittedly rare part of psychiatric practice and the *Kaimowitz* court may have overstated the issue somewhat, hospitalization, even when voluntary, may have coercive influences on patients. Hospitalized patients are more vulnerable than usual, due to the condition of illness. They are further placed in an environment that induces regression and fosters dependency by making the patient entirely dependent on others for his needs. Components of the doctor–patient relationship also lend weight to the physician's views, and these may color even seemingly *neutral* statements. This factor requires the physician to be aware of the subtle aspects of persuasion such as tone of voice, manner, and the positive or negative valence with which information is framed, so as to minimize *threatening* the patient.

Some of the coercion in the doctor–patient relationship may be unconscious. From a psychodynamic perspective, much of the motivation behind human behavior lies beyond conscious knowledge and control. All behaviors are determined by a multitude of conscious and unconscious influences, which together challenge the notion of free choice. Physicians, knowing that the boundaries of voluntariness are so difficult to define, should strive to limit their role to persuasion, while minimizing the coercive elements of medical practice (Faden and Beauchamp, 1986).

There are two situations in psychiatric practice in which the degree of voluntariness of a patient's consent is frequently at issue. The first is in consent to psychiatric hospitalization. Though a number of studies have challenged the competency of patients to admit themselves voluntarily (Appelbaum et al, 1981; Olin and Olin, 1975), few have systematically examined the coercion attendant to this process. Anyone who has worked in an emergency room, however, is aware of the tremendous pressure that psychiatrists can exert when attempting to persuade patients to sign in to the hospital. This pressure is maximized when the patient is clearly in need of hospitalization but does not quite meet the criteria for involuntary admission. Family members may be clamoring for admission and the clinician may be wary of the clinical and legal consequences (Rachlin and Schwartz, 1986) of failing to admit. There is a tendency in such a circumstance to leave the patient with the impression that failure to agree to hospitalization will be met with commitment; the patient thus feels threatened and cannot resist. One study found that many hospitalized patients believed that their only alternative to voluntary hospitalization was to be hospitalized involuntarily (Gilboy and Schmidt, 1971).

An analogous situation exists with the patient who refuses treatment on an inpatient service who is informed that he can choose between "voluntarily" accepting medication or receiving it involuntarily. A range of treatment options for psychotic and uncooperative psychiatric inpatients exists, but most are coercive, and the choice presented may be a sham. The patient's clinical condition may have deteriorated to the extent that an emergency exists; he will be medicated against his will if he objects. When the patient, understanding this condition, agrees to accept the medication, he may be acting responsibly but certainly not voluntarily.

In sum, voluntariness is a condition toward which we can aspire, while knowing it cannot be reached. Psychiatrists can maximize the voluntariness of patient choice by keeping a close eye on the many institutional and interpersonal influences that diminish it and by dropping the pretense of voluntary patient choice in those situations that are clearly involuntary (coercive).

Competency

"The search for a single test of competency is a search for a Holy Grail," wrote Roth and colleagues in 1977. There is no single accepted definition of incompetency, in part because the courts, unable to balance competing values and complex social pressures with any single set of legal rules, have spoken vaguely on the subject (Meisel, 1979). Another source of confusion about competency is vocabulary. Unless determined otherwise by a court, all adults are considered competent as a matter of law (*de jure*); prior to the age of consent, minors are considered *de jure* incompetent. *De jure* incompetency usually refers to "general" or "global" incompetency. Thus, minors are legally disqualified from a variety of significant decisions, such as making contracts, marrying, or deciding about medical care (Roth, 1982). Though all adult patients are presumed *de jure* competent until adjudicated otherwise, a patient may be in fact (*de facto*) incompetent. Despite a patient's *de jure* competency, his consent to treatment may be considered invalid if he was *de facto* incompetent at the time of consent due to mental disease, disorder, or retardation (Roth, 1982). In medical practice, the question of a patient's *de facto* competency generally arises around the ability to make a specific treatment decision or set of decisions. The competency to make a specific treatment decision is referred to as decisional capacity, partial or clinical competency, or specific competency.

In the absence of firm guidance from the courts, we can only review the criteria for assessing competency that the courts and clinicians appear to use and attempt to place these criteria in an ethical framework. Roth et al (1977) have summarized the criteria by which competency is usually assessed, as follows: whether the patient 1) evidences a choice; 2) makes a choice that leads to a reasonable outcome; 3) chooses rationally; 4) has the ability to understand the information related to the decision; or 5) actually understands the information. The ability to appreciate has been suggested as a still more stringent standard (Appelbaum and Roth, 1982; Drane, 1985). These criteria focus on four aspects of decision-making relevant to competency assessment: choosing, understanding, reasoning, and appreciating (Appelbaum and Roth, 1982). The standard chosen in any particular case to assess incompetency reflects the balance that is struck between the values of autonomy and health (Meisel, 1979).

The standard seemingly most protective of autonomy is the *evidencing a choice* or *presence of decision* standard. By this test, anyone who indicates a choice is competent, and only patients who do not communicate a choice (by virtue of coma or catatonia, for example) are judged incompetent. Some have argued that any more rigorous evaluation of competency, evaluations that examine reasoning and understanding, for instance, are unacceptably paternalistic (Goldstein, 1978). This argument simplistically equates the *stated wish* with autonomous decision-making and ignores the erosion of autonomy psychotic conditions can produce (Schwartz et al, 1988). The evidencing a choice standard is seldom used alone.

The criterion that stands farthest at the health end of the autonomy versus health spectrum is the reasonableness of outcome standard. Reasonableness, of course, is to be judged by someone other than the patient decision-maker and by definition requires that the evaluator bring his own values to the judgment. Application of this standard could theoretically subject the patient to a finding of incompetency whenever patient and evaluator disagree. This standard may rob the patient of even a pretense of autonomous decision-making (Meisel, 1979) and is biased in favor of decisions to consent to treatment (Appelbaum et al, 1987). This test is used more often than clinicians and the courts might like to admit (Roth et al, 1977). In psychiatric practice the reasonableness of outcome standard is commonly used in conjunction with the evidence of a choice standard in accepting patients' decisions to voluntarily admit themselves for hospitalization. Appelbaum and Bateman (1980) have suggested that courts abandon the "legal fiction" that all voluntary patients are competent, perhaps by adopting a standard of agreement to admission based on mere assent rather than consent.

The "reasonableness of outcome" standard can clearly be abused, but it cannot be abandoned altogether if physicians are to fulfill other obligations to patients. To clarify its use, "reasonableness of outcome" should be clearly demarcated as an element the evaluator subjectively brings to the assessment of competency. This standard then becomes a threshold test. Though "unreasonable" decisions are not by definition incompetent, beyond a certain degree of unreasonable outcome, all decisions qualify for further competency assessment (President's Commission, Volume 1, 1982). This is consonant with the tendency of the courts to scrutinize competency most closely when life and limb seem needlessly at risk.

A more stringent standard for assessing competency is one that focuses on the process of decision-making by examining reasoning. By this standard, decisions based on delusional reasoning could be judged incompetent. This test is problematic for several reasons. First, there is no legal requirement that decisions be rational. Second, it is often difficult to establish that the delusional reasoning is, in fact, the primary determinant of the patient's decision. Third, reliance on such a standard can too easily lead to the equation of psychosis with incompetency (Roth et al, 1977). Thus it is best to consider examination of a patient's reasoning process as a building block in the assessment of understanding or appreciation, rather than as a sufficient test in and of itself.

Understanding and Appreciation

The patient's ability to understand the risks, benefits, and alternatives to treatment is the test that seems most consistent with the intent of the courts. In fact, the courts often equate competency and understanding with language indicating that patients who "know" or "comprehend" the disclosed risks and benefits are competent (Meisel, 1979). The courts also tend to use the words "inform" and "understand" interchangeably, reflecting a simplistic assumption that understanding is the natural and expectable consequence of adequately informing an individual (Meisel, 1977; Meisel and Roth, 1983). A further blurring occurs in the distinction between the ability to understand and actual understanding. Although the courts appear to be satisfied when adequate information is provided to an individual with the capacity to understand it, there is as yet no clear legal obligation to ascertain the patient's actual degree of understanding. Here, legal obligations and ethical imperatives part company. It is our belief that the presence of understanding is indisputably the most substantial element of competent decision-making, and the demonstration of actual understanding should be sought whenever possible (Schwartz and Blank, 1986). The requirement of understanding best strikes a balance between the protection of autonomy and health.

As with the other tests, theoretical problems attach to understanding when it is a criteria for competency. As a practical matter, there are clearly times when it is inadequately or overly stringent. The first theoretical problem revolves around the absence of a universally acceptable definition of understanding. Closely related are the difficulties inherent in measuring understanding (Meisel and Roth, 1983). A majority of studies examining the degree of actual understanding of disclosed information which patients can demonstrate reveal a disappointingly low level of understanding (Meisel and Roth, 1981; Meisel and Roth, 1983). A growing number of studies have concluded that psychiatric patients demonstrate poor understanding of the elements necessary to decide about voluntary hospitalization (cited above) or medication (Beck and Staffin, 1986). However, before we are tempted to abandon the understanding test as impossible to achieve, we must acknowledge that the "assessment-of-understanding" literature is flawed by two methodological issues so serious that we can only conclude that we know very little about the ability of patients to understand (Roth et al, 1982b). The first flaw arises because most of these studies have focused on recall as though it were synonymous with understanding, when, in fact, what patients remember about disclosure is only one element of what they may have understood about it. The second flaw in this research derives from a general failure to control for disclosure (Meisel and Roth, 1983). Thus, understanding is tested by examining the recall of information that may not have been provided or may have been inadequately provided to begin with. Other criticisms of the understanding test focus on the degree to which factual comprehension standards favor patients with good verbal skills and recall and are biased against inarticulate patients of lower intelligence (Stanley, 1983) and nonverbal determinants of decisions such as unconscious motivation (Zeichner, 1985).

The most vigorous test by which competency can be assessed is *appreciation* (Appelbaum and Roth, 1982). Appreciation, which has both cognitive and emotional components, can be thought of as the highest degree of understanding (Drane, 1985). The requirement for such a test is illustrated by the patient who employs massive denial about illness and the need for treatment (Roth et al, 1982a). Such a patient may have a circumscribed delusional disorder and may have an actual understanding of the facts of his case and the capacity to reason rationally, but for the denial of illness. Thus, the patient may understand all that is explained but be unable to appreciate the meaning of the facts for him. This standard is heavily weighted toward the preservation of health at the risk of autonomy and must be used with great caution.

Given the lack of definitive guidance about tests of competency, it is vital that clinicians come to understand the issues involved and uniformly apply standards that are ethically and legally justifiable. To that end, in Table 1 we have reformulated the tests of competency in a step-wise hierarchy that can be used to approach all competency assessments.

Choosing a Criterion

The legal presumption is one of competency until proven otherwise. However, when competency does come to be at issue, a standard or combination of standards for assessing it must be chosen. Given the degree of subjectivity within individual standards such as understanding, some method for choosing how stringently a criterion will be applied must be developed. Roth and colleagues (1977) have proposed a model for competency assessment, based on the risk/benefit ratio of treatment, which has influenced the competency literature profoundly. They proposed that, when the risk/benefit ratio of treatment is favorable and the patient consents to treatment, a lower test of competency can be applied. A low test should also be applied when the risk/benefit ratio is

Table 1. A Hierarchy of Tests of Competency (with highest on bottom)

1. *Making a Decision*

Evidences a choice:
not necessarily competent but allows the evaluator to proceed along the hierarchy of tests

Does not evidence a choice:
not competent except when a specific waiver of decision-making has been made

2. *Reasonableness of Outcome*
A threshold test, not strictly an assessment of competency, which looks to the effect the decision is likely to have

Outcome is reasonable:
may suggest competency but does not prove it; proceed with assessment depending on considerations such as the degree of risk which attaches to the decision

Outcome is unreasonable:
may suggest incompetency but not necessarily; obligates the evaluator to proceed with the competency assessment

3. *Reasoning*
Examines the patient's mental condition, capacity to reason in a rational fashion, and the process of decision-making

Reasoning is unimpaired:
may suggest competency but does not prove it; serves as a building block for the demonstration of knowing

Reasoning is impaired:
formal thought disorder and delusions do not necessarily imply incompetency but may have bearing on knowing

4. *Knowing*
Encompasses the increasingly stringent criteria of capacity to understand, actual understanding, and appreciation

Has capacity to understand:
generally competent but not necessarily (e.g., denial, uninformed)

Lacks capacity to understand:
almost always incompetent

Understands:
usually competent but not necessarily (e.g., denial of meaning)

Lacks understanding:
usually incompetent

Appreciates:
competent

Lacks appreciation:
may be incompetent for high risk decisions

unfavorable and the patient refuses. Conversely, a high test of competency should be required when patients refuse treatments with a favorable risk/benefit ratio or consent to treatments with an unfavorable one. Such a model reflects the bias of the courts and clinicians toward facilitating treatments considered medically necessary and protecting patients from treatments thought to be risky or of speculative value. The authors emphasized that, when competency is not clear, it is not inappropriate to factor the desired medical and social values into the decision. Drane (1985) reworked this model into a sliding scale in which, as the consequences of a patient's decision to consent or refuse treatment become more serious, the criteria for assessing competency become more stringent. The principle of linkage between the criterion chosen to assess capacity and the consequences of the decision has been endorsed by the President's Commission for the Study of Ethical Problems in Medicine and Biomedical and Behavioral Research (1982). Drane urges that reasonableness pertains at all levels and that evidencing a choice that is reasonable to the evaluator is a sufficient test for treatments that are clearly safe and effective. Moderately serious treatment decisions would call for the capacity to understand. As treatment decisions become increasingly serious, they would call for tests of rationality and appreciation. Schwartz and Blank (1986) propose a model highlighting the notion of *shifting competency*. They emphasize that judgments about clinical competency are derived from two factors—the patient's mental status (and hence his ability to choose, reason, and know) and the nature of the decision he is being asked to make. Clinical competency is never static; rather, it is subject to shifts in both of these conditions during the course of treatment. Thus, competency is subject to continual reassessment. Different combinations of clinical conditions, proposed treatments, and risk/benefit ratios lead to the choosing of more or less stringent criteria for competency assessment as treatment proceeds. Given the lack of legal guidance in this area, it is vital that clinicians carefully document the basis for their decisions.

EXCEPTIONS TO INFORMED CONSENT

There are circumstances other than patient incompetency when informed consent need not or cannot be obtained. Informed consent doctrine views patients, not physicians, as the final decision-makers about treatment. Therefore, patients may choose not to receive information about treatment or may decide "not to decide," but instead to let the physician decide; "waivers" may be of information, decision, or both. It is no violation of patients' rights to permit waiver, so long as the physician ascertains that this approach to decision-making is what the patient truly desires.

In other circumstances, informed consent to treatment is neither sought nor required. The best known exception is that of *emergency*. In health or mental health emergencies, when life or limb are at stake and there is danger of imminent harm to the patient or others (suicide, mutilation, extreme physical deterioration, or assault on another), treatment may be given to contain the emergency. Thus, virtually every right-to-refuse-treatment court case (see Chapter 21) has permitted emergency treatment, even for legally competent patients, when such is necessary. Inevitably, there has been much controversy about the scope and definition of emergency within psychiatry. Do psychiatric emergencies include not only preventing imminent harm to self or others, but also acting for pater-nalistic reasons; that is, preventing or relieving imminent psychological distress in psychotic conditions? These matters are reviewed by Swartz (1987), with model definitions provided. Central to the conceptualization of the emergency is that patient consent is *implied*, admittedly at times a legal fiction. The time necessary to obtain informed consent can place the patient or others at unac-ceptable risk. Also, in many emergencies, patients are truly incompetent and unable to decide. The *emergency exception* to informed consent permits treatment, but usually only for a very brief period of time—hours to a few days—during which time other treatment approaches should be considered, while procedures are initiated to permit continued forced treatment.

Finally, mental health has long recognized a so-called *therapeutic privilege*. Physicians may withhold information from a patient, particularly information about risks, when to inform the patient would cause such a high degree of psychological distress that the decision-making process itself would be badly compromised (Meisel, 1979). The scope of the therapeutic privilege exception continues to be debated. This exception to informed consent does not sanction the withholding of information merely because to learn the information might change the patient's decision or cause him to refuse treatment. However, when patients are very upset, when the transmission of information clearly causes distress, then the physician may choose to invoke the therapeutic privilege and withhold information, at least on a temporary basis. Generally, the matter should not end here. Under these circumstances, it is only prudent for the physician to discuss relevant treatment information, withheld from the patient, with the patient's relatives or friends. This approach permits a variant of *substituted judg-ment* (see below) and also secures the agreement of others that withholding information is truly in the patient's best interest. When such an approach is followed, it is frequently possible to arrive at other strategies. For example, family and friends can also play a role in information disclosure to distressed patients. They can assist the physician to understand how best to approach the patient the next time, etc. The therapeutic privilege exception, like other excep-tions, usually permits physicians to balance autonomy and health needs of patients in a clinically sensitive fashion.

SUBSTITUTE DECISION-MAKING

Patients who are incompetent must have decisions made for them by substitute or proxy decision-makers. The choice of decision-maker is often made informally (without recourse to the courts), in which case it is usually a family member, a close friend, the physician, or other member of the hospital staff. It may also be made by a court, in which case the judge will either make the decision or appoint a guardian, conservator, or committee to do so.

The vast majority of incompetency decisions are made by physicians (without recourse to the courts) who, by medical tradition, rely on family members to make decision for patients who are incapacitated (Appelbaum et al, 1987). In recent years, controversy about who should decide for incompetent patients and how these decisions should be made has mushroomed, leading the Presi-dent's Commission for the Study of Ethical Problems in Medicine and Biomedical and Behavioral Research (Volume 1, 1982) to endorse the continued involvement of families as substitute decision-makers. There are, unfortunately, no clear guidelines indicating when such *de facto* determinations and reliance on family are appropriate and when more formal procedures are necessary. Though reliance on a family member is often most practical, there are numerous situations in which family dynamics or conflicts of interest make this problematic.

In a growing number of cases, the courts have ruled that such informal procedures inadequately protect patients' rights. The right to refuse treatment cases are an example. In Massachusetts, the court has delegated such decisions to itself, working in conjunction with a court-appointed guardian *ad litem*, whose role is to monitor the treatment that the court orders (*Rogers vs. Okin, 1984*). In New York, the courts have ruled that only a judge can make a determination of incompetency to refuse medication and of the need for treatment (*Rivers v. Katz, 1986*). Court cases involving the termination of life-sustaining treatment (reviewed in Regan, 1987) have been another vehicle for the debate about who should decide for incompetent patients and by what standards the decisions should be made. It is imperative that physicians and hospital staff inform themselves of the statutory requirements and case law in their jurisdiction and that hospitals develop formal guidelines for incompetency determinations and substitute decision-making.

Historically, substitute decisions were to be made according to the *best interests* of the patient. For a generation now, this theory of substitute decision-making has been challenged by the theory of *substitute judgment*, in which the surrogate attempts to decide as the patient would, based on the patient's values and wishes to the extent that they can be reconstructed (President's Commission, Volume 1, 1982). Though substituted judgment decisions would seem to be most protective of patient autonomy, they can be extremely difficult to implement for patients who have never been competent, who have never articulated their values or wishes, or who have done so in a conflicted and ambivalent manner (Gutheil and Appelbaum, 1985). Advance directives, such as living wills or durable powers of attorney, are likely to have increasing importance as a means of extending one's choice when competent to circumstances in which future decisional capacity is lost. Legal sanctions for their use, however, remain unclear in most jurisdictions.

OBTAINING CONSENT: THE INFORMED CONSENT DIALOGUE

In a simplistic model of informed consent, the doctor and patient come together at a single point in time. Information is transmitted to an apparently competent patient, who then rationally chooses a course of treatment and gives his consent, and treatment ensues. Though this model does conform to the legal requirements, it does not conform to what we know about how treatment decisions are really made (Lidz et al, 1984). Appelbaum et al (1987) have referred to this as the *event model*. They propose in its place a *process model*, in which informed consent is viewed as a continuous process with an ongoing exchange of information throughout the course of the physician-patient relationship. We refer to this process as a *dialogue*, to emphasize that there are (at least) two parties engaged in an ongoing process of decision.

Any approach to truly informed consent begins with the attitudes a physician brings to the first encounter with a patient. Does the treatment environment encourage independent thinking or dependency? Has sufficient time been set aside to encourage a real dialogue? Does the physician convey an interest in discussion with the patient or a rushed authoritarianism? Does the physician develop rapport with the patient? How far the informed consent dialogue can go will be established through these means, before either party has spoken a word.

As the informed consent dialogue begins, the physician should present information to the patient in a discussion-like format, encouraging questions. Katz (1984) has emphasized that patients should be given an opportunity to discuss their values and preferences, before the physician makes recommendations. In this way, the physician begins to understand the rationale for the patient's choices before precluding their expression. The patient is then asked to make a final choice only after hearing the physician's explanation of the recommendations. The patient should understand the rationale behind the doctor's choices. The physician should be prepared to return to the subject in future discussions, acknowledging the patient's need to reconsider what has been learned, consult with family and friends, and have additional questions answered. As treatment proceeds, modifications of the original decision may occur.

In presenting information, the physician should attend to the patient's level of sophistication and intelligence and tailor information to the patient's needs (Stanley, 1983). Technical information should be framed in an intelligible fashion. The informed-consent doctrine has never meant that all risks, regardless of how remote, should be disclosed, and it is vital to avoid a defensive medicine posture, in which a litany of risks is presented to the patient on the erroneous theory that this is necessary to avoid liability.

The way in which information about risks is disclosed can significantly influence the way the risks are perceived. For example, emphasizing the probability of success of a treatment has a very different effect than emphasizing the likelihood of failure (McNeil et al, 1982). Risks should be presented in such a way that patients can meaningfully compare then, and physicians should question the patient's understanding of disclosed information to monitor problems in communication. It is often appropriate to enlist the aid of family members or close friends in the decision-making process.

Consent forms, which are notoriously overcomplicated, should be as readable as possible, and patients should be given time to review them. One study of five surgical consent forms found them to be written at the level of advanced undergraduate or graduate students (Grunder, 1980). A study of patients in a state psychiatric hospital found that hospital documents demanded an ability to read far beyond the literacy skills of most patients (Berg and Hammitt, 1980). Comprehension increases when consent forms are simplified and shortened and when they are left with the patient for several days (Bergler et al, 1980). Miller and Willner (1974) propose a two-part consent form, in which the second part consists of a list of questions the patient must answer regarding information disclosed in the first part. Thus the consent form becomes an educational instrument testing deficiencies in understanding and leading to further dialogue. Other teaching and review methods can be devised, such as psychoeducational videotapes and pamphlets, medication groups, or other educational materials.

A few more words about consent forms are in order. The informed consent process is too readily reduced to the ritual of getting the patient's signature on the form. This is because physicians and patients believe the primary purpose of the consent form is to protect doctors from lawsuits (Harris et al, 1982). In fact, insufficient legal protection may be provided by a signed consent, if adequate information has not been disclosed orally or if a discussion has not been documented in the chart. In psychiatry, the use of consent forms has generally been limited to electroconvulsive treatment (ECT), sodium-amytal interviews, and experimental treatments, but in recent years, proposals have arisen to require consent forms for neuroleptics (Deveaugh-Geiss, 1979). Model consent forms have been published (Klein et al, 1984), and California has enacted legislation requiring their use. However, an emphasis on form-signing deemphasizes the importance of discussion; consent forms are a sign of, not the substance of, informed consent.

CONSENT IN PSYCHIATRIC PRACTICE

The Psychiatrist Consultant in Competency Assessments

Psychiatrists are commonly asked to assess the competency of medical and surgical patients who refuse treatment. That such a consultation is requested implies that the patient's physician is alarmed by this choice and questions the patient's competency to make it. Appelbaum and Roth (1982) have outlined a number of considerations vital to such consultations. First, it is critical to know what information has been presented to the patient because it is impossible to evaluate the patient's understanding without knowing the accuracy and completeness of what has been disclosed. This task may be complicated by the involvement of multiple clinicians caring for the patient, as each may be unclear about how much responsibility for disclosure other staff members are taking (Munetz, 1985).

When assessing competency, the patient's mental status should be evaluated over time in several interviews. Competency is a fluid phenomenon, and it can fluctuate with the courses of illness and treatment (Schwartz and Blank, 1986). Following the initial interview, it is often necessary to confirm the information provided by the patient. Patients with circumscribed delusions, for example, will often appear quite intact unless accurate historical data is provided by others.

The most important contribution the psychiatrist can make in such consultations is consideration of psychodynamic factors that may be contributing to the patient's apparent incompetency. The proposed treatment may have a special meaning to the patient, conscious or unconscious, that produces a regression to primitive defense levels, thus preventing understanding. A brief therapeutic intervention may resolve the crisis. Recommending medication may also help.

The obligation for obtaining informed consent should remain that of the physician requesting the consultation. It is generally useful to work in tandem with the patient's primary physician, asking him or her to reexplain the procedure to the patient in the consultant's presence. This helps keep lines of responsibility clear and provides the consultant with knowledge of information disclosed, creating a framework within which to understand the patient's confusion or distortion.

Hospitalization

At least one state legislature has sought to promote voluntary consent by explicitly prohibiting doctors from inducing patients to sign in voluntarily under the threat of commitment (Brakel et al, 1985). A number of state legislatures have embodied other informed consent provisions into the mental health statutes governing admission into the hospital. For example, the New York Mental Hygiene Law (1978, Supp. 1988) requires that:

> In order for a person to be suitable for admission to a hospital as a voluntary or informal patient, or for conversion to such status, he must be notified of and have the ability to understand the following:
> (1) that the hospital to which he is requesting admission is a hospital for the mentally ill
> (2) that he is making an application for admission
> (3) the nature of the voluntary or informal status, as the case may be, and the provisions governing release or conversion to involuntary status

A Pennsylvania statute goes still farther by requiring that the patient shall be informed of the types of treatments he may receive and any restraints or restrictions to which he may be subject (Pa. Stat. Ann., 1978).

Medication

The symptoms with which psychiatric patients present can create special problems in the implementation of informed consent for medications. Impaired cognition, affect, and volition may all compromise patient decision-making. Nevertheless, the presumption of patient competency initially applies. During the 1950s and 1960s, the law came to recognize that even involuntary commitment to a psychiatric hospital did not necessarily mean that the patient was legally incompetent. This development paved the way for later development of a *right to refuse treatment* not only for outpatients, but also for inpatients, and laid the groundwork for extension of the informed consent doctrine to every area of psychiatric practice.

The most common psychiatric intervention for which consent is required is the administration of psychotropic medication. Of the various classes of psychotropics, the neuroleptics are of greatest concern because of the risk of tardive dyskinesia, and because they are often introduced when the patient's decisional capacity is impaired by psychosis. The disclosure of information about antipsychotic medication should begin with a description of the patient's condition and of the likely course and outcome of psychosis, with and without treatment. The level of detail will necessarily vary as a function of patient motivation, intelligence, and previous treatment experience. Alternative treatments (such as ECT) should be discussed when the therapist believes them to be credible options. Common side effects, such as sedation, hypotension, akinesia, akisthesia, and acute dystonic reactions, should be mentioned, as well as the risk of tardive dyskinesia.

It is often impossible to meaningfully discuss these issues with acutely psychotic, agitated, and disorganized patients. While it generally remains useful to attempt discussion of acute side effects (for example, dystonic reactions that will have immediate treatment and compliance implications), the exceptions to informed consent generally permit some delay in full disclosure. For severely disturbed patients, a delay of a few weeks (until the acute disorganization has resolved) may be justified before discussing tardive dyskinesia, but in general, further delay is not clinically, ethically, or legally supportable (Roth, 1983; Halleck, 1980). While there is no single right way to handle disclosure about tardive dyskinesia, failure to disclose the risk creates a potential liability that could be considerable, given the number of patients on long-term neuroleptic treatment (see Chapter 19 and Wettstein, 1985). The obstacles to such discussions, created by institutions, therapists, and patients alike, remain great (Munetz, 1985). Therapist resistance to discussing tardive dyskinesia is high (Lidz et al, 1984), probably out of concern that such discussions will threaten the working alliance with paranoid, hostile, ambivalent, or negativistic patients (Munetz, 1985). Although some patients may use such information to rationalize their medication refusal, these patients are generally noncompliant to begin with and the little research done on the subject indicates that informing patients about tardive dyskinesia does not lead to increased noncompliance with neuroleptics (Munetz and Roth, 1985).

The clinical considerations which bear on informing patients about tardive dyskinesia and other neuroleptic-induced movement disorders illustrate the need for a process (ongoing dialogue) model of informed consent. Empirical studies point to a pattern of omission and denial about this subject, as if both doctor and patient collude to keep it from discussion. In his review, Wettstein (1988) notes that patients minimize or deny these side effects, and they fail to remember clinicians' disclosures about them. At the same time, physicians fail to recognize extrapyramidal syndromes (Weiden, 1987) and inadequately disclose information about these risks to patients (Lidz et al, 1984). The need for an ongoing dialogue, with repeated disclosures and assessments, is clear. Such discussions should heighten the clinician's awareness of side effects, as well as the patient's need for more information, and lead to dosage or other treatment adjustments as an integral part of the ongoing dialogue (Schwartz, 1986). In this model, the patient learns more about medication through experience, while the physician learns more about the impact of medicine on the patient's life. As the therapeutic alliance grows, compliance may be enhanced.

Electroconvulsive Therapy

ECT is indisputably one of psychiatry's most effective treatments (Weiner, 1979). Though it is the treatment of choice in a number of clinical situations and may be the only effective treatment available, its use is associated with risks of medical complications and memory loss, which must be disclosed in the informed-consent process. Informing patients about ECT can be a difficult process, complicated by the gravity of mental illness that ECT candidates often experience and by the complexity of the procedure. Nevertheless, the law is clear: Legally competent patients must give informed consent for ECT. The refusals of competent patients must be honored, and most statutory regulation requires that, when competency is in question, clinicians must turn to the courts. Though ECT can be administered involuntarily in an emergency in some jurisdictions (Brakel et al, 1985), doing so requires the utmost attention to documentation of medical urgency.

Because ECT is considered a procedure and requires the administration of anesthesia, virtually all institutions require written consent forms. The American Psychiatric Association's *Task Force Report on Electroconvulsive Therapy* (1978) provides a model of information disclosure that can be modified to the needs of individual patients.

Psychotherapy

Psychiatrists and other psychotherapists have not traditionally engaged patients in discussions of the risks and benefits of psychotherapies. In part, this omission reflects the rarity of malpractice actions against therapists engaged solely in verbal therapies. This reluctance is also rooted in a psychoanalytically based theoretical tradition (Robitscher, 1978). The patient's need for extensive information may be viewed as resistance, and it is feared that extended discussions early in the course of treatment will contaminate the development of the transference. Still another explanation lies in the uncertainty surrounding the prediction of risks, benefits, and prognosis of any particular treatment, and the difficulties doctors face in disclosing uncertainty (Katz, 1984). As research on differential therapeutics and psychotherapy outcomes progresses, the requirements for disclosure about verbal therapies will more closely approximate those for somatic treatments.

In our experience, it is best to provide basic information about psychotherapy during the initial evaluation period. Such discussions should touch on the nature of the treatment process, the length of treatment, prognosis, cost, and other similar factors. The psychiatrist should encourage and answer the patient's questions, even though some may be overdetermined or idiosyncratic or may become the subject of later therapeutic scrutiny (Simon, 1982). Possible adverse consequences, such as the development of regressive dependency states, untoward transference reactions, or other dysfunctional reactions, should be discussed when the therapist believes they are likely to occur (Simon, 1982). Robitscher (1978) discusses the distorting effects such discussions can have on the process of psychoanalytic psychotherapies.

The limits of confidentiality is another issue requiring attention. Any situation where the psychiatrist's loyalties are divided (for example, school or military psychiatrists may be required to convey clinical information to the organization) should be revealed before the patient discloses information to the clinician. The *Tarasoff* case, and others that followed, have focused attention on the therapist's duty to balance the protection of the patient's confidentiality against the therapist's obligation to protect third parties, who may be harmed by the patient (Roth and Meisel, 1977). When a therapist suspects that a patient may reveal a confidence the therapist will be unable to keep, the patient should be so advised. Such an informed-consent discussion may allow the therapist to share the dilemma with the patient, leading to other constructive resolutions that maintain confidentiality while satisfying the *duty to protect* (Roth and Meisel, 1977). The *Tarasoff* duties are discussed in greater detail by Dr. Wettstein in Chapter 19.

Patients who test positive for human immuno deficiency virus (HIV) and refuse to inform their sexual partners pose an analogous dilemma for their physicians. If all efforts to persuade the patient of his or her moral responsibilities fail, the physician arguably has an ethical obligation to protect an unwitting partner. Yet such breaches of confidentiality, if anticipated, may discourage patients from seeking HIV testing and counseling and ultimately pose a greater risk to public health. Every effort must be made to help patients face their responsibilities in such cases. Though no firm case law is available to guide us, we believe that, when all else fails, clinicians have an ethical obligation to advise the sexual partners of HIV-infected individuals. The American Psychiatric Association (1988) has also concluded that such warnings are ethically permissible.

Research

It is beyond the scope of this chapter to discuss the special considerations that apply to informed consent for research, but excellent reviews of the subject are available elsewhere (Appelbaum and Roth, 1982; Appelbaum et al, 1987). It is important to note, however, that research is a unique condition, generating special requirements for consent that are intended to protect the rights of patient/ subjects. The structure of research projects is such that therapeutic and research objectives are easily intermixed and confused, and patient/subjects tend to operate under a *therapeutic misconception* (Appelbaum et al, 1982); they come to believe, despite explanation, that procedures or treatments not intended to be of benefit to them are actually of therapeutic value. Investigators should apply themselves to careful and complete disclosure of the risks and benefits of participation in a research project to dispel such misunderstanding and the consequent risk of invalid consent.

CONCLUSION: THE FUTURE OF INFORMED CONSENT

In contemplating the future of informed consent as a clinical practice, two factors loom as most influential: practitioners' attitudes and the structure of the health-care delivery system. In an excellent essay on informed consent within the British National Health Service, Schwartz and Grub (1985, p. 23) argue that ". . . there is no informed consent where the patient-consumer cannot have a choice of health care options." The British system, dependent on prospective funding and marked by rigidly limited resources, requires strict limitations on patient choice and hence on informed consent. There is, for example, little discussion of maintaining life support for terminally ill and comatose patients, and decisions to deny dialysis are routinely made by physicians without discussion with the patient. Of note, British courts have rejected the "American" expansion of informed consent and have supported restrictions on disclosure.

The conditions of medical care in Britain remind us that the individualism and autonomy promoted by informed consent are relative, not absolute, values, balanced not only by the value of health but by a myriad of economic and social considerations that reflect culture. Changes in the structure of health-care delivery in the United States, for example the growth of prepaid health maintenance organizations (HMOs) and the implementation of diagnostic related groups (DRGs), are intended to cut costs by limiting the choices of both patients and physicians. The inexorable growth and influence of cost containment measures pose alarming threats to the evolution of informed consent in the United States.

The challenge posed by economic constraints may well require an accommodation of the threshold for individual choice in medical care. Promoting the value of informed consent in this environment will require a commitment to the value of individual autonomy for its own sake and for its value in health. To nurture these values will require an ongoing process of physician education and socialization.

The legislation and litigation underlying the development of informed consent as a legal doctrine have proven inadequate to the task of significantly influencing physician attitudes and behavior. Informed consent as envisioned by the courts remains all too frequently absent from the clinical setting (Meisel and Roth, 1983; Lidz et al, 1984). Resistance to informed consent has many roots, but concern that it is just another trap to ensnare the unwary physician in liability is not supported by the small number of suits that have to date been based on failure to obtain informed consent (Slawson, 1984). Perhaps central to physicians' concerns is the belief that informed-consent doctrine requires that the practitioner value autonomy more than health. This is an unfortunate misconception, for, "while physicians may have a responsibility to foster the autonomy of patients by adhering to the doctrine of competent informed consent, they have a primary obligation to see that their interpretation of this doctrine, like all their efforts on patients' behalf, leads to a reasonable clinical outcome" (Schwartz and Blank, 1986, p. 1260). The future of informed consent will rest in large part on the educational efforts made to correct these misconceptions, as well as on the value society places on individual autonomy and free choice in an age of cost-containment.

REFERENCES

Alfidi RJ: Controversy, alternatives, and discussions in complying with the legal doctrine of informed consent. Radiology 1975; 114:231–234

American Psychiatric Association: Task Force Report 14: Electroconvulsive Therapy. Washington, DC, American Psychiatric Association, 1978

American Psychiatric Association: Policy statement: AIDS policy: confidentiality and disclosure. Am J Psychiatry 1988; 145:541

Appelbaum PS, Bateman AL: Competency to consent to voluntary hospitalization: a theoretical approach. Bull Am Acad Psychiatry Law 1980; 7:390-399

Appelbaum PS, Lidz CW, Meisel A: Informed Consent: Legal Theory and Clinical Practice. New York, Oxford University Press, 1987

Appelbaum PS, Mirkin SA, Bateman AL: Empirical assessment of competency to consent to psychiatric hospitalization. Am J Psychiatry 1981; 138:1170–1176

Appelbaum PS, Roth LH: Clinical issues in the assessment of competency. Am J Psychiatry 1981; 138:1462–1467

Appelbaum PS, Roth LH: Competency to consent to research: a psychiatric overview. Arch Gen Psychiatry 1982; 39:951–958

Appelbaum PS, Roth LH, Lidz CW: The therapeutic misconception: informed consent in psychiatric research. Int J Law Psychiatry 1982; 5:319–329

Beck JC, Staffin RD: Patients' competency to give informed consent to medication. Hosp Community Psychiatry 1986; 37:400–402

Benson PR, Roth LH: The evolution of social controls over biomedical research, in Law and Mental Health: International Perspectives. Edited by Weisstub DN. New York, Pergamon Press, in press

Berg A, Hammitt KB: Assessing the psychiatric patient's ability to meet the literacy demands of hospitalization. Hosp Community Psychiatry 1980; 31:266–268

Bergler JH, Pennington AC, Metcale M, et al: Informed consent: how much does the patient understand? Clin Pharmacol Ther 1980; 27:435–439

Brakel SJ, Parry J, Weiner BA: The Mentally Disabled and the Law, third edition. Chicago, American Bar Foundation, 1985

Canterbury v. Spence, 464 F 2d 772, 787 (1972)

Cobbs v. Grant, 502 P 2d 1 (1972)

Devaugh-Geiss J: Informed consent for neuroleptic therapy. Am J Psychiatry 1979; 136: 959–962

Drane JF: The many faces of competency. Hast Cent Report 1985; 15:17–21

Faden RR, Beauchamp TL: A History and Theory of Informed Consent. New York, Oxford University Press, 1986

Gilboy O, Schmidt O: "Voluntary" hospitalization of the mentally ill. Northwestern University Law Review 1971; 23:429–453

Goldstein J: On the right of "institutionalized mentally infirm" to consent to or refuse to participate as subjects in biomedical and behavioral research. Research Involving Those Institutionalized as Mentally Infirm, DHEW Publ. No. (OS) 78-0006, 2.1-2.39, 1978

Grunder TM: On the readability of surgical consent forms. N Engl J Med 1980; 302:900–902

Gutheil TG, Appelbaum PS: The substitute judgment approach: its difficulties and paradoxes in mental health settings. Law, Medicine and Health Care 1985; 13:61–64

Halleck SL: Law and the Practice of Psychiatry. New York, Plenum Press, 1980

Harris L, Boyle JM, Bromsetin PJ: Views of informed consent and decision-making: parallel surveys of physicians and the public, in Making Health Care Decisions: The Ethical and Legal Implications of Informed Consent in the Patient-Practitioner Relationship. President's Commission for the Study of Ethical Problems in Medicine and Biomedical and Behavioral Research, volume two: Appendices, Empirical Studies of Informed Consent. Washington, DC, Superintendent of Documents, 1982

Kaimowitz v. Michigan Department of Public Health. Div no 73-19434-AW, Cir Ct of Wayne County, Mich. 1973. Reprinted in Law, Psychiatry and the Mental Health System. Edited by Brooks AD. Boston, Little, Brown and Co., 1974

Katz J: Why doctors don't disclose uncertainty. Hast Cent Report 1984; 14:35–44

Klein JI, Macbeth JE, Onek JN: Legal Issues in the Private Practice of Psychiatry. Washington, DC, American Psychiatric Press, Inc., 1984

Lankton JW, Batchelder BM, Ominsky AJ: Emotional responses to detailed risk disclosure for anesthesia, a prospective, randomized study. Anesthesiology 1977; 46:294–296

Lidz CW: The weather report model of informed consent: problems in preserving patient voluntariness. Bull Am Acad Psychiatry Law 1980; 8:152–160

Lidz CW, Meisel A, Zerubavel E, et al: Informed Consent: A Study of Decisionmaking in Psychiatry. New York, Guilford Press, 1984

McNeil BJ, Panker SG, Sox HC, et al: On the elicitation of preferences for alternative therapies. N Engl J Med 1982; 306:1259–1262

Meisel A: The expansion of liability for medical accidents: from negligence to strict liability by way of informed consent. Nebraska Law Review 1977; 56:51–152

Meisel A: The "exceptions" to the informed consent doctrine: striking a balance between competing values in medical decisionmaking. Wisconsin Law Review 1979; 2:413–488

Meisel A, Kabnick L: Informed consent to medical treatment: an analysis of recent legislation. University of Pittsburgh Law Review 1980; 41:407–564

Meisel A, Roth LH: What we do and do not know about informed consent. JAMA 1981; 246:2473–2477

Meisel A, Roth LH: Toward an informed discussion of informed consent: a review and critique of the empirical studies. Arizona Law Review 1983; 25:265–346

Meisel A, Roth LH, Lidz CW: Toward a model of the legal doctrine of informed consent. Am J Psychiatry 1977; 134:285–289

Mill JS: On Liberty. Chicago, H. Regnery, 1955

Miller, R, Willner HS: The two-part consent form: a suggestion for promoting free and informed consent. N Engl J Med 1974; 290:964–966

Munetz MR: Overcoming resistance to talking to patients about tardive dyskinesia. Hosp Community Psychiatry 1985; 36:283–287

Munetz MR, Roth LH: Informing patients about tardive dyskinesia. Arch Gen Psychiatry 1985; 42:866–871

Natanson v. Kline, 300 P. 2d 1093, 1104, 1106 (1960)

Olin GB, Olin HS: Informed consent in voluntary mental hospital admissions. Am J Psychiatry 1975; 132:938–941

Pa. Stat. Ann. Tit. 50 §7101 (Purdon 1978)

Pernick MS: The patient's role in medical decisionmaking: a social history of informed consent in medical therapy, in President's Commission for the Study of Ethical Problems in Medicine and Biomedical and Behavioral Research: Making Health Care Decisions: The Ethical and Legal Implications of Informed Consent in the Patient-Practitioner Relationship, volume two: Appendices, Empirical Studies of Informed Consent. Washington, DC Superintendent of Documents, 1982

President's Commission for the Study of Ethical Problems in Medicine and Biomedical and Behavioral Research: Making Health Care Decisions: The Ethical and Legal Implications of Informed Consent in the Patient-Practitioner Relationship, volume one. Washington, DC, Superintendent of Documents, 1982

Rachlin S, Schwartz HI: Unforeseeable liability for patients' violent acts. Hosp Community Psychiatry 1986; 37:725–731

Regan JJ: Withholding life support from the elderly, or learning to live with high-tech death, in Geriatric Psychiatry and the Law. Edited by Rosner R, Schwartz HI. New York, Plenum Press, 1987

Rivers v. Katz, 495 NE 2d 337 (N.Y. 1986)

Robitscher J: Informed consent for psychoanalysis. J Psychiatry Law 1978; 6:363-370

Rogers v. Okin, 478 F. Supp. 1342 (D. Mass), aff'd in part and rev'd in part, 634 F. 2d 650 (1st Cir. 1980), vacated and remanded 457 U.S. 291 (1982), opinion on certification sub nom. *Rogers v. Commissioner of the Department of Mental Health*, 458 N.E. 2d 308 (Mass., 1983), and on remand *Rogers v. Okin*, 738 F 2d (1st Cir. 1984)

Roth LH: Competency to consent to or refuse treatment in psychiatry, in Psychiatry 1982: The American Psychiatric Association Annual Review. Edited by Grinspoon L. Washington, DC, American Psychiatric Press, Inc., 1982

Roth LH: Is it best to obtain informed consent from schizophrenic patients about the possible risk of drug treatment, for example, tardive dyskinesia, before initiating treatment or at a later date? J Clin Psychopharmacol 1983; 3:207–208

Roth LH: Informed consent and its applicability for psychiatry, in Psychiatry. Edited by Michels R, Cavenar J, Brodie HKH, et al. Philadelphia, J.B. Lippincott, 1985

Roth LH, Appelbaum PS, Sallee R, et al: The dilemma of denial in the assessment of competency to refuse treatment. Am J Psychiatry 1982a; 139:910–913

Roth LH, Lidz CW, Meisel A: Competency to decide about treatment or research: an overview of some empirical data. Int J Law Psychiatry 1982b; 5:29–50

Roth LH, Meisel A: Dangerousness, confidentiality and the duty to warn. Am J Psychiatry 1977; 134:508–511

Roth LH, Meisel A, Lidz CW: Tests of competency to consent to treatment. Am J Psychiatry 1977; 134:279–284

Salgo v. Leland Stanford Junior University Board of Trustees 317 P. 2d 170, 181 (1957)

Schloendorff v. Society of N.Y. Hospital, 211 N.Y. 125, 105 N.E. 92 (N.Y. 1914)

Schwartz HI: Legal and ethical issues in neuroleptic non compliance. Psychiatric Annals 1985; 16:588–595

Schwartz HI: Do-not-resuscitate orders: the impact of guidelines on clinical practice, in Geriatric Psychiatry and the Law. Edited by Rosner R, Schwartz HI. New York, Plenum Press, 1987

Schwartz HI, Blank K: Shifting competency during hospitalization: a model for informed consent decisions. Hosp Community Psychiatry 1986; 37:1256–1260

Schwartz HI, Rachlin S: Patient access to mental health records: impact on clinical practice, in Legal Encroachment on Psychiatric Practice. Edited by Rachlin S. San Francisco, Jossey-Bass Inc., 1985

Schwartz HI, Vingiano W, Berzerganian-Perez C: Autonomy and the right to refuse treatment: patients' attitudes after involuntary medication. Hosp Community Psychiatry, 1988; 39:1049–1054

Schwartz R, Grubb G: Why Britain can't afford informed consent. Hastings Cent Rep 1985; 15:19–25

Simon RI: Psychiatric Interviews and Malpractice: A Primer for Liability Prevention. Springfield, MA, Charles C Thomas, 1982

Slater v. Baker and Stapleton, 95 Eng. Rep. 860 (K.B. 1767)

Slawson PF: The clinical dimension of psychiatric malpractice. Psychiatric Annals 1984; 14:358–364

Stanley B: Senile dementia and informed consent. Behav Sci Law 1983; 1:57–71

Stone AA: Informed consent: special problems for psychiatry. Hosp Community Psychiatry 1979; 30:321–327

Strull WM, Lo B, Charles G: Do patients want to participate in medical decision making? JAMA 1984; 252:2990–2994

Swartz MS: What constitutes a psychiatric emergency: clinical and legal dimensions. Bull Am Acad Psychiatry Law 1987; 15:57–68

Weiden PJ, Mann JJ, Haas G, et al: Clinical nonrecognition of neuroleptic-induced movement disorders: a cautionary study. Am J Psychiatry 1987; 144:1148–1153

Weiner RD: The psychiatric use of electrically induced seizures. Am J Psychiatry 1979; 136:1507–1515

Wettstein RM: Legal aspects of neuroleptic-induced movement disorders, in Legal Medicine 1985. Edited by Wecht CH. New York, Praeger, 1985

Wettstein RM: Informed consent and tardive dyskinesia. J Clin Psychopharmacol, 1988

Zeichner B: The role of unconscious conflict in informed consent. Bull Am Acad Psychiatry Law 1985; 13:283–290

Chapter 21

Involuntary Treatment

by Steven K. Hoge, M.D., Paul S. Appelbaum, M.D., and Jeffrey L. Geller, M.D., M.P.H.

Every branch of medicine at times employs involuntary care and, as in the right to die controversy, can become embroiled in the legal and ethical conundra with which it is associated. But no field is more involved—perhaps inextricably so— than psychiatry. The very nature of mental illness, affecting the rational and emotional functioning of the mind, results in many afflicted individuals who do not recognize their predicament and, consequently, are too often unwilling to seek treatment; coercive measures become necessary if they are to receive care. American society throughout our history has sanctioned—and at times demanded—the imposition of involuntary care for a significant number of the mentally ill (Appelbaum, 1985). Even in the present era of deinstitutionalization and expanded patient rights and with great emphasis placed on encouraging patients to accept care, approximately 300,000 patients per year are civilly committed in the United States (National Institute of Mental Health, 1985).

In the not distant past, society granted psychiatrists wide latitude in providing involuntary treatment to the mentally disabled, a natural outgrowth of the paternalistic basis for civil commitment. Historically, this paternalism has been the predominant rationale for involuntary treatment: the state, through its agents, psychiatrists, intervened to provide help to patients. Wide discretion, it was reasoned, should be allotted to psychiatrists in the exercise of professional judgment in order to maximize patients' benefit. An improved quality of life and individualized treatment would be patients' quid pro quo.

More recently, however, the public has been wary of ceding broad discretion to professionals for involuntary psychiatric care. Society has placed greater emphasis on the freedom of individuals to make decisions based on personal value systems, rather than on the notion that another, more *objective* set of values should dictate treatment decisions. This has resulted in a marked decrease in the deference shown professionals in the legal arena, where laws now set strict operational criteria for commitment decisions, and due process requirements are imposed that assure judicial oversight at significant junctures of the decision-making process.

A second major legal development, the evolution of the doctrine of the *least restrictive alternative*, has set a high standard for assessing the acceptability of the degree of government intrusion: in choosing means to effect legitimate government policies, the state must employ the one that least infringes on constitutional rights to personal liberty. This doctrine was applied first to civil commitment decisions in *Lake v. Cameron 1976* and has been used since that time to scrutinize virtually every aspect of involuntary care. Legislators and judges have applied the doctrine to ensure that statutes are formulated and implemented in the narrowest fashion to accomplish their goals. The outcome has been further limitation of professional discretion.

In this chapter we review the major areas of involuntary treatment in psychiatry: involuntary hospitalization and involuntary treatment with medication. In addition, we explore the development of involuntary outpatient commitment, an innovation that has attracted considerable attention.

INVOLUNTARY HOSPITALIZATION

Civil commitment laws have undergone cyclic periods of reform, with alternating calls for more and less restrictive statutes. When there arose optimism that active treatment held the promise of recovery for the mentally ill, as in much of the first two-thirds of this century, commitment laws reflected this hope: wide latitude was granted to commit those *in need of treatment*, with the expectation that psychiatrists and courts would use this discretion wisely. Oversight of commitment procedures was loose, and commitment laws were grounded in the state's *parens patriae* powers (literally state as father) which apply when individuals are unable to act in their own best interests. Under in need of treatment standards and lax procedures for civil commitment, institutionalization reached its zenith in the mid-1950s, when more than 550,000 patients populated state mental-health facilities (Appelbaum, 1985).

By the 1960s, the in need of treatment standard and relaxed commitment procedures were under attack. Popular media exposed institutional abuse of patients, both intentional and neglectful, and brought to public attention the committed mentally ill who were warehoused without effective treatment. Civil libertarian reformers assailed the states' power to confine patients for long periods under the vague in need of treatment standard, and critics emerged from within the psychiatric profession, primarily from the community psychiatry movement, whose opposition to institutional care was based on the belief that patients could be better cared for in the community. These forces converged at a time of widespread skepticism of governmental benevolence and intrusion into individuals' lives. The result was a rejection of paternalistic grounds for commitment in favor of police power principles and criminalized procedures: the focus of commitment laws shifted from the patients' treatment needs to the likelihood that behavior dangerous to the patient or others would occur (Livermore, et al, 1968).

Both legislative initiatives and appellate cases have played important roles in the adoption of dangerousness-oriented commitment criteria. In 1969, California enacted the Lanterman-Petris-Short Act, which required that a person be, by reason of mental illness, dangerous to self or others, or so gravely disabled as to be at risk of physical harm in the community in order to be involuntarily committed (California Welfare and Institutions Code Sec. 5150). This emphasis on dangerousness was carried to its fullest limit in *Lessard v. Schmidt*, decided in Wisconsin in 1972, which specified similar grounds for commitment but required as demonstration of dangerousness an overt act within 30 days of filing for commitment. The *Lessard* court also set strict procedural guidelines for commitment proceedings, many borrowed from criminal law: proof beyond a reasonable doubt, notice, adversarial hearings. Virtually every jurisdiction subsequently tightened its procedures and adopted a dangerousness-oriented standard (Brakel et al, 1985).

In contrast to the mood that was pervasive during the 1970s, when most civil commitment laws were last revised, the current perception is that commitment statutes are too narrow in scope and fail to satisfy society's legitimate interests in caring for the mentally disabled. Although it is difficult to draw firm conclusions about the effects of tighter commitment statutes from existing empirical studies (Appelbaum, 1984), opinions abound. Families of the mentally ill have emerged as critics of dangerousness-oriented commitment criteria that require them to abandon their loved ones or to suffer violence at their hands before help can be obtained (Dunham, 1985). The plight of the homeless mentally ill has led many people to question the ability of some mentally ill individuals, now outside the reach of commitment standards, to care adequately for themselves or to exercise their new-found civil liberties in a meaningful way (Lamb, 1984). Psychiatrists have voiced objections to a standard requiring that they act as agents of social control, rather than practitioners who treat their patients (Lamb and Mills, 1986). Finally, the entire enterprise can be called into question because the ability of mental health professionals accurately to predict violent behavior has been difficult to demonstrate (Monahan, 1981). The result has been numerous proposals for change.

Recent Changes in Commitment Criteria

State legislatures have been receptive to some of the many proposals for reform, generally broadening commitment criteria and relaxing procedural requirements. The following are among the major legislative changes in the past several years.

Addition of a deterioration standard. A few states have sought to broaden commitment standards by creating a criterion of likely "substantial deterioration"—similar to one proposed in the American Psychiatric Association's (APA) Model Law on Civil Commitment (Stromberg and Stone, 1983)—that is, more permissive than the usual gravely disabled criterion, which requires a likelihood of physical danger as a result of an inability to care for self. This change grows out of the frustration voiced by many clinicians and family members over prevailing standards that often postpone commitment of seriously ill individuals clearly on their way to being gravely disabled, thereby prolonging their suffering; that preclude treatment of some patients who decompensate into chronic illnesses, but who fall short of meeting dangerousness-oriented standards because they are able to subsist on their own in the community (many of the homeless mentally ill are thought to fall into this category); or that force families to abandon the ill in order to demonstrate their inability to provide for their basic needs (Wasow, 1986).

Typically, the new statutes specify that mental deterioration must be associated with a significant impairment in judgment, reason, or behavior or, alternatively, repeated and escalating loss of cognitive or volitional control over actions. Hawaii allows civil commitment of patients who are "obviously ill" (Hawaii Rev. Stat. Sec. 334-60.2, 1986). Texas combines a requirement that the patient be "unable to make a rational and informed decision" about treatment with its severe-deterioration criterion (Texas Stat. Ann. Art. 5547-33, 1983).

The addition of a deterioration criterion injects a greater measure of paternalism into the commitment statutes, while granting psychiatrists and the courts wider discretion in the employment of involuntary hospitalization. In the only empirical study of the deterioration standard, Durham and colleagues reported on the experience in the state of Washington; introduction at a time of great public support for broadening the commitment statute led to a massive increase in the number of committed patients, placing a severe strain on the mental health system's capacity to deliver services (Durham, 1985; Durham and LaFond, 1985). Though Durham has recommended caution to policymakers in adopting similar standards, since that time other states have undertaken comparable changes in commitment laws without reported problems. This suggests that the social and political climate may play a larger than expected role in how civil commitment authority is exercised.

Expansion or creation of gravely disabled criteria. Some states, in moving to dangerousness-oriented standards, did not create a *gravely disabled* criterion, relying solely on dangerousness to self and others to define the population subject to civil commitment. Although in practice or by case law many of these states have stretched the existing criterion of danger to self to encompass gravely disabled patients, some have perceived the need to amend their statutes to allow explicitly commitment of those patients (Hawaii Rev. Stat. Sec. 334-60.2, 1986). Oklahoma, for example, has made provision for this population in a standard that also requires a recent act demonstrating grave disability (Oklahoma Stat. Ann. tit. 43A, Sec. 3 [West 1978]). This stipulation indicates a continuing concern about how the gravely disabled criterion will be applied. One state, Minnesota, in its new mental health code, eliminated the phrase "failure to protect self from exploitation" from possible justifications for invoking its gravely disabled standard (Minn. Stat. Ann. Chap. 253B.02, Subd. 13 [West 1982]). This may reflect legislators' concerns about how such a vaguely worded criterion could be used or misused in practice.

Relaxation of the recent overt act requirement. The requirement for a recent, overt act demonstrating dangerousness, initially articulated in *Lessard*, operationalizes the dangerousness-oriented standard so that the prediction of future dangerousness—a clinically elusive task—is anchored by a demonstrable past event. Such a criterion undoubtedly reduces clinician-to-clinician variability in the application of civil commitment standards and gives clear guidelines to the judicial system. Nonetheless, this requirement has been subjected to criticism for not allowing hospitalization of patients who have threatened violence or who seem to be moving toward violent action. Various states have amended their statutes to relax the overt act criteria. For example, Alaska has broadened its criteria to include recent threats as well as acts, and eliminated the 30-day time limit for the dangerous to others criterion (Alaska Stat. Sec. 47.30.915 [1984]), and Arizona has done away with similar provisions in its civil commitment code (Ariz. Rev. Stat. Ann. Chap. 36-501 [1986]). Once again the effect of these revisions is to grant greater freedom to the committing psychiatrist and the adjudicating judge to determine how the commitment standards should be applied. Minnesota, in fine-tuning its commitment code, allowed either acts or threats in its danger to self and danger to others criteria, whereas prior to this only an actual attempt to harm would suffice for the danger to others criterion; simultaneously, however, the new code required that these acts or threats be recent, making the overall impact of the changes on the scope of civil commitment unclear (West 1982).

Other changes. One criterion of incompetency has attracted considerable interest and has been a component of treatment-oriented commitment reform proposals

(Stone, 1975; Treffert, 1985). The APA Model Law on Civil Commitment, which consists of both dangerousness- and treatment-oriented criteria, requires incompetency (Stromberg and Stone, 1983). An incompetency criterion, if applied rigorously, is likely to narrow the scope of the state's commitment authority. Some studies have found that one treatment-oriented commitment standard is more restrictive—largely due to the criterion of incompetency—than current dangerousness-oriented statutes; restricts commitment to a subset of more seriously ill patients from the group of patients now committable; and allows commitment of few new patients (Hoge et al, 1988, in press). Equally significant is the demonstration that treatment-oriented criteria may be more effective in restricting the scope of commitment and eliminating arbitrary decisionmaking than dangerousness-oriented criteria. This may be a function of reliance on clinical concepts familiar to the average psychiatrist as the bases for making commitment decisions, rather than on difficult-to-accomplish predictions of dangerousness. While no state has made incompetency necessary for involuntary hospitalization, Texas has restricted the use of "grave disability" to this group of potential patients (Texas Stat. Ann. Art. 5547-33, 1983). Kansas defines mental illness, for the purpose of civil commitment, as including patients who are incompetent or who refuse treatment; the latter requirement voids much of the significance of the incompetency provision (Kan. Stat. Ann. Art. 29, Sec. 59-2902 [1982]).

Some states have chosen to make subtle modifications in existing civil-commitment standards to effect policy changes. Alaska, for example, has eliminated the requirement that harm to self or others be "imminent and substantial," leaving the threshold for commitment to the trial judge's discretion. Washington and Alaska now allow for commitment on the basis of "danger to property," clearly broadening the scope of their statutes (Alaska Stat. Sec. 47.30.915 [1984]; Wash. Rev. Code Ann. Chap. 71.05.020, [1979]).

While the focus of this chapter is on standards for civil commitment, it should be noted that commitment procedures are equally important. Many states have changed some of their procedures, usually in the direction of facilitating the commitment process. Recently, the National Center for State Courts (1986) has issued extensive guidelines for lawyers, mental health professionals, and judges involved in the commitment process. The guidelines note steps that can be taken to improve the functioning of the commitment system, regardless of the statutory framework and without the need for legislative reform.

The Clinical Approach to Civil Commitment

Whether the consideration of civil commitment arises during the course of ongoing treatment or in the context of emergency evaluation, the imposition of involuntary care is a crisis point for the therapeutic relationship. The manner in which clinicians handle civil commitment may have lasting effects on patients' attitudes toward treatment. Furthermore, civil commitment represents a substantial curtailment of individual liberty and is typically initiated by the clinician rather than the court. Although legal protections are triggered quickly, patients may be involuntarily hospitalized in some jurisdictions for several weeks before due process produces a judicial hearing. Psychiatrists should therefore employ their commitment power after careful assessment of the applicability of the governing commitment standard and only after efforts to enlist the patient's cooperation have failed.

Commitment is often the terminal event in a series of involuntary or coerced intrusions, as for example, when patients are brought to psychiatric attention unwillingly by police, family, or friends. At such times, the evaluation itself may require that clinicians breach confidentiality, over their patients' objections, to gather information relevant to clinical and commitment decision-making from third parties. Clinicians face the challenge of conveying to reluctant, oppositional, or frankly hostile patients that their interests are being placed foremost in these endeavors.

In many cases, particularly where a prior treatment relationship is lacking and the reliability of informants unknown, psychiatrists will face some uncertainty about whether the commitment standard has been met. Largely, this is a consequence of dangerousness-oriented standards requiring prediction of violent acts. In unclear circumstances, psychiatrists should err on the side of safety and initiate emergency commitment. Further evaluation and observation in the hospital will provide a broader database and the opportunity for consultation, which will enhance decision-making. Ultimately, it is the responsibility of the judicial system to determine whether or not the commitment standard has been met, and psychiatrists are advised to act in the clinical interests of their patients at all times.

Conclusions

For the time being, legislatures have chosen to make relatively modest changes in their statutes. In general, these changes reflect a small swing of the pendulum back toward a paternalistic commitment code and increased discretionary power for psychiatrists and judges. The APA Model Law on Civil Commitment and its precursor, the Stone model, have been influential in reintroducing incompetency as a criterion, thereby holding out the possibility that ethical and legal problems associated with coercive treatment of competent individuals will no longer trouble the mental health field.

INVOLUNTARY TREATMENT WITH MEDICATION

Until the last decade, psychiatrists routinely exercised their authority to impose treatment on committed patients. The recently recognized right of civilly committed patients to refuse medication has diverse origins that can best be understood in historical perspective. Under the traditional commitment standards, patients were confined because they were "in need of treatment"; legally, ethically, and clinically, to allow patients to refuse the care for which they have been committed made little sense.

Necessary to the dramatic change in this practice was the maturation of the informed-consent doctrine, which altered the negotiation of care between all patients and their physicians. While competent—and, in psychiatric hospitals, voluntary—patients previously had been asked to consent to treatment after being told only the nature of the proposed procedure, informed consent required physicians to further divulge the relevant benefits, risks, side effects, and alternatives. This requirement grew from the recognition that individuals, facing similar medical decisions and provided with the same information, would make different choices based on personal circumstances and values. Informed consent, by emphasizing the value-laden nature of decision-making, undermined the idea that the choice of treatment was based on scientific objectivity and thereby weakened the authoritarian position of the doctor in forcing treatment. The doctor's role was to recommend treatments; the patient had the discretion to choose among options, including the option of no treatment (Appelbaum et al, 1987). Simultaneously, the doctrine suggested a means of analysis—the risk-benefit ratio—by which laymen could evaluate treatments.

The right to refuse treatment also arose from concerns about the quality of care in institutions. Over time, it had become apparent that antipsychotic medications were neither a panacea for mental illness nor risk free. Some patients were refractory or only partially responsive to treatment and, because of their intractability, remained on state hospital wards. For these patients, the advantages of long-term antipsychotic treatment were, at best, unclear. The recognition that tardive dyskinesia was a potential consequence of treatment with antipsychotics created concerns, even when antipsychotics proved effective; its potential for irreversibility made refusal seem a reasonable reaction to some. Some advocates charged, in addition, that underfunded and understaffed state hospitals used antipsychotics for their nonspecific, sedating properties to control patients—even, in some cases, to punish them—rather than for their specific, psychosis-ameliorating effects (Plotkin, 1977). It was further alleged that many institutions lacked sufficient, trained psychiatrists to supervise patients' pharmacotherapy. These allegations, undoubtedly accurate in some cases, fueled public concern that punitive motives predominated in public institutions. Further, constitutional questions were raised about the "mind-altering properties" of antipsychotics, and the implications of forced treatment for freedom of thought and expression (Gutheil and Appelbaum, 1983).

The birth of the right to refuse treatment awaited the change in the fundamental basis for civil commitment previously discussed. Under the new dangerousness-oriented criteria, the state sought commitment to avert the probability that harm would befall patients or others. But because treatment needs were no longer the basis for commitment, advocates began to question whether, once patients were confined, the state had the authority to medicate them involuntarily.

The Right to Refuse Treatment

In the late 1970s, two cases were initiated that delineated the two major approaches courts would subsequently take in sanctioning a right to refuse treatment: one a treatment-driven model, the second, rights-driven. In *Rennie v. Klein* (1983), the federal courts ultimately focused on quality-of-care concerns and required institutions to assure the appropriateness of proposed care by obtaining independent psychiatric opinions in cases of treatment refusal. By contrast in *Rogers v. Commissioner of the Department of Mental Health* (1983), the Massachusetts Supreme Judicial Court placed as the overriding concern the right of patients to determine their own treatment when competent to do so, absent an emergency. An informed consent analysis was thus adopted by this court requiring that the state, to override refusal, first demonstrate the patient's incompetency to make informed treatment decisions. Even then, a guardian could not make the decision to medicate with antipsychotics by the usual best interests standard; the Supreme

Judicial Court imposed a substituted judgment standard, whereby the court itself would make treatment decisions consonant with its understanding of the decisions the patient would have made if competent.

The psychiatric community greeted the right to refuse treatment with dire predictions that mental hospitals would collapse as untreated and unmanageable patients created new Bedlams; the safety of all patients and staff would be compromised (Gill, 1982). The prospect of committing patients who could not be treated also raised ethical considerations for psychiatrists and left many to question, in the absence of treatment, what distinguished hospitals from prisons (Gutheil, 1980). Furthermore, they argued that the quality of care would suffer as doctors shuttled back and forth to court while patients were left unattended and untreated at the hospital. Hospital administrators questioned the economic impact of delays in recovery brought about by the right to refuse treatment in an era of cost containment. On the other side, advocates of the right to refuse treatment believed that this right offered the best impetus for reform of institutional care; appropriate treatment would be guaranteed, along with respect for patients' rights (Schwartz, 1986). Now, more than a decade later, the impact of the right to refuse treatment can be assessed.

The Clinical Impact of Treatment Refusal

The frequency of treatment refusal in extant research varies with the definition of refusal episodes, patient populations, and methods for identifying refusers. Taken as a whole, the studies suggest that many patients, from 20 percent to 50 percent, refuse treatment at some time during their hospitalization (Appelbaum and Gutheil, 1980; Callahan, 1986; Hargreaves and Shumway, 1985). Most episodes of refusal either will not come to the clinician's attention at all, as when patients "cheek" medications, or will somehow be resolved, for example, through negotiation between patient and clinician.

Why do patients refuse antipsychotics? This is an issue of great importance, as advocates of the rights-based approach believe that refusal usually stems from a rational weighing of risks and benefits. Recent research, however, indicates that refusal is equally or more likely to be a result of the effects of illness, as with psychosis that can include denial of illness (Callahan, 1986; Hoge et al, 1988).

On most demographic parameters, refusers do not differ from patients who accept antipsychotics (Hoge et al, unpublished data). A few studies have, however, found that refusers may be more likely to suffer from bipolar disorder or schizoaffective disorder, but patients who persist in their refusal may be more likely to have a schizophrenic disorder (Zito et al, 1985).

Treatment refusers have been shown to have less insight into their illness and to exhibit more negative attitudes to hospitalization and past, present, and future treatment (Hoge et al, unpublished data). One study found that, though the degree of psychopathology measured by the Brief Psychiatric Rating Scale (BPRS) did not differ between groups, refusers rated significantly higher on subscales of conceptual disorganization, hostility, uncooperativeness, unusual thought content, excitement, and grandiosity; refusers also had lower scores on the guilt and depressed-mood subscales (Hoge et al, 1988). These findings support earlier reports that refusers were more likely to have formal thought disorder and delusions, but not hallucinations or paranoia (Marder et al, 1983; Marder et al, 1984). They also support the findings of Van Putten et al (1976) that patients whose psychoses incorporate ego-syntonic grandiosity are more likely to refuse treatment than are those who experience dysphoric or depressive affects.

As previously mentioned, most refusals are short-lived; in one study, 53 percent resolved within one week and 71 percent within 15 days, without recourse to formal means of adjudication (Hoge et al, 1988). However, documented cases of refusal extending beyond one year do exist (Geller, 1982), and crude outcome measures favor treatment acceptors: in the hospital, treatment refusers are more likely to be secluded or restrained than treatment acceptors (Appelbaum et al, unpublished data). Other studies have reported that refusers, compared to acceptors, have longer hospitalizations; in some samples the increased time in the hospital has been related to the length of refusal (Bloom et al, 1984; Hassenfeld and Grumet, 1984). Another study found that when the groups were controlled for diagnostic differences, there were no differences in length of hospitalization (Zito et al, 1986). Yet another study found refusers' increased length of hospitalization could not be accounted for by the length of treatment refusal or by diagnostic differences (Appelbaum et al, unpublished data).

Ultimately the impact of the right to refuse treatment rests on the long-term outcome of refusers. More research is necessary to delineate the courses of treatment refusers, both those who are eventually treated and those who escape involuntary care.

Recent Legal Developments

Every state has addressed the issue of the right to refuse treatment, some by statute or regulation, but major developments continue to evolve from court cases (Callahan, 1983). Most cases have followed the lead of *Rennie* or *Rogers* and can be classified into treatment-driven and rights-driven models (Appelbaum, 1988).

Treatment-driven models have been devised by courts that view patients' interests as limited to freedom from inappropriate care. The mechanisms devised to implement this right leave the discretionary authority to override refusal in professionals' hands, either those of the treating psychiatrist, the medical director, or an independent psychiatrist. Jurisdictions that have accepted this approach rely on informal procedures or a second opinion to screen out abuses of medications and support psychiatrists as the best decision-makers. Clinicians tend to favor such models because they minimize the likelihood that patients who need medications will go untreated. Administrators accept this model because it is economical, diverting little of psychiatrists' time from clinical responsibilities. Legal advocates often oppose these mechanisms, however, arguing that they are not sufficiently protective of individuals' rights because they allow involuntary treatment of competent patients.

Rights-driven models operate on an informed consent paradigm: competent patients—regardless of commitment status—have the absolute right to make treatment decisions, absent an emergency. In these jurisdictions the focus of inquiry becomes the capacity of the refusing patient to make treatment decisions; treatment needs are peripheral until a patient has been adjudicated incompetent. Jurisdictions that have adopted a rights-driven approach have rejected psychiatrists' ability to curb past abuses of discretion, and they cite the competing interests of institutions in maintaining order, discharging patients, or pleasing family members. The necessity of competency determinations, and secondarily, the need to balance competing interests, lead to judicial mechanisms of adjudication. Psychiatrists are leary of rights-driven adjudication because they fear that mentally ill patients will be denied needed treatment. Hospital administrators oppose rights-driven models because considerable clinical time must be devoted to preparation for and participation in court hearings; further, more resources must be diverted from patient care to legal representation.

In practice, the outcomes of these two different models are remarkably similar. In both cases, treatment refusal is infrequently upheld (Appelbaum and Hoge, 1986; Hoge et al, 1987), and the highest rates of refusal upholding are found in systems where the ultimate decision-making authority is in the hands of the clinician (Zito et al, 1984; Callahan, 1986). There is reason to believe that treatment needs are of primary importance, regardless of the official mechanism for adjudicating treatment refusal (Appelbaum, 1988). In rights-based systems, judges at the trial level are frequently most interested in the effectiveness of the treatment. Rigorous judicial models, however, can lead to caregivers reticent to seek to override refusals. Some patients who would benefit by treatment may not be taken to the adjudication phase due to time and staff constraints. (Hoge et al, 1987).

The Clinical Approach to Treatment Refusal

Treatment refusal arises in a wide variety of clinical contexts. In most cases, barring an emergency, psychiatrists initially should eschew overriding their patients' refusal in favor of thorough exploration of the motivating factors. Such an approach frequently leads to an uncovering of meaningful clinical material, facilitating negotiation of an end to refusal and a strengthening of the treatment alliance (Appelbaum and Gutheil, 1982).

Psychiatrists should begin with the assumption that the patient's refusal is reality-based. Antipsychotics can cause sedation, cognitive disturbances, dysphoria, akathesia, and akinesia (which may be subtle in presentation). Impotence, retrograde ejaculation, and other sexual dysfunctions should be specifically explored, as patients are often embarrassed to complain about them. Medication adjustments may be all that are necessary to regain the patient's compliance.

Patients often have fears about medication that are unfounded. Taking time to review recognized risks and side effects may reassure the patient. Of course, some risks, such as tardive dyskinesia, are quite real and cannot and should not be explained away. Nonetheless the patient is entitled to a full explanation of the attendant risks to treatment and may be relieved that the treating psychiatrist openly discusses them.

Secondary gain, interpersonal difficulties with caregivers, and transference can be manifested in the refusal of treatment and are amenable to therapeutic intervention. Some chronic patients refuse treatment as a nonspecific means of expressing distress or gaining staff attention. Mental illness itself can lead directly to treatment refusal; denial, projection, excessive guilt, mania, and delusions underlie much refusal. In some instances a consistent supportive stance will convince the patient to accept medication.

Conclusions

The future of case law on the right to refuse treatment is clouded (Appelbaum, 1988). The U.S. Supreme Court had the opportunity to hear both the *Rogers* and *Rennie* cases but preferred to return them for reconsideration to lower courts— the former, in light of another state mental health case, the latter, in light of *Youngberg v. Romeo (1982)*. In *Youngberg*, the U.S. Supreme Court found that, although patients had constitutionally protected interests at stake in care involving loss of liberty, the exercise of professional judgment is sufficiently protective of these rights and no formal judicial review is required. Federal courts have generally taken the *Youngberg* decision as an endorsement of treatment-driven models (as did the *Rennie* court); examples of these are *Project Release v. Prevost (1983)* and *Stensvad v. Reivitz (1985)*. State courts have tended to adopt rights-driven models, at times effectively overruling federal cases to do so; examples are *Rivers v. Katz (1986)* and *State ex rel. Jones v. Gerhardstein (1986)*. These courts, finding that individual autonomy trumps economic and treatment interests, are attracted to the informed-consent analysis. Current practices, however, suggest that, regardless of the views of appellate courts, quality of care considerations will dominate trial courts' concerns; this tension between theory and practice suggests that the capacity to provide involuntary treatment eventually will be brought into line with civil commitment authority, perhaps by requiring a finding of incapacity to make treatment decisions before allowing commitment.

INVOLUNTARY OUTPATIENT TREATMENT

In recent years, much attention has centered on involuntary outpatient commitment. The interest generated by outpatient commitment has two wellsprings, both derived from the conviction that the typical dichotomous commitment scheme—in which patients are either wholly at liberty or are confined to institutions—inadequately serves the chronic mentally ill. Disagreement exists, however, on whether outpatient commitment should be predicated on treatment-related issues or patients' rights.

Treatment-related concerns date to the introduction of antipsychotic medications in the 1950s, which opened the asylum doors to many for the first time. Administrators were encouraged by economic pressures to embark on deliberate policies of deinstitutionalization. Nearly a generation later, sober reflection on the efficacy of the new mental health system led to mixed conclusions. While many patients have benefited from acute, short-term hospitalization and outpatient care, others seem destined to frequent re-admissions through the "revolving door," often because they failed to take antipsychotic medications as outpatients (Geller, 1986a). The high rate of relapse has contributed to community intolerance of the mentally ill, due in part to public misconceptions about their dangerousness. This has complicated the development of outpatient programs and further undermined chances of successful adjustment for many former inpatients. The public's fears are compounded by the high visibility of the mentally ill and the adverse attention that relapse inevitably generates. There has been a growing consensus among psychiatrists that the ultimate success of community treatment may rest on the system's ability to insure that patients continue to take their medications as outpatients (Appelbaum, 1986). Many psychiatrists and families feel that involuntary outpatient treatment would enable these patients to spend more time outside of institutions and free from psychosis (Scheid-Cook, 1987).

Alternatively, patient-rights advocates have favored outpatient commitment as a means of limiting inpatient civil commitment. In this view, commitment to outpatient treatment would be an inpatient-treatment alternative to be preferentially employed by the courts under the doctrine of the least restrictive alternative (National Center for State Courts' Guidelines for Involuntary Civil Commitment, 1986).

Although superficially the goals of these two groups are similar—both aim to decrease the time patients spend in hospitals—proponents of outpatient commitment who are primarily concerned with treatment tend to conceptualize a system that exerts controls over more of the mentally ill; those who view outpatient commitment as a less restrictive alternative to routine commitment see it as a way of limiting those subject to more extensive controls.

Standards for Involuntary Outpatient Treatment

At present, statutory provisions for involuntary outpatient commitment are explicit in 27 states and the District of Columbia. The remaining states implicitly permit judges to commit patients to outpatient settings, often under the least restrictive alternative doctrine, with the sole exception of New York, whose civil commitment statute refers only to inpatient treatment (Brakel et al, 1985; Keilitz and Hall, 1985; Schwartz and Costanzo, 1987). Similar results can be effected for incompetent patients through guardianship proceedings available in all jurisdictions.

Among the states that make explicit provision for outpatient commitment, a diversity of approaches is taken. Most states make no distinction between the criteria for commitment to inpatient and outpatient treatment. A few of these jurisdictions restrict the application of outpatient commitment to a subset of chronic patients, usually defined by frequent, past, inpatient commitments. More recently there have been a few states (North Carolina, Hawaii, Georgia, Tennessee; N.C. Gen. Stat. Sec. 122C [1985], Hawaii Rev. Stat. Sec. 334 [1985], Tenn. Code Ann. Sec. 33 [1986], Ga. Code Ann. Sec. 37 [1986]) that have created commitment criteria, solely for outpatient commitment, that depart from the typical dangerousness-oriented standards. These statutes seem intended to broaden the scope of civil commitment or, at least, to target a different group of potential patients; they require a finding that outpatient commitment is necessary to prevent a relapse that would result in dangerousness—placing the imminence of the predicted behavior one step further removed from the time of assessment (Stefan, 1987). In two states, Hawaii and North Carolina, these predictions are anchored by the requirement that patient histories indicate a pattern of dangerous behavior when unmedicated. Both of these states also require a finding of impaired competence.

The American Psychiatric Association Task Force on Involuntary Outpatient Treatment has issued a report that may influence future legislative efforts. Under this proposal, the outpatient commitment standard would be the same as those recommended for inpatient commitment; that is, involuntary outpatient treatment could be ordered for those patients with a severe mental disorder who meet dangerousness-oriented criteria or who are likely to suffer deterioration, and who are adjudicated as incompetent to make treatment decisions. In addition, the proposal requires a detailed plan for treatment and monitoring, a finding that the proposed treatment is likely to be effective, and agreement by the outpatient psychiatrist or facility to accept responsibility (APA Task Force, 1988).

Effectiveness of Involuntary Outpatient Treatment

Considerable enthusiasm has been generated in the psychiatric community by case studies reporting dramatic improvements in the courses of patients under outpatient commitment (Geller, 1986b; Schneider-Braus, 1986; Owens, 1985). The research literature, however, is scant and conflicting: Uncontrolled studies have documented—as expected—that not all patients are compliant with outpatient commitment; consequently, some will be subject to involuntary hospitalization (Hiday and Goodman, 1982; Miller and Fiddleman, 1984). The methodology of other studies makes conclusions difficult (Appelbaum, 1986; Bursten, 1986). Zanni and deVeau (1986), in the most encouraging study, found that involuntary outpatient treatment resulted in a reduction in frequency and duration of subsequent hospitalizations compared to the previous course.

Considering how little is known about the effectiveness of outpatient civil commitment, it is not surprising that many psychiatrists and advocates have reservations about employing it. It follows that statutes have not been vigorously implemented, and, in the absence of research and extensive experience, clinical approaches to patients committed to outpatient treatment, while undoubtedly sharing features with approaches to inpatient commitees, have not fully evolved.

The most fundamental issue is one of funding. In many states, outpatient services are inadequate to meet the needs of the population presently served. Introduction of outpatient commitment—which requires active follow-up and monitoring—places additional strains on already overburdened delivery systems and may divert resources from voluntary patients. Legislative initiatives to establish outpatient commitment are likely to fail unless outpatient programs are sufficiently funded to provide essential services.

Success is also dependent on outpatient treatment systems that are invested in involuntary treatment. Many are not: outpatient clinicians, seeing their mission as serving only those who seek therapy, tend to philosophically oppose involuntary treatment. Such intangibles could significantly affect the efficacy of outpatient commitment and may account for the remarkable, but ungeneralizable, successes of a few devoted clinicians. Treatment models in which patients are cared for by the same team regardless of inpatient or outpatient status may mitigate these problems, as well as reported difficulties involving outpatient caregivers in devising treatment plans (Owens, 1985; Zanni and deVeau, 1986).

Implementation of outpatient commitment has been inhibited by the failure of most states to provide statutory means for ensuring compliance and effecting inpatient civil commitment if necessary. Some clinicians have felt that, without such provisions, they are placed in the position of being duplicitous with patients when informing them that outpatient commitment orders mean they "have to" take prescribed medication (Geller, 1986c). Perhaps for both practical and ethical reasons, this defect has resulted in outpatient commitment being largely ignored, except in the relatively few states—all having enacted outpatient-commitment statutes in recent years—that specify how enforcement is to occur. Without such provisions, outpatient commitment differs little from guardianship procedures that ultimately rely on the resourcefulness and initiative of the guardian in ensuring that treatment takes place.

Liability concerns have contributed to psychiatrists' reluctance to accept the responsibility attendant to outpatient commitment. To date, the scope of liability is unknown. Such concerns are well founded in jurisdictions where outpatient commitment is based on dangerousness-oriented criteria; in the event of an adverse outcome the patient's situation may be readily seen—with the benefit of retrospection—to have warranted inpatient care. Separating patients whose dangerousness can be managed safely as outpatients from those who require hospitalization may be too fine a distinction to reasonably expect clinicians to make. Some states have foreseen this problem and granted limited immunity to psychiatrists making these decisions (N.C. Gen. Stat. Sec. 122C [1985], Or. Rev. Stat. Sec. 426.130 [1983]). Fears of increased liability are greater in those jurisdictions where the means of enforcement are unclear.

Legal Concerns in Involuntary Outpatient Treatment

Considerable concern exists over the erosion of privacy stemming from outpatient commitment. While inpatient commitment has clear boundaries because it is defined by confinement to a *place*, outpatient commitment involves a general obligation to accept *treatment* that is not sharply delimited. Questions have been raised about which treatments are to be considered appropriate for outpatient committees, the duration of commitment, and the need for periodic judicial review. What criteria should govern the termination of outpatient commitment is also unclear. Improvements in functioning that follow outpatient commitment can readily be attributed to the effects of medication. The patient may perpetually face this irrebuttable presumption, making it difficult to prove that further commitment is unnecessary. Arbitrary commitment periods have the advantage of setting clear limits, but subsequent noncompliance may reduce the value of outpatient commitment to trivial increases in time spent on the outpatient side of the revolving door.

Defining acceptable treatments that can be ordered under outpatient commitment may be the most important boundary yet to be made explicit. Commentators agree that involuntary treatment with medication is central to the idea of outpatient commitment, not only because antipsychotics are important in the treatment of chronic mental patients, but because they are easily administered and can be effective without patients' cooperation. However, while outpatient commitment has come to be equated with involuntary medication treatment, most statutes do not limit its application to this treatment. (Hawaii and North Carolina are anomalous in specifically excluding involuntary medication.) Some have expressed concern that the expectation that outpatient commitment will involve forcible injections and perhaps involuntary monitoring of blood values sets a high tolerance for intrusion into personal privacy. This tolerance could pave the way, it is argued, for superficially less intrusive measures such as individual, family, or behavioral psychotherapy that could be applied to lesser problems than psychosis and have the potential of infiltrating every aspect of life.

Commentators have pointed out that outpatient commitment has a high risk for social control abuses (Mulvey et al, 1987). Like parole and probation systems that initially had therapeutic and rehabilitative goals, outpatient commitment, if inadequately funded, could degenerate into simple monitoring and control. There is some evidence that outpatient commitment is subject to such abuses. In North Carolina, Hiday and Scheid-Cook (1986) found that many patients committed to outpatient treatment did not meet statutory criteria; in the same jurisdiction, Miller et al (1984) found that outpatient commitment often occurred following a plea-bargaining process at the behest of judges, and that many patients were clinically inappropriate for such care.

Patients' legal advocates will face practical problems resulting from the looser structure of outpatient commitment. It will be more difficult to provide legal advice and to monitor for potential abuses in outpatient treatment, where care is decentralized and patients dispersed to various settings.

Enforcement of outpatient commitment is complicated by the ability of patients to cross state lines to avoid commitment. While return to the initial jurisdiction could be simplified by the negotiation of an amendment to the interstate compact currently covering inpatient escapees, there are troubling implications for individual freedom to travel.

Conclusions

Involuntary outpatient commitment has attracted the interest of patients' advocates, psychiatrists, administrators, and policy makers in the last few years. That this innovative form of involuntary care has been able to stir representatives of a broad range of perspectives is perhaps a result of its unrealized nature: outpatient commitment is a Rorschach blot in which each group finds what it will. It seems likely that outpatient commitment will fail to meet some, if not all, expectations. Those who see outpatient commitment as a cost-efficient alternative to hospitalization are likely to be severely disappointed. Providing a diverse range of outpatient services is expensive, and to provide them involuntarily, with appropriate monitoring to prevent abuses, is even more costly. It is not clear that society is prepared to make that investment. Those who believe outpatient commitment promises an extension of rights may find that, in fact, it results in a curtailment of rights. Those who seek to treat a carefully delimited patient population may find themselves saddled by the courts with a wide range of inappropriate new commitees. Those who believe outpatient commitment will lower state hospital censuses may find its impact negligible.

On the other hand, outpatient commitment may solve some of the problems society faces in its struggle to serve the young, adult, chronic patients, the homeless mentally ill, and the revolving-door patients. Much empirical work needs to be done before we know whether outpatient commitment can play a positive role for a significant percentage of patients, whether the course of the chronically mentally ill can be improved, and which patients are most likely to benefit.

SUMMARY

The legal framework governing involuntary treatment affects our entire society. Many citizens have strong opinions about the legitimate scope and purposes of government's intrusion into private lives; indeed, these are bedrock issues echoing back to the founding of our nation. Yet the majority expect the government to provide care and services, even involuntarily, for those unable to provide for themselves, as is demonstrated by current concern over the homeless mentally ill. Laws regulating involuntary treatment—inpatient and outpatient—reflect society's balancing of these competing values. Public perceptions of the quality and effectiveness of psychiatric care have frequently tipped the balance. Clearly, the pursuit of involuntary means of administering psychiatric treatment will be for naught unless those in charge of policy provide the funds necessary to guarantee that any involuntary care is quality care.

REFERENCES

Alaska Stat. Sec. 47.03.915, 1984

American Psychiatric Association: Task Force Report on Outpatient Civil Commitment. American Psychiatric Association, Washington, DC, 1988

Appelbaum PS: Standards for civil commitment: a critical review of empirical research. Int J Law Psychiatry 1984; 7:133–144

Appelbaum PS: Civil commitment, in Psychiatry. Edited by Michels R, Cavenar JO. Philadelphia, J.B. Lippincott, 1985

Appelbaum PS: Outpatient commitment: the problems and the promise. Am J Psychiatry 1986; 143:1270–1272

Appelbaum PS: The right to refuse treatment with antipsychotic medication: retrospect and prospect. Am J Psychiatry, 1988; 145:413–419

Appelbaum PS, Gutheil TG: Drug refusal: a study of psychiatric inpatients. Am J Psychiatry 1980; 137:340–346

Appelbaum PS, Gutheil TG: Clinical aspects of treatment refusal. Compr Psychiatry 1982; 23:560–566

Appelbaum PS, Hoge SK: The right to refuse treatment: what the research reveals. Behavioral Science and the Law 1986; 4:279–292

Appelbaum PS, Lidz CW, Meisel A: Informed Consent: Legal Theory and Clinical Practice. New York, Oxford University Press, 1987

Ariz. Rev. Stat. Ann. Chap. 36–501, 1986

Bloom JD, Faulkner LR, Holm VM, et al.: An empirical view of patients exercising their right to refuse treatment. Int J Law Psychiatry 1984; 7:315–328

Brakel SJ, Parry J, Weiner BA: The Mentally Disabled and the Law. Chicago, American Bar Foundation, 1985

Bursten B: Posthospital mandatory outpatient treatment. Am J Psychiatry 1986; 143:1255–1258

Callahan LA: Changing mental health law: butting heads with a billygoat. Behav Sci Law 1986; 4:305–314

Callahan LA, Longmire DR: Psychiatric patients' right to refuse psychotropic medication: a national survey. Mental Disability Law Reporter 1983; 7:494–499

Dunham AC: APA's model law: protecting the patient's ultimate interests. Hosp Community Psychiatry 1985; 36:973–975

Durham ML: Implications of need-for-treatment laws: a study of Washington State's Involuntary Treatment Act. Hosp Community Psychiatry 1985; 36:975–977

Durham ML, LaFond JQ: The empirical consequences and policy implications of broadening the statutory criteria for civil commitment. Yale Law and Policy Review 1985: 2:395–446

Ga. Code Ann. Sec. 37, 1986

Geller JL: Sustaining treatment with the hospitalized patient who refuses treatment. Am J Psychiatry 1982; 139:112–113

Geller JL: In again, out again: preliminary evaluation of a state hospital's worst recidivists. Hosp Community Psychiatry 1986a; 37:386–390

Geller JL: Rights, wrongs, and the dilemma of coerced community treatment. Am J Psychiatry 1986b; 143:1259–1264

Geller JL: The quandaries of enforced community treatment and unenforceable outpatient commitment statutes. J Psychiatry Law 1986c; 2:149–158

Gill MJ: Side effects of a right to refuse treatment lawsuit: the Boston State Hospital experience, in Refusing Treatment in Mental Health Institutions—Values in Conflict. Edited by Doudera AE, Swazey JP. Ann Arbor, MI, AUPHA Press, 1982

Gutheil TG: In search of true freedom: drug refusal, involuntary medication, and "rotting with your rights on." Am J Psychiatry 1980; 137:327–328

Gutheil TG, Appelbaum PS: "Mind control," "synthetic sanity," "artificial competence," and genuine confusion: legally relevant effects of antipsychotic medication. Hofstra Law Review 1983; 12:77–120

Hargreaves WA, Shumway M: The Jamison-Farabee consent decree: an attempt to protect the right of involuntary psychiatric patients to refuse antipsychotic medication. Unpublished paper presented at the Annual Meeting of the American Psychiatric Association, Dallas, Tex, 1985

Hargreaves WA, Shumway M, Knutsen EJ, et al.: Effects of the Jamison-Farabee consent decree: due process protection for involuntary psychiatric patients treated with psychoactive medication. Am J Psychiatry 1987; 144:188–192

Hassenfeld IN, Grumet B: A study of the right to refuse treatment. Bull Am Acad Psychiatry Law 1984; 12:65–74

Hawaii Rev. Stat. Sec. 334–60.2, 1986

Hiday VA, Goodman RR: The least restrictive alternative to involuntary hospitalization, outpatient commitment: its use and effectiveness. J Psychiatry Law 1982; 10:81–96

Hiday VA, Scheid-Cook T: The North Carolina experience in outpatient commitment; a critical appraisal. Presented at the XII International Congress of Law and Mental Health, Montreal, June 20, 1986

Hoge SK, Appelbaum PS, Greer A: An empirical comparison of the Stone and dangerousness criteria for civil commitment. Am J Psychiatry (in press)

Hoge SK, Sachs G, Appelbaum PS, Greer A, Gordon C: Limitations on psychiatrists' discretionary civil commitment authority by the Stone and dangerousness criteria. Arch Gen Psychiatry 1988; 45:764–769

Hoge SK, Gutheil TG, Kaplan E: The right to refuse treatment under *Rogers v. Commissioner*: Preliminary empirical findings and comparisons. Bull Am Acad Psychiatry Law 1987; 2:163–169

Kan. Stat. Ann. Art. 29, Sec. 59–2902, 1982

Keilitz I, Hall T: State statutes governing involuntary outpatient civil commitment. Mental and Physical Disability Law Reporter 1985; 9:378–397

Lake v. Cameron, 364 F. 2d 657 (1966)

Lamb HR (ed): The Homeless Mentally Ill, American Psychiatric Association, Washington, DC, 1984

Lamb HR, Mills MJ: Needed changes in law and procedure for the chronic mentally ill. Hosp Community Psychiatry 1986; 37:475–480

Lessard v. Schmidt, 349 F. Supp. 1078 (E.D. Wis. 1972); vacated and remanded on other grounds, 414 U.S. 472 (1974); judgment reinstated, 413 F. Supp. 1318 (E.D. Wis. 1976)

Livermore JN, Malmquist CP, Meehl PE: On the justification for civil commitment. U Penn Law Rev 1968; 117:75–96

Marder SR, Mebane A, Chien CP, et al.: A comparison of patients who refuse and consent to neuroleptic treatment. Am J Psychiatry 1983; 140:470–472

Marder SR, Swann E, Winslade WJ, et al.: A study of medication refusal by involuntary psychiatric patients. Hosp Community Psychiatry 1984; 35:724–726

Miller RD, Fiddleman PB: Outpatient commitment: treatment in the least restrictive environment? Hosp Community Psychiatry 1984; 35:147–151

Miller RD, Maher R, Fiddleman PB: The use of plea bargaining in civil commitment. Int J Law and Psychiatry 1984; 7:395–406

Minn. Stat. Ann. Chap. 253B.02, Subd. 13, West 1982

Monahan J: The Clinical Prediction of Violent Behavior. National Institute of Mental Health, Rockville, MD, 1981

Mulvey EP, Geller JL, Roth LH: The promise and peril of involuntary outpatient commitment. Am Psychol 1987; 42:571–584

N.C. Gen. Stat. Sec. 122C, 1985

National Center for State Courts' Guidelines for Involuntary Civil Commitment. Mental and Physical Disability Law Reporter 1986; 10:409–514

National Institute of Mental Health: Mental Health, United States, 1985. DHHS Publication No. (AMD) 85–1378. National Institute of Mental Health, Rockville, MD, 1985

Oklahoma Stat. Ann. Tit. 43A, Sec. 3, West 1978

Or. Rev. Stat. Sec. 426.130, 1983

Owens J: Involuntary Outpatient Commitment: An Exploration of the Issues and Its Utilization in Five States. Bethesda, MD, National Institute of Mental Health, 1985

Plotkin R: Limiting the therapeutic orgy: mental patients' right to refuse treatment. Northwestern Law Review 1977; 72:461–525

Project Release v. Prevost, 551 F. Supp. 1298 (E.D.N.Y. 1982); 722 F. 2d 960 (2nd Cir.) 1983

Rennie v. Klein, 462 F. Supp. 1131 (D.N.J. 1978), 476 F. Supp. 1294 (D.N.J. 1979), aff'd in part, 653 F.2d 836 (3rd Cir. 1981), vacated and remanded, 102 S.Ct. 3506 (1982), 700 F.2d 266 (3rd Cir. 1983)

Rivers v. Katz, 495 N.E. 2d 337 (N.Y. 1986)

Rogers v. Commissioner of the Department of Mental Health, 458 N.E. 2d 308 (Mass. 1983)

Scheid-Cook TC: Commitment of the mentally ill to outpatient treatment. Community Ment Health J 1987; 23:173–182

Schneider-Braus K: Civil commitment to outpatient psychotherapy: a case study. Bull Am Acad Psychiatry Law 1986; 14:273–279

Schwartz SJ: Equal protection in medication decisions: informed consent, not just the right to refuse, in The Right to Refuse Antipsychotic Medication. Edited by Rapoport D, Parry J. American Bar Association, Washington, DC, 1986

Schwartz SJ, Costanzo CE: Compelling treatment in the community: distorted doctrines and violated values. Loyola of Los Angeles Law Review 1987; 20:1329-1429

State ex rel. Jones v. Gerhardstein, No. 85-1718 (Wis. Ct. App. Oct. 28, 1986)

Stefan S: Preventive commitment: the concept and its pitfalls. Mental and Physical Disability Law Reporter 1987; 4:288-302

Stensvad v. Reivitz, 601 F. Supp. 128 (W.D. Wis. 1985)

Stone AA: Mental Health and Law: A System in Transition. Department of Health, Education and Welfare, Publication ADM 75-176. U.S. Government Printing Office, Washington, DC, 1975

Stromberg CD, Stone AA: A model state law on civil commitment of the mentally ill. Harvard Journal on Legislation 1983; 20:275-396

Tenn. Code Ann. Sec. 33, 1986

Texas Stat. Ann Art. 5547-33, 1983

Treffert DA: The obviously ill patient in need of treatment: a fourth standard for civil commitment. Hosp Community Psychiatry 1985; 35:259-264

Van Putten T, Crumpton E, Yale C: Drug refusal and the wish to be crazy. Arch Gen Psychiatry 1976; 35:1443-1446

Wash. Rev. Code Ann. Chap. 71.05.020, 1979

Wasow M: The need for asylum for the chronic mentally ill. Schizophr Bull 1986; 12:162-167

Youngberg v. Romeo 457 U.S. 308 (1982)

Zanni G, deVeau L: A research note on the use of outpatient commitment. Hosp Community Psychiatry 1986; 37:941-942

Zito JM, Hendel DD, Mitchell JE, et al.: Drug treatment refusal, diagnosis, and length of hospitalization in involuntary psychiatric patients. Behavioral Science and the Law 1986; 4:327-337

Zito JM, Lentz SL, Routt WW, Olson GW: The treatment review panel: a solution to treatment refusal? Bull Am Acad Psychiatry Law 1984; 12:349-358

Zito JM, Routt WW, Roerig JL: Clinical characteristics of psychotic patients who refuse antipsychotic drug thearpy. Am J Psychiatry 1985; 142:822-826

Chapter 22

Criminal Responsibility

by Seymour L. Halleck, M.D.

CRIMINAL RESPONSIBILITY

In the criminal law, the ascription of responsibility implies blameworthiness for past conduct. Although this is only one of several meanings of the term *responsible* (Hart, 1968), it is the only one that will be considered in this chapter. Those designated as blameworthy are viewed as fit subjects for punishment. The ascription of responsibility is closely allied to the idea of choice; thus, if a person commits a harmful act when non-harmful alternatives are available, society usually assumes that he had a choice and is blameworthy (Halleck, 1984).

The criminal justice system attempts to minimize the incidence of social harm by blaming and usually punishing those who violate its laws. Every civilized society, however, has developed mechanisms for excusing from legal blame those who appear unable to exercise choice. It is generally acknowledged that offenders who lack understanding of their actions or who appear unable to control them are not blameworthy (Sendor, 1986). Those who commit crimes as a result of a legally recognized *mistake* or *duress* may also be excused, as are infants (children below the age of seven years). The legal system further acknowledges that some offenders have mental disorders that so impair their understanding or impulse control that their criminal conduct cannot be viewed as chosen. These offenders may not be held responsible for their criminal conduct. This chapter is a review of the manner in which our criminal justice system currently conceptualizes and deals with mentally disordered people who have committed illegal acts and who might be viewed as nonresponsible. Emphasis will be placed on the psychiatrist's role in determining who shall be found nonresponsible and how these individuals should be managed.

Definitions of Crime

Psychiatrists cannot expect to understand the conceptual issues involved in ascribing responsibility in the criminal justice system unless they have a rudimentary knowledge of how criminal acts are defined. Criminally prohibited acts and omissions (failures to act) are very carefully and precisely defined. The definitions are made up of *elements* or conditions under which acts (or omissions) are perpetrated; these elements relate both to the nature of the harmful act and the state of mind of the actor. For a criminal act to exist, there must be a wrongful act (*actus reus*) and an evil or guilty mind (*mens rea*) (Perkins, 1969). Neither alone will suffice. A wrongful or harmful act committed without a guilty mind (*mens rea*) is not a crime.

To meet the requirements of the *actus reus*, the offender's conduct must not only be harmful, it must be voluntary—the act must be the offender's own; he is not culpable if he is pushed against another person who is subsequently harmed—and it must be expressly prohibited by law. The concept of *mens rea* is much less precise, and it has been subject to varying meanings throughout the history of jurisprudence.

In its most restrictive or narrow sense, *mens rea* is restricted to consideration of the intent of the actor. *Intent*, in a legal sense, is judged to be present if the actor is aware of his conduct, the circumstances under which it is committed, and its probable consequences. Under this view, *mens rea* is a mental state that may actually be inferred from the circumstances under which the crime is committed (Sendor, 1986). The motivations of the offender, which in many social contexts would be relevant to his blameworthiness, are not considered. Under this view, the mercy killer may be found to have the same *mens rea* as the paid assassin. At various times in the history of jurisprudence, however, *mens rea* has been defined more broadly. In its larger sense, *mens rea* can include much more than the issue of intent and implies moral culpability (Golding and Roesch, 1987). Here, it is possible to consider how aspects of an individual's mental disorder might have precluded his having a guilty mind.

Under the narrow or strict view of *mens rea*, evidence of mental impairment has limited relevance in establishing nonresponsibility. Those mental disorders that would preclude an individual being aware of his conduct or its consequences would, of necessity, have to be severe and limited to disorders associated with major perceptual impairment. (For example, the man who strangles his wife while believing he is squeezing a lemon might not be committing an intentional act under the narrow view. Most other impairments, however, would not be relevant to negating the existence of *mens rea*.) Under the broader view of *mens rea*, evidence of mental disorder becomes much more relevant to negating the existence of an evil or wicked mind. Delusional systems that might impair an individual's ability to know or appreciate the wrongfulness of his conduct or volitional impairments that might interfere with his control of his conduct could negate the presence of *mens rea*.

During periods in the history of jurisprudence when broader concepts of *mens rea* predominated, the same mental disabilities that exculpate under the insanity defense might have been considered when determining the presence of *mens rea*. Current Anglo-American law, however, is dominated by the more restrictive view (Dix, 1984). Psychiatric testimony directed at negating the existence of the *mens rea* element of crime is now used infrequently. It is much more common in the modern era for defendants to argue that their mental disorder should excuse them from responsibility because it has made them insane. Defendants who plead insanity may acknowledge their intent to have committed a harmful act (and thereby acknowledge the existence of *mens rea*), but they claim that they should not be held responsible because their mental impairment deprived them of the capacity for choice. Thus, the insanity defense, while closely related to that broader view of *mens rea* which requires moral culpability, is *not*, under current Anglo-American law, directed at negating proof of the existence of the mental elements of the crime. The insanity defense is rather an affirmative defense in which the defendant acknowledges that the *actus reus* and *mens rea* are provable, but his emotional state was such as to have provided him with a legally recognized excuse (Hermann, 1983).

Partial and Complete Criminal Responsibility

While the idea of criminal responsibility is usually conceptualized as an "all or none" phenomenon in which those found nonresponsible are acquitted and those found responsible are guilty, there are some instances in which the criminal justice system allows for grading of responsibility. The state may diminish the degree of punishment, as measured in terms of length of prison confinement, in instances when it believes that an individual's mental illness makes him less responsible for a similar offense than those who are not mentally disabled. Conceptually, the attribution of partial responsibility can be viewed two ways: first, it is a device the court can use to maintain that an individual is not responsible for the crime for which he was charged but is responsible for a lesser crime (Arenella, 1977). Second, it can be a judgment, made at the time of sentencing, that an offender had "less choice" or "harder choices" than others who committed the same crime and should, therefore, receive less punishment (Dix, 1984).

An understanding of the idea that an individual may not be responsible for a crime for which he was charged but is responsible for a lesser crime requires a reexamination of the subjects of *mens rea* and the definition of crimes. As noted above, offenders whose perceptual disturbances might be so severe that they do not intend their act could be acquitted for lacking the *mens rea* for any crime. When this happens, the defendant is completely or totally nonresponsible and innocent. The concept of *mens rea*, however, may also allow for finding some mentally disturbed offenders responsible only for a lesser offense than the one they were originally charged with. This can happen because many offenses that produce similar harms are graded, in terms of the severity of the culpable (legally defined) mental state required, and carry different penalties. For example, in crimes involving homicide, terms such as *premeditation, deliberation,* or *malice* are used to define the mental states (or the requisite *mens rea*) associated with greater or lesser penalties. In most jurisdictions, the mental element of premeditation or deliberation is required if the defendant is to be found guilty of murder in the first degree. If this element is not present, the offender may still be guilty of second degree murder. For both first and second degree murder, the mental state of malice must be present if the individual is to be found guilty. If malice is not present, the individual is still likely to be guilty of voluntary manslaughter.

In general, efforts to use evidence of psychiatric disability to negate the existence of legally defined mental elements and reduce culpability to that appropriate for a lesser offense have been limited in Anglo-American jurisprudence. Many states do not permit such testimony on the grounds that it would confuse jurors or produce too much leniency (Shah, 1986). It is also unclear how states of mind described by such terms as *deliberately* or *with malice* can be understood to be negated by the presence of mental disability (Dix, 1984). A notable effort to surmount this difficulty was made in California during the 1960s and 1970s. A series of judicial decisions in that state led to a redefinition of premeditation and malice in terms that expedited the use of psychiatric testimony in negating the presence of these elements. This approach enabled the state to avoid finding certain youthful offenders guilty of capital murder when they did not meet the criteria for the insanity defense but did have severe emotional disturbances

(Winslade and Ross 1983). Thus, for a time, homicidal offenders in California could receive a much-reduced sentence if they were mentally impaired, but public concern over such leniency gradually increased. That concern escalated to a sense of outrage following the trial in San Francisco of Daniel White for the murders of Mayor George Moscone and Supervisor Harvey Milk. When psychiatric testimony was used to negate the mental elements of deliberation and malice and White was convicted of only voluntary manslaughter (with a six-year sentence), the public demanded that this approach be abolished, and, in 1981, California passed legislation prohibiting its use (Krausz, 1983).

Another approach that allows an individual to be held responsible only for a lesser crime involves statutory provisions for reducing murder to manslaughter if a homicide is committed under extreme mental or emotional disturbance. Currently, ten states have statutes allowing the introduction of psychiatric testimony leading to conviction and punishment for a lesser offense (Shah, 1986). Lesser degrees of responsibility may also be ascribed at the time of sentencing. Traditionally, the criminal-court judge has had the power to consider evidence of mental disability as a factor that limits the offender's responsibility and justifies a lesser sentence. While a jury may find that the defendant could have chosen not to commit the crime, the judge may conclude that illness made such a choice difficult.

Until recently, evidence of mental impairment at the time of sentencing was considered only on an informal basis, but in the last two decades, formal consideration of mental disability in the sentencing process has received greater emphasis because of two major trends: the first applies in cases of first degree murder for which the death penalty can be imposed. A hearing is now constitutionally required following a conviction for first degree murder in which aggravating and mitigating circumstances will determine whether the individual receives the death penalty or life imprisonment. Mental impairment is generally admissable as a mitigating factor, and such constitutionally mandated individualization of the sentencing process frequently results in the use of mental health testimony to determine whether to impose the ultimate penalty (American Psychiatric Association, 1984). Second, the new emphasis on presumptive sentencing, in which the judge must consider both mitigating and aggravating circumstances to determine the length of sentence, allows mental illness at the time of the crime to be considered a mitigating circumstance (Dix, 1984). Increased use of presumptive sentencing should result in more instances where formal testimony of psychiatric impairment will influence the degree of responsibility and punishment.

While the relationship of mental disorder to partial responsibility is an interesting and complex aspect of the overall problem of criminal responsibility, the most common and most important means of determining the relationship between mental illness and nonresponsibility is the insanity defense. Offenders who successfully plead insanity are relieved of all responsibility for their crimes. It should be clear, however, that while they are not subjected to criminal sanctions, they do not routinely obtain freedom. As a rule, the need for public protection is invoked to subject acquittees to indeterminate periods of hospitalization. The remainder of this chapter will deal solely with the insanity defense.

THE NATURE OF THE INSANITY DEFENSE

The insanity defense attracts scholarly attention from lawyers, mental health professionals, and philosophers and seems to elicit emotional reactions from almost everyone. The reason for this concern is not immediately apparent, because in terms of its impact on any significant proportion of criminal offenders, the insanity defense is relatively unimportant. It is rarely raised and is successful in less than one percent of all felony cases tried. The best explanation for the amount of interest the insanity defense engenders is that it touches upon concerns all people have about the nature of responsibility and the extent to which mental impairment may negate blameworthiness or obligation. Goldstein is probably correct in pointing out that the trial of this defense "is treated as if it were a contemporary morality play revolving around the issues of sickness and guilt" (Goldstein, 1967).

The emotionalism surrounding the insanity defense is highlighted by the discrepancy between the volume of verbal and written statements made about it and the amount of actual research into its impact on our society. Research on how the administration of the insanity defense influences the criminal justice system was almost nonexistent until this decade (Pasewark, 1981). As a result, many ordinary citizens and professionals mistakenly overestimate its influence. Widespread fears that the insanity defense allows dangerous offenders to avoid punishment they deserve and that such leniency encourages criminality and compromises public safety abound. The little research available, however, tells us that acquittals are extraordinarily rare, and those acquitted spend a substantial amount of time in confinement. Claims that this defense favors the affluent are not supported by the data; nor is the use of the defense restricted to violent or sensational crimes. Public perceptions that the insanity defense regularly results in a battle of psychiatric experts before a jury are also incorrect—the majority of insanity verdicts are uncontested (Steadman and Cocozza, 1978).

The purposes of the insanity defense have been viewed as both moral and utilitarian, with the majority of commentators emphasizing its moral purpose—to provide a means of not punishing those who are not truly responsible for their harmful acts. Perhaps the most succinct statement of the purpose of the insanity defense is Judge David Bazelon's statement in *Durham vs. United States, 1954:* "our collective conscience does not allow punishment where it cannot impose blame." Most students of the insanity defense conclude that our cultural sense of *fairness* and *justice* requires an option that excuses those whose mental condition renders them unable to choose the criminal act for which they have been charged. Even those who recommend abolition of the insanity defense would retain some device for limiting the culpability of the severely mentally disordered by allowing evidence of major disability to negate proof of *mens rea*.

The utilitarian arguments for the insanity defense are less persuasive, but they raise interesting questions about the nature of criminal conduct and the structure of the criminal justice system. Some have argued that the utilitarian value of punishment as a deterrent may not influence the severely mentally disordered and thus punishing them serves no purpose. This argument is countered by those who fear that, while the insane offender may not be deterred by punishment, his acquittal might encourage others to commit crimes in the belief that they too will be acquitted (Hart, 1968).

Invoking a different type of utilitarian interpretation, Alan Stone (1975) has argued that the insanity defense preserves the integrity of the criminal justice system. Punishment is based on the premise of free-will; when the court is confronted with an individual who is so severely disturbed and bizarre that the premise of free will seems inappropriate, the very integrity of the judicial system is threatened. Stone argues that the insanity defense provides criminal law with an escape hatch, which further allows the law to assume that every defendant who is not found insane does have free will. He notes, "thus, the insanity defense is in every sense the exception that proves the role. It allows the court to treat every other defendant as someone who chose 'between good and evil' " (Stone, 1975). Halleck (1986a) has elaborated upon this thesis and notes that our criminal justice system could not function in its present form if it did not limit the extent to which it considered psychological variables in assessing liability and punishment. Because the insanity defense is an "all or none" doctrine that excuses only a few, it helps to create a powerful demarcation point that allows the criminal justice system to avoid considering the psychological disabilities of many others who may be almost as gravely impaired (Halleck, 1986a).

Standards for Determining Insanity

The task of a legal tribunal that must determine when an individual's mental impairment rises to a level negating the capacity for choice and responsibility is greatly facilitated by a standard that clarifies what facts are relevant to that determination. From the early part of the sixteenth century to the present, Anglo-American jurists have struggled to determine what instruction should be given the jury as to the nature and degree of mental impairment that exculpates defendants from criminal liability. No constitutional standard has emerged in the United States, and, as a result, the 62 United States jurisdictions (50 states, the District of Columbia, and 11 Federal Circuit Courts) do not have identical standards. The two most common standards are the M'Naghten test and the American Law Institute (ALI) test.

According to the M'Naghten test (M'Naghten's Case, 1843):

> Every man is presumed to be sane and . . . to establish a defense on the ground of insanity it must be clearly proved that at the time of the committing of the act the party accused was laboring under such a defect of reason from disease of the mind, as not to know the nature and quality of the act he was doing or if he did know it, that he did not know he was doing what was wrong.

The quest for an excuse here can be paraphrased as "I did not know what I was doing" or "I did not know what I did was wrong."

According to the American Law Institute test (American Law Institute, 1962):

> A person is not responsible for criminal conduct if at the time of such conduct as a result of mental disease or defect, he lacked substantial capacity either to appreciate the criminality of his conduct or to conform his conduct to the requirements of the law.

This test includes elements of "I didn't know what I was doing or that it was wrong," but it also adds the volitional element, "I couldn't control my behavior."

The ALI test also differs from the *M'Naghten* test in using two terms susceptible to more broad interpretation, namely, *substantial* and *appreciate*. It does not demand a finding of total lack of appreciation for exculpation but only a *substantial lack of capacity*. By using the term *appreciate* rather than *know*, it allows for consideration of emotional incapacities that may influence understanding. Presumably an individual might be intellectually aware of (know) the wrongfulness of an act, but various emotional disorders might compromise his moral judgment of its wrongfulness. Some commentators believe that this term facilitates the consideration of evidence of delusional or affective states in determining the responsibility of defendants who cannot empathize with the impact of their behavior on others.

That the nature of the insanity standard would ultimately influence the frequency of acquittal seems logical, and some evidence supports this view. During the 1950s, when the "liberal" Durham Rule was the standard in the District of Columbia, there was a noticeable increase in acquittals (Brooks, 1974). The Durham Rule stated that an accused is not criminally responsible if his unlawful criminal conduct was the product of a mental disease or mental defect. This standard survived for only a few years because it was believed to provide too much power to psychiatrists, who influenced jurors by creating arbitrary definitions of mental illness. It is not clear, however, whether the broader ALI test actually results in the presentation of more information to the jury and more acquittals than the *M'Naghten* test (Dix, 1984). In many *M'Naghten* jurisdictions, psychiatrists are allowed to present information about emotional aspects of "knowing" to the jury. Jurors may also pay more attention to other variables, such as the severity of the defendant's illness, rather than the actual standard for determining responsibility.

The search for a "best" standard for determining insanity generally reflects society's uncertainty regarding the extent to which it wishes to allow mental illness to be an exculpatory factor. The history of the insanity defense suggests that when the public is deeply concerned with crimes of violence, it views the insanity defense as a possible impediment to effective law enforcement and favors a more narrow standard. Following the acquittal of Daniel M'Naghten (who was acquitted on a standard different from the one carrying his name), the British House of Lords was stimulated by the groundswell of public uproar and Queen Victoria's indignation to come up with the more restrictive *M'Naghten* test (Walker and McCabe, 1973). The John Hinckley case appears to have had a similar effect in the United States. Prior to the Hinckley trial, a tendency to liberalization of insanity tests had prevailed, with many jurisdictions replacing the *M'Naghten* with the ALI standard. Since Hinckley's acquittal, two states (Idaho in 1982 and Utah in 1983) have, in effect, abolished the insanity defense by allowing testimony of mental disorder only with regard to the *mens rea* for the particular crime (Shah, 1986). Other states have made efforts to abolish the insanity defense, and several states have moved towards a return to the *M'Naghten* standard. In 1982, the American Psychiatric Association drafted a statement on the insanity defense endorsing the following standard, which is very close to *M'Naghten*:

A person charged with a criminal offense should be found not guilty by reason of insanity if it is shown that as a result of mental disease or mental retardation he was unable to appreciate the wrongfulness of his conduct at the time of the offense. . . . (American Psychiatric Association, 1982).

The Insanity Defense Reform Act of 1984 (part of the Comprehensive Crime Control Act of 1984) brought about major changes in the federal criminal code and narrowed the standards for determining insanity in the federal courts. The new federal test states:

It is an affirmative defense to a prosecution under any federal statute that, at the time of the commission of the acts constituting the offense, the defendant, as a result of severe mental disease or defect was unable to appreciate the nature and quality or the wrongfulness of his acts (Comprehensive Crime Control Act, 1984).

This is essentially a return to a *M'Naghten* standard, with the term *appreciate* being substituted for the word *know*.

Saleem Shah (1986) notes that there are three basic elements to any insanity test:

1. There must be a mental disorder which is legally defined. The key term here is *legal*. A system of psychiatric nomenclature cannot be viewed as providing the requisite legal threshold for determining responsibility by the criminal justice system.
2. A legally relevant impairment in functioning must be shown to have resulted from the mental disorder. These impairments or incapacities pertain generally to various cognitive or volitional functions.
3. There must be a demonstration of a clear and direct causal connection or relationship between the behavioral impairment resulting from the mental disorder and the criminal act. The mental disorder must be viewed as a necessary or "but-for" cause of the criminal act.

Throughout the history of the insanity defense, those mental processes viewed as relevant to the question of responsibility have been conceptualized as cognitive or volitional. The term *cognitive* refers to mental functions involved in the act or process of knowing. It includes mental functions such as perception, memory, capacity to reason, and understand. As cognition is powerfully influenced by the individual's emotional state, a cognitive standard may, and generally does, allow the jury to consider how emotional states might have impaired the defendant's capacity to choose. Because it appears clear to most people that a lack of rational understanding of the nature and quality of what one is doing or its wrongfulness would clearly subvert the will, the use of cognitive standards assist the court to ascribe responsibility is not generally controversial.

The term *volition* refers to the act of willing, choosing, or resolving. Volitional standards, such as those in the second part of the ALI standard or in irresistible-impulse standards (a few states add a clause to the *M'Naghten* standard which allows for exculpation if the crime was the result of an irresistible impulse) are more controversial, and this has been particularly true since the Hinckley acquittal (Dix, 1984). Volition is also described in terms of a person's capacity to control oneself or to conform one's conduct to the requirements of the law. It is never entirely clear whether a statement that one lacked capacity to conform his conduct to the requirement of the law is anything more than a statement that we do not wish to blame him. Nor is it entirely clear what mental processes other than cognitive processes must be disordered if volition is to be impaired. It would appear that, when clinicians find volitional impairment, it is closely linked to disordered cognition or related to some motivation aberrance. Bizarre, excessive, or out-of-awareness motivation have all been invoked as impairing capacity to choose (Halleck, 1984).

The idea of excusing based on volitional impairment also raises the possibility of circular reasoning. A statement that a behavior was not controlled because it was uncontrollable may not be much more than an argument for not assigning blame because there is no scientific means of determining the degree of impulse or mental disability that renders an act uncontrollable (APA, 1982). Jurists who oppose the volitional prong in standards for insanity fear that psychiatrists will testify that some defendants lack volitional capacity without sufficient data or that, even without definitive psychiatric testimony, jurors might use an overly lenient, common sense approach to deciding whether defendants had the capacity to conform.

Psychiatric Evaluation for the Defense of Insanity

The psychiatrist's task when examining a patient who may wish to plead criminal responsibility is one of the most difficult evaluative functions in psychiatry. He is asked to comment on the nature of the defendant's capacities to behave, perceive, think, and feel at some time in the past, often many months after the crime has taken place. The task is complicated by the likelihood that the defendant's mental condition at the time of the crime was probably quite different from that which he demonstrates at the time of the examination. In fact, by the time the psychiatric examination is initiated, treatment of the defendant may have already begun. Even if the defendant has been institutionalized without treatment, the hospital environment may have profoundly affected his mental status. Thus, evaluation of the defendant's current mental status may not provide insights as to what he was like at the time of the crime.

The details of forensic evaluation in general are discussed in Chapter 24. The following material deals only with special issues that arise when evaluating insanity: As a rule the primary sources of information available to the clinician are 1) what the patient is willing or able to tell about his mental status at the time of the crime, and 2) reports by third parties, including the police, as to how he behaved before, during, and after the crime. The clinician's task is somewhat easier if the defendant's current mental status is consistent with a chronic mental disorder. Such evidence enables the clinician to postulate that the defendant might have been under the influence of that disorder at the time of the crime. Findings of chronic organic brain disease, for example, may strongly suggest that the individual was impaired at the time of the crime.

Even if a great deal of data is available and the clinician can define with some precision exactly what impairments the defendant might have had at the time of the crime, it is rarely possible to know exactly how these disabilities influenced the defendant's behavior. Psychiatric clinicians regularly evaluate patients' capacities and use these evaluations to make predictions of how patients will behave in various settings. In making these judgments, they are also aware of how such incapacities have influenced the patient's past conduct. Whether the psychiatrist is concerned with future or retrospective capacities, however, he can rarely do much more than make a probability statement as to how the patient's disability either predicts future or explains past behavior (Monahan, 1981; Halleck, 1986a).

A number of efforts have been made to gain reliability and minimize error in the evaluation process of insanity defendants by using structured or standard-ized interview techniques. Slobogin and colleagues (1984) have sought to make mental state at the time of the offense (MSO) evaluations more relevant both legally and forensically. They have described a loosely structured interview technique that relies heavily on legal criteria. Golding and Roesch (1987) have described a five-stage evaluation process that begins with creating rapport and a contractual understanding with the defendant. This is followed by a thorough review of the patient's history, a review of his present mental state (when possible) and of his mental state at the time of the offense, and a reconciliation of the above data with other data sources, including consultation with other professionals who have evaluated the defendant.

Rogers and Cavanaugh (1981) attempted to develop a semistructured inter-view schedule, entitled the Rogers Criminal Responsibility Assessment Scales, for the evaluation of insanity with a set of scales. The test directs the clinician to rate a defendant on 25 scales grouped into five areas: reliability of report, organicity, psychopathology, cognitive control, and behavioral control. The examiner then rates whether the disturbance is attributable to the assessed, organic, or psychopathological conditions and makes a final rating of legal insan-ity (Rogers and Cavanaugh, 1981). It is of some interest that Rogers scale includes criteria for assessing volitional capacity (since it is directed toward the ALI standard). Rogers insists that with use of his scale, there is high reliability in clinician's judgments of cognitive and volitional impairment (Rogers and Cavan-augh, 1981). Many of the criteria they suggest for assessing volitional capacity, however, are more properly viewed as cognitive functions.

Halleck (1986b) has warned of the dangers of tautological thinking, particu-larly in the discussion of the volitional impairment, and has suggested that impairments can best be conceptualized in terms of a benefit-risk alternative model of assessing behavior. The clinician is asked to consider any cognitive or motivational factors that minimize or exaggerate benefits or risks or that impair the perception of alternatives. The defendant's capacity to weigh risks against benefits is also considered.

In conducting an examination of a defendant who is seeking to plead insanity, the psychiatrist must also be aware of how the information gained during the evaluation process will be used. On occasion, insanity defense examinations may be requested by the court even if the defendant has not raised the insanity defense. In such examinations the defendant is at risk of providing information to the psychiatrist that is relevant to his possible future dangerousness. If the insanity defense is not raised or is unsuccessful and if the case is one of capital murder, the psychiatrist could end up testifying about the defendant's danger-ousness at the constitutionally mandated trial to determine whether the death penalty should be imposed. The Supreme Court has held that information, obtained by a psychiatrist in a situation in which the defendant has not raised the insanity defense and has not been advised by counsel, cannot be utilized in death-sentencing hearings because it was obtained in violation of the defendant's Fifth Amendment rights against self-incrimination and Sixth Amendment right to counsel (*Estelle v. Smith, 1981*). In one case, however, information reflecting adversely on a defendant's claim of innocence that was obtained in an examination by a federally employed psychiatrist *which was requested by the defendant* was allowed to be retained in testimony by a federal appellate court (*United States v. Byers, 1984*).

A related legal issue concerns the accuracy of both adverse and positive information gained by defense, prosecution-employed, or state-employed psychiatrists. In a dissenting opinion in *United States v. Byers, 1984*, Judge David Bazelon suggested that the insanity evaluation be videotaped and that these tapes be made available to both the defense and prosecution, that this might assist the fact finders in evaluating the accuracy of the psychiatrist's report.

The Defendant and the Psychiatrist in Court

Perhaps one reason why so few defendants are acquitted by reason of insanity is that the degree of illness they may have manifested at the time of the offense is not apparent at the time of trial. Months or years may have elapsed between the time of the offense and the trial. During that time the defendant has changed and his mental condition has more than likely improved. Before the trial takes place, the defendant must meet the standards of competency to proceed in the criminal justice process. While the standards for determining this capacity are different from those used for determining insanity, they nevertheless presume a certain degree of cognitive proficiency and freedom from impairments that could prevent his assisting in his own defense. In effect, whatever symptoms of mental illness may still be present are not likely to be apparent to the jury. The defense may thus have a difficult time convincing jurors that the relatively normal-looking defendant was actually so disturbed as to be incapable of not choosing criminal conduct at some remote time (Goldstein, 1967).

The most troubling issue with regard to psychiatric testimony is whether the expert witness should be allowed to answer the "ultimate question," that is, should they be allowed to answer "yes" or "no" to the questions posed by either the *M'Naghten* or ALI standards. This issue is considered in Chapter 24.

THE DISPOSITION OF ACQUITTEES

A person who has been found not guilty by reason of insanity has been absolved of all responsibility for his crime; as noted previously, however, he is not likely to be set free. Society remains concerned that the acquittee is a person who is at high risk of harming others and, therefore, dangerous. Historically, acquittees in England were confined to jail or prison immediately following acquittal. Most of them, including Daniel M'Naghten, spent the rest of their lives in confinement. In the United States, acquittees have generally been confined in security or forensic hospitals. The time spent thus confined is likely to parallel the amount of time they would have spent in prison if they had been convicted of the crime for which they were charged.

The confinement of individuals, charged with and tried for committing a criminal act, but who have been acquitted, requires special legislation. Most state legislatures have framed statutes to facilitate the process of examining acquittees and determining if they should be committed to hospitals, usually security hospitals, for an indeterminate period of time following acquittal (Bloom and Bloom, 1981). A period of restraint is usually imposed upon the offender until the examination is completed. As a general rule, requirements for commitment of an individual who has been found not guilty by reason of insanity are less stringent than those required for ordinary civil commitment of the mentally ill. Dangerousness is likely to be assumed from the nature of the crime, and mental illness is often assumed from the fact that the individual has successfully invoked the insanity defense.

It is also more difficult for the insanity acquittee to obtain release from a mental hospital than it is in ordinary civil commitment. Some states, for example, California, require that sanity be completely restored before release is possible. Under this criterion, even offenders who are no longer viewed as dangerous can be restrained. Other states, for example, Delaware, continue to restrain offenders who are no longer insane but who are still viewed as dangerous. Thus, offenders viewed as still dangerous or still mentally ill may be retained. This contrasts with release procedures for civilly committed individuals, who are eligible for release if they are either "safe" or "sane" (Morris, 1983).

Courts also regulate the hospital treatment of insanity acquittees and can influence how much security is imposed on them in the hospital, whether they receive passes or leaves of absence from the hospital, and when they are allowed conditional release. Unlike civilly committed patients, insanity acquittees in many jurisdictions cannot be released when their psychiatrist or hospital superintendents conclude that they no longer need hospitalization. The court may retain control of the release and may overrule the psychiatrist's recommendation. Some states require the prosecutor or district attorney who tried the original case to participate in any release hearing initiated by the acquittee (Dix, 1984). A 1983 Supreme Court ruling in *Jones v. United States, 1983* has substantially increased the power of state legislatures to impose more stringent limits in the management of acquittees found not guilty by reason of insanity.

The Psychiatrist's Role in the Treatment and Release of Insanity Acquittees

Psychiatrists who work in hospitals that treat insanity acquittees utilize all traditional modes of psychiatric treatment. As a rule, these patients are characterized by mixed diagnoses, with some symptoms of psychosis and some symptoms of severe personality disorders. Most often, it is the presence of psychosis that leads to a finding of insanity. The presence of a personality disorder is more likely to be associated with criminal tendencies. Given the availability of treatment facilities in hospitals where insanity acquittees are housed, it is likely that the most effective psychiatric interventions will be directed at psychosis. Effective treatment of an acquittee's personality disorder is more difficult. This poses certain obvious management and release decision problems for the psychiatrist. Offenders successfully treated for psychosis may still retain personality characteristics associated with criminality. Their criminal propensities may be better controlled when the psychosis is in remission, but they may not be entirely absent. When the acquittee's psychosis is controlled largely through the use of medication, there is a risk that he will commit new antisocial acts if placed in situations where he might stop taking his medication.

Most criminologists agree that the person acquitted by reason of insanity carries a higher risk of subsequent involvement in criminal conduct than other mentally ill individuals, and some data support this belief (Halleck, 1986a). Acquittees, therefore, may require more control when they are in the hospital setting, and decisions involving receipt of passes or conditional discharges must be made with great caution. Where psychiatrists assume sole obligation for determining how much freedom these patients may have, they are at considerable risk of malpractice litigation if the acquittee commits a violent crime while free.

Psychiatrists have generally welcomed an increasing trend on the part of the courts to become involved in decisions involving the release of acquittees (APA, 1982). They have also welcomed programs that provide for a trial release period and extensive monitoring, as well as continued treatment of the acquittee in the community. The most promising model, currently in use in Oregon, requires that authority for discharge be delegated to a special review board whose members represent the viewpoints of the criminal justice system and the lay public, as well as those of mental health professionals. This board makes release decisions and continues to monitor the acquittee's behavior and treatment in the community. Provisions are available for immediately returning the acquittee to an institution if his conduct suggests that continued dangerous behavior is likely (Bloom et al, 1986). Programs similar to the one in Oregon have recently been developed in Maryland and Connecticut, and they have been met with the general approval of the public, the judiciary, and the medical profession.

THE GUILTY BUT MENTALLY ILL ALTERNATIVE

Even before the Hinckley acquittal, the state of Michigan had provided an alternative to the traditional verdicts of guilty, not guilty, or not guilty by reason of insanity. The Michigan statute provided the jury with the option of finding defendants who have raised the insanity defense, *guilty but mentally ill*. This doctrine, which appears to have been originally proposed by Queen Victoria in the nineteenth century (Bloom et al, 1986), appears to accomplish two purposes: It recognizes as different from the ordinary offender the defendant who has been adjudicated guilty but mentally ill. At the same time, it allows for sentencing under the ordinary criminal code and makes it possible to impose a lengthy sentence. Recognition of the special status of these offenders is accomplished by a requirement that, once sentenced, they receive some type of mental health treatment while serving their prison term. The addition of this alternative to the jury gives them the opportunity to identify defendants who have severe enough disorders to be categorized differently from other defendants while at the same time not having to come up with a verdict that might set them free.

The guilty but mentally ill verdict was considered by many state legislatures after the Hinckley acquittal, and ten states very quickly passed statutes allowing its use. Most observers feel that the intent of these laws was clearly to diminish the number of acquittals by reason of insanity by making it easier for the jury to acknowledge that some defendants were mentally ill, even though they were fit subjects for punishment (Halleck, 1986a). While this alternative has met with approval from many in the criminal-justice system, particularly prosecutors and those involved with law enforcement, it has been criticized by attorneys and mental health professionals (Golding and Roesch, 1987). These critiques can be stated as follows:

1. The guilty but mentally ill alternative dilutes the moral power of the insanity defense. It can provide the jury with an easy way to avoid grappling with the more difficult moral issues inherent in adjudicating guilt or innocence.
2. Little reason exists to believe that offenders sentenced as guilty but mentally ill will in fact be treated differently than ordinary offenders. Mental health treatment has, in theory, always been available to those found guilty and sentenced to prisons. The guilty but mentally ill alternative offers no new advantages to offenders. It can hardly be distinguished from an ordinary criminal conviction unless it is accompanied by a firm commitment on the part of the state to expand its treatment resources and provide offenders with adequate care. So far there is little evidence that this is happening. (Grostic, 1978).

PSYCHIATRISTS AND CRIMINAL RESPONSIBILITY

In the aftermath of the Hinckley trial, the psychiatric profession's involvement in the adjudication of criminal responsibility was severely criticized by public officials, journalists, and other physicians. Many psychiatrists agreed with some of these critiques. Currently, psychiatrists hold to a variety of differing viewpoints as to the proper role of psychiatry in the criminal-justice process and particularly in the process of ascribing responsibility. Such disagreement is certainly understandable, but our profession would be better served if dialogue on this issue were based on appreciation of a few realities: First, the criminal justice system will always be concerned with the question of how mental impairment may modify or preclude responsibility. Second, the criminal justice system will continue to seek the assistance of psychiatrists in dealing with the issue of criminal responsibility. Third, the issue of criminal responsibility is incredibly complex, and, although many scholars have devoted much of their careers to understanding and explaining it, the debate will go on. Psychiatrists who wish to voice opinions about criminal responsibility will contribute little unless they have taken the time to study its many legal and psychological parameters.

REFERENCES

American Law Institute: Model Penal Code. Philadelphia, The American Law Institute, 1962

American Psychiatric Association: Statement on the Insanity Defense. Washington, DC, American Psychiatric Association, 1982

American Psychiatric Association: Issues in Forensic Psychiatry. Washington, DC, American Psychiatric Association, 1984

Arenella P: The diminished capacity and diminished responsibility defenses: two children of a doomed marriage. Columbia Law Review 1977; 77:827–872

Bloom JD, Williams MH, Roger JL, et al: Evaluation and treatment of insanity acquittees in the community. Bull Am Acad Psychiatry Law 1986; 14:231–244

Bloom JL, Bloom JD: Disposition of insanity defense cases in Oregon. Bull Am Acad of Psychiatry Law 1981

Brooks A: Law, Psychiatry and the Mental Health System. Boston, Little, Brown and Co, Inc, 1974

Comprehensive Crime Control Act of 1984 (Public Law 98–473)

Dix G: Criminal responsibility and mental impairment, in American Criminal Law: Response to the Hinckley Acquittal, in Historical Perspective in Law and Mental Health: International Perspectives, volume one. New York, Pergamon Press, 1984

Durham v. United States, 2/4 F. 20 862 (D.C. Cir., 1954)

Estelle v. Smith, 451 U.S. 454 (1981)

Golding SL and Roesch L: The assessment of criminal responsibility: a historical approach to a current controversy, in Handbook of Forensic Psychology. Edited by Weinder IB, Hess AK. New York, Wiley, 1987

Goldstein A: The Insanity Defense. New Haven, CT, Yale University Press, 1967

Grostic JM: The Constitutionality of Michigan's Guilty But Mentally Ill Verdict. Journal of Law Reform 1978; 12:188

Halleck SL: The assessment of responsibility in criminal law and psychiatric practice, in Law and Mental Health: International Perspectives: volume one. New York, Pergamon, 1984

Halleck SL: The Mentally Disordered Offender. National Institute of Mental Health, DHH8 Pub No (Adm) 86–1471. US Government Printing Office, Washington, DC, Superintendent of Documents, 1986a

Halleck SL: Responsibility and excuse in medicine and law: a utilitarian perspective. Law and Contemporary Problems 1986b; 49:127–146

Hart HL: Punishment and Responsibility; Essays in the Philosophy of Law. New York, Oxford University Press, 1968

Hermann D: The Insanity Defense. Springfield, IL, Charles C. Thomas, 1983

Jones v. United States, 103 S. Ct. 3043 (1983)

Krausz FR: The Relevance of Innocence: Proposition 8 and the Diminished Capacity Defense. California Law Review 1983

M'Naghten's Case, 10 C1 and F. 200, 8 Eng. Ref. 718, 1843

Monahan J: The Clinical Prediction of Violent Behavior. National Institute of Mental Health, DHHS Pub. No. (ADM) 81–921. US Government Printing Office, Washington, DC, Superintendent of Documents, 1981

Morris G: Acquittal by Reason of Insanity, in Mentally Disordered Offenders. Edited by Monahan J, Steadman I. New York, Plenum Press, 1983

Pasewark R: The insanity plea: a review of the research literature. Journal of Psychiatry and Law 1981; 357–401

Perkins R: Perkins on Criminal Law, 2nd edition. Mineola, New York, The Foundation Press, 1969

Rogers R: American Psychiatric Association's position on the insanity defense: empiricism versus emotionalism. Am Psychol 1987; 840–848

Rogers R, Cavanaugh SL: Roger's Criminal Responsibility Assessment Scales. Illinois Medical Journal 1981; 160:164–169

Sendor BB: Crime as communication: an interpretive theory of the insanity defense and the mental elements of crime. Georgetown Law Journal 1986; 74:1372–73, 1394–1494

Shah SA: Criminal Responsibility in Forensic Psychiatry and Psychology. Edited by Curran MO, McGarry AL, Shah SA. Philadelphia, FA Davis, 1986

Slobogin C, Melton GB, Showalter CR: The Feasibility of a Brief Evaluation of Mental State at the Time of the Offense. Law and Human Behavior 1984; 8:305–321

Steadman HO, Cocozza JS: Selective repeating and the public's misconceptions of the criminally insane. Public Opinion Quarterly 1978; 14:523

Stone A: Mental Health and Law: A System in Transition. National Institute of Mental Health. DNEW Pub. No. (Adm) 75–176. U.S. Government Printing Office, Washington DC, Superintendent of Documents, 1975

United States v. Byers, 760 F. 2d 1104 (D.C. Cir 1984)

Walker N, McCabe S: Crime and Insanity in England. Scotland, Edinburgh, University Press, 1973

Winslade WJ, Ross JW: The Insanity Plea. New York, Charles Scribner's, 1983

Chapter 23

Child Psychiatry and the Law

by Diane H. Schetky, M.D.

OVERVIEW

The law has had significant influence on the practice of child and adolescent psychiatry over the past two decades, with increased emphasis on children's rights and related adversarial proceedings. In turn, the rapidly expanding field of child forensic psychiatry has influenced the way in which courts make decisions concerning children. The origins of child forensic psychiatry go back to the roots of the child guidance movement. Public concern over juvenile delinquency around the turn of the 20th century led to the founding of child-guidance clinics to study and treat delinquency, and to the establishment of the juvenile court. The early juvenile courts operated in an atmosphere of benevolence but soon failed to live up to expectations, as they were often lacking in dispositional options and ineffectual in dealing with repeat juvenile offenders. In more recent years, juvenile courts have opted for waiver of certain dangerous juvenile offenders to the adult courts. Psychiatrists have continued to consult to the juvenile courts on matters of diagnosis, disposition, competency, and recently waiver and have actively pursued research in the area of juvenile delinquency.

A second wave of interest in matters concerning child psychiatry and the law has related to custody issues. Until the 20th century, custody was almost always awarded to fathers, as children were viewed as property and little heed was paid to any special needs or interests they might have. In the early 20th century, father-preference gave way to the tender-years presumption, and it was deemed that mothers were the more appropriate care givers, at least during the child's early years. In 1925, in the case of *Finlay v. Finlay* (p. 629), the court's role in custody cases was defined as to serve as *parens patriae* and do "what is in the best interests of the child." In 1973, Goldstein and colleagues published *Beyond the Best Interests of the Child* and attempted to put forth guidelines for making custody recommendations. While some (Awad, 1984) have criticized the rigid thinking of these authors, the book remains a milestone in terms of its application of psychoanalytic principles and insights to the legal arena. It has also been an impetus for further refinement of guidelines and has stimulated professional interest in custody issues. With the rise in the number of divorcing families in the past 50 years and in the number of contested custody cases, psychiatrists have increasingly been requested to help courts resolve the question of the child's best interests.

Although child abuse and neglect have been with us since early mankind, it was not until 1974 that mandatory child abuse reporting laws were established. Child psychiatrists are often involved in detecting and intervening in these cases. They may provide consultation to protective services agencies in regard to evaluating children in foster care, assessing parenting skills and potential, participating in permanent planning for foster children, and terminating parental rights when reunification is not feasible. Media attention to the battered child has been eclipsed in the 1980s by the sexually abused child. A new concern has been the phenomenon of false allegations of sexual abuse arising during custody litigation. The psychiatric profession has been caught off guard without guidelines as to how to evaluate these complex cases. Other paraprofessionals have stepped in to fill the void, many lacking adequate training in child development, family dynamics, and interviewing skills, with results that are often disastrous to child and family. Child psychiatrists have become involved in the fray and are often called into court to testify on a variety of issues, such as delayed disclosure in sexual abuse, false retraction, and false allegations, as well as determining a child's competency to be a witness (Quinn, 1986). However, the admissibility of expert testimony in matters related to child sexual abuse remains highly controversial (Cohen, 1985; Serrato, 1988).

The field of child forensic psychiatry continues to expand, and one of the newer issues we now face is civil litigation cases claiming damages related to psychic trauma (Terr, 1980; Malmquist, 1985). Questions are put to the expert witness regarding extent of damages, liklihood of future suffering, and need for treatment. Such cases are bound to increase, given the prevalence of child sexual abuse and the fact that the statute of limitations in many states runs until the age of majority. We are also seeing more professionals being sued for failure to diagnose, erroneous diagnosis of sexual abuse, faulty evaluations, and even abusive practices. In malpractice cases, we may be called upon to testify as to the standard of practice, breach of the standard of care, as well as assessment of damages.

Another, new area is that of intervention with children who have witnessed violence. Eth and Pynoos (1984, 1985; Pynoos and Eth, 1986) have developed protocols for working with children traumatized by violence and important liaisons with law enforcement agencies. The pioneering work of Terr (1979, 1983, 1985) on psychic trauma in children continues to yield new insights to aid the clinician working in this area. Fetal forensics is the newest horizon in child forensic psychiatry, and we are now having to grapple with moral and ethical issues related to high-technology reproduction, fetal rights, and surrogacy, for which we have no absolute answers.

Training has failed to keep pace with the demand for our services in child forensic psychiatry. Many practicing child psychiatrists feel ill-equipped to do child forensic evaluations and assiduously avoid going to court (Benedek, 1986). Those child psychiatrists who are active in the field are largely self-taught, have learned from mentors, or are in continuing medical education courses. Training in child forensic psychiatry remains woefully inadequate in most fellowships, and, as of this writing, there is only one fellowship offered in forensic child psychiatry, at the University of Michigan. This is lamentable, given the fact that the field is an extremely challenging one that utilizes all of our skills and training as diagnosticians, therapists, consultants, researchers, and educators. It also allows us to have some input into public policy, and is a natural extension of our role as advocates for children and educators.

The following discussions will review current trends and issues in child psychiatry and the law. This chapter is intended to familiarize general psychiatrists with the issues and new developments and help them recognize when a referral to a child psychiatrist with specialized skills and training in these areas might be indicated. For the child psychiatrist, the chapter offers guidelines for involvement in these cases, references for further readings, and hopes to encourage their involvement in forensic child psychiatry.

CHILD CUSTODY

Changing Trends

The number of divorces and number of children affected by divorce has continued to decline in the United States since 1982 (United States Department of Health and Human Services, 1987). Nonetheless, over one million children are involved in divorce each year. It is estimated that 45 percent of all children born in the United States in 1983 will experience divorce of their parents. Of these children, 35 percent will experience remarriage and 23 percent a second divorce (Wallerstein, 1985a). Women continue to receive custody in about 90 percent of divorces; however, in contested custody cases, fathers win custody in two out of three cases (New York Times, B8, March 17, 1986). Joint custody or shared parenting has become increasingly popular: about half of the states now have joint-custody laws, and several states have legal presumptions favoring joint custody (Folberg, 1984). Another trend has been toward the use of mediation services to resolve custody issues outside of court. In several states, such as Maine and California, mediation is now mandatory, and successful settlements are attained in 55 percent to 85 percent of cases (Wallerstein, 1985a).

Concern over the number of children languishing in foster care has led to mandatory, periodic, court review of children in foster care in most states. Greater emphasis has been placed upon either returning children to their homes as part of a parental reunification plan or, when this is not feasible, freeing these children for adoption. The trend has been toward increased accountability on the part of social service agencies, who must outline goals to parents whose children have been removed and document efforts made toward helping such parents regain their children. In 1982, the standard of evidence required for removing children from home and for terminating parental rights was raised from *preponderence of evidence* to *clear and convincing evidence*, making it more difficult to remove children from home and to terminate parental rights (*Santosky v. Kramer, 1982*).

Recognizing that foster care is only a temporary solution and that children need homes to call their own, greater emphasis has been placed upon finding permanent homes for older and hard-to-place children, such as physically and emotionally handicapped or biracial children. Adoptability now tends to be defined in terms of who will have the child in question. With freer use of birth control and abortion, and the trend for many single mothers to keep their babies, the market of healthy white newborns has practically dried up. Infertility has increased among American women, due to venereal disease, use of contraception, and postponement of childbearing. Couples eager to adopt infants must often look abroad or consider taking an infant with special needs. Many agencies are relaxing their standards for adoptive parents, when it comes to hard to place children, and are now willing to consider single parents, as well as parents with alternate life styles. Private adoptions continue and are often controversial, as when they involve inadequate screening, questionable financial deals, and lack of supervision.

Divorce Research

Research on the aftermath of divorce is beginning to yield important and troubling data. Wallerstein (1986) conducted a 10-year follow-up of children and parents undergoing divorce in California. She found that the quality of life for parents postdivorce improved for both parents in only 10 percent of cases and that in 20 percent of cases it worsened. Females were more likely than males to experience an improved quality of life emotionally, whereas the majority of males remained psychologically unchanged. Women who were over 40-years-old at the time of divorce fared less well than younger women; they were less likely to remarry, and more likely to experience loneliness and financial hardship. Men were four times more likely than women to experience financial security postdivorce. Wallerstein (1986) notes that anger remained high in both parents and that, in 20 percent of cases, the mother's anger spilled over to the child and interfered with the father–child relationship.

Regarding the long-term effects of divorce on children, Wallerstein (1984, 1985b) found that, although preschool children experienced the most stress during the divorce, they tended to fare better in the long run than older children. Boys appeared to be more vulnerable to the acute effects of divorce, whereas girls experienced more difficulty later, as adolescents. However, both had significant adjustment problems at follow-up. Father-yearning persisted in all children; half of the children felt paternal rejection, and most of them had poor relationships with their father at the 10-year follow-up. The father's psychological stability seemed to be a significant factor in visiting patterns. In spite of poor relationships with their fathers, many children opted to change custody and live with their fathers as teens. Although most fathers fared well financially, only half of them provided adequate financial help to their college-age children. Heatherington and associates (1985) studied the long-term effects of divorce and remarriage on children. They found that divorce had more adverse effects on the adjustment of boys and that remarriage was more disruptive for girls. They also noted that boys tended to exhibit more externalizing behaviors, whereas girls tended to internalize more.

Another study, by Cooney and colleagues (1986), looked at the immediate effects of divorce on young adults and found that father–daughter relationships were particularly vulnerable to disruption. Following divorce of their parents, many college-age women experienced positive changes in relationship to their mothers, whereas frequency of contacts with their fathers diminished. The women in the study tended to be more angry with their fathers than the males, whereas both groups experienced significant loyalty conflicts.

Special Issues

Joint Custody. Joint custody involves parents having shared responsibility and authority for their children, implies that fathers are viewed as equally important to their children, and usually involves alternate living in both parental homes. It does not necessarily imply that each parent is granted equal time with the child, and developing visitation schedules tends to be individualized according to the child's age and school schedule, locations of parents' homes, and parents' work schedules. Joint custody has been popular with parents and attorneys, as neither party emerges the loser and it promotes parental access to children. There has been the presumption that joint custody might cut down on parental conflict postdivorce, although data on this are mixed (Ilfeld et al, 1982; Ash and Guyer, 1986b), and, as noted by Derdeyn and Scott (1984), joint custody per se does not necessarily promote parental cooperation. Joint custody has been shown to be psychologically beneficial to fathers and to promote their involvement with their children postdivorce (Grief, 1979).

In terms of the effects of joint custody on children, Steinman (1981, 1985) found that one-third of the children in her study were having trouble adjusting to it, and that joint custody arrangements often broke down when the children reached adolescence. Shiller (1986) concluded that joint custody seemed to have a beneficial effect for latency-aged boys and their parents though cautioned that it was not clear whether this reflected on the strengths of parents who sought joint custody or the arrangement itself. Most authors agree that, for joint custody to work, parents need to be capable of communicating, cooperating, putting aside marital and divorce engendered anger, and building new boundaries. Further, there is general consensus that joint custody should not be imposed upon parents who do not want it (Steinman, 1985; Awad, 1983; Tibbets-Kleber, 1987).

Father custody. The number of single-parent fathers has increased dramatically in recent years, and courts seem to be overcoming their biases against fathers as custodial parents. According to a preliminary study by Turner (1984), fathers who seek custody tend to have been quite involved in the care of their children or else do so out of a concern for their former wives' ability to parent. Some may be angry over refusal to be allowed access to their children, or they may be vindictive. Studies of single-father caretakers reveal them to be generally well educated and financially and socially stable. They tend to be nurturing, confidant, well organized, well adjusted, and capable of using community supports (Berry, 1981). Research on infants raised by fathers who were the primary nurturing parent indicates fathers were capable of forming strong nurturing attachments and that infants thrived under their care (Pruett, 1983). One study suggests that children living with the same sexed parent may fare better than those living with the opposite sexed parent (Santrock and Marshak, 1979).

Homosexual parents. Much prejudice has surrounded awarding custody or even visitation to homosexual parents. A more recent concern raised by some parents has to do with fears of exposing children to AIDS (New York Times, p. A18, April 28, 1987; New York Times, p. 11, September 21, 1987). Courts have tended to operate under biases that homosexual parents are maladjusted, that their lifestyle is contagious, or that contact with the child would be harmful (Hitchens and Kirkpatrick, 1985). The few studies conducted on parenting by lesbian mothers show them to be quite comparable to heterosexual mothers in their parenting styles (Hoeffer, 1981). Similarly, children raised by lesbian mothers are comparable to children raised by heterosexual mothers in most parameters. The exceptions are that boys of lesbian mothers score higher on sensitivity and girls of lesbian mothers score higher on leadership and adventuresomeness (Hoeffer, 1981). No differences in sex-role traits have been noted (Hoeffer, 1981; Kirkpatrick et al, 1981). Very little has been written about homosexual fathers, but one study suggests that many encounter difficulty reconciling their homosexual identity with fatherhood (Bozett, 1981).

The Psychiatrist's Role in Custody Disputes

Child custody evaluations differ from diagnostic evaluations in several regards. Communications are not confidential, as a verbal or written report to the attorneys and the court will be expected from the expert. This should be explained to all participants in the initial meeting, and informed-consent and release forms should be signed. These evaluations tend to be highly adversarial, and the psychiatrist needs to remain allied with the child's best interests and avoid pressures from various parties and attorneys to take sides. It is preferable to enter into these evaluations as court appointed, as this confers more neutrality. However, one is just as likely to enter into these disputes by request from one party or the other, their respective attorneys, or the guardian *ad litem* for the child. In such cases, it is important to have equal access to all parties and to avoid making judgments on parties not seen. It is essential to ascertain at the start precisely what the legal questions at hand are and address them in the evaluation and report. Prior to seeing any parties, fees should be discussed, and it is becoming customary for psychiatrists to expect payment in advance of rendering an opinion or report.

These evaluations tend to be very time consuming, and it is important not to take short cuts. Given that parental perceptions of events may be skewed or self-serving, it is often necessary to get corroborating information from outside sources. A thorough, fair, and persuasive evaluation may often lead to an out-of-court settlement or at least to the judge following the evaluator's recommendations (Ash and Guyer, 1986a). In contrast, an inadequate or biased report may be discredited, and the family is then forced to go through an entire evaluation again. It is beyond the scope of this chapter to discuss the process of the child-custody evaluation, which is extensively described elsewhere (APA Task Force on Child Custody, 1984; Benedek and Schetky, 1985a; Benedek and Benedek, 1980; Parry et al, 1985; Solnit and Schetky, 1986; Weiner et al, 1985; Weithorn, 1987).

Countertransference issues tend to run high in custody cases, and the expert needs to avoid rescue fantasies or overidentification with one parent or the other or with the child. One needs to be aware of possible biases toward homosexual parents or fathers seeking custody. Questions regarding motivation for seeking custody, the parent–child relationship, and parenting skills should be the same, regardless of the parent's gender or sexual identity.

The psychiatrist also needs to be tolerant of parents' lifestyles and value systems, when they differ from his or her own, providing they do not endanger the child. A final caveat has to do with the need to separate the functions of evaluator and therapist in custody cases. The treating psychiatrist is not in a position to do an objective evaluation for custody and should refer the child or parent elsewhere if a custody evaluation is indicated. This also serves to preserve confidentiality. Likewise, having rendered an opinion in a custody case, one is no longer neutral vis-à-vis parents, and this may interfere with working in a therapeutic modality with the family.

CHILD SEXUAL ABUSE

Child sexual abuse has been with us throughout recorded history (Schetky, 1988a). However, it was not until the 1970s that the full extent of the problem began to surface. Increased media attention to child sexual abuse, the women's movement, victims more willing to speak out, and more responsiveness on the part of professionals have all resulted in greater intolerance for child sexual abuse and efforts toward intervention and prevention. The number of reported cases of child sexual abuse continues to rise at a staggering rate, with a 57.4 percent increase between 1983 and 1984 (Report of the Select Committee on Children, Youth, and Families, 1987). However, the majority of reported cases of suspected child abuse remain unsubstantiated (American Humane Society Statistics, 1984, personal communication) and are not prosecuted for lack of evidence.

There is much ongoing research in the area of child sexual abuse which has identified risk factors (Finkelhor, 1986) and the acute effects of sexual abuse on children (Gomes-Schwartz et al, 1985), as well as long-term effects of sexual abuse. Although there are many flaws in the existing research, there is general consensus on the damaging long-term effects of child sexual abuse (Schetky, in press). Common findings include depression, increased likelihood of psychiatric hospitalization, substance abuse, self-destructive behavior, posttraumatic stress disorder, dissociative disorders and multiple personality disorder, revictimization, and impaired interpersonal relationships. Among children who have been sexually abused, many become eroticized, have learning difficulties, and as teens may be prone to acting-out behaviors. The long-lasting negative effects of childhood sexual abuse appear to be correlated with abuse by a father or step-father, use of force, being unsupported by a close adult, and sexual activity which is intrusive and of long duration (Schetky, in press).

The Psychiatrist's Role

Child psychiatrists are frequently called upon to assess and validate allegations of child sexual abuse. As with child custody evaluations, these cases are often minefields frought with difficulties. The clinician needs to approach them from a framework that takes into consideration developmental factors, family dynamics, prior abuse, exposure to adult sexuality, and other stressors that might account for behavioral changes (American Academy of Child and Adolescent Psychiatry, 1988; Benedek and Schetky, 1987). There are no behavioral signs that are pathognomonic for child sexual abuse, though eroticized behavior may be highly suggestive (Yates, 1987). Physical findings may be more explicit (Finkel, 1988); however, absence of physical findings does not mean absence of sexual abuse. Factors enhancing a child's credibility include the child's description in childlike vocabulary as described from her point of view, good recall of details including idiosyncratic and sensorimotor ones, reenactment of the trauma in play or drawings, sexual themes in drawings and play, consistency of core of allegations over time, absence of secondary gain, and behavioral changes related to the alleged abuse. Anatomically correct dolls have become a popular way of evaluating child sexual abuse, but they do not constitute a litmus test for sexual abuse, nor should they be substituted for a more thorough evaluation. They may be useful to clarify a child's sexual vocabulary or to allow her to demonstrate what happened, but they can readily be misused, as when the clinician offers suggestions to the child about what transpired. There has been great pressure to develop techniques that will facilitate the evaluation of these complex cases. As with new medication, initial enthusiasm needs to be tempered with caution, until the evidence of the efficacy of new diagnostic techniques such as anatomically correct dolls and penile plethysmography for offenders has been proven. California, in 1987, ruled that testimony based on the use of anatomically correct dolls may not be used until such a time that the "procedure has been generally accepted as reliable in the scientific community in which it was developed" (*In the Matter of Amber B and Teela B, 1987*).

The psychiatrist needs to be alert to the possibility of false allegations, particularly if charges arise in the midst of custody or visitation disputes. False allegations are more likely to be lodged by parents rather than the child. Often they stem from an anxious mother's misinterpretation of events; for example, a father bathing or toileting a young child during visitation. In more extreme cases, they may involve parents with borderline or paranoid features that affect their reality testing or vindictive parents who are trying to exclude their former spouses from their child's life (Benedek and Schetky, 1985b; Green, 1986). Other situations in which false allegations may arise include children, previously abused by others, who misinterpret the actions of adults around them or use allegations spitefully or for secondary gain. Occasionally, there may be contamination, as when children in nursery-school situations are exposed to other children's allegations, and a bandwagon effect ensues. Teens may sometimes make false allegations out of anger or to cover up their own sexuality. Finally, given the increased public awareness of the problem, some well-meaning individuals may overreact, as when daycare workers misinterpret diaper rash, urinary-tract infections, or masturbation for sexual abuse.

The clinician performing evaluations for suspected sexual abuse needs to approach them without bias and attempt to maintain an objective stance. Interview techniques using suggestion, reinforcement, or coercion should be avoided. Given the magnitude of the allegations and serious implications for all involved, there is no room for short-cuts. If intrafamilial abuse is alleged, the psychiatrist should attempt to see all parties involved. If allegations are brought against a parent during a custody dispute, it may be helpful to see the child with the accused parent, if the child is willing and the psychiatrist feels it would not be harmful to the child (Awad, 1987; Benedek and Schetky, 1985b; Green, 1986).

Upon completing an evaluation of suspected sexual abuse, the clinician needs to formulate an opinion and recommendations that will protect the child from future abuse. Often, the most immediate question will be whether or not it is safe to allow the child to return home. Such a decision must weigh the parents' abilities to protect the child and their willingness to believe her, the child's wishes, and whether the offender, if in the home, is willing to take responsibility for the abuse and enter into treatment. It should be emphasized that, by law, all cases of suspected child abuse must be reported, and the firm backup of the law is often essential to the offender's cooperating with a treatment plan. Treatment decisions will need to be made for various family members, and these will often be determined by what is available in the community. Usually, a variety of treatment modalities will be employed, including family, individual, and group therapy. Group therapy is particularly useful for adolescent victims, and play therapy for the needs of younger children (Schetky, 1988b). Recently, concern has been expressed about the pressing need for treatment programs for adolescent sex offenders, as studies have noted that many pedophiles begin as adolescents (Becker and Caplan, 1988; Fehrenback et al, 1986).

If allegations of sexual abuse are felt to be unfounded, the clinician needs to come forth with a psychodynamic explanation for the charges. Impressions should be shared with parents, who may react with relief, or, in some cases, by escalating the charges and seeking yet another opinion. In some instances, it may not be possible to determine whether abuse occurred because the child is too young, the case has been contaminated by too many interrogations, or the child's memory has faded with time. In such cases, one must create a plan that protects the child but also preserves parent–child ties. This may involve supervised visitation, therapy for the child, or periodic reevaluation.

THE CHILD AS A WITNESS

Statutory law regarding the child as witness did not come into effect until the late 18th century in England (*Rex v. Brasier, 1779*), whereas prior to this time children were barred from giving testimony. In the United States, children were freely permitted to give testimony during the Salem witch trials and leading questions such as "How long hast thee been a witch?" (Upham 1969, p. 207) were permitted. It was not until 1895 (*Wheeler v. U.S.*) that any attempts were made to define competency to be a witness. In this case it was noted that "competency depends upon the capacity and intelligence of the child, his appreciation of the difference between truth and falsehood, as well as duty to tell the former" (*Wheeler v. U.S., 1899*, p. 524). In the ensuing years, statutory requirements for children to be witnesses have remained similar to these in most states. Competency is usually determined by the judge on a case-to-case basis. No minimum age for competency exists, and the trend has been for younger and younger children to be put on the stand, particularly in cases of child sexual abuse. Since *Wheeler*, the elements of testimonial capacity have become more refined and, as outlined by Stafford (1962), these include:

1. The child's capacity to communicate, observe, and remember matter about which testimony is being sought
2. The child's mental capacity at the time of the occurrence in question and ability to observe and register such occurrence
3. Memory sufficient to retain an independent recollection of the observations made
4. Capacity to translate into words the memory of such events

Unfortunately, the legal criteria for competency do not take into consideration emotional factors that may complicate the child's ability to testify. These include temperament, loyalty conflicts, emotional stability, and ego impairment. The child's fears and anxiety level will also affect how she conducts herself on the witness stand. Children commonly fear that they will not be believed, that they are on trial, and that the defendent may seek retaliation, and older children often feel humiliated or embarrassed if asked to give intimate details of sexual abuse. On the other hand, with proper support, many children do well on the witness stand, and depending on the outcome, the experience may be constructive.

Recent research suggests that children's memories are more fragmented than adults' (Johnson and Foley, 1984) but, when given external cues, they perform well on recall (Kobasigawa, 1974). Children are more likely to have difficulty with facial recognition than adults (Chance and Goldstein, 1984) and may be more susceptible to leading questions and misleading information than adults (Dale et al, 1978). Goodman and colleagues (1984) found that jurors were reluctant to judge a person's guilt or innocence solely on a child's testimony.

Changes in the Treatment of Child Witnesses

Courtrooms were not designed for children and can be very intimidating to the child witness, as is the prospect of confronting the offender and being cross examined. In efforts to render the process of giving testimony less traumatic, numerous states have permitted the use of videotaped testimony, at least during the Grand Jury and sometimes during the actual trial. The biggest obstacle to the use of videotaped testimony is the confrontation clause of the Sixth Amendment, which provides the accused "the right to be confronted with the witness against him." One way around this is the use of two-way, closed-circuit television, wherein defendent and witness can see each other but are in separate rooms. In spite of the popularity of electronic testimony, there is no evidence that such testimony is any more reliable, and many have concerns as to how jurors react to it.

Simpler efforts to accommodate child witnesses have included familiarizing the child with the courtroom ahead of time, the use of child-sized furniture, providing the child with drawing materials, allowing a trusted but neutral adult to be with the child, and recognizing the child's physiological needs and short attention span with frequent breaks and snacks.

The American Academy of Child and Adolescent Psychiatry (1986) has made recommendations for children undergoing abuse investigations and testimony and urges limiting the number of times a child can be interviewed, coordinating agency efforts, using child psychiatrists to evaluate and interpret to the courts, and prioritizing child sexual abuse cases on court dockets. In addition, the Academy has urged modification of hearsay rules in these cases and excluding the press and spectators from these trials.

LEGAL ISSUES IN PRACTICE

Consent

In as much as minors are not capable of giving consent in most states, it must be obtained from their parents or guardians in matters pertaining to evaluation and treatment. Exceptions exist in some states, such as Michigan, where individuals over the age of 14 may enter into psychotherapy without parental permission. For consent to be informed, the consentor needs to be made aware of the nature of the condition being treated, treatment alternatives, and foreseeable risks and benefits. In cases of divorce, consent must be obtained from the custodial parent. If joint custody exists, one needs to be aware of what the custody decree states regarding consent for medical procedures, as these can vary. It is usually best to include both parents in decisions where joint custody is in effect, even though it may not be legally necessary, as shared decision-making is one of the underpinnings of joint custody.

Exceptions to the need for parental consent include emancipated minors, information pertaining to birth control, the treatment of venereal diseases and substance abuse, and certain emergency situations. Psychiatrists are likely to encounter more difficulty in getting paid than with liability for entering into contracts with minors, though technically they could be charged with battery if they enter into treatment without proper consent.

Reporting Child Abuse

Psychiatrists are mandated reporters, and any reasonable suspicion of the physical or sexual abuse of a child must be reported even if the patient is in treatment. The intent of the law is to protect children at risk, and a therapist would be naive to think that he or she could handle an abuse situation single-handedly. If abuse is within the family, the report should be filed with protective services agencies, otherwise the local District Attorney's or sheriff's office should be notified. The patient should be informed that a report will be filed.

Confidentiality

This is not likely to be an issue with young children, and the psychiatrist's judgement will determine how much to share with parents. With adolescents, the rules of confidentiality should be spelled out in the initial session. Generally, the psychiatrist will adhere to confidentiality unless the patient is in danger of harming himself or others. When parents are contacted, the psychiatrist should inform the patient and give him or her an idea of what will be discussed or offer to include the patient. If it is necessary to breach a confidence, the patient may be given the option of being first to inform the parents; the patient should always be informed of the therapist's intent to disclose.

When releasing information about adolescents, consent from a parent or guardian is required. However, it is often advisable to get the patient's assent and inform her or him, as well as the parents, as to what information is to be shared and with whom.

A troubling issue for many psychiatrists is when attorneys attempt to subpoena records of patients in treatment to be used in divorce litigation. The psychiatrist's duty remains to the patient, and efforts should be made to quash such a subpoena, through appealing to the lawyers involved or to the judge and spelling out why it is not in the patient's interest for the psychiatrist to testify or release information. The psychiatrist may further recommend that an independent psychiatrist be appointed for purposes of performing a custody evaluation and providing the court with the information needed.

NEW ISSUES

The Rights of Juveniles

Defining the rights of juveniles has increasingly occupied the U.S. Supreme Court. In the last 10 years, the court has considered the abortion rights of minors (New York Times, p. B32, November 4, 1987), the rights of parents to voluntarily institutionalize their children (*Parham v. J.R., 1979*), the execution of persons for crimes committed as juveniles (*Thompson v. Oklahoma, 1987*), and freedom from search and freedom of speech within the schools. Regarding the latter, the U.S. Supreme Court sided with school officials to allow search of students as long as "reasonable grounds" exist (New York Times, p. 1, January 16, 1985), and to censor school newspapers and "school sponsored expressive activities" (New York Times, p. 1, 1988). The court has also upheld preventative detention of juveniles (*Schall v. Martin, 1984*).

Historically, the law has moved from viewing children as nonentities, to property, to persons with special needs and rights. Presently, the law treats them more as adults in conjunction with due process rights in delinquency proceedings (*In re Gault, 1967*), the right to an attorney in certain custody proceedings, and the right to make decisions independent of their parents in matters of birth control and venereal disease treatment. At the same time, the law offers them more protection in areas of child abuse and termination of parental rights and, as noted, has sided with schools and family autonomy in matters of how much control they may exert over juveniles.

Waiver is another example of how the law has come to regard certain juveniles more like adults. There has been a trend toward juveniles committing more violent crimes, and this has led to greater use of waiver of juveniles to the adult court, where they are likely to receive harsher and more prolonged sentences. A study on the use of waiver in the state of New York over a 10-year period failed to show that it had any deterrent effect on juvenile crime (New York Times, p. B6, February 4, 1987). In some states, another trend has been toward legislation that allows juveniles to be emancipated from their parents, if they are competent and capable of supporting themselves. This often involves juveniles freeing themselves from difficult home situations, although parents occasionally divorce themselves from out-of-control teens.

Psychiatrists may be requested to evaluate juvenile offenders in regard to waiver or competency to stand trial (Benedek, 1985; Palombi, 1980). The issues involved in competency determinations are similar to those for adults; namely, ability to understand the charges and the nature of the proceedings and to participate in one's own defense.

Surrogacy

Surrogacy has become a topic of great public and professional interest and has generated much attention from the media. Surrogacy has pitted the right to privacy against the state's interests, the interests of infertile couples against potential interests of surrogate mothers, and the right of the child to be raised in a relatively conflict-free environment. It has also introduced moral and ethical concerns over "baby selling." Feminists, taking afront, argue that surrogacy exploits women and renders them a "commodity in the reproductive marketplace" (New York Times, p. B3, July 31, 1987). Many are puzzled by this opposition coming from the same group that has advocated for women's rights to control their own bodies and make their own decisions. Strong opposition also comes from the Vatican, which opposes embryo transfer and any artificial means of fertilization (New York Times, p. A14, March 11, 1987). Several states now have legislation pending that would prohibit surrogacy, and Britain has already outlawed commercial surrogacy (New York Times, p. A13, September 1, 1987).

Similar questions and problems arise "in the brave new world of egg donation" that have yet to be resolved (New York Times, p. 1, January 18, 1988). It is apparent that many have been caught off-guard by rapid advances in reproductive technology and have not yet fully considered the ethical and moral implications, nor have they developed reasonable guidelines for these procedures.

Psychiatrists may become involved in screening potential surrogate mothers and parental applicants. Parker (1984) discusses the ethical and moral dilemmas in these consultations and provides guidelines for screening. The psychiatrist may also become involved in helping to assure that consent is both informed and voluntary. Provocative questions have been raised as to whether participants in surrogacy can give truly informed consent when they can not anticipate how they will react to something they have never experienced (Parker, 1984). Psychiatrists may also become involved when surrogacy contracts are breached and a custody battle ensues, as was the case in the famed Baby M case (*In the Matter of Baby M, 1987*). Issues at this point are likely to focus on whether consent was informed, the relative fitness and lifestyles of parents, and the father's interest versus the mother's, with relatively less emphasis on the child's ties, given her young age.

Fetal Forensics

Interest in ethical and forensic issues involving newborns and fetuses was highlighted by the Baby Doe case in 1984, which pitted right-to-life organizations and the Reagan administration against the abilities of physicians and parents to make treatment decisions concerning severely handicapped infants. The impact of this case was considerable and led to widespread development of hospital-ethics committees and a policy statement by the American Academy of Pediatrics regarding the "best interests of children" being a determining factor in decisions not to treat (Lantos, 1987).

Following Baby Doe, cases focusing on liberty interests of pregnant women versus fetuses emerged, which raised issues such as can a pregnant woman be forced to follow medical advice? and how can a fetus be treated without curtailing a mother's liberty? Typically, issues involved Caesarean sections, fetal transfusions or treatments, and the problem of what to do with a mother whose lifestyle endangers her fetus. In one case, criminal charges were brought against a woman for conduct harmful to her fetus, but they were later dismissed (Newsweek 1987). Sixteen states have now passed laws making it a crime to cause the death of an unborn child (Newseek, 1987). Attempts to override maternal treatment refusal have been on "dubious legal grounds" (Kolder et al, 1987, p. 1184). However, *Roe v. Wade* (1973), which prohibited the abortion of a fetus of viable age, decisions ordering procedures on pregnant women, and malpractice claims for prenatal injury or death, have all tended to support claims on behalf of personhood of the fetus (Robertson, 1983). We are now witnessing the advent of attorneys and guardians ad litem being appointed for fetuses. At this time, fetal rights appear to be subordinate to the health and safety of the pregnant female (*Thornburgh v. American College Obstetricians & Gynecologists, 1986*); however, several cases have involved keeping brain-damaged pregnant women alive to preserve the life of fetuses (New York Times, p. 39, March 8, 1987; Washington Post, September 23, 1988). Contradictions continue to abound, and, notes Newsweek (1987), "How can it be legal to abort a baby one week and illegal to deny it proper care the next?"

Presently much controversy exists over the medical use of tissues from aborted fetuses for research or transplants to treat Parkinson's disease (New York Times, p. 1, August 16, 1987; New York Times, p. B13, January 7, 1988). Concerns that a market for fetuses may arise have been voiced, and ethical issues about using anencephalic newborns as organ donors have been raised (New York Times, p. A18, December 14, 1987).

Psychiatrists may be called upon to assess a mother's competency to refuse medical procedures or to determine whether she needs to be restrained if her lifestyle is endangering her fetus. They may also serve on hospital ethics committees dealing with neonatal clinical and research issues. Eventually, we shall have to deal with the matter of what children should be told about their origins if they resulted from surrogacy or other artificial means of insemination, and parents will be wanting answers to questions of how these new reproductive techniques affect the future child and the rest of the family.

SUMMARY

The law is exerting increasingly significant influences on the ways in which we practice medicine and make decisions concerning children and their families. Hospitals now routinely employ attorneys on-staff to guide us in making ethical and moral decisions. Awareness of legal issues and their impact on psychiatry has become critical to the practice of psychiatry. Rapid developments in the field of psychiatry and law have made it difficult to keep abreast of all of the issues we may be asked to address. As suggested by Dietz (1987), child forensic psychiatry may soon become a specialty unto its own. In the meantime, we must at least give careful thought to the critical issues in this field, and, if in doubt about legal issues arising in our practices, seek consultation from a forensic psychiatrist or an attorney.

REFERENCES

American Academy of Child Psychiatry: Statement on Protecting Children Undergoing Abuse Investigations and Testimony. American Academy of Child Psychiatry, Washington, DC, 1986

American Humane Society: Personal Communication, 1984.

American Psychiatric Association Task Force on Child Custody: Child Custody Consultation in Issues in Forensic Psychiatry. Washington, DC, American Psychiatric Association Press, Inc, 1984

Ash P, Guyer M: The functions of psychiatric evaluation in contested child custody and visitation cases. J Am Acad Child Psychiatry 1986; 25:554–561

Ash P, Guyer M: Relitigation after contested custody and visitation evaluations. Bull Am Acad Psychiatry Law 1986; 14:323–330

Awad J: Joint custody: preliminary impressions. Can J Psychiatry 1983: 28:41–44

Awad G: Beyond the best interest of the child: ten years later. Can J Psychiatry 1984; 29:258–262

Awad G: The assessment of custody and access disputes in cases of sexual abuse allegations. Can J Psychiatry 1987; 32:539–544

Becker J, Caplan M: Sex offenders, in Child Sexual Abuse: A Handbook for Health Care and Legal Professionals. Edited by Schetky DH, Green AH. New York, Brunner/Mazel, Inc, 1988

Benedek EP: Waiver of juveniles to adult court, in Emerging Issues in Child Psychiatry and the Law. Edited by Schetky DH, Benedek EP. New York, Brunner/Mazel, Inc, 1985

Benedek EP: Forensic child psychiatry: an emerging subspecialty. Bull Am Acad Psychiatry Law 1986; 14:295–300

Benedek EP, Benedek R: Participating in child custody cases, in Child Psychiatry and the Law. Edited by Schetky DH, Benedek EP. New York, Brunner/Mazel, Inc, 1980

Benedek EP, Schetky DH: Custody and visitation: problems and perspectives. Psychiatric Clin North Am 1985a; 8:857–873

Benedek EP, Schetky DH: Allegations of sexual abuse in child custody and visitation disputes, in Emerging Issues in Child Psychiatry and Law. Edited by Schetky DH, Benedek EP. New York, Brunner/Mazel Inc, 1985b

Benedek EP, Schetky DH: Problems in validating allegations of sexual abuse. J Am Acad Child Adolesc Psychiatry 1987; 26:912–921

Berry KK: The male single parent, in Children of Separation and Divorce. **Edited by ???.** New York, Van Nostrand Reinhold Co, 1981

Bozett FW: Gay fathers: evolution of the gay-father identity. Am J Orthopsychiatry 1981; 51:552–559

Chance JE, Goldstein AC: Face-recognition memory: implication for children's eyewitness testimony. J Soc Issues 1984; 40:69–85

Cohen A: The unreliability of expert testimony on the typical characteristics of sexual abuse victims. Georgetown Law Review 1985; 74:429–456

Cooney TM, Smyer MA, Hagestad GO, et al: Parental divorce in young adulthood: some preliminary findings. Amer J Orthopsychiatry 1986; 56:470–477

Dale PS, Loftus EF, Rathburn E: The influence of the form of the question on the eyewitness testimony of preschool children. J Psycholinguist Research 1978; 7:269–277

Derdeyn A, Scott E: Joint Custody: A critical analysis and appraisal. Amer J Orthopsychiatry 1984; 54:199–209

Dietz P: The forensic psychiatrist of the future. Bull Am Acad Psychiatry Law 1987; 15:217–228

Eth S, Pynoos R: Developmental perspectives on psychic trauma in childhood, in Trauma and its Wake. Edited by Figley CR. New York, Brunner/Mazel, Inc, 1984

Fehrenbach P, Smith W, Manastersky C, et al: Adolescent sex offenders: offenders and offense characteristics. Am J Orthopsychiatry 1986; 56:225–233

Finkel M: The medical evaluation of child sexual abuse, in Child Sexual Abuse: A Handbook for Health Care and Legal Professionals. Edited by Schetky DH, Green A. New York, Brunner/Mazel, Inc, 1988

Finkelhor D: Sourcebook on Child Sexual Abuse. Beverly Hills, Sage Publications, 1986

Finlay v. Finlay, 148 NE 624 N.Y., 1925

Folberg J: Custody overview, in Joint Custody and Shared Parenting. Edited by Folberg J. Washington, DC: Bureau of National Affairs, 1984

Gomes-Schwartz B, Horowitz JM, Sauzier M: Severity of emotional distress among sexually abused preschool, school-age, and adolescent children. Hosp Community Psychiatry 1985; 36:503–508

Green A: True and false allegations of sexual abuse in child custody disputes. J Am Acad Child Psychiatry 1986; 25:449–456

Grief J: Fathers, children and joint custody. Am J Orthopsychiatry 1979; 49:311–319

Goldstein J, Freud A, Solnit A: Beyond the Best Interest of the Child. New York, The Free Press, 1973

Goodman GS, Golding JM, Haith NM: Jurors' reactions to child witnesses. J Soc Issues 1984; 40:139–156

Heatherington EM, Cox M, Cox R: Long-term effects of divorce and remarriage on the adjustment of children. J Amer Acad Child Psychiatry 1985; 24:518–530

Hitchens D, Kirkpatrick M: Lesbian Mothers/Gay Fathers, in Emerging Issues in Child Psychiatry and the Law. Edited by Schetky DH, Benedek EP. New York, Brunner/Mazel, Inc, 1985

Hoeffer B: Children's acquisition of sex-role behavior in lesbian-mother families. Am J Orthopsychiatry 1981; 51:536–544

Ilfeld FW, Ilfeld HZ, Alexander JR: Does joint custody work? A first look at outcome data of relitigation. Am J Psychiatry 1982; 139:62–66

In the Matter of Baby M: Sup. Ct. N.J. IM 25314–86 E (March 1987)

In Amber B and Teela B: Solano, County Superior Court, No. 18488, 1987

In the Matter of Gault. 2287 U.S. 1, 1967

Johnson MK, Foley MA: Differentiating fact from fantasy: in reliability of children's memories. J Soc Issues 1984; 40:33–50

Kirkpatrick M, Smith C, Roy R: Lesbian mothers and their children: a comparative survey. Am J Orthopsychiatry 1981; 51:545–551

Kobasigawa K: Utilization of retrieval cues by children to recall. Child Development 1974; 45:127–134

Kolder V, Gallagher J, Parson M: Court-ordered obstetrical interventions. N Engl J Med 1987; 316:1192–1196

Lantos J: Baby Doe five years later: implications for child health (editorial). N Engl J Med 1987; 317:444–447

Malmquist C: Children who witness violence: tortious aspects. Bull Am Acad Psychiatry Law 1985; 13:221–232

Newsweek: The question of fetal rights, in On Health. Spring 1987

New York Times, p. B8, March 17, 1986

New York Times, p. A18, April 28, 1987

New York Times, p. B11, September 21, 1987

New York Times, p. B32, November 4, 1987

New York Times, p. B21, December 10, 1987

New York Times, p. B6, December 4, 1986

New York Times, p. B3, July 31, 1987

New York Times, p. A14, March 11, 1987

New York Times, p. A13, September, 1987

New York Times, p. A1, January 18, 1988

New York Times, p. A3, March 8, 1987

New York Times, p. 1, August 16, 1987

New York Times, p. B13, January 7, 1988

New York Times, p. A18, December 14, 1987

Palombi J: Competency and criminal responsibility, in Child Psychiatry and the Law. Edited by Schetky DH, Benedek EP. New York, Brunner/Mazel, Inc, 1980

Parker P: Surrogate motherhood, psychiatric screening and informed consent, baby selling and public policy. Bull Am Acad Psychiatry Law 1984; 12:21–40

Parham v. J.R., 422 U.S. 584, 1979

Parry R, Broder E, Schmitt E, et al: Custody Disputes: Evaluation and Intervention. Lexington, MA, Lexington Books, 1986

Pruett K: Infants of primary nurturing fathers, in Psychoanalytic Study of the Child. Edited by Solnit A, Eissler R, Neubauer P. New Haven, Yale University Press, 1983

Pynoos R, Eth S: Children traumatized by witnessing acts of personal violence: homicide, rape or suicide behavior, in Post-Traumatic Stress Disorder in Children. Edited by Eth S, Pynoos R. Washington, DC, American Psychiatric Press, Inc, 1985

Pynoos R, Eth S: Witness to violence: the child interview. Journal of the American Academy of Child Psychiatry 1986; 25:306–319

Quinn K: Competency to be a witness. Bull Am Acad Psychiatry Law 1986; 14:311–322

Report of the Select Committee on Children, Youth, and Families. U.S. House of Representatives. Washington, DC, U.S. Government Printing Office, 1987

Rex v. Brasier, 1 Leach 199 68 Eng. Rep 202, 1779

Robertson JA: Procreative liberty and the control of conception, pregnancy and childbirth. Virginia Law Review 1983; 69:405–463

Roe v. Wade, 410 U.S. 113, 1973

Santosky v. Kramer, 50 USAW U.S. Mar 4, 1982

Santrock J, Marshak R: Father custody and social development in boys and girls. Journal of Social Issues 1979; 35:112–125

Schall v. Martin, USLW 4681, 1984

Schetky, DH: Child Sexual Abuse in History, Mythology and Religion, in Child Sexual Abuse: A Handbook for Health Care and Legal Professionals. Edited by Schetky DH, Green AH. New York, Brunner/Mazel, Inc, 1988a

Schetky DH: The treatment of child sexual abuse, in Child Sexual Abuse: A Handbook for Health Care and Legal Professionals. Edited by Schetky DH, Green AH. New York, Brunner/Mazel, Inc, 1988b

Schetky DH: The long-term effects of childhood sexual abuse, in Incest-Related Syndromes of Adult Psychopathology. Edited by Kluft R. Washington, DC, American Psyciatric Press, in press

Serrato V: Expert testimony in child sexual abuse prosecution: a spectrum of issues. Boston University Law Review 1988; 68:155–192

Shiller V: Joint versus maternal custody for families with latency age boys: Parents' characteristics and child adjustment. Am J Orthopsychiatry 1986; 56:486–489

Solnit A, Schetky DH: In the best interests of the child: an overview, in Psychiatry, vol VI. Edited by Michels R, Cavenar J. Philadelphia, JB Lippincott Co, 1986

Stafford CF: The child as a witness. Washington Law Review, 1962; 37:303–324

Steinman S: The experience of children in a joint custody arrangement. Am J Orthopsychiatry 1981; 51:403–414

Steinman S: Joint custody: the need for individual evaluation and service, in Emerging Issues in Child Psychiatry and the Law. Edited by Schetky DH, Benedek EP. New York, Brunner/Mazel, Inc, 1985

Terr L: Children of Chowchilla: a study of psychic trauma. Psychoanalytic Study of the Child 1979; 34:552–623

Terr L: Personal injury to children: the court suit claiming psychic trauma, in Child Psychiatry and the Law. Edited by Schetky DH, Benedek EP. New York, Brunner/Mazel, Inc, 1980

Terr L: Children of Chowchilla revisited: The effects of psychic trauma four years after a school bus kidnapping. Am J Psychiatry 1983; 40:1543–1550

Terr L: Psychic trauma in children and adolescents. Psychiatric Clin North Am 1985; 8:815–835

Thompson v. Oklahoma, 108 Supreme Court 2687, 1988

Thornburgh v. The American College of Obstetricians and Gynecologists, 106 S. Ct 2169, 1983

Tibbets-Kleber AL, Howel RH, Kleber DJ: Joint custody: a comprehensive review. Bull Am Acad Psychiatry Law 1987, 15:27–43

Turner J: Divorced fathers who win contested custody of their children, an exploratory study. Am J Orthopsychiatry 1984; 54:498–501

Upham CW: Witchcraft at Salem Village. New York, Frederick Ungar, 1969

United States Department of Health and Human Services, National Center for Health Statistics: Monthly Vital Statistics Report, 1986; 35:1

Wallerstein J: Children of divorce: preliminary report of a ten-year follow-up of young children. Am J Orthopsychiatry 1984; 54:444–458

Wallerstein J: Children of divorce: emerging trends. Psychiatric Clin North Am 1985a; 8:837–856

Wallerstein J: Children of divorce: preliminary report of a ten-year follow-up of older children and adolescents. Journal of the American Academy of Child Psychiatry 1985b; 24:545–553

Wallerstein J: Women after divorce: preliminary report from a ten-year follow-up. Am J Orthopsychiatry 1986; 56:65–77

Wallerstein J: Children of divorce: report of a ten-year follow-up of early latency age children. Am J Orthopsychiatry 1987; 75:199–211

Washington Post, p. C1, September 23, 1988

Weiner B, Simons V, Cavanaugh J: The child custody dispute, in Emerging Issues in Child Psychiatry and the Law. Edited by Schetky DH, Benedek EP. New York, Brunner/Mazel, Inc, 1985

Weithorn L (ed): Psychology and Child Custody Determinations. Lincoln, Neb, University of Nebraska Press, 1987

Wheeler v. United States, 159 U.S. 523, 1895

Yates A: Psychological damage associated with extreme eroticism in young children. Psychiatric Annals 1987; 17:257–261

Chapter 24

The Psychiatrist in Court

by C. Robert Showalter, M.D., and W. Lawrence Fitch, J.D.

Roughly two million *forensic* mental-health evaluations are conducted annually in the United States (Curran and McGarry, 1986). Many of these evaluations are performed by psychiatrists who specialize in the application of psychiatry to the law. Many more, however, are conducted by psychiatrists in general practice (Rappeport, 1982). It is for the general psychiatric practitioner who must occasionally appear in court that this essay is intended.

Psychiatric expertise may be sought on a range of legal issues. In the criminal area, the accused's competency to stand trial and criminal responsibility are frequent referral questions. Ironically, in the years since John Hinckley was acquitted by reason of insanity of shooting then-President Ronald Reagan—as unpopular as that verdict was and as much as psychiatry has been criticized for its role in the case—the presence of psychiatry in the criminal arena has grown considerably. Indeed, in 1985 the United States Supreme Court ruled for the first time that criminal defendants whose "sanity" at the time of a crime is likely to be a "significant factor" at trial are constitutionally entitled to "competent psychiatric assistance" on questions of criminal responsibility (*Ake v. Oklahoma, 1985*). More recent decisions have recognized a right to psychiatric assistance on other criminal justice issues as well (see *Ford v. Wainwright, 1986*).

The growing involvement of psychiatry in the adjudication of death penalty cases is particularly noteworthy. A number of courts have held that the failure of the defense attorney to seek psychiatric assistance in a capital case constitutes *ineffective assistance of counsel*, in violation of the defendant's Sixth Amendment right to counsel. Such decisions virtually guarantee psychiatry a role in death penalty determinations.

The ethical problems psychiatrists face in capital cases, of course, are enormous (Showalter and Bonnie, 1984; Appelbaum, 1986). Should psychiatrists predict future dangerousness in the face of laws recognizing dangerousness as a predicate for imposition of the death penalty? Should they offer their expertise on questions of competency to be executed? Should they provide treatment of death-row inmates to assure competency to be executed?

Issues psychiatrists routinely address in Juvenile and Family Court cases also can be thorny: At what point should the Juvenile Court abandon its *therapeutic* jurisdiction and order transfer of a child to be tried as an adult? What constitutes parental unfitness warranting removal of a child from one or both of its parents? Under what circumstances may an individual be deemed unable to make a procreative choice and be involuntarily sterilized?

Even psychiatrists practicing entirely outside the forensic speciality—psychiatrists who have no interest in participating in the legal process—may, on occasion, find themselves pressed to share their expertise in court. Questions of involuntary hospitalization, legal guardianship, and competency to refuse medical care face nearly all practicing psychiatrists. Psychiatric opinion may also be sought on questions of a patient's mental disability proceedings to determine eligibility for disability benefits or in the course of a lawsuit in which money damages are sought for disability suffered by the patient as a result of the wrongful behavior of another. Finally, and regrettably, psychiatrists increasingly are being called on to review the work of their colleagues in cases in which psychiatric malpractice has been alleged.

As psychiatry's involvement in legal concerns has grown in recent years, professional organizations in psychiatry and law have proliferated and an impressive, specialized literature has emerged. Institutes in psychiatry and law can be found in a number of major universities, and postresidency forensic psychiatric fellowships and other specialty training programs are available throughout the country (Rosner, 1982). Indeed, the field of forensic psychiatry has grown so rapidly and in so many directions that at least one noted scholar has called for specialization within the field (Dietz, 1987). No longer, he contends, is it reasonable to expect "forensic psychiatrists to retain proficiency in the full spectrum of potential activities."

Of course, psychiatry's rush to embrace the forensic specialty is not without risk. Concerned members of the profession have for years objected to the unsavory image of psychiatrists cavorting with assassins and babykillers. The specter of psychiatric experts engaged in courtroom battle is viewed by some as particularly horrific (Talbott, 1984). Moreover, there is the risk that as forensic specialists turn their attention away from traditional psychiatric endeavors toward the narrower confines of the law, their value as experts in psychiatry will be diminished:

> There is a danger that, if the [specialty's] efforts at professionalism continue to take the course of attaining more legal knowledge and practicing diagnostic skills with legal ends in mind, these attempts to become more credible may result in the loss of those very skills for which psychiatrists' opinions were sought in the first place. . . . In the process of [expert] testimony . . . the reality of the clinical inquiry which exists in virtually every patient's situation is lost, and with it the richness and subtlety which lie at the heart of the real contribution which psychiatry has to make to the law . . . (Kaplan and Miller, 1986, p. 463).

Certainly, it is incumbent on psychiatrists who participate in legal cases to retain their professional identity. The "hardened" specialist whose practice is limited to addressing narrow legal issues is no doubt at risk for having his or her clinical sensibilities atrophy. But, at the same time, the traditionalist who refuses to bend at all to the requirements of the law will likely encounter frustration in any effort to influence legal decision-making. Clearly, the most well-adjusted forensic psychiatrist is the one who is well grounded in his or her science and who also understands and can communicate meaningfully within the boundaries the law imposes on the involvement of psychiatrists as experts.

CHARACTERISTICS OF FORENSIC PSYCHIATRY

Forensic psychiatry differs fundamentally from traditional, *therapeutic* psychiatry in that its purpose ordinarily is not to provide treatment but, rather, to inform legal decision-making (Rappeport, 1982). Except perhaps in cases in which the psychiatrist's participation is solely for the purpose of satisfying some legal prerequisite to a patient's treatment (for example, civil commitment), the psychiatrist who conducts a clinical assessment for legal consumption enjoys no doctor–patient relationship with the subject of the assessment (Monahan, 1980). There can be no expectation of privacy. The psychiatrist may or may not communicate his or her findings to the subject of the assessment, but invariably a report will be made to the subject's attorney, and, of course, the potential exists for the psychiatrist's findings to be shared in open court. Moreover, these findings may do nothing to improve the patient's psychological lot. That is not their purpose.

Because the forensic psychiatrist serves ends other than treatment, it is critical that he or she guard against the phenomenon of transference. It is to be expected that individuals who come into contact with psychiatrists will feel some degree of trust, even in the face of warnings about the constrained nature of the relationship (Stone, 1984). Moreover, the techniques employed by psychiatrists have an inherently seductive quality (Halleck, 1984). Of course, the psychiatrist must maintain some level of rapport if he or she is to elicit meaningful information with which to support credible conclusions, but at the same time, he or she must not allow the evaluee to lose sight of the purpose of the evaluation or the limits on confidentiality.

The forensic psychiatrist in the evaluative role must also guard against countertransference. Because the forensic evaluation is typically requested to explore some psychological question pertaining to the subject's legal predicament, the subject may present quite differently from clients presenting for treatment. Depending on the circumstances of the referral, the subject may oversubscribe or undersubscribe to the symptoms of mental disorder. Some may tell outright lies, and a few may even be hostile. Others may be highly sympathetic, appearing as victims of unfortunate circumstance. The phenomenon of countertransference is natural in such cases.

Countertransference also may derive from the clinician's philosophical beliefs (for example, paternalistic versus libertarian) or particular social or political views. In certain kinds of cases—death penalty cases, child molestation cases—some psychiatrists are particularly susceptible to countertransference. If significant countertransference develops and the psychiatrist cannot function objectively, he or she is obliged to withdraw from the case (Schetky and Colbach, 1982).

Just as the forensic psychiatrist's role is highly circumscribed, so, too, is his or her contact with the individual whose mental condition is at issue. The psycholegal issue the psychiatrist is asked to address may be quite specific, encompassing only a narrow band of psychological functioning. Thus, the psychiatrist may ignore many areas that, in therapy, could be of critical significance. Of course, the forensic psychiatrist is not expected to abandon his or her therapeutic instincts altogether. If, for example, the subject of a forensic assessment is in acute distress, perhaps is suicidal, it is incumbent upon the psychiatrist to refer the individual for treatment. It may not be an adequate defense to a charge of malpractice—or a charge of unprofessional behavior—that 'as a forensic psychiatrist, it wasn't my job to intervene' (*Ahnert v. Wildman, 1978*). First and foremost, the psychiatrist is a healer. But, it must be emphasized, therapeutic intervention is not part of the psychiatrist's *forensic* role.

Because the role of the forensic psychiatrist is essentially nontherapeutic, it may be inappropriate for a psychiatrist already in a treatment relationship with an individual to take on the role of forensic evaluator (Miller, 1984). Particularly in criminal cases, where the evaluation findings may run counter to the subject's therapeutic interests, the roles of evaluator and therapist inexorably conflict.

TERMS OF INVOLVEMENT

The psychiatrist whose expertise is sought in a legal matter may be expected to serve any of several functions. The psychiatrist may be employed to serve one side or the other in the case (plaintiff or defense in a civil case; prosecution or defense in a criminal case) or may be appropriated as an *amicus* expert to serve as a *friend of the court* and offer neutral advice. The psychiatrist may serve exclusively as a consultant to one of the attorneys, offering guidance on the preparation and conduct of the case, or may develop expert opinion for presentation in court.

While, of course, maintaining clinical objectivity and adhering to professional standards, the psychiatrist may be expected to devote some degree of loyalty to the party offering the employment. Indeed, depending on the terms of involvement, the psychiatrist's legal status may be that of *agent* to the party. As an agent, the psychiatrist may be expected to maintain a trusting, fiduciary relationship with the party. In its opinion in *Ake v. Oklahoma (1985)*, the United States Supreme Court made it clear that such a relationship should characterize dealings between the defense and its expert in a criminal case (Fitch, 1985). Given such a relationship, the circumstances under which the psychiatrist's findings may be communicated to third parties may be quite narrow, perhaps only if the psychiatrist is called to testify. Thus, to properly discharge one's responsibility, it is imperative that the psychiatrist clarify the terms of involvement at the time of employment.

CONSTRAINTS ON THE USE OF PSYCHIATRIC OPINION

Ordinarily, the testimony of the witnesses in a legal proceeding must be limited to the recounting of the perceptions of the witness as they bear on some fact at issue in the case. Lay witnesses ordinarily are not permitted to offer opinion testimony. However, if a witness has "scientific, technical, or other specialized knowledge [which] will assist the trier of fact [the judge or jury] to understand the evidence or to determine a fact in issue . . ." (Rules of Evidence for the United States Courts and Magistrates Rule 702, p. 267), the witness may be qualified as an "expert" to offer an opinion. Witnesses may be qualified as experts on the basis of knowledge, skill, experience, training, or education (Federal Rules of Evidence, Rule 703). In some states, depending on the issue to be addressed, the law specifies particular educational credentials that must be held before the witness will be accepted as an expert. Also, in a growing number of states, the law requires specialized training and experience in the particular area of psycholegal expertise at issue (see, for example, Virginia Code Ann., 1950, Supp. 1987, Sec. 19.2–169.5).

In many states, not only must it be shown that the witness has specialized knowledge or skill that can assist the trier of fact, but it also must be shown that the particular scientific principles or hypotheses that support the expert's conclusions "have gained general acceptance in the particular field to which

[they] belong" (*Frye v. United States*, 1923, p. 1014). This test, the so-called *Frye* test, for years was the governing standard for determining the admissibility of expert opinion. The test is responsible for the exclusion of testimony concerning polygraph results (*Frye*), psychological voice-stress analysis to determine whether a person is lying (*Barrel of Fun, Inc. v. State Farm Insurance Company*, 1984), and a casual link between compulsive gambling disorder and specific criminal conduct (*United States v. Gould*, 1984).

In recent years, however, the *Frye* test has come under attack. Indeed, at least one Federal Circuit Court has rejected the *Frye* standard in favor of a *helpfulness* standard, under which two factors are balanced: ". . . (1) the reliability of the scientific principles upon which the expert testimony rests, hence the potential of the testimony to aid the jury in reaching an accurate resolution of a disputed issue; and (2) the likelihood that introduction of the testimony may in some way overwhelm or mislead the jury . . ." (*United States v. Downing*, 1985, p. 1237). In this opinion, the United States Court of Appeals for the Third Circuit overruled a trial court judge's exclusion of expert testimony concerning the reliability of eyewitness identification.

For psychiatrists, even under the relatively restrictive *Frye* test of admissibility, expert opinion concerning most clinical diagnoses—for example, those appearing in DSM-III-R—is routinely admitted (assuming, of course, that the opinion is *relevant* to some fact at issue in the case). Only when dealing with more novel diagnoses, such as rape trauma syndrome, or psychodynamic speculation should the expert anticipate serious challenge. And, even here, depending on the nature of the legal proceeding, many courts welcome the psychiatrist's input. Indeed, some courts are so happy to admit psychiatric testimony that the burden must fall on the profession of psychiatry to guard against an overextension of psychiatric expertise (Wasyliw et al, 1985; Aber and Reppucci, 1987; Bloom and Rogers, 1987). The further psychiatric experts stray from traditional psychiatric technique, the more the discipline is open to charges that it is *pseudo-science* (Morse, 1978).

As suggested above, it is often the expert's personal biases that most seriously threaten the objectivity and reliability of the expert's opinion:

> There is no objection to forensic experts making statements of informed and concerned opinion on important issues. It is rather the lack of differentiation between legitimate scientific deduction and personal value judgement, which constitutes a critical vulnerability of the scientist as an expert witness and which, in one manner or another, has added to much of current criticism (Wasyliw et al, 1985, p. 149).

Perhaps the most hotly debated question having to do with the overextension of psychiatric expertise in legal matters is whether psychiatrists should present opinion testimony on the *ultimate issue* before the court. Of course, in some cases, the ultimate issue is clearly within the scope of psychiatric expertise; for example, whether a psychiatrist charged with malpractice met professional standards of care. In many cases involving psychiatric testimony, however, the ultimate issue is only partly psychiatric. Whether, for example, a mother's parental rights should be terminated because she is unfit to function as a parent may have a clinical dimension, but, ultimately, the question is laden with moral, political, and philosophical values. Psychiatrists may comment quite credibly on the influence of the subject's mental and emotional condition on her ability to exercise good parental judgment, but whether the degree to which her ability is compromised is so great as to justify this intervention is clearly a social value judgment. To allow the expert to tell the jury that the science of psychiatry has the answer is not only to invade the province of the jury, but also to mislead the jury as to the legitimate boundaries of psychiatric expertise.

It is in the criminal area that the question of ultimate-issue testimony has received its greatest attention. While, no doubt, the majority of practicing forensic psychiatrists are accustomed to offering their conclusions regarding the criminal responsibility (that is, *sanity*) of defendants they have examined, such ultimate-issue opinion testimony has long been criticized (Roche, 1958; Halleck, 1971) and in recent years has become a subject of escalating debate (Morse, 1978; Bonnie and Slobogin, 1980; Morse, 1982). In the wake of John Hinckley's trial, in which prominent psychiatrists, while in agreement on many clinical questions, were squarely opposed on the question of Hinckley's criminal responsibility, both the American Bar Association (ABA), in its carefully considered *Criminal Justice/Mental Health Standards* (1984), and the American Psychiatric Association (APA), in its *Statement on the Insanity Defense* (1982), have recommended against psychiatric testimony on the ultimate issue in insanity cases:

> When . . . 'ultimate issue' questions are formulated by the law and put to the expert witness who must then say 'yea' or 'nay,' then the expert witness is required to make a leap in logic. He no longer addresses himself to medical concepts but instead must infer or intuit what is in fact unspeakable, namely, the *probable relationship* between medical concepts and legal or moral constructs such as free will (APA Statement, 1982, p. 19).

This bold position, embraced by the leading organizations of both the legal and psychiatric professions, has not gone unnoticed. Indeed, laws in many jurisdictions, including all federal courts, have been amended in accordance. The psychiatrist retains a significant role in insanity defense cases in these jurisdictions—to assess whether or not the accused suffered from a mental disorder at the time of the alleged crime and to describe the effects, if any, of the mental disorder on the defendant's thoughts and behavior at that time— but the expert is proscribed from going on to conclude whether the accused's mental impairment was so great as to negate responsibility.

In many states, the law continues to allow (in some states, require) psychiatrists to address the ultimate question of criminal responsibility. And many respected forensic specialists continue to argue in support of such ultimate-issue testimony (Ciccone and Clements, 1987), but clearly the tide has turned.

THE CLINICAL EVALUATION FOR COURT USE

In most cases, what the psychiatrist has to offer in a legal matter will be based on a forensic evaluation. The cornerstone of the forensic evaluation is the direct examination of the subject. The examination, however, must always be supplemented by an assessment of other available data.

In the forensic evaluation context, there are always competing agenda. As suggested above, the person undergoing the evaluation may have a strong motivation either to "look good" or to "look bad," depending on his or her perceptions of the way in which the results of the evaluation may influence legal outcome. Accordingly, the evaluation process must become both more investigative and more confrontive in nature than is customary in therapy. Ultimately because the psychiatrist may be called upon to explain why he or she chose to believe or disbelieve what the subject had to say, every effort must be made to marshall available data to determine whether the subject's story is fabricated, distorted (consciously or unconsciously), or honestly reported.

Psychiatric conclusions offered in the adversarial setting have long been criticized as impressionistic and capricious, and lacking clear connection between raw clinical data, psychiatric inference, and psycholegal opinion (Morse, 1978). In recent years, the field of forensic psychiatry has responded to this criticism by developing more rigorous evaluative paradigms, designed to help the examiner organize and objectify relevant data in a systematic fashion. At a general level, it now is customary to recognize that virtually every forensic evaluation entails three basic phases: 1) the *investigative phase*, in which potential sources of third-party information are contacted and background information is collected; 2) the *clinical examination phase*, in which the subject is interviewed, tested, and otherwise examined; and 3) the *clinical opinion formation phase*, in which the various data are reviewed and explained in terms that address the psycholegal question at issue.

Phase One: The Investigation

The investigatory phase of the evaluation ordinarily should begin prior to any direct clinical contact with the subject. Indeed, one of the primary purposes of this investigation is to establish meaningful parameters for the clinical examination.

As a first step, the psychiatrist must ascertain the specific psycholegal question(s) to be addressed. Simply reviewing the contents of a referral letter or court order will not suffice. Too often, such documents fail to identify the particular question of concern. Moreover, the question posed may contemplate a particular legal standard that requires definition. Accordingly, the psychiatrist always should begin by clarifying the referral question directly with the referral source. During this contact, the terms of the psychiatrist's involvement—as consultant or expert witness, serving on a partisan or *amicus* relationship—also must be resolved. Finally, the reasons the referral source believed an evaluation was indicated and the anticipated uses to which the expert's findings might be put should be discussed.

Next, the psychiatrist should begin to assemble a social history, typically including:

1. developmental information
2. history of medical or psychiatric illnesses
3. family history
4. education, employment, and military history
5. psychosexual history (including marital adjustment, if married)
6. information concerning social skills
7. information concerning previous maladaptive behavior

This social history, of course, will be most complete and credible if family members or significant others are interviewed in addition to the subject.

The investigative phase of the evaluation is completed with the review of any relevant ancillary information that may exist, derived from as many authoritative and credible sources as possible (medical records, court records, school records, military records, attorneys' notes, statements of witnesses, copies of prior accounts given by the subject, police reports, etc.). Any media accounts of the incident precipitating the referral should also be examined.

Some observers emphasize the importance of statistical information that may help generate insight into the behavior of a person with a particular set of characteristics (Saks and Kidd, 1980). Caution must be exercised, however, against yielding to the seductive power of such "hard," statistical data in the legal case. Indeed, the specifics of each individual case ultimately must outweigh group statistics, lest the individual be adjudicated on the basis of his or her psychological *profile* rather than the merits of the case (Loftus and Monahan, 1980; Anderten et al, 1980).

Phase Two: The Clinical Examination

It is during the examination phase that the forensic evaluation best approximates traditional psychiatric endeavor. Even here, however, differences exist. While the subject of any psychiatric interview ordinarily should be encouraged to be open and forthcoming, it must be emphasized, as discussed above, that the subject of a forensic assessment should never be allowed to assume that a prototypic doctor–patient relationship has been established. The psychiatrist bears an ethical burden to advise the subject of the purposes of the assessment and the limits on confidentiality (Ciccone and Clements, 1984). Such a warning may be legally required as well (Estelle v. Smith, 1981; Slobogin, 1982).

Interviews with the subject, in addition to addressing general clinical concerns, must directly and thoroughly explore all aspects of the referral question. For example, in criminal cases in which the subject's responsibility—legal insanity—is at issue, the evaluation must focus in depth on the defendant's thoughts and behaviors around the time of the offense. In cases raising the question of competency to confess, the evaluation must focus on the defendant's understanding of his or her rights at the time of the police interrogation and the defendant's susceptibility to the techniques used by the interrogators.

Depending on the results of the clinical interview, it may be necessary to arrange for specialized neurological or other medical examinations. Such procedures should not be regarded as routine but rather should be employed only to clarify diagnostic impressions that may have been ambiguous during the interview. If, for example, signs or symptoms of organic illness are observed during the interview, metabolic studies, endocrine profiles, EEG, CT scanning, or magnetic resonance imaging may be indicated (Tancredi and Volkow, 1988; Brown et al, 1987). Such hard data, of course, are rarely dispositive of the psycholegal issue in the case, but they may enable the psychiatrist to reach his or her conclusions with a greater degree of confidence.

Psychological testing also has its place in the forensic evaluation. Some forensic psychiatrists rely heavily on the results of psychological testing as *objective* data that enhances the credibility of psychiatric opinion. Others believe it is too vulnerable to attack by the savvy cross-examiner (Elwork, 1984; Ziskin, 1981).

Of course, some psychological tests are more useful than others. The Wechsler Adult Intelligence Scale–Revised or Wechsler Intelligence Scale for Children–Revised may provide valuable data concerning the individual's level of cognitive functioning and will help establish the parameters of intellectual capacity. The Minnesota Multiphasic Psychological Inventory (MMPI), in addition to helping the clinician systematically assess levels of symptomatology, can be powerfully useful in detecting whether the evaluee is oversubscribing or undersubscribing to the symptoms of psychopathology; elevated L scales and F-K scales on the MMPI have been shown to be reliable indicators of deception (Rogers, 1984). Finally, neuropsychological testing, including the Halstead-Reitan and Luria-Nebraska tests, may be indicated when the subject's symptoms suggest organic impairment.

Projective instruments, such as the Rorschach and the Thematic Apperception Test, may be less useful to the forensic psychiatrist, as attorneys are quick to attack the results of such tests, due to their apparent subjective quality. Accordingly, projective testing in the forensic evaluation should be limited to refining diagnoses made primarily on other bases.

Psychological tests administered as part of a retrospective evaluation—that is, one focusing on the subject's mental condition at some time in the past—are of particularly limited value. The longer the interval between the time in question and the time the test was administered, the less applicable the findings (Melton et al, 1987). Finally, it is important for the psychiatrist to recognize that, if psychological testing contributes to the psychiatrist's opinion in a case, it may be necessary to have the psychologist who conducted the testing appear in court to explain the test results. Clearly, the interpretation of psychological test data is beyond the special expertise of most psychiatrists.

The problem of amnesia is encountered with some frequency in the forensic evaluation process, particularly in criminal cases. The vast majority of valid amnesias seen in criminal defendants, of course, are psychogenic in nature, that is, they are induced by repression of egodystonic events. Thus, the defendant's memory may be subject to retrieval or enhancement. Because the defendant's recollection of his or her thinking and behavior at the time of the offense may be critical to any meaningful assessment of criminal responsibility, in some cases the psychiatrist may feel obliged to attempt such enhancement.

Hypnosis is a tool that sometimes is used to enhance memory. Not only has hypnosis been used to enhance the memory of criminal defendants, it has also been used with witnesses and victims and to aid recall by plaintiffs in accident cases (Greene, 1986). In 1985, however, the Council on Scientific Affairs of the American Medical Association (AMA) issued a report in which the use of hypnosis in the medicolegal context was uniformly discouraged. The substantial risk of obtaining confabulated data and *pseudomemories* (Dywan and Bowers, 1983; Orne, 1985) was offered as the primary basis for this position.

The courts have expressed significant ambivalence concerning the testimony of witnesses who have explored a matter in question while under hypnosis. Some courts flatly exclude such testimony. Others ban testimony concerning posthypnotic recollections but not recollections registered prior to hypnosis. Still others impose no special restrictions. In 1987, the United States Supreme Court ruled that to deny a *criminal defendant* the opportunity to present hypnotically refreshed testimony may violate the defendant's constitutional rights to be heard and offer testimony (Rock v. Arkansas, _____ U.S. _____ , 55 U.S.L.W. 4925, June 22, 1987). At least one Federal Circuit Court since has recognized the right of a criminal defendant to the assistance of a competent hypnotist where a witness for the prosecution testified about events recalled under hypnosis (Little v. Armontrout, _____ U.S. _____ , 56 U.S.L.W. 2382, January 19, 1988).

Another technique sometimes employed to enhance memory is narcoanalysis. The use of a short-acting barbiturate, such as sodium amytal or brevital, is considered by some clinicians to yield refreshed recollections less likely to be contaminated by confabulation or pseudomemory than those retrieved through hypnosis (Ruedrich et al, 1985). Moreover, narcoanalysis not only may help to refresh recollection, it may also stimulate significant emotional abreaction in the subject.

It has been suggested that the mechanism of response to an intravenously injected, short-acting barbiturate follows the principle of *in vino veritas* (Herman, 1985). Of course, unlike self-induced intoxication, the narcoanalytic process is environmentally controlled and designed to minimize distractions to truthful reporting. Nevertheless, as with hypnosis, most courts view information obtained through narcoanalytic technique with significant reservation (Kadish et al, 1986).

A relatively recent innovation in forensic psychiatry is the development of *forensic assessment instruments*. Forensic assessment instruments differ from traditional clinical constructs in that they center on an operational definition of the psycholegal condition in question, focusing quite narrowly on the particular functional abilities that pertain thereto. Ultimately, their purpose is to help the evaluator bridge the conceptual gap between behavioral science constructs and legal constructs. Because, as discussed above, in most cases psycholegal questions ultimately require some social value judgement (often entailing consideration of factors completely independent of the individual's mental or emotional condition), we believe forensic assessment instruments should never be relied on to produce a *score* of the individual's psycholegal *condition*. However, they can be extraordinarily useful in structuring the evaluation and focussing the evaluator's attention on factors that may have legal relevance.

The pioneering work in the development of forensic assessment instruments was done in the early 1970s by McGarry and Associates at the Laboratory of Community Psychiatry, Harvard Medical School (McGarry et al, 1973; Lipsitt, 1971). Two instruments designed to assess competency to stand trial were developed by this group, the Competency Fitness Test and the Competency Assessment Instrument. These instruments have been used extensively by psychiatrists throughout the country and have served as models for the development of more sophisticated forensic-assessment instruments dealing with a range of psycholegal issues, including legal insanity (Slobogin et al, 1984; Rogers, 1984), competency to consent to treatment (Roth et al, 1982), parental fitness (Shure and Spivack, 1978; Helfer et al, 1978), competency to waive rights (Grisso, 1981), competency to care for oneself (Anderten-Loeb, 1986), and, again, competency to stand trial (Golding et al, 1984). Synopses of two forensic assessment instruments are presented as appendices. These instruments and more are examined in some detail in an extraordinarily smart volume by Grisso (1986).

Phase Three: Clinical Opinion Formation and Reporting

In the opinion-formation phase of the forensic evaluation, the psychiatrist must organize and synthesize the various data generated in both the investigative and clinical examination phases and develop a clinical opinion addressing factors pertaining to the applicable legal standard. Care must be taken to identify a factual basis for all inferences drawn and opinions reached. "[An opinion] is only as good as the *investigation*, the *facts* and the *reasoning* that underlie it" (Bazelon, 1978, p. 143).

A psychiatric diagnosis by itself rarely is of much utility to a legal decision-maker. Relating psychiatric symptoms to functional and behavioral impairments that have significance for the applicable legal standard becomes the crux of effective clinical opinion formation and subsequent expert testimony. In performing this task, the psychiatrist must remain mindful of the fact that the consumer of the product—an attorney, the judge, or the jury—will require an explanation employing lay terminology and sensible reasoning. Unless the psychiatrist's conclusions lend themselves to such explanation, they are likely to be of limited value.

Immediately upon completion of the evaluation, the psychiatrist ordinarily should reduce his or her findings and conclusions to writing. Not only will prompt reporting yield the most accurate record of the examiner's conclusions, but a properly prepared report can go far toward obviating the need for courtroom testimony (for example, by providing a basis for effective pretrial negotiation of the case). While the psychiatrist must, of course, rely on the referring attorney to identify particular issues to be addressed in the report, the psychiatrist should never permit the attorney to dictate the report or materially alter the psychiatrist's conclusions. Such behavior on the attorney's part constitutes unprofessional conduct for which the attorney may be subject to disciplinary sanction (Fitch et al, 1987).

THE PSYCHIATRIST AS EXPERT WITNESS

While, of course, some forensic evaluations inevitably result in courtroom testimony (for example, those to assess civil committability), most probably do not. In studies conducted in Virginia, mental health professionals responsible for providing evaluation services in criminal cases reported testifying in approximately 10 percent of cases evaluated (Institute of Law, Psychiatry and Public Policy, unpublished, 1986, 1987). The vast majority of criminal cases are resolved by a guilty plea, usually obviating the need for expert testimony. Similarly, many civil cases—particularly those in which money damages are sought for another's negligence (*tort* cases)—are settled out of court.

Of course, any psychiatrist whose practice includes a forensic component will find himself or herself in court on occasion. For the psychiatrist who is unaccustomed to the nature of the legal process, the experience can be highly traumatic. In the legal arena, controversies are resolved by an adversarial process. The parties to the controversy, in an effort to persuade the judge or jury, present evidence favoring their positions and attempt to discredit evidence that is unfavorable. Evidence that is deemed untrustworthy, for example because it was reported second-hand (*hearsay*), is excluded from consideration. Similarly, evidence that does not bear directly on the question before the court (*irrelevant* evidence) is excluded. The theory of the adversary system is that, if all of the competent, relevant evidence that can be marshalled by those interested in the case is presented and both sides are given a meaningful opportunity to demonstrate for the trier of fact the strengths and weaknesses of this evidence, then justice will be done and the truth will best be approximated.

For the psychiatrist who, as a scientist, is accustomed to ascertaining truth in a collaborative, inquisitorial manner (Gutheil and Applebaum, 1982), the adversarial process may seem arcane, unsophisticated, and unfriendly. In an effort to discredit unfavorable testimony, trial attorneys may attempt to distort, malign, or otherwise attack conclusions offered by the psychiatrist in the best of faith. While many psychiatrists resent such treatment and believe it distracts the fact-finder from the truth, such an attitude may be short-sighted.

It is important for psychiatrists to recognize that psychiatric opinion, even when based on accepted professional practice, does not necessarily represent truth (Wallace, 1988). Indeed, the manner in which psychiatrists reach opinions is, in a sense, adversarial:

> The psychiatrist functions as a scientist, and, as a scientist, the psychiatrists's method involves the establishment and 'proof' of hypotheses. Claim and counterclaim and argument and counterargument are developed as each hypothesis is tested. Ultimately, one hypothesis is accepted, but rarely will the thoughtful psychiatrist regard this hypothesis as a statement of factual 'truth' (Showalter and Fitch, 1987, p. 184–185).

The fallibility of psychiatric opinion has been acknowledged by the profession (Zusman and Simon, 1983). Explanations that have been suggested for the unreliability of psychiatric opinion include criterion variance (that different psychiatrists may recognize different criteria in clinical decision-making), evaluator variance (that different psychiatrists may have different professional orientations they bring to bear on a case or may have personal biases that affect their objectivity), subject variance (that the mental condition of the subject may vary over time so that the subject presents differently to two different psychiatrists conducting evaluations at two different points in time), and information variance (that different evaluators may have access to different sets of background information in the case) (Morse, 1978).

Given that psychiatric opinion can never be relied on for absolute accuracy, it should not be surprising that the law insists it be subject to adversarial scrutiny in court. In *Ake v. Oklahoma* (1985, p. 1096), the United States Supreme Court explicitly affirmed the right of criminal defendants to partisan psychiatric assistance: "[W]ithout the assistance of a psychiatrist to conduct a professional examination on issues relevant to the defense, to present testimony, and to assist in preparing the cross-examination of a State's psychiatric witness, the risk of an inaccurate resolution of sanity issues is extremely high." One year later, in *Ford v. Wainwright* (1986, p. 2604), the Supreme Court declared: "Cross-examination of the psychiatrists . . . would contribute markedly to the process of seeking truth in sanity disputes by bringing to light the bases for each expert's beliefs, the precise factors underlying those beliefs, any history of error or caprice of the examiner, any personal bias with respect to the issue . . . , the expert's degree of certainly about his conclusion, and the precise meaning of ambiguous words used in the report."

The expectation that psychiatric expertise will be shared within the context of an adversarial proceeding has significance for the role the expert should play. Indeed, as suggested earlier, it is clear, given the *Ake* decision, that the expert assigned for the defense in a criminal case must serve as an agent for the defense. Accordingly, the expert should not regard himself or herself as a neutral examiner with allegiance only to the court. It must be understood, however, that, while the expert may owe allegiance to one party or the other, this should in no way affect the objectivity of the psychiatrist's opinion (Appelbaum, 1987; Showalter and Fitch, 1987). It simply means that the psychiatrist's objective expertise is to be made available exclusively for the use of the party to whom the psychiatrist is assigned.

Some observers question whether psychiatrists reasonably can be expected to remain objective under these partisan circumstances (Gorman, 1983; Diamond, 1973). Inevitably, they argue, the psychiatrist, out of a psychological need to triumph, will become caught up in the advocacy of the case. Others believe objectivity can be assured by adhering to one of several professional standards: the *good clinical practice standard*, which suggests psychiatrists simply remain true to the traditional evaluative and diagnostic techniques used in other areas of practice; the *standard of science*, which suggests psychiatrists avoid value-laden judgements in forensic work, relying instead on provable, *scientific facts* as the basis for clinical decision-making; or the *standard of truth*, which allows for consideration of subjective as well as objective insights and emphasizes thoroughness and an acknowledgement of the strengths and weaknesses of the various interpretations the data suggest (Stone, 1984; Watson, 1984; Applebaum, 1984).

The standard of truth, if adhered to rigorously, is particularly well suited to the adversarial process. Because the psychiatrist's opinion is always subject to challenge in an adversarial setting, the psychiatrist must be prepared to present and explain not only his or her findings and conclusions, but also the scientific paradigm used in data analysis and opinion-formation process. Under these circumstances, the psychiatric expert arguably will provide maximum benefit to the process of legal decision-making, because he or she may function openly as an *educator* with respect to the meaning and application of psychiatric technique. The conceptualization of the expert as an educator casts the expert's role in a light that should allow the expert to function not only most effectively but also most comfortably (Showalter and Fitch, 1987).

FORENSIC PSYCHIATRY IS PSYCHIATRY AFTER ALL

The psychiatrist in court is first a psychiatrist and will function in a manner consistent with his or her training and clinical experience. Although psychiatry emphasizes a scientific approach to diagnostic and treatment decision-making, in which the practitioner draws on an established behavioral science database, each clinical decision must be made by considering the relevant facts in the specific case. This process of bridging the gap between the features of the specific case and a more general scientific database is the crux of the psychiatrist's decision-making skill. The same phenomenon occurs in forensic psychiatric decision-making except that, because the ultimate psycholegal question may not be one that is exclusively clinical (that is, it may require some degree of social value judgement), the psychiatrist's opinion may by necessity be less conclusive. The effective psychiatric expert will learn to become comfortable with this limitation on his or her role. This interplay with and dependence on lawyers and the law should not provoke an identity crisis for the psychiatrist in court.

The training and experience that shape the specialty of forensic psychiatry focus on principles of legal philosophy, purpose, and procedure. These insights are not intended to change the intrinsic nature of the psychiatrist's clinical function. Rather they are meant to provide a grounding in the methodology of a different discipline—the law—which, in spite of its many signals of ambivalency, relies heavily on traditional psychiatric expertise to enhance the quality of its decision-making. Thus, any well-trained psychiatrist, sensitive to the tasks and methods of the law, can enter the courtroom as an expert, assured that his or her clinical observations will be of value. Moreover, it is likely that the closer the expert adheres to basic psychiatric theory and technique, the more credible (and, hence, more useful) his or her input will be. Forensic psychiatry is psychiatry after all.

APPENDIX I

Synopsis of Community Competency Scale (Anderten-Loeb, 1986)

The Community Competence Scale was developed to assist in the assessment of the ability of the elderly to care for themselves and/or their property. It consists of 16 subscales, including a total of 124 items. The subscales and selected items from 7 of these subscales are as follows:

1. *Emergencies*—If you heard a loud scream name two things that you would expect it to be.
2. *Compensate for incapacities*—If you had a difficult time remembering appointments, what would you do and why?
3. *Manage Money*—Do you use checks or money order? Please fill out this check (money order) for fifteen dollars payable to the telephone company.
4. *Communication*—Show me how you call the police. (Use nearby telephone receiver left on hook.)
5. *Adequate memory*—Suppose you had to take medication three times a day. How would you remember to take your medication and how much to take?
6. *Mobility*—Go through the motions of putting on a pair of slacks, a shirt and a pair of shoes.
7. *Judgment*—Suppose you lived in a rented apartment and it's summertime. Your refrigerator-freezer doesn't work; it doesn't keep things cold. You have talked to your landlord about it a number of times, but nothing has happened. What would you do, and why?

8. Care of Medical Needs	13. Maintain Household
9. Satisfactory Living Arrangement	14. Utilize Transportation
10. Proper Diet	15. Acquire Money
11. Sensation	16. Verbal-Math Skills
12. Personal Hygiene	

The number of items within each subscale varies and ranges from 4 for sensation to 20 for communication. Items which require the subject to perform a task or provide factual information (75 items) are scored as 0 or 1 point. Items in which the subject must provide a response requiring judgment or reasoning (49 items) are scored as 0, 1 or 2 points depending on the quality of the reasoning demonstrated.

Apparatus such as a telephone book, blank checks and money orders, an envelope and play money are required for some test items. All of the items are read aloud by the examiner who also records the subject's response. Administration of this form of the CCS requires approximately one hour. Guidelines for scoring have been developed.

APPENDIX II

The Mental State at the Time of Offense Screening Examination (Slobogin, Melton, Showalter, 1984)

In this screening examination, questions should be phrased to elicit data that will facilitate tentative conclusions on (1) the five historical categories outlined in Part I, (2) the degree of mental impairment at the time of the offense as outlined in Part II, and (3) assessment of current (present) mental status (Part III).

I. Historical information (from interview with defendant and available records)
  A. Does the defendant have a history of prolonged bizarre behavior [i.e., association with delusions, hallucinations, looseness of association of ideas (thought processes incoherent and illogical), or disturbance of affect (behavior disorganized, aggressive, intensely negativistic or withdrawn)]? If not, exclude:
    1. Organic brain syndromes of a progressive or chronic nature
      a. Dementia
      b. Organic personality syndrome
    2. Psychoses
      a. Schizophrenias
      b. Paranoid disorders
      c. Schizophreniform disorders
      d. Affective disorders
  B. Does the defendant have a history of convulsive disorder (e.g., "fits" or "seizures")? If not, exclude most forms of epilepsy.
  C. Has the defendant ever experienced a brief period of *uncharacteristic* bizarre behavior (i.e., association with delusions, hallucinations, sudden alterations in consciousness or motor functioning, sudden aggressive

affectual discharge), not associated with psychoactive substance use? If not, exclude:

1. Brief reactive psychosis
2. Intermittent or isolated explosive disorder
3. Automatism
   a. Postconcussion syndrome
   b. Temporal lobe (psychomotor) epilepsy
   c. Cerebral anoxia
4. Dissociative disorders
   a. Psychogenic fugue
   b. Sleepwalking
   c. Post-traumatic stress disorder

D. Does the defendant have a history of *episodic*, uncharacteristic bizarre behavior [i.e., association with delusions, hallucinations, looseness of association of ideas (thought processes incoherent and illogical), or disturbance of affect (behavior disorganized, aggressive, intensely negativistic or withdrawn)], associated with psychoactive substance use? If not, exclude:

1. Withdrawal syndrome
2. Delirium or delusional disorder
3. Hallucinosis

E. Does the defendant exhibit signs of moderate or severe mental retardation? If not, exclude mental retardation.

If all of the above disorders are excluded, there is probably no evidence of "significant mental abnormality" approaching legal relevance, but further, more detailed evaluation regarding the degree of functional impairment at the time of the offense should always be performed. If one or more of the above disorders does or did exist, it is still necessary to determine whether it played a role in *significantly* impairing cognitive or volitional functioning at the time of the offense (i.e., insanity, diminished capacity, or automatism defense).

II. Offense information
   A. From the defendant
      1. Defendant's present "general" response to offense
         a. Cognitive perception of offense
         b. Emotional response
      2. Detailed account of offense
         a. Evidence of intrapsychic stressors
            1. delusions
            2. hallucinations
         b. Evidence of external stressors
            1. provoking events
            2. fear of panic stimulants
         c. Evidence of altered state of consciousness
            1. alcohol-induced
            2. drug-induced
         d. Claimed amnesia
            1. partial
            2. complete

3. Events leading up to offense
    a. Evidence of major changes in environment
        1. change in job status
        2. change in family status
    b. Relationship with victim
    c. Preparation for offense
4. Post-offense response
    a. Behavior following act
    b. Emotional response to act
    c. Attempts to explain or justify act
B. From extrinsic sources
    1. Indictment, information, or complaint
    2. Confessions, preliminary hearing transcripts, statements to the police
    3. Witness accounts
    4. Attorney's notes
    5. Autopsy reports (if relevant)

The above information will probably be sufficient to ascertain the existence of significant mental abnormality at the time of the offense; however, assessment of present mental status may provide a more complete picture of the defendant's general level of psychological functioning.

III. Present Mental Status Examination
    (Here an outline of a typical mental status examination is followed.)

REFERENCES

Aber MS, Reppucci ND: The limits of mental health expertise in juvenile and family law. Int J Law Psychiatry 1987; 10:167–184

Ahnert v. Wildman, 376 N.E. 2d 1182, Ind. App, 1978

Ake v. Oklahoma, 105 S. Ct. 1087, 1985

American Bar Association: Criminal Justice/Mental Health Standards. Washington, DC, American Bar Association, 1984

American Medical Association, Council on Scientific Affairs: Scientific status of refreshing recollection and the use of hypnosis. JAMA 1985; 253:1918–1923

American Psychiatric Association: Statement on the insanity defense, in Issues in Forensic Psychiatry. Washington, DC, American Psychiatric Press, 1984

Anderten P, Staulcup V, Grisso T: On being ethical in legal places. Professional Psychology 1980; 11:764–773

Anderten-Loeb P: Community competency scale, in Evaluating Competencies: Forensic Assessments and Instruments. Edited by Grisso T. New York, Plenum Press, 1986

Appelbaum PS: Psychiatry ethics in the courtroom. Bull Am Acad Psychiatry Law 1984; 12:225–231

Appelbaum PS: Competency to be executed: another conundrum for mental health professionals. Hosp Community Psychiatry 1986; 37:682–683

Appelbaum PS: In the wake of Ake: the ethics of expert testimony in an advocate's world. Bull Am Acad Psychiatry Law 1987; 15:15–25

Barrel of Fun, Inc. v. State Farm Insurance Co., 739 F.2d 1028, 5th Cir., 1984

Bazelon DL: The role of the psychiatrist in the criminal justice system. Bull Am Acad Psychiatry Law 1978; 6:139–148

Bloom D, Rogers JL: The legal basis of forensic psychiatry: statutorily mandated psychiatric diagnosis. Am J Psychiatry 1987; 144:847–853

Bonnie R, Slobogin C: The role of mental health professionals in the criminal process: the case for informed speculation. Virginia Law Review 1980; 66:427–522

Brown RS Jr, Fischman A, Showalter CR: Primary hyperparathyroidism, hypercalcemia, parnoid delusions, homicide and attempted murder. J Forensic Sci 1987; 32:1460–1463

Ciccone JR, Clements C: Forensic psychiatry and applied clinical ethics: theory and practice. Am J Psychiatry 1984; 141:395–399

Ciccone JR, Clements C: The insanity defense: asking and answering the ultimate question. Bull Am Acad Psychiatry Law 1987; 15:329–338

Council on Scientific Affairs, American Medical Association: Scientific status of refreshing recollection and the use of hypnosis. JAMA 1985; 253: 1918–1923

Curran WJ, McGarry AL: The psychiatrist as expert witness, in Forensic Psychiatry and Psychology. Edited by Curran WJ, McGarry AL, Shah AS. Philadelphia, F.A. Davis Co., 1986

Diamond BL: The psychiatrist as advocate. Journal of Psychiatry and Law 1973; 1:5–21

Dietz PE: The forensic psychiatrist of the future. Bull Am Acad Psychiatry Law 1987; 15:217–227

Dywan J, Bowers KS: The use of hypnosis to enhance recall. Science 1983; 222:184–185

Elwork A: Psychological assessments, diagnosis, and testimony: a new beginning. Law and Human Behavior 1984; 8:197–263

Estelle v. Smith, 101 S. Ct. 1866 (1981)

Fitch WL: Ake v. Okkahoma: new directions for forensic evaluation. Developments in Mental Health Law 1985; 5:1–23

Fitch WL, Petrella RC, Wallace J: Legal ethics and the use of mental health professionals in criminal cases. Behavioral Sciences and the Law 1987; 5:105–117

Ford v. Wainwright, 106 S. Ct. 2595, 1986

Frye v. United States, 293 F. 1013, 1014, D.C. Cir., 1923

Golding S, Roesch R, Schreiber J: Assessment and conceptualization of competency to stand trial: preliminary data on the inter-disciplinary fitness interview. Law and Human Behavior 1984; 8:321

Gorman WF: Are there impartial psychiatric witnesses? Bull Am Acad Psychiatry Law 1983; 11:379

Greene E: Forensic hypnosis to lift amnesia: the jury is still out. Behavioral Sciences and the Law 1986; 4:65–72

Grisso T: Juveniles' Waiver of Rights: Legal and Psychological Competence. New York, Plenum Press, 1981

Grisso T: Evaluating Competencies: Forensic Assessments and Instruments. New York, Plenum Press, 1986

Gutheil TG, Appelbaum RS: Clinical Handbook of Psychiatry and the Law. New York, McGraw-Hill, 1982

Halleck SL: Psychiatry and the Dilemmas of Crime. Berkeley, CA, University of California Press, 1971

Halleck SL: The ethical dilemmas of forensic psychiatry: a utilitarian approach. Bull Am Acad Psychiatry Law 1984; 12:279–288

Helfer R, Hoffmeister J, Schneider C: A manual for use of the Michigan screening profile of parenting. Boulder CO, Test Analysis and Development Corporation, 1978

Herman M: Amytal and the detection of deception, in Critical Issues in American Psychiatry and the Law, Vol. II Edited by Rosner R. New York, Plenum Press, 1985

Kadish MJ, Brofman RA, Peskin S, et al: The polygraph, hypnosis, truth drugs, and the psychological stress evaluator: admissibility in a criminal trial. American Journal of Trial Advocacy 1986; 4:593

Kaplan LV, Miller RD: Courtroom psychiatrists: expertise at the cost of wisdom? Int J Law Psychiatry 1986; 9:451–468

Lipsitt P, Lelos D, McGarry AL: Competency to stand trial: a screening instrument. Am J Psychiatry 1971; 128:105

Little v. Armontrout, _____U.S. _____, 56 U.S.L.W. 2382, January 19, 1988

Loftus E, Monahan J: Trial by data: psychological research as legal evidence. Am Psychol 1980; 35:270

McGarry AL, Curran WJ, Lipsitt PD, et al: Competency to Stand Trial and Mental Illness. Department of Health, Education and Welfare, DHEW Publication No. (ADM) 77–103, Washington, D.C., 1973

Melton GB, Petrila J, Poythress NG, et al: Psychological Evaluations for the Courts. New York, Guilford Press, 1987

Miller RD: The treating psychiatrist as forensic evaluator. J Forensic Sci 1984; 29:825–830

Monahan J: Who Is the Client? Washington, DC, American Psychological Association, 1980

Morse SJ: Crazy behavior, morals, and science: an analysis of mental health law. S Cal L Rev 1978; 51:527–654

Morse SJ: Failed explanations and criminal responsibility: experts and the unconscious. Virginia Law Review 1980; 68:971–1084

Orne MT: The use and misuse of hypnosis in court, in Critical Issues in American Psychiatry and the Law, Vol. II. Edited by Rosner R. New York, Plenum Press, 1985

Rappeport J: Differences between forensic and general psychiatry. Am J Psychiatry 1982; 1139:331–334

Roche P: The Criminal Mind. New York, Farrar, Straus & Cudahy, 1958

Rock v. Arkansas, _____U.S. _____, 55 U.S.L.W. 4925, June 22, 1987

Rogers R: Towards an empirical model of malingering and deception. Behavioral Sciences and the Law 1984; 2:93–111

Rogers R: Rogers Criminal Responsibility Assessment Scales. Odessa, Fl., Psychological Assessment Resources, 1984

Rosner R: Accreditation of fellowship programs in forensic psychiatry: the development of the final report on standards. Bull Am Acad Psychiatry Law 1982; 10:281–287

Roth L, Lidz C, Meisel A, et al: Competency to decide about treatment or research: an overview of some empirical data. Int J Law Psychiatry 1982; 5:29–50

Ruedrich SL, Chu CC, Wadle CU: The amytal interview in the treatment of psychogenic amnesia. Hosp Community Psychiatry 1985; 36:1045–1046

Saks MJ, Kidd RF: Human information processing and adjudication: trial by heuristics. Law and Society Review 1980; 15:123–160

Schetky DH, Colbach EM: Countertransference on the witness stand: a flight from self? Bull Am Acad Psychiatry Law 1982; 10:115–121

Showalter CR, Bonnie RJ: Psychiatry and capital sentencing: risks and responsibilities in a unique legal setting. Bull Am Acad Psychiatry Law 1984; 12:159–167

Showalter CR, Fitch WL: Objectivity and advocacy in forensic psychiatry after Ake v. Oklahoma. J Psychiatry Law 1987; (Summer):177–188

Shure M, Spivack G: Problem Solving Techniques in Child Rearing. San Francisco, CA, Jossey-Bass, 1978

Slobogin C: Estelle v. Smith: the constitutional contours of the forensic evaluation. Emory Law Journal 1982; 31:71–138

Slobogin C, Melton G, Showalter C: The feasibility of a brief evaluation of mental state at the time of the offense. Law and Human Beahvior 1984; 8:305–320

Stone AA: The ethical limits of forensic psychiatry: a view from the ivory tower. Bull Am Acad Psychiatry Law 1984; 12:209–219

Talbott JA: Response to the presidential address: psychiatry's unfinished business in the 20th century. Am J Psychiatry 1984; 141:927–930

Tancredi LR, Volkow N: Neural substrates of violent behavior: implications for law and public policy. Int J Law Psychiatry 1988; 11:13–49

United States v. Downing, 753 F.2d 1224, 3d Cir., 1985

United States v. Gould, 741 F.2d 45, 4th Cir., 1984

Wallace ER IV: What is truth? Some philosophical contributions to psychiatric issues. Am J Psychiatry 1988; 145:137–147

Virginia Code Ann., 1950, Supp. 1987, Section 19.2–169.5

Wasyliw OE, Cavanaugh JL, Rogers R: Beyond the scientific limits of expert testimony. Bull Am Acad Psychiatry Law 1985; 13:147–158

Watson AS: Response from a straw man. Bull Am Acad Psychiatry Law 1984; 12:221–224

Ziskin J: Coping with Psychiatric and Psychological Testimony, third edition. Venice, CA, Law and Psychology Press, 1981

Zusman, Simon J: Differences in repeated psychiatric examinations of litigants to a lawsuit. Am J Psychiatry 1983; 140:1330–1304

Afterword

by Paul S. Appelbaum, M.D.

To the clinician it must sometimes seem as though there are as many legal rules governing psychiatric care as there are diagnoses in *DSM-III-R*—and that the diagnostic categories, whatever their failings, are easier to apply than the ever-changing jumble of statutes, regulations, and case law with which we are all confronted. I trust that having completed this condensed survey of recent developments in law and psychiatry, the reader feels somewhat more in charge of this body of material. For it is unquestionable that, just as the driver needs to know the laws governing the operation of motor vehicles, the psychiatrist cannot remain ignorant of the legal rules that regulate his or her practice.

Given the degree of regulation that we experience, there is a tendency, to which we all succumb at times, to believe both that psychiatry is particularly disfavored by the legal system and that each new layer of regulation threatens to overwhelm our precarious systems of psychiatric care. In fact, though they are natural-enough conclusions, each is the result of somewhat egocentric misperception.

The laws governing psychiatric practice, both clinical and forensic, have multiplied enormously since mid-century. But psychiatry is not alone in this experience. The demands of all of us for greater fairness and greater protection from those stronger than we—in a word, for justice—are behind this huge growth of legal regulation. (A slim volume by the distinguished legal historian Lawrence Friedman [1985] entitled *Total Justice*, is well worth perusing for some perspective on this phenomenon.) Whenever we join in expressing the belief that "there ought to be a law . . .," we too contribute to its proliferation. Of course, this is not necessarily bad. Our society is in many ways fairer, especially for the disadvantaged, than it was 30 years ago.

There are negative aspects to increased legal regulation, however, and even when we resist the temptation to feel especially beleaguered by the legal system, it is sometimes difficult to keep the positive and negative consequences of any new law or rule in perspective. Major new legal developments in psychiatry often lead to outcries of anguish and prophecies of the destruction of psychiatry or psychiatric care. It seems difficult to resist this role of Cassandra. I have fallen victim to it, as have most other psychiatrists I know.

In the wake of the abandonment of need for treatment statutes for civil commitment in the early 1970s and their replacement by dangerousness-based laws, many psychiatrists announced that it would no longer be possible to care adequately for the severely mentally ill. When the duty to protect potential victims of patients' violent acts was first promulgated in California in the mid-1970s, the doom of psychotherapy was pronounced. As courts began to adopt the right to refuse treatment with antipsychotic medications in the late 1970s and early 1980s, it was predicted that institutional psychiatry, particularly in the public sector, would be destroyed. When Congress passed an act prohibiting psychiatrists from testifying to the ultimate legal issue in insanity defense proceedings in federal courts, many forensic psychiatrists bemoaned the end of their abilities to provide useful information in criminal trials.

Actually, none of these new legal rules was followed by the disaster that had been predicted. This is not to deny that some of them had significant negative consequences. But despite restrictive commitment laws, studies suggest that the vast majority of patients who need hospitalization are admitted; in the face of greater pressure to protect potential victims, patients still seek psychotherapy; even with the right to refuse treatment, most patients who really need medication get it; and regardless of restrictions on psychiatric testimony, the assistance of psychiatrists in criminal cases is more highly valued than ever.

How can we account for the inaccuracy of predictions of doom in the face of enormous, often negative, legal pressures? Several factors are involved here. First, when we cry wolf at the sight of new legal regulations, we frequently underestimate the resiliency of psychiatry and of the systems of psychiatric care. Creative approaches often develop, enabling us to find ways to address the legal mandates within the context of delivering good clinical care. The duty to protect is a case in point here, as psychiatrists rapidly accepted their legal responsibilities and found ways of minimizing the negative impacts on patient care.

A corollary is that we often misjudge the flexibility of the law. In studies of dangerousness-based commitment statutes, it has been difficult to identify substantial numbers of persons who appeared to be seriously in need of hospitalization, but who were released to the streets because of restrictive statutes. Although no one doubts that such cases occur on occasion, their infrequency is probably due to the leeway that even narrow dangerousness-based statutes afford in defining dangerous behavior, particularly in the category of inability to meet basic needs.

In addition, our doomsaying often focuses on the most extreme legal statements of a new rule, as if that position will become the norm. Rarely is this the case. Legal regulations that lead to widespread dysfunction of the regulated system have a relatively short half-life. They tend to be replaced, within a few years, by more reasonable statements of the legal rule. That process appears to be going on now with both civil commitment—as less restrictive statutes are introduced—and the duty to protect—as good statutes and court decisions are, in general, driving out the bad.

Finally, there is a tendency for people to act rationally even in the face of irrational laws. Regardless of rules limiting psychiatric testimony, most judges admit the evidence that is likely to help them or the jury make a decision. While judicial willingness to commit severely ill patients who do not meet strict dangerousness criteria has been decried by civil libertarians for many years, it too represents a reasonable response to unreasonable legislation. Most people involved with the mental-health system display remarkably good common sense, which has a decided homeostatic influence on the system as a whole.

This is not to say that bad court decisions should be embraced or irrational statutes welcomed. Clearly there is value in fighting for the best law we can get when it comes to regulating psychiatric practice. But neither is undue pessimism warranted. Rather, the challenge is to find ways to make the laws with which we live compatible with our aspirations for excellent psychiatric practice.

REFERENCE

Friedman L: Total Justice. New York, Russell Sage Foundation, 1985

V

Difficult Situations in Clinical Practice

Contents

Section V

Difficult Situations in Clinical Practice

Foreword

by William H. Sledge, M.D., Section Editor

NATURE OF PRACTICE

Psychiatric practice has evolved and developed as the underlying knowledge base has expanded. Modern psychiatric practice is complex, drawing on different intellectual paradigms to give conceptual meaning to the disorders faced and the solutions employed. There is no single paradigm that can claim complete truth or therapeutic efficacy. To remain current and up-to-date is a challenge to the busy practitioner.

The work of psychiatric practice is generally very rewarding for the intrinsic qualities of close contact with individuals and the variety of clinical phenomena that provide diversity and interest. However, this diversity can also be a source of strain. And just as psychiatric practice can be so satisfying because of the proximity to the subjectivity of others, so it can also be extremely difficult. In no other branch of medical care is the practitioner so exposed to the strain of emotionally wrought people, frequently in difficult situations and sometimes with chronic, severe illnesses that not only may be tragically limiting but also be dangerous to the patient and to others.

Another source of potential strain for psychiatric practitioners is the fact that the practitioner's work life is full of intense, affective states. In order to remain sensitive and responsive to the emotional lives of patients, the clinician uses his own subjectivity as an access to and measure of the patient's experience. The clinician may find himself responding to a wide range of affective states and intensities. Such a use of the self requires discipline and forebearance in order to avoid the imposition of the inevitable biases that characterize all people, including those who work as psychiatric clinicians, onto the patient. These biases have broad cultural features as well as idiosyncratic personal elements. For instance, changing roles and expectations based on gender require the practitioner to constantly be aware of his or her own gender-linked stereotypes so as not to confuse his or her reality with that of the patient.

DIFFICULT PATIENTS IN DIFFICULT SITUATIONS

The mental health practitioner frequently feels placed between Scylla and Charybdis in a sea of seemingly contradictory choices. On the one hand, the practitioner is enjoined to be sensitive and responsive to the experience of troubled and suffering people who seek help; on the other hand, such sensitivity can be the source of considerable difficulty for the practitioner. Many of our patients live at the extremes of human existence. Sometimes they are physicially dangerous and direct violence toward themselves or others. More insidious (but no less demanding) is that some patients may persistently demand and require all (and then some) of the clinician's energy, attention, skill, knowledge, patience, and generosity. People who are in trouble either acutely or chronically may make particular demands on those around them, especially those who are trying to help them. This is true for life in general, but it is particularly true if people have some condition that either affects their characteristic ways of experiencing and behaving, or if their characteristic ways of behaving are problems in themselves. Many people who consult psychiatrists have problems with their life situations as well as problems with their mental life. These difficult life problems can be felt as a strain for the psychiatrist.

ACTUAL/FANTASIED THREATS

Patients may pose a physical threat to the practitioner. Patients with psychotic conditions and those with certain character disorders may become unpredictably violent. These patients tend to be seen more often in the public sector; however, they populate the private practice of psychiatry as well. Although psychiatrists are less likely to be sued than are other medical specialists, there is, nevertheless, the additional threat of tort action in the ebb and flow of clinical work.

Much more common, however, are patients who present a psychological threat to the clinician's professional self-esteem because they fail to improve. Practitioners may base their sense of effectiveness on the outcome of their therapeutic work. In psychiatric practice this may be problematic. Some patients have conditions that cannot be expected to improve very much—keeping them at status quo or reducing the rate of decline in such situations should be considered a success. Other patients have an unconscious need to fail; and therefore, the success of treatment is in itself a source of considerable threat to them. Still other patients sense the psychiatrist's wish for them to get better and are fearful of this kind of involvement and the implications it has for their sense of self, so they unwittingly fail the treatment as well. These sources of failed treatments can become confounded with other causes of failed treatments such as technical errors based on faulty skills and knowledge, and on negative countertransference reactions. These potential sources of failure produce a veritable professional minefield for the unwitting practitioner who bases his or her professional self-esteem too exclusively on the explicit manifestations of success from patients.

THE STRAIN OF DEALING WITH ENTITLED PEOPLE

Dealing with people who are generally convinced that life (and, in particular, the clinician) owes them something can be very wearisome work—particularly if on some level (usually unconscious) the clinician believes it is appropriate (and necessary for a feeling of competence and self-worth) to satisfy this special need. Entitled people can be even more difficult when they have the resources in the form of prestige, power, and/or wealth to transcend the usual bonds of social reality, or when they have the bitterness and tenacity to use legal action in the face of real or imagined failings on the part of the clinician. Treating the

VIP patient, for example, requires particular skill and clarity on the clinician's part concerning his or her own motivations and needs.

THE STRAIN OF DEALING WITH TRANSFERENCE

Another source of strain for the clinician is the burden of being the object of transference projections for so many different people for so much of the time. In exploratory forms of psychotherapy where the aim is an attempt to make explicit and understandable unconscious mental processes, the projection of transference paradigms onto the therapist is highly desirable and comprises the core of the work. However, when these projections are negative or have contents related to warded off and/or feared aspects of the therapist's personality, then dealing with them can be a particular strain for the therapist.

DIFFICULT EMOTIONAL REACTIONS TO THE WORK

Bearing witness to the pain of others, allowing oneself to be influenced by others, and coming into daily contact with realistic life problems and the problems of past history evokes emotional reactions in the therapist. The degree of comfort with these trials is intimately related to how the clinician has come to terms with his or her own past history, and the degree to which the therapist can know and acknowledge warded off aspects of his or her own personality. It is inevitable, however, that a serious, competent practitioner will have, at some point, difficult emotional reactions to aspects of the work. If not corrected, these reactions could lead to a failed or seriously flawed treatment. If the therapist is able to acknowledge his or her problematic reactions, then such reactions can become the occasion to extend an understanding of the patient and enrich the therapy.

IDENTIFICATION WITH PATIENTS

It is characteristic of many good things (psychiatric practice included) that the features that enliven and deepen it are also the potential source of problems. So it is with the ubiquitous tendency (even necessity) of therapists to identify with their patients. A fleeting "trial identification" is probably an essential component of effective empathy. A lasting, unwitting identification with patients is an occupational hazard that can cause the therapist undue difficulty and interfere with the proper use of technique. Therapists may find themselves negotiating between the feeling of intense overinvolvement with their patients and the feeling of detached uninvolvement. Obviously, the middle ground of disciplined yet genuine interest serves both the patient and therapist best. This disciplined position may be hard to achieve.

RESPONSIBILITY/ACCOUNTABILITY

In addition to the personal aspects of the strain of psychiatric practice noted above, there are important and sometimes ambiguous social responsibilities that can add to some of the difficulty of clinical practice. Clinical and legal responsibility for patients with severe and dangerous conditions is full of contradictions for practitioners. Matters of confidentiality versus duty to warn, and protection of civil rights versus duty to protect society from the dangerous mentally ill, are a few of the conflicts that face psychiatrists today. Clinicians work with people to help them take responsibility for their own lives, yet we are expected to take responsibility for those who go beyond a socially defined level of responsibility.

PROBLEMS WITH MEANS/ENDS RELATIONS

The final source of strain that I will identify concerns the uncertain relationship between the means (the application of psychiatric knowledge and treatments) for effecting cure and relieving suffering, and the outcome resulting from the use of these means. Practitioners must constantly struggle with an imperfect mastery of what is generally known; in addition, what is universally known is imperfect. In other words, even if someone could have available all the psychiatric knowledge, the outcome of applying this knowledge energetically and vigorously would still be variable and uncertain. Given this ambiguity of means/ends relationships, there is the occasion for strain and magical thinking.

This section is an exploration of some of the prominent sources of difficulty in the conduct of psychiatric practice. These topics share the feature of addressing problematic aspects of psychiatric practice and giving recommendations for ways to cope with these issues. The chapters focus on ways to cope with the problem when it affects the reader, as well as on ways to help others cope with the problem when it affects them. There is a decidedly psychodynamic orientation to the work reported here, mostly because psychodynamic theory has been the dominant clinical theory for psychiatric practice.

Each chapter is a separate entity and stands alone as an independent work. However, all chapters relate to one another, and to gain maximum benefit from this section, they should be read together. While the chapters address discrete problems in psychiatric practice, the principles enumerated can be applied more generically. At the center of any consideration of problems in psychiatric practice is the concept of countertransference. Those intense and bothersome emotional reactions to patients as well as those silent, yet inhibiting, unknown tendencies, are documented and discussed in Chapter 25, by Drs. Victor Altshul and William Sledge. They provide a formulation for understanding countertransference and suggest ways to incorporate this understanding into practice.

In Chapter 26, Dr. Sara Charles describes the experience of being sued and identifies features of the situation that are sources of difficulty for the defendant physician. Her formulation is of help to the physician being sued, as well as to the clinician who may treat a sued physician. She also provides an overview of the differences between the judicial and clinical situation in terms of responsibility and accountability.

Dr. William Reid, in Chapter 27, provides an overview of the causes of violence, gives an apt account of the legal and treatment issues surrounding violent behavior, and describes ways in which the clinician can anticipate and cope with violence and threats of violence.

In Chapter 28, Dr. Michael Sacks discusses suicide from the position of the therapist of the dead patient. His account is a fresh perspective on the issue of accountability and responsibility, and provides a model for considering accountability and responsibility in all clinical relationships.

Dr. Richard Munich presents an updating of the understanding and treatment of the VIP patient in Chapter 29, and in doing so focuses attention on the phenomenon of entitlement, a process that has applicability far beyond the understanding and treatment of the VIP.

In the final chapter of this section, Chapter 30, Dr. Dianna Hartley presents a fine discussion of the issue of therapeutic stalemate, and provides the reader with a reformulation of the negative therapeutic reaction from the point of view of the interaction between therapist and patient.

Chapter 25

Countertransference Problems

by Victor A. Altshul, M.D., and William H. Sledge, M.D.

COUNTERTRANSFERENCE DEFINED

Among psychotherapy issues, countertransference is a controversial, conceptually complex matter. Some writers have regarded countertransference as the empathic, mostly conscious reactions of the therapist to the patient's transference (Abend, 1986; Freebury, 1979; Heimann, 1950; Kernberg, 1976; Langs, 1976; Loewald, 1986; Searles, 1965). Others have viewed it as the inappropriate reactions of the therapist, transferred from his or her own past, to the patient (Reich, 1960; Brenner, 1985). These two views broadly correspond to the ways in which these emotional reactions are regarded; namely, as important, useful data about the patient that enhance therapeutic understanding, or as an unwanted, albeit omnipresent, interference with the therapist's understanding of the patient and use of technique.

The broad clinical discussion that follows does not require us to delimit the concept in these ways. For our purposes we will define countertransference as encompassing all the emotional reactions of the therapist toward the patient, since we believe that dichotomization invites the reader to choose one or the other alternative and to risk premature closure.

Individual psychoanalytic psychotherapy is an emotionally alerted and charged relationship between two people with the intent to produce change in the patient's emotional life. What each person feels toward and from the other matters to himself and to the other. Each person's feelings about the self, the other, and the relationship between them is relevant to the psychology of both, but by mutual agreement and consistent with the task, it is the psychology of the patient that receives explicit focus. The purpose of this focusing is to allow the patient to experience his or her past in the present, to perceive the connections between ostensibly disconnected realms of experience, and thus to understand and experience one's psychology more deeply and richly than has been possible before. A state of emotional involvement, in which two people's feelings about themselves and each other arise with a sense of heightened intensity and importance, is essential to the process (Langs, 1976; Loewald, 1986). The interaction creates an emotional valence in which the patient is free to react with conviction and intensity to what is happening between them.

In this alerted state, the therapist should be as free as the patient to experience a full range of feelings, thoughts, and fantasies about the patient. Ideally, the therapist does not struggle against or suppress these inner experiences. When they are not too intense, he or she can comfortably accept them and use them as a major tool in the effort to understand the patient deeply (Heimann, 1950;

All of the clinical material reported here derives from the authors' clinical experience, supervision of trainees, or peer supervision.

Loewald, 1986; Segal, 1977) and to identify attitudes or reactions of the therapist that may impede the emotional development of the patient.

Familiar examples come readily to mind. A therapist who feels sexually aroused, after scanning his or her emotional landscape for possible idiosyncratic responses and obtaining confirmatory data from memories of past interactions, may draw conclusions about the unconscious seductive intent of the patient. A therapist who finds himself feeling hateful or contemptuous toward, let us say, a paranoid patient, may come to understand his reactions, as they become more differentiated, as reflections of the way the patient feels about himself—feelings which he may have been unable to convey to the therapist in any other way. Similarly, states of anxiety or depression that arise in the therapist should be noted, "savored," and pondered, since in most cases they will bear importantly on aspects of the patient's conflict or character that is not being otherwise expressed.

The range of such normative countertransference reactions is enormous. Some authors have particularly emphasized the centrality of the therapist's emotional reactions in working with severely disturbed, nonneurotic patients (Kernberg, 1976; Searles, 1965). One ambulatory schizophrenic patient complained that he was unable to develop relationships beyond the most superficial level. He would go to dances by himself, strike up conversations with women, and after some initial pleasantries, find that he was utterly unable to think of anything to say. This was particularly so if the woman showed any interest in him. The paralysis of thought and speech would be accompanied by debilitating anxiety. Feeling that he was not interested in the woman anyway, he would turn away from her in an apparent effort to not recognize that she had already begun to turn away from him.

Some of the dynamics of the problem were intuitively obvious to the therapist. In the face of a threat of human closeness the patient would become disorganized and disoriented, unable to locate within himself a structured feeling or perception from which to generate a response. He was terrified of exposing the extent of his debility and nonachievement, of which he was deeply ashamed. Moreover, he knew that if he opened up to the woman, he would show her his looseness and disorientation, which would seem crazy to her.

The therapist understood that the patient confronted the same dilemmas in the transference. He was prepared for the patient's blocking, his circumstantiality, and his repeated denigration of the therapy. However, he had an unforeseen personal response to the patient's behavior. In the face of the looseness, the quick changes of subject, the derisive and inappropriate hoots of laughter, he would often have a sense of having lost his place, of feeling anxious and confused, and of not knowing how to respond. Ordinarily never at a loss for words, the therapist felt uncharacteristically tongue-tied and stymied.

His state of mind was identical to the state of mind about which the patient had been complaining. When the therapist recognized he had been responding to the patient by allowing himself to experience the patient in this fashion, he felt that he understood the patient far more profoundly than a simple perception of the verbal material would have allowed. When he found a tactful way of telling the patient about his reactions, the patient said that he finally felt understood and was able to speak of his confusion with far greater fluency.

The process by which the therapist comes to have strong or unusual emotional reactions to patients is broadly conceived as arising within the therapist (Brenner, 1985; Reich, 1951) or through the interaction with the patient (Altshul, 1977; Bigras, 1979; Heimann, 1950; Langs, 1979; Loewald, 1986, Racker, 1953; Tyson, 1986). Brenner, writing about psychoanalysis, discusses countertransference as the breakdown of a series of compromise formations that are part of every analyst's defensive adaptation to the work. He emphasizes the internal state within the analyst as the major component of the countertransference reaction.

Other authors emphasize the interaction between the patient and the therapist (Langs, 1976, 1977). Money-Kryle (1956) believes normal countertransference is a function of trial identification; Segal (1977) accounts for it as a form of projective identification. Arlow (1985) differentiates between normal empathy, which is based on a brief and fleeting identification with the patient, and countertransference, which in his view is based on a fixed identification with the patient. Abend, 1986, presents the intriguing formulation that empathy is countertransference when it is accurate and that countertransference is empathy when it is wrong.

There are times when countertransference can be a prognostically favorable event (Searles, 1965). Thus, one therapist who for years had felt no discernible human feeling toward a particular schizophrenic woman, was astonished to find himself feeling aroused in her presence. This event was the first sign that there was any affective connection between them at all. The therapist did not feel threatened by his arousal, felt no temptation to act on it, and came to welcome it as a sign of her improvement.

Most authors believe countertransference reactions are an inevitable and perhaps even desirable part of the work of psychotherapy and psychoanalysis (Abend, 1986; Arlow, 1985; Heimann, 1950; Loewald, 1986). With this extra channel of input, the therapist is able to register and use data from a greater number of sources. But the willingness to make use of this expanded source of data may prove burdensome to the therapist (Abend, 1986). Many therapeutic circumstances require the therapist to delay action in the face of uncomfortable inner experience. The more closely some of these sources tap deep feeling within the therapist, the greater the tension and pressure for discharge.

PROBLEMATIC COUNTERTRANSFERENCE

In problematic countertransference, the therapist experiences conscious reactions to the patient that interfere with or even shatter the alerted state of evenly hovering attention and interest, thus paralyzing his or her capacity for synthetic, imaginative, and therapeutically neutral work. While the causes of problematic countertransference are many and complex, manifestations may be thought of as belonging to three major types, which we will designate as follows: turning away, activated, and unconscious enactment.

The Turning Away Countertransference

The first of these types of conscious countertransference may be broadly referred to as the "turning away" countertransference. It includes states of boredom, indifference, apathy, depression, sleepiness, repugnance, and forgetfulness. While these states may be descriptively dissimilar, they share the common property of involving an intense form of turning away from the patient, an inability to allow oneself to feel engaged or touched by him, which is inevitably felt by the therapist to be distressing and accompanied by a paralysis of empathy. Individual therapists may experience the turning away countertransference in ways that are particular for them. Thus one therapist may respond characteristically with smug withdrawal, another with sleepiness, a third with disgust, and so on. Or a given therapist, depending on circumstances, may have many of these reactions available to him.

A 33-year-old mother of two was referred to a psychiatrist by a colleague who was seeing her husband. The colleague had also seen the wife in consultation and was impressed by her chronic depression and intense phobic anxiety, which seemed to be jeopardizing her marriage and which were clearly interfering with her satisfaction in living.

As soon as the psychiatrist began treating her, he felt an appalling boredom that made it impossible to listen to her, or even to look at her. When he tried to force himself to attend to her, he felt anxiety and dread; these feelings would not abate until he let himself begin to tune out again.

He tried to consider what he could take in about her in order to figure out what was going on. He found her immensely unattractive; indeed, in grooming and dress she seemed to be making a point of appearing almost offensively so. In her speech she had a habit of telling him what she did not feel. She would carefully, if monotonously, describe a situation, and when she seemed on the verge of coming to some point about it, she would list all the things that did not happen and all the things she did not think about it. This pattern drove the therapist to the point of anxious desperation. When she told him about a party in which she was allowing herself to flirt with a strange man, only to reveal that nothing had come of it and that the two of them had walked away from each other in mid-sentence, he had all he could do to refrain from running out of the room himself.

Of course, he had not really heard the deeper meaning of her story. He had been so upset by his aversive responses to her that he was unaware that she had identified him with the stranger and had unconsciously perceived her effect on him. He was aware, however, of his own confusion. His body seemed to be telling him that he was being overstimulated, while his mind was saying that he was being understimulated, even deprived of stimulation. He grew even more bored with her, increasingly intolerant of his own reactions. For her part, she seemed increasingly bored herself, and the two were eventually unable to disguise their feelings. The termination was not overtly hostile, but it was clear that neither felt that anything positive had happened.

A week following the termination, the psychiatrist encountered the colleague who had referred the patient. "A complete turn-off," said the latter. "That's interesting. Had I mentioned that when I saw her in consultation, she described a whole set of elaborate, exciting sadomasochistic fantasies about every strange man she sees?" He had not, of course.

What had happened here? Three mutually compatible formulations seem possible. The woman had buried all her sexual and, particularly, sadomasochistic urges and made herself appear so drab that no one, not even she, could think she had any erotic wishes at all. Or suddenly and outside the therapist's conscious awareness she communicated these urges to him, and he responded with such aversion that no one, not even he, could think he was aroused by them. Or she enacted her sadomasochistic fantasies within the therapeutic relationship; by being at once titillatingly flirtatious and maddeningly bland, she invited her therapist to have sadistic wishes toward her, from which he defensively withdrew into boredom and somnolence.

It is not only repressed excitement in the patient that may lead to a turning away countertransference. Often a sense of excitement directly expressed may threaten to overstimulate a therapist and cause him to repond aversively. One of the authors (Altshul, 1977), reported a case in which a young man was struggling energetically to sort out the details of a complicated family history of which he had been given contradictory versions. The very richness of the material he was producing tended to make it indigestible, and the therapist responded with a sense of anxious and fidgety boredom.

Many therapists have observed that when they examine the occasions in which boredom, fidgetiness, drowsiness, and other such affects arise, they often do so just before a significant insight bursts into their awareness. The aversive feelings appear to be an effort to fight off the awareness of the insight. One therapist described a case in which he regularly had turning away feelings just before he became aware of his patient's sexual feeling toward him. Another therapist reported a case of a male patient who was having an exhilarating affair, which was causing him to feel wonderfully attractive, competent, and brilliant. The therapist felt a similar exhilaration when the patient was talking about the affair, but found himself losing interest when the patient started to talk about anything else. He began to realize that he would feel bored whenever the patient tried to tell him that he felt fundamentally inept and unsure of himself when he was not diverting himself with the affair. The therapist finally had to realize that, owing to uncomfortable identifications he was making with the patient, he did not really want to hear about the underlying feelings of ineptitude. This insight led to a richer understanding of the patient's hidden conflicts and defenses.

The genesis of the turning-away countertransference may also be related to a way of handling anger in relation to needs of the therapist, which are unrecognized, unacknowledged, and inappropriate to the therapy. The young man with the tangled family history, for instance, was so absorbed in the conflicting accounts of his past that the therapist did not seem to exist for him as a person in the present or as a transference object. The pattern seemed to conform to Kohut's mirror transference (Kohut, 1971), in which the therapist is called upon simply to murmur admiring affirmations of the patient's insight and wisdom. The therapist came to understand his boredom as a warding off of his resentment at being treated as a nonperson. He had had an unacknowledged need for recognition by the patient, which had led to symptomatic countertransference until it could be acknowledged and mastered.

A depressed young woman who seemed determined not to be understood by her therapist revealed the following story. Her father had been a glib, superficially charming, alcoholic, emotionally shallow, unsupportive, and dismissive of communications to him as jokes. He had also been openly seductive, walking around the house nude, barging into the patient's bedroom when she was naked, and fondling her at will.

The patient seemed to enact conflicts aroused by this relationship in the transference. Early in the therapy, she showed a repetitive pattern of behavior. Although she and her male therapist clearly had good rapport, she appeared to take flight whenever she felt in danger of being understood. Typically she would begin to talk meaningfully about an important issue. Empathically in tune with her, the therapist would start to feel on the verge of a significant insight. Regularly at this point she would veer off into a volley of superficial chatter and hide her experience behind a mask of impersonal friendliness. The therapist responded to this behavior with feelings of annoyance and boredom, and because of these feelings, it was some time before he felt he understood what she was doing. Her life-long perception of feeling forced to cater to the wishes of a voyeuristic father was being revived in the transference. For her, to be understood by her therapist meant to titillate him by exposing secret and shameful parts of herself. The abrupt retreats into superficial chatter were her way of clothing herself, and by eliciting boredom in her therapist, she was able to keep him from being too interested in her. At the same time, she was titillating him by partly unclothing herself and refusing to take off the rest.

The therapist's boredom and annoyance could be understood as defenses against the overstimulation aroused by the patient's unconsciously seductive behavior, as well as angry reactions to the consistent thwarting of his need to understand her. It is well for therapists to recognize that their need to understand arises from a series of sublimations or compromise formations (Brenner, 1985) that may become disrupted. At the same time, this example can be understood as an instance of the therapist's participation in an unwitting interaction with the patient through the mechanism of projective identification, whereby the therapist enacts a role in accordance with the patient's inner objects. In this case the therapist reacts with boredom, presumably in reaction to his sadistic response to the patient's representation of him as a dangerously intrusive figure. Such a disruption may intensify narcissistic needs, but, of course, it is inappropriate for the patient to be expected to gratify them or to be under any obligation to do so as a result of the interaction with the therapist (Altshul, 1977).

There are many kinds of needs that therapists can have of their patients without clearly understanding that they have them. The needs to be recognized, appreciated, connected, liked, not alone, and helpful are all related, but each is slightly different from every other. If these needs are not met or modified through self-analysis, each can have a hidden effect on the therapist's feelings about the patient, depending on what is happening in his or her life in and out of the office, and on how these needs are being processed (Brenner, 1985; Abend, 1986).

The Activated Countertransference

Another general type of problematic countertransference we label as "activated" countertransference, which in turn has two components. In this reaction empathy is hampered by impulses opposite to the turning away reaction. These two components are distinguished by the valences of the feelings (positive or negative) and have in common a state of arousal. Positive activated countertransference reactions include sexual desire, admiration, or rescue fantasies, in which the therapist responds by imagining him- or herself on intimate terms with or even fused with the patient. This kind of excited overidentification interferes with empathy by obliterating distance, by converting empathy into sympathy, and by causing the therapist to restrict his perception of dynamic possibilities in the interest of protecting his own vulnerabilities and experiencing his own needs, either in fact or fantasy. The constructed intimacy with the patient may range from the experience of siding uncritically with the patient, as in a conflict with a spouse, to states of intense sexual longing.

Negative activated countertransference reactions take the form of aroused aggressive feelings toward the patient, such as anger, intimidation, and rage, and center around fantasies of attacking or harming the patient. Manifestations of this kind of reaction may be undue argumentation with the patient, wishing to be rid of the patient, or behaving in a tactless fashion.

Neither a turning away nor activated countertransference is necessarily pathological, and its intensity alone does not cause it to become so. It becomes problematic only when the therapist loses track of his or her emotional state. The therapist then loses the sense of "hold" on the therapeutic relationship and begins to feel (usually unconsciously) that he or she is there for a different reason. In the face of the patient's wish for him to behave in a certain way or to be something he is not, he develops a blind spot to the source of his own emotional responses and treats as socially real a set of feelings that should have an "as if" character. Thus, for example, a patient's request for solace may be taken as an invitation to mature love, or his raging, contempt, or devaluation may be heard as valid judgments of the therapist's competence or character. When the therapist loses this vital perspective on what the patient is saying and on what he is feeling in return, the therapy is imperiled. If he can restore the therapeutic perspective, he will have achieved a much richer appreciation of the patient's difficulties.

In this discussion we are assuming a therapist who is competent under ordinary circumstances to understand and deal constructively with his or her own responses. This therapist is trained to follow simultaneously the patient's and his or her own associations, and to perceive the connections between them and his or her emotional reactions to the patient. This therapist is presumed to have no major enduring blind spots. We make these points to illustrate that even the most psychologically attuned and reflective therapist can be expected to develop episodic transient countertransference problems. It no longer seems appropriate to dismiss such aberrations as manifestations of fixed pathology in the therapist.

In the positive activated countertransference, we are referring to an excited response of sufficient intensity to cause the therapist to forget that it has arisen in a therapeutic context, to cease thinking about it in a therapeutic way, and to deal with it as if it were socially "real"; that is, as if it originated outside the therapeutic relationship and therefore had a more compelling claim on the totality of his emotional life. He finds himself beginning to live within and for the feeling. He begins to look forward to the sessions and to the excitement he anticipates from them. He starts to think of therapy as a treat, as if it existed for his pleasure rather than as a service to the patient. Often the patient will sense the therapist's excitement, and, delighted at the impact he or she is having, will intensify the behaviors that are provoking it. Thus, the patient too may lose the sense that the therapy is for him- or herself, but on a superficial level the patient does not resent the loss because he or she feels amply compensated by the pleasure he or she is giving the therapist. Feeling loved, valued, and effective, the patient may thus obtain considerable symptomatic relief. This may be confused with genuine progress, and neither patient nor therapist may feel motivated to discontinue the pathological interaction.

One subset of the activated countertransference, the eroticized countertransference, has recently been the focus of much attention as an ethical issue. To deal with the question of sex between therapist and patient in ethical terms is a welcome direction in our profession, but this should not blind us to the fact that sexual arousal in a therapist is also a highly complicated countertransference issue. Obviously it is vital to distinguish between sexual arousal, which is not unethical, and sexual behavior, which is—though, interestingly, this elementary distinction is often blurred, and the blurring inhibits thoughtful discussion of the topic.

It is our impression that sexual arousal in the therapist occurs in the context of a complex interaction in which both patient and therapist play important roles. It is possible to think of it as lying along a continuum. At one end the patient's conflicts seem unusually prominent—as, for example, when the patient is openly seductive and suggests a sexual relationship. At the other end, the therapist's issues are in the forefront, as, for instance, when he mistranslates a request for solace or a longing for support as primary communications of sexual feeling and feels aroused in response. In our experience, most instances lie between these extremes. Let us remember that under ordinary circumstances erotic arousal, like other countertransference affects, is commonplace and is worked with as a way of understanding the patient. It is when the response interferes with the therapeutic perspective of the relationship that it becomes problematic.

Just as a turning away countertransference can arise as a vicissitude of anger and frustration because of needs that are unmet and unacknowledged, so an activated countertransference can occur in the wake of an implied promise of their fulfillment. From their supervisory and therapeutic experience the authors are aware of cases in which eroticized countertransference took this form and reached dangerous levels of intensity before they were resolved. In both cases the patients were reported to be directly and energetically seductive from the outset, conveying considerably less interest in therapy than in consummation. Superficially the patients appeared to be causing the relationships to take on a sexual character. On closer inspection, however, it seemed probable that the therapists were unconsciously sending subliminal signals to the patients about their vulnerability to seduction. Each therapist appeared to have long-standing difficulties with self-esteem regulation, and each was currently going through a divorce.

In both instances the patient appeared to be a kind of savior, offering relief of intensely felt needs for love and solace which had been acknowledged previously and which seemed to take the therapist utterly by surprise. To his own therapist or supervisor, the therapist emerged as a lovelorn bungler completely deserted by his therapeutic acumen and in serious danger of abandonment by his professional superego. Lacking guideposts, disoriented, and confused, he genuinely saw the patient as offering all that his life had been denying him. Without quite being aware of the process by which it had evolved, he experienced himself as being in the midst of an authentic love relationship.

Fortunately, each therapist was able to make use of his supervision or therapy to pull back from the danger and to reestablish his therapeutic "hold" on the relationship. It is our impression that too many such cases have less fortunate outcomes. Many therapists go through periods of substantial difficulty in their lives, in which they may be inadequately prepared to deal with such assaults on their vulnerabilities and inadequately aware of the manner in which they may be inviting them. In the present censorious climate, it may be hard for a therapist to present himself for therapy or supervision when he finds himself sexually drawn to a patient. Moreover, supervision during his training will probably not have dealt openly with the emergence of such temptations and with their meaning and management, and will not have prepared him to deal with them in the isolation of his practice. These observations offer obvious implications for improved training and supervision throughout a therapist's professional lifetime.

There is a darker side to the matter of eroticized countertransference which is sometimes lost on less experienced therapists. The conditions of conducting therapy—the abstinence, the buildup of instinctual pressures, and the loneliness—may seem intolerable to a needy therapist; he may respond by hating the therapy, which is depriving him of discharge and gratification. To whatever extent he alters its parameters to allow for more personal gratification, he attacks the very therapy the patient needs. Thus, the conversion of any therapy into a personal relationship, particularly a sexual one, is invariably a hostile attack on the patient. This is likely to be so even after the formal termination of the therapy, no matter how the therapist may try to rationalize his behavior.

Many cases of excited countertransference can be problematic even for gifted, experienced psychotherapists. A countertransference of one form may be a defensive reaction against that of another form. A therapist found himself feeling erotically stimulated by a patient who was decidedly not behaving in a seductive way. She was a middle-aged woman of reasonable attractiveness, but drab of dress and bizarre of manner. As an infant, she had repeatedly been left alone for what seemed an eternity. Her earliest memories were of screaming loudly, of having nobody come in to comfort her, and of seeing the walls and objects in the room swim about and change their shapes in terrifying ways. She retained a lifelong vulnerability to separation; and when separated from her therapist, she would deal with her disorientation and terror by imagining herself to be the same person as he. Thus she could pretend there was no separation at all; she could sit in wordless comfort, in or out of the session, while he would understand every nuance of her feeling without her having to say a word.

In spite of her lack of overt seductiveness, and in spite of his recognition that her longings were pregenital in origin and character, the therapist felt clear sexual arousal. At first he could not account for it. He considered the possibility that he was responding to the indirect seductiveness of her flattery of him, but did not think that this factor could account for the intensity of his response. Finally he concluded that his genital response to the patient's pregenital stimulus was defensive. It served to ward off primitive affects that were even more disruptive to him than sexual feeling, in particular a terrifying longing for and temptation toward dedifferentiation and fusion which were raging in both people. When the therapist finally understood the nature of his fears, he was able to face them more directly, and the sexual feelings subsided. We speculate that these dynamics may occur with some regularity and that many cases of sexual acting-out may represent defensive miscarriages of impulses to offer solace to patients whose needs are primarily pregenital.

Some kinds of activated countertransference may not involve overt sexual arousal but may take the form of advocacy for the patient. This process is charmingly depicted in the operetta *Trial by Jury*. In this work, W. S. Gilbert satirizes the supposed impartiality of British jurisprudence. In the beginning, the judge, jury, and lawyers sing of their profound respect for the even-handedness of the law. But when Angelina, suing Edwin for breach of promise, sings her tale of woe, they all burst into tears of pity and love. By contrast, when poor Edwin enters, he can barely sing a note before the jury has leapt to its feet, pointing fingers at him in furious denunciation. In the end the judge resolves the dispute: He will marry Angelina himself.

Like the judge and jury, we may find ourselves vigorously taking a patient's side in a conflict with a lover or spouse. Or, in a more subtle form of the same process, we may place ourselves squarely at one pole of a patient's internal conflict, energetically urging him to see the matter our way. We would be hard pressed to think of a single instance in which this kind of countertransference reaction, in its extreme form, does not primarily serve the defensive needs of the therapist. It reflects a denial of the complexity of the patient's world and an intolerance of the anxiety the therapist would feel if he were to consider broader and more sophisticated notions about what he is hearing. For his part, the patient may respond with superficial gratitude, but on a deeper level, he is likely to feel misunderstood and abandoned.

An attractive woman in early middle age came into therapy when her marriage of 10 years began to unravel. She was a dependent person with an overpowering need to please others and a pronounced fear of asserting herself lest she lose the other's love. These traits had led her to form many relationships, including her marriage, in which she was dominated, bullied, ungratified, and hurt. She was unable to locate a sense of self; she was often incapable of standing up to others because she did know what she felt herself. She was aware of many of these qualities and disliked them in herself, but felt unable to change them without help.

Although the patient might not have agreed, her therapy was initially compromised by the therapist's intense positive countertransference. He was appalled by the husband's scurrilous conduct and infantile demandingness, which reminded him of everything he had ever read about Caligula. In spite of himself, he found himself vigorously persuading the patient to adopt a more negative view of her husband than she had allowed herself to do. He rationalized his approach as one of helping her to get in touch with more intense affects he supposed she must have had. In response, the patient behaved gratefully and flatteringly.

With the help of supervision, the therapist came to realize that he had been reenacting with the patient the pattern of all her other relationships. Like her husband, he, too, had been dominating and bullying her. He began to see that through subtle displays of helplessness, she had been stimulating his rescue fantasies and unconsciously manipulating him to dominate her. In time he came to understand that he had been reluctant to recognize her dependency, obsequiousness, and self-abasement, since he was revolted by these traits when he sensed them in himself.

Other issues had also informed the therapist's initial distorted response. He himself had recently undergone a divorce and had not yet worked out a balanced view of what had happened; he preferred to believe that his wife's character traits had been responsible for all the difficulties. By taking a one-sided view of the patient's marriage, he protected himself from the recognition that all marital conflicts are many-sided. By taking the position that the man in his patient's marriage was entirely responsible, he worked off some unconscious guilt about his own marriage without having to own up directly to his contribution to its failure.

Unconscious Enactments

The third form of problematic countertransference entails the acting out of a technical failure without the experience of a particularly problematic conscious reaction. We call this phenomenon unconscious countertransference enactment. A therapist forgot a second appointment with a new patient. Initially, he was at a loss to understand why; there were no particular indentifiable features of the patient that troubled him or made him uncomfortable. Self-scrutiny suggested that perhaps he was intimidated or revolted by her cloying dependency. He had been also particularly busy lately, an explanation that seemed reasonable. As the therapy progressed, however, it came to be known that the patient had been severely neglected by a parental figure in her past. Characteristically, this parental figure had acted as if the patient did not exist. After several months of therapy, it became clear that the patient had managed to evoke at the first meeting a psychological field that replicated the sense of being a helpless victim in which the therapist had been an unwitting participant by forgetting the second session. Part of the motivation for forgetting the session was the wish to avoid the rage and reproach of the patient while at the same time complying with a particular dynamic role, which in this case was the neglectful parent.

Jacobs (1986) has called attention to the subtle manifestations of countertransference attitudes by which normal aspects of psychoanalytic work become imbued with countertransference meanings, such as how one listens to patients, how the session is characteristically terminated, and so on. Arlow (1986) has written about how analysts can have countertransference reactions toward some aspect of the conditions of the therapy itself. Wile (1972) has related the general sense of therapist discouragement and pessimism as possibly related to countertransference issues.

Another aspect of countertransference enactments in the form of attitudes that should be mentioned briefly is the use of cultural stereotypes to carry the unacknowledged feelings and attitudes. Guttman (1984) has examined issues of transference between female therapists and male patients and notes that certain cultural images are commonly used for expressing countertransference reactions in these situations.

CONCLUSION

Countertransference is a forceful, living reality that informs our minute-by-minute experience with our patients, whether we choose to recognize it or not. At best it is a powerful, indispensable tool for understanding the patient on the deepest levels. It becomes problematic when its quality leads us to lose track of its subordinate position within the therapeutic relationship. We then lose a secure sense of our primary function in the therapy; we may feel we are there for a reason other than that of treating the patient psychotherapeutically. In this case the problematic countertransference distorts the therapist's capacity for empathy and effective technique so that it remains problematic even if it is not directly acted out.

At the risk of being schematic, we will conclude with a suggested approach to the issue of problematic countertransference that is composed of the process of recognizing that a problem exists, diagnosing the cause of the problem, and intervening once the problem is recognized and diagnosed.

Recognizing the Problem

Of course, a major challenge in dealing with problematic countertransference is to recognize there is a problem before the therapy becomes irretrievably compromised. Countertransference feelings of a nonproblematic nature are familiar as strong or unusual feelings or attitudes that are out of place or unusual. Problematic countertransference feelings may also be manifested as strong feelings of either a positive or negative nature or as unusual attitudes for the therapist, but these feelings usually are rationalized as being appropriate for the reality of the therapist, or as being caused by something else. Signs of the problematic nature of such countertransference reactions may be the presence of a parapraxis, particularly in the therapy, the absence or marked diminution of feeling, the presence of unusually strong negative or positive feelings, a break in routine without a clear reason, or a break in some general technical rule. If these kinds of phenomena begin to occur, the therapist should adopt a skeptical attitude toward whatever kind of quick explanation he may make to himself. The difficult task is to recognize and admit to himself that there is a problem.

Diagnosis

The important diagnostic issues are twofold: 1) to recognize the unmet needs of the therapist that are being aroused by the work with the patient, and 2) to identify the patient's contribution to the countertransference. The identification of the unmet needs of the therapist is the first step in reestablishing the therapeutic perspective. The understanding of the countertransference phenomenon in terms of the patient's psychology is the second step.

Intervention

When previously disavowed countertransference reactions become known to the therapist, he or she will have to make the decision as to whether and how to communicate something of this new knowledge to the patient. It is very important for the therapist not to overreact through a feeling of guilt with an intrusive, tactless confession. Although each instance is unique and requires a thoughtful, measured response, probably it is best to listen carefully for references to what constituted the therapist's previously unacknowledged countertransference and facilitate the patient's speaking of it. Certainly, the therapist should acknowledge errors and obvious lapses in technique and understanding. But even this acknowledgement must be made from the perspective of what is best for the goals of the psychotherapy. Knowledge gained by the therapist from the understanding of a problematic countertransference, if it is to be shared with the patient, must be shared in a careful, tactful fashion. One countertransference enactment does not offset another; the main correction the therapist can make is to reestablish a therapeutic perspective.

Of course the best intervention is prevention through sound basic clinical training, the development of the capacity for self-scrutiny and reflection—perhaps best achieved through a personal psychotherapy or psychoanalysis, supervision past the time of formal training, and the use of peers. We are particularly enthusiastic about on-going peer supervision. We have participated in such a peer group that has met for many years. Many of our ideas about countertransference have come directly from discussions generated by informal presentations in this group.

REFERENCES

Abend SM: Countertransference, empathy, and the analytic ideal: the impact of life stresses on analytic capability. Psychoanal Q 1986; 55:563–575

Altshul VA: The so-called boring patient. Am J Psychother 1977; 31:533–545

Altshul VA: The hateful therapist and the countertransference psychosis. Journal of the National Association of Private Psychiatric Hospitals 1980; 11:15–23

Arlow J: Some technical problems of countertransference. Psychoanal Q 1986; 54:164–174

Bigras J: The interminable analysis of countertransference. Psychoanal Rev 1979; 66:311–322

Brenner C: Countertransference as compromise formation. Psychoanal Q 1985; 54:155–163

Freebury DR: Clinical aspects of the countertransference. Can J Psychiatry 1979; 4:71–74

Guttman HA: Sexual issues in the transference and countertransference between female therapist and male patient. J Am Acad Psychoanal 1984; 12:187–197

Heimann P: On countertransference. Int J Psychoanal 1950; 31:81–84

Jacobs TJ: On countertransference enactments. J Am Psychoanal Assoc 1986; 34:289–307

Kernberg O: Transference and countertransference in the treatment of borderline patients, in Objects Relations Theory and Clinical Psychoanalysis. Edited by Kernberg O. New York, Jason Aronson, 1976

Kohut H: The analysis of the self, a systematic approach to the psychoanalytic treatment of narcissistic personality disorders. New York, International Universities Press, 1971

Langs R: The therapeutic interaction, vol. 2. New York, Jason Aronson, 1976

Langs R: The therapeutic interaction, a synthesis. New York, Jason Aronson, 1977

Levy ST: Countertransference aspects of pharmacotherapy in the treatment of schizophrenia. Int J Psychoanal Psychother 1977; 6:15–30

Loewald HW: Transference–countertransference. J Am Psychoanal Assoc 1986; 34:275–287

Money-Kryle RE: Normal countertransference and some of its deviations. Int J Psychoanal 1956; 37:360–366

Racker H: The countertransference neurosis. Int J Psychoanal 1953; 34:313–324

Reich A: On countertransference. Int J Psychoanal 1951; 32:25–31

Reich A: Further remarks on countertransference. Int J Psychoanal 1960; 41:389–395

Searles H: Oedipal love in the countertransference, in Collected Papers on Schizophrenia and Related Subjects. Edited by Searles H. New York, International Universities Press, 1965

Segal H: Countertransference. Int J Psychoanal Psychother 1977; 6:31–37

Tyson RL: Countertransference evolution in theory and practice. J Am Psychoanal Assoc 1986; 34:251–274

Wile D: Negative countertransference: therapist discouragement. Int J Psychoanal Psychother 1972; 1:36–67

Chapter 26

Stress Associated with Medical Malpractice Litigation

by Sara C. Charles, M.D.

MEDICAL MALPRACTICE LITIGATION AS A STRESSOR

The education of the physician involves not only the acquisition of medical knowledge and skills but also the development of a professional sense of responsibility. When the patient contracts for the doctor's expertise, a clear fiduciary obligation arises which has certain legal ramifications. This includes not only the duty to "do no harm," but also the duty to adhere to the standards of medical practice for a given specialty in a given geographical area. If a patient sustains an injury while under medical treatment and determines that the injury resulted from a failure to meet those standards, then the patient may use the law of torts to initiate a malpractice complaint. The patient thereby sets into motion a process aimed at establishing fault; that is, showing that, more likely than not, the doctor or health care facility, either by omission or commission, deviated from this standard of care, thereby directly causing the injury for which damages are claimed.

A Short History

The law of torts establishes the rules and procedures whereby injuries, which occur to either person or property as a result of contacts between persons and things, are compensated. Tort law has traditionally been influenced by the social and philosophical climate in which it functions so that changes in cultural mores and social conditions contribute to its development and refinement. Until the late 19th century, the concept of strict liability applied, which means that to achieve compensation it was necessary only to establish a relationship between an injury and "a person or thing." Fault was not an issue. In 1843, a New York court ruled that a person who used ordinary care and foresight was not liable for injury or accident and that the injury, therefore, was "the misfortune of the sufferer, and lays no foundation for legal responsibility" (Schwartz, 1974). This introduction of fault into tort law occurred when the Industrial Revolution was in full force and when the Spencerian Darwinism philosophy of "survival of the fittest" permeated the American scene. In this instance, the courts moved to protect emerging industrial enterprises from financial ruin while shifting to the individual worker and citizen the burden of proof for establishing the origin of the negligence which directly caused the injury.

Liability insurance also came into broader use around the end of the 19th century and provided an additional layer of protection for burgeoning industries. Claims for injuries which were rejected or disputed necessitated that individuals seek recourse in the law in order to gain access to the insurance funds.

As individuals became more vulnerable to injury from the multitude of potential disasters inherent in "modern society" at the same time that the courts demanded that fault be established, state and national legislatures observed the growing inequities. Driven by the philosophical concerns about life in the modern world, they began to devise ways of assuring compensation for individuals who were subject to an increasing number of life's inevitable vicissitudes. They reasoned that if modern society increased the individual's risk for tragedy, then society should shoulder the burden of recompense for the injuries that eventuated. As legal scholar Bernard Schwartz observed, "The law of torts has steadily moved from a fault to a social insurance basis" (Schwartz, 1974).

Despite significant and increasing technological developments in medical care with their concomitant incremental risk for individuals already compromised by illness and/or old age, the social insurance concept does not yet apply to injuries sustained in the health care sector. As efforts to obtain compensation for injury intensify, there is growing tension between tort law and insurance interests. At the center of the dispute is the individual practitioner or health care facility, the insured parties, against whom fault must be alleged if any avoidable or unavoidable injury occurs. This is so because, lacking other mechanisms, this action is the principal means of obtaining access to insurance funds.

The System: Distortions and Ambiguities

A commonly held perception is that this system, by imposing sanctions on "bad doctors," acts as a deterrent to future negligent behavior, effectively enforces adherence to the standards of medical practice, and protects the public. Outcome statistics, one measure of the system's effectiveness, suggest that most malpractice claims do not involve true negligence. Nationally, an estimated 57 percent of the 73,472 medical malpractice claims closed in 1984 resulted in no payment to the plaintiff (U.S. GAO, 1987). In Illinois alone, the physician-owned insurance company has closed approximately 12,000 claims since 1976, and 84 percent resulted in no payment to the plaintiff (ISMIE, 1988). These cases lacked sufficient merit so that they were dismissed, dropped, or the doctor won at trial. Nor are settlements or jury awards necessarily indicative of poor medical practice. In cases of severe injury, it may mean that the negligence criteria were relaxed (Danzon, 1982). Illustrative is the California case in which a $667,550 award to an injured patient was accompanied by a court order stating that "the judgment rendered here does not relate to a breach of integrity or any lack of professional competency or training on the part of the defendant" (Carlova, 1983).

The civil justice system which determines fault and awards compensation has faced increasing criticism (Bowen, 1987). Danzon, an economist, argues that the system can only be rationalized on the basis of its deterrent effect and not as a means of compensation (Danzon, 1985). Legal scholars argue that the original and direct intent of the law is not to discipline erring doctors but to compensate individuals for losses (Keeton, 1984).

Originally, the stimulus to tort action was patient injury. This has been broadened to include both avoidable and unavoidable adverse outcomes, patient dissatisfactions, poor doctor–patient relationships, societal rage, and a host of displacement phenomena. The system now serves as an objective target for transferences common to the doctor–patient relationship and which extend far beyond actual physical injury caused by negligence. In addition, the scope of tort actions and theories of recovery broaden continuously so that "perfectly good medicine today may be malpractice tomorrow" (Rapp, 1988).

Although the majority of physicians accused of malpractice are found not negligent, many often have remained under the cloud of accusations of fault and embroiled in legal processes for many years prior to their vindication. Good doctors, even the best doctors, rather than the so-called bad doctors, are the principal objects of malpractice actions. At the core of their reactions is this accusation of fault, a legal concept not always indicative of or equivalent to clinical negligence and/or moral fault.

Psychiatrists and the System

Psychiatrists are among the least sued of medical professionals and consequently may have minimal contact with this facet of the legal system (See Table 1). The full impact of, and knowledge about, the problem, therefore, may not be sufficiently appreciated.

MALPRACTICE LITIGATION AS A STRESSFUL LIFE EVENT

The Emotional History of a Malpractice Suit

For almost every physician presented with a summons, there is an immediate, albeit usually temporary, intense emotional response. Initially, the doctor feels stunned, denies the reality of the complaint, and disavows the content of the allegations. As contacts with the insurer and lawyer begin, the stunned reaction

Table 1. Physicians' Claim Experience in Three Time Periods by 10 Specialty Categories (Percent of Physicians Sued at Least Once)

	Career	1981–1985	1985
All Physicians	36.5	25.4	8.5
Specialty			
General/Family Practice	34.4	20.2	5.3
Internal Medicine	28.7	20.6	5.5
Surgery	49.5	36.4	13.4
Pediatrics	27.7	17.4	6.9
Obstetrics/Gynecology	64.0	48.3	21.0
Radiology	38.8	27.1	11.1
Psychiatry	15.8	10.3	2.4
Anesthesiology	35.6	26.3	6.5
Pathology	16.5	11.8	3.1

Source: AMA Socioeconomic Monitoring System (AMA's survey data generally indicates a lower number of claims than insurance industry sources, probably because some physicians do not report claims that do not ripen into suits).

quickly gives way to expressions of rage. The doctor feels narcissistically injured by accusations of having "failed" to discharge the duty due the patient and commonly expresses feelings of "devastation." As a result, the insurance and legal counsel, as well as the spouse, family, professional associates, and the system, often become the objects for this displaced rage. Horowitz's paradigm for describing reactions to serious life events is useful in understanding these reactions. The event generates an initial outcry followed by a pattern of both intrusive and denial experiences, some of which may be of pathological intensity and expressed as despair, impaired work functions, social withdrawal, or substance abuse. There follows a period of working through the experience, which may be accompanied by pathological expressions of anxiety, depression, and physiological disruptions before a relative completion of the response is effected (Horowitz, 1986).

A critical dimension of the litigation experience is its chronicity. Although the average case is closed in approximately 30 months, cases that go to trial may take as many as six or more years (Sonderby, 1987), and posttrial activities commonly extend the process even longer. In addition, litigation is not just a single event but consists of a series of discrete events. For example, the process of working through the stressor of the initial summons may be almost completely resolved when a respected expert gives a highly critical deposition. This unanticipated but related new stressor may exacerbate all the initial reactions. The period of emotional disruption may therefore disappear within a few weeks after the initiation of the suit, persist for many months, diminish and recur periodically in concert with the amount of involvement with the process, or remain unrelieved until the case is resolved.

Common Emotional and Physical Reactions

Little literature exists on the emotional effects on any group of subjects in reaction to any type of litigation. Our studies suggest that approximately 33 percent of sued doctors report, at some time during the process, a symptom cluster which resembles a major depressive disorder as defined by The *Diagnostic and Statistical Manual of Mental Disorders, Third Edition, Revised (DSM-III-R)* (American Psychiatric Association, 1987; Charles, 1984, 1985, 1987). The fact that many doctors who have been threatened by litigation, but never actually sued, report a similar cluster of symptoms (Charles, 1985) needs to be interpreted in the light of those studies which document the vulnerability of certain physician groups to affective symptoms, especially depressive disorders (Pearson and Strecker, 1960; Valko and Clayton, 1975; Jones, 1977).

Our studies also reveal that an average 26 percent of sued doctors experience a second cluster of symptoms, determined to be an adjustment disorder, characterized by pervasive anger accompanied by at least four (an arbitrarily chosen number) of eight symptoms: depressed mood, inner tension, frustration, irritability, insomnia, fatigue, gastrointestinal symptoms, or headache (Charles, 1984, 1985, 1987). A significantly greater number of sued than nonsued doctors report this symptom cluster and, currently, it is more frequently reported among sued doctors than is the depression cluster (Charles, 1985, 1988). This may be related to the greater availability of social support. In 1982, only 10 percent of sued doctors reported talking to their peers about their litigation experience as compared to over 70 percent of sued doctors in 1986 (Charles, 1988). Additionally, legal tactics have changed naming multiple defendants rather than a sole defendant in a single suit. This may decrease the feelings of isolation as well as diminish the perception that being sued identifies one as "bad." Doctors, therefore, may experience greater anger and frustration directed externally toward the system, and less guilt, shame, lowered self-esteem, and depression, which are internally directed and which were so commonly experienced by sued physicians just a few years ago.

Approximately 16 percent of the doctors studied reported the onset or exacerbation of a physical illness (Charles, 1984, 1985, 1987). These were generally stress-related illnesses such as coronary artery disease, colitis, duodenal ulcer, and hypertension. In addition, seven percent acknowledged excessive drinking and fewer than one percent reported the abuse of drugs, while three percent cited suicidal ideation as a reaction to litigation (Charles, 1984, 1985, 1987).

This reported symptomatology needs to be put into perspective. As noted earlier, only an estimated three to four percent of malpractice cases go to trial and more than one-half of all cases filed and closed result in no payment to the plaintiff (ISMIE, 1988). According to our data, the major impact of the litigation experience, in terms of physical, emotional, and behavioral changes, results from the allegation rather than the outcome of the suit (Charles, 1988). This is *the* event that generates the majority of stress response syndromes. This suggests that the majority of the emotional disruption resulting from these suits is related to cases found to be without merit.

Among multiply sued doctors, each suit has its own stress valence; that is, the degree of stress experienced relative to each suit is a function of a variety of unique factors. The third suit filed rather than the first may be the most stressful and productive of symptoms. In addition, we found no significant differences in self-reported symptomatology between doctors who won their trials and those who lost, although the latter were significantly more likely to feel that the plaintiff's case was justified, to report lack of social support, and tended to report more feelings of guilt (Charles, 1988).

The majority of doctors also implemented a variety of changes in the way they conduct their medical practices, generally aimed at defending themselves against further malpractice suits. They may refuse to do certain procedures even though fully trained to do so; change the way they relate to patients, most frequently through distancing behaviors; and refuse to see certain kinds of patients they perceive as presenting specific risks (Charles, 1988). For psychiatrists, this latter most commonly involves the exclusion of patients with suicidal tendencies and/or threats, patients who are prone to develop negative transferences, and those with impulse disorders.

CONTRIBUTING FACTORS TO THE STRESS OF LITIGATION

Medicine: A Stressful Profession

Renee Fox has argued that medical work *is* different from other kinds of work and, because it deals with some of the most transcendent aspects of the human condition, it is "morally and existentially serious." Physicians derive pressure from their need to "define their work as limitless in time and potential urgency," as well as from the "uncertainties that stem from how much and how little they know." She maintains that no matter how much training or experience doctors have, the "basic, human condition-associated stresses and dilemmas . . . cannot be eliminated" (Fox, 1979).

Our recent study of stressors in medical practice supports the findings of previous researchers (McCue, 1982; Mechanic, 1975; Mawardi, 1979; McCranie et al, 1982; Anwar, 1983; Clarke et al, 1984; and Linn et al, 1985) that doctors identify time constraints and working with patients and their families as the most stressful aspects of practice. The rapidly changing economic scene in health care, as well as changes in the social structure of medicine and in the role of the physician, generated some frustration and complaint. Litigation, however, was considered a stressful life event and was identified by 23 percent of sued physicians as the most stressful event of their entire life (Charles, 1987).

The Personality of Physicians

The key variable in the consideration of the origins of stress in physicians' lives arises from the unique characteristics of the physician's personality (Roeske, 1981). Although within the physician population there exists a broad spectrum of personality styles and a certain degree of psychiatric symptomatology, there are also commonly shared personality characteristics that render them vulnerable to the litigation experience. The normal physician has been called the compulsive physician, characterized by the triad of self-doubt, guilt feelings, and an exaggerated sense of responsibility (Gabbard, 1985). These can be adaptive as well as maladaptive in that the same traits that assure the best of medical care and concern for the patient can, for sued physicians, contribute to a destructive personal outcome.

Self-doubt, for example, is a stimulus for diagnostic rigor which leads physicians to extend themselves beyond ordinary expectations, and to consider "outside" diagnostic and therapeutic possibilities. Medical training promotes "ever-increasing compulsivity" and "newer developments in the theory of medical practice requiring more time to study, harder work and more risk taking" solidify these tendencies for practitioners (Krakowski, 1982). These external professional demands are fueled by the increased focus on malpractice litigation; the propensity of even the most competent of doctors to be sued exacerbates the internal personality pressures already operative.

Institutional pressures also play on this characteristic of self-doubt and generate role strain so that physicians believe that they must function at a maximum level of competence at all times (Roeske, 1981). The underlying message of institutional efforts to improve care, to encourage risk management education, to establish standards of practice, and to strengthen disciplinary actions against physicians is that "you (physicians) are not quite good enough."

Doctors' vulnerability to guilt feelings is exacerbated by any suggestion of failure. This often results in symptoms of anxiety, irritability, and depression and may be intensified when there is an *allusion* of fault (Krakowski, 1982). Clarke, in a study of neonatologists, found that it was extremely difficult for the latter to deal with the death of infants even though their patients were high risk and therefore likely to succumb (Clarke et al, 1984). To be sued for an event that has already been experienced as a personal failure and has already caused sleepless nights and emotional disruption further deepens the feelings of guilt.

Feelings of an exaggerated sense of responsibility are intensified by propatient developments that emphasize the concept of "shared responsibility." Theoretically, the doctor is absolved from complete responsibility as control over medical decisions is shared with patients. When an untoward outcome occurs, however, the weight of responsibility shifts to the doctor, the final determination of which is often played out in the courtroom. Doctors who hold themselves responsible even for events which they could not have foreseen and over which they could not possibly exert control find themselves in a bind between maintaining control and sharing it with their patients.

Practice situations over which doctors feel insufficient control often generate anxiety, especially among doctors who have already been sued (Charles, 1987). Emergency and high risk situations, therefore, can lead to behaviors that may not only be maladaptive but also a source of decreased competence or avoidant behaviors. These conceivably could generate greater problems and contribute to the development of a malpractice suit.

The Doctor–Patient Relationship and Litigation

Insurance and legal counsel, as well as many physicians, maintain that the failure of doctors to manage the relationship plays a significant role in a patient's decision to sue (Welch, 1975; Vacarrino, 1977; Wright, 1984). Among the few empirical studies, plastic surgeons showed no significant relationships between the time the surgeon spent with each patient, the physician–patient dialogue, the sharing of responsibility for decision making, and the number of times the surgeon had been sued for malpractice (Wright, 1980). Another study found that the performance of the variables they used to measure patient–doctor relationships had no significant direct bearing on decisions to sue or not sue (May and DeMarco, 1986). A major deterrent to establishing the facts about this subject is the admonishment not to discuss the case with anyone other than legal and insurance counsel in order to preserve the defensibility of the case. This, however, establishes a legal embargo on access to either party's experience until the action is resolved.

Not every doctor–patient dyad functions optimally. Most observers place the primary burden of responsibility for a satisfactory relationship on the doctor, and Katz's book on informed consent is among a number of recent publications that reassess their mode of relationship with patients (Katz, 1984).

This relationship is most stressed when a poor or untoward outcome occurs. Ideally, a full discussion should precede the event and anticipate any poor outcome, which may also diminish the doctor's exposure to litigation (Gutheil, 1984). What often occurs following an untoward event is that doctors react by increasing their hard work and perfectionistic behavior (Krakowski, 1982) and by engaging in distancing and withdrawal from the patient (McCue, 1982) rather than managing their own compulsive feelings and the negative feelings of the patient. Withdrawal of the physician at a time when the patient and/or family is most in need of a truthful explanation of an untimely death or complication is sometimes the first stimulus to legal action. The doctor should be available and accessible to the patient and the family and, for example, willing to make whatever fee adjustments or restitutions may be appropriate if this becomes an issue. The challenge to be forthright about problems that, foreseen or not, have arisen is especially threatening in some areas of the country in which legal action is often the first, rather than last, step in seeking redress. In these instances, the doctor can be forthright and honest about the source of the clinical problems and at the same time cognizant of the legal climate of medical practice.

The Meaning of the Event

Charges of negligence and incompetence are a direct assault on a professional's sense of self and integrity; as a result, they are disruptive to the sense of cohesiveness experienced in relationship to self and to others in the same social structure.

Doctors we have studied assigned to the event a variety of meanings that made the experience particularly stressful (Charles, in press). For some, it was that the plaintiff was a long-standing patient or relative of a friend so that a lawsuit was unanticipated. For others, it was the widespread publicity about the doctor's competence. For those whose suits were eventually dropped or settled for insignificant awards, the event was often perceived as a "nuisance" generating feelings of frustration and irritability.

The Degree of Control

The degree of control a person has over the event has been a factor used to determine or predict the degree of morbidity that results. Fairbank and Hough (1979) suggest that it is not the events that are beyond the individual's control that are linked with illness but rather those for which the person is partially responsible. Dohrenwend's work on stressful life events supports this conclusion (1974). In the case of litigation, the accusation suggests that the doctor is at fault while the doctor's defense is usually that the event was "beyond control." If a jury verdict against the doctor is the measure of "degree of control," our limited studies suggest that neither determines the illness outcome since the proportion of symptomatology between those who won and those who lost is not significant. The relationship between the stressor, the development of illness, and degree of control, while complex, may appear oversimplistic in the light of new discoveries of alterations in immunocompetence following stressful life events (Calabrese, 1987).

COPING WITH MALPRACTICE LITIGATION

The doctor's feeling of well-being is a key variable in determining the quality of care delivered to patients (Editorial, Family Practice, 1985). How the doctor reacts to and copes with the litigation experience, therefore, is of concern not only because of its negative impact on an individual doctor but also because of its long-term effects on the quality of health care.

Adaptive coping mechanisms commonly used by doctors in response to ordinary stressors include intellectual involvement in the subject matter, detached concern, suppression, and humor (Fox, 1979). McCue suggested that they emotionally withdraw from loved ones and isolate themselves from the non-medical world (McCue, 1982). Vaillant noted their use of reaction formation, hypochondriasis, and altruism (Vaillant, 1972). Some suggest that an individual's personality traits are the best predictor of coping response (Cohen and Lazarus, 1973). Situation-oriented researchers suggest that the wide range of coping strategies used are in large part a function of the specific stressor (Lazarus and Folkman, 1984). More recent empirical studies suggest that doctors do not cope in unique ways but use a variety of positive and negative mechanisms that vary from doctor to doctor (Krakowski, 1982; Linn et al, 1985).

Lazarus and Folkman's conceptualization of the coping process is useful in evaluating doctors' responses to litigation and identifying specific interventions. They describe two types of coping mechanisms which are both operative, the proportion of each determined in part by how the person appraises the stressor (Lazarus and Folkman, 1984). Emotion-focused coping consists of cognitive processes that are directed at lessening the emotional distress; it includes avoidance, minimization, distancing, selective attention, and wresting positive value from negative events. Their goal is to maintain hope and optimism. Problem-focused coping mechanisms are aimed at defining the problem, generating alternative solutions, choosing among them, and acting on them. Their goal is to change, or get rid of, the source of stress. How the doctor appraises the event is critical; that is, how the meaning and significance of the event is evaluated in terms of what might and can be done. If a situation is appraised as having few possibilities for change, coping mechanisms tend to be emotion-focused. If it is appraised as amenable to change, problem-focused coping predominates.

In our studies, those doctors who appraised litigation as the most stressful event in their entire life tended to use emotion-focused coping in contrast to those doctors who appraised it as stressful but not as much as some other life event (Charles, 1988). The former self-rated their coping responses as less effective than did the latter. This suggests that the relative stressfulness of litigation to other life events as well as the perception that "nothing can be done" about it is a critical factor for devising interventions.

EVALUATION AND TREATMENT OF THE SUED PHYSICIAN

An estimated 10 to 15 percent of sued doctors and/or their families will seek formal consultation with a psychiatrist. Another undetermined number will approach their psychiatric colleagues by utilizing the "curbstone" or hospital corridor mode of consultation. Others will contact medical and specialty society programs which use psychiatrists as consultants in efforts to provide social support for sued doctors. Underlying all these requests for help is the fact that litigation, as a lengthy process, requires varying degrees of personal involvement until it is resolved (see Table 2). In one study, 51.6 percent of sued doctors indicated that the entire process, or a combination of its stages, was most stressful while 20.3 percent mentioned the period surrounding notification of the suit and 15.6 percent identified the trial itself (Charles, 1988).

Informal Consultation with the Sued Doctor

The most common contact with sued physicians is a short informal conversation immediately following their receiving the summons and complaint or just prior to their going on trial. Psychiatrists should be aware of physicians' resistances and their tendency to minimize the extent of their symptomatology. Psychiatrists should be alert to the opportunity to encourage more formal consultation, if indicated.

Formal Psychiatric Consultation

This may consist of a well conducted evaluation that is in itself a therapeutic interview. It may comprise only one session in which primary goals are: the expression of empathy, supportive measures of ventilation, and strengthening and supporting of the doctor's ego-adaptive functioning. In addition to the routine evaluation, specific themes and areas of concern should be explored.

A Thorough Psychiatric History

Integral to this is a precise history of family illness, past and present medical history, past and present use of prescribed medications, past psychiatric consultation or treatment, and a history of recreational drugs and/or alcohol use. A thorough discussion of symptomatology should be included.

Personality Traits of the Physician-Patient

It is not uncommon for doctors to judge themselves harshly for failing in their treatment of a patient. The psychiatrist needs to clarify whether the guilt is real

Table 2.   The Litigation Process

- *The summons*—This formal legal document, issued by the clerk of the court and usually served by the sheriff, is notification that a suit has been filed.
- *The complaint*—This accompanies the summons and tells in legal terms the nature of the complaint. It may be preceded or followed by a notice in the local newspaper.
- *The pleading stage*—Shortly after the complaint is filed, the attorney begins to communicate with the court by filing *motions*, a request addressed to the court to do something.
- *The discovery stage*—A process designed to discover information relevant to the case. This includes *interrogatories* (written questions) and *depositions* (oral questions and verbal responses taken before a person empowered to take testimony under oath). The discovery may also request *inspection of documents* and/or *physical and mental examinations*. For the psychiatrist, this stage often raises conflicts about confidentiality issues.
- *Expert witnesses*—A case proceeds only if each side presents experts who will given an opinion about whether the facts relevant to the case represent a deviation from the accepted standard of medical care.
- *Summary judgment*—This is a decision entered by the judge when it is clear that all the facts indicate that one or other side of the case should win. If a judgment is issued, the case is resolved.
- *The trial*—This may be preceded by a series of pre-trial maneuvers which may or may not contribute to a resolution of the case by settlement or some other method. If these fail, the case goes to trial before a judge or a judge and jury as determined by laws in a given location.
- *The verdict*—This is the decision reached by the deciding body.
- *Posttrial activities*—If a participant fails to receive a favorable verdict, the law permits a number of procedures to appeal the outcome. A *posttrial motion* must be submitted within a prescribed period of time and is a request to the court to void the verdict usually on technical grounds. A formal *appeal* may also be initiated to overturn the verdict on legal grounds.

---

or neurotic. In doing so, objective data are not always immediately available because the accusation·generating the guilty feelings may take many years to resolve. If neurotic guilt is present, it can be explored and treated effectively. Psychiatrists, however, should not permit themselves to be manipulated into giving legal opinions about the degree of guilt at issue, particularly since legal guilt is not necessarily indicative of or equated with moral guilt.

If the doctor-patient appears to be actually responsible for the event in question, has been flagrantly negligent as confirmed by expert opinion, and has been advised to settle, the psychiatrist should help the doctor come to as realistic a decision as is possible about defending the case. A guilty physician does not make a good defendant in a deposition or at trial. If the case is defensible but the doctor's emotional state prohibits him or her from functioning well in court, the proceedings should either be delayed until the symptoms can be resolved in therapy or some other acceptable compromise can be effected.

Two potential outcomes of medical malpractice suits may be stimuli for psychiatric consultation. A doctor who has performed competently and responsibly may be urged to settle for very good economic and/or legal reasons. Although a settlement assesses no guilt and resolves the suit legally, it often prevents the doctor from feeling vindicated or absolved. As a result, many doctors continue to suffer from lingering feelings of guilt and shame which can no longer be resolved by any external action. In another scenario, a physician who loses at trial often tends to have persistent guilt feelings for a longer period of time than a physician who is vindicated.

Differential Diagnosis

The most commonly experienced illness suffered by sued doctors are the depression and the adjustment clusters described previously.

Although some have suggested that symptoms of posttraumatic stress disorder can occur, we have not found the full-blown syndrome in doctors we have studied. This may be related to the nature of the stressor, in that litigation is not associated with threat to one's physical person. This idea is supported by an epidemiologic study, which found that although some symptoms of posttraumatic stress disorder occurred commonly among the general population, the full syndrome was common only among veterans wounded in Vietnam (Helzer et al, 1987).

Based on our studies, drug and alcohol abuse as a response to litigation among physicians is infrequent (Charles, 1984, 1985, 1987). This may represent an underestimation and we have no firm data on substance abuse in these subjects prior·to litigation. There is no evidence that physician impairment plays a role in the etiology of a malpractice suit. Anecdotal evidence suggests that impaired physicians tend to see fewer patients and refrain from high-risk work in general so that their liability is less than that of the average well-functioning practitioner.

Suicide

The well-known data on suicide rates among physicians, including psychiatrists, are relevant (Rich and Pitts, 1980). The sketch of the suicide prone physician as one who seeks treatment for emotional problems, is depressed, has a history of physical and mental health problems, self-medicates or abuses drugs or alcohol, has suffered recent financial losses, and gives a history of difficult childhood and/or troubled family of origin, serves as a useful guideline (AMA Council on Scientific Affairs, 1987). The role of a malpractice suit in the final equation of a successful suicide is not well researched, although numerous anecdotal accounts have been documented. In the AMA/APA Physician Mortality Project, for example, the most common problem or loss *ever* experienced by these suicide victims was a malpractice claim (AMA Council on Scientific Affairs, 1985).

Changes in Practice Behaviors

The psychiatrist should document closely strategies the physician-patient has developed to deal with the anxieties generated by the suit, particularly those which directly affect patient care. In one of our studies, the number of practice changes introduced was significantly and positively correlated with the number of symptoms reported (Charles, 1988). Such changes, especially if related to a formerly satisfying aspect of medical practice, may generate role strain (Roeske, 1981), thus increasing the stressfulness of the doctor's daily practice.

Countertransference Awareness

Physician patients may contribute to burdensome feelings within the psychiatrist because they may demand greater attention and/or accountability. Conflicting with these are the positive feelings that arise from being chosen to treat a physician, especially one that is highly esteemed. Often the doctor-patient is presumed knowledgeable, so that portions of the history, psychiatric exam, or physical history may be insufficiently explored, overlooked, or avoided. Marzuk's (1987) review of how doctors manage issues of privacy, control, and supportiveness in reference to their physician-patients is pertinent.

The psychiatrist's preconceived notions about the meaning of being sued for malpractice are also relevant. Premature assumptions about the relative "guilt" of the accused doctor may confound the psychiatrist's unconscious attitudes toward the specific patient. Psychiatrists need to be cognizant of how closely their own personality traits resemble those of their colleagues, in whom self-criticism is often externalized as criticism of others. The sued doctor also represents a direct threat in that, as practicing physicians, psychiatrists are themselves vulnerable to the unanticipated malpractice suit. An informed construct of the malpractice problem, as well as healthy denial, can aid in maintaining the objectivity required to treat these physician-patients.

The Psychiatrist-Patient

Sued psychiatrists are more similar than dissimilar to their physician colleagues. Unlike the ordinary physician, the psychiatrist is more cognizant of transferences, especially negative ones, and is better equipped to deal with them directly. When a malpractice suit occurs, however, this same advantage becomes a liability. The psychiatrist is supposed to be the preeminent "manager" of the doctor–patient relationship. A malpractice suit, whatever its focus, represents a disruption in that relationship and a narcissistic failure for the psychiatrist.

Treatment Considerations

Pharmacological and/or psychotherapeutic treatment may be indicated. Although not explored in this chapter, marital and family problems resulting from the litigation experience may also require specific referrals. Conditions necessitating immediate referral include severe depression, suicidal ideation, a major psychiatric illness, or alcohol or drug abuse. The psychiatrist may also play a principal role in enabling the physician to obtain an appropriate medical referral, especially when resistance is evident.

Psychotherapy

This is especially indicated for those physicians for whom the stress of litigation activates latent conflicts and/or pathology and in whom the stress response syndrome persists. Although not confined to the psychotherapeutic process, Horowitz has identified at least nine themes common to the working-through phase subsequent to a serious life event (Horowitz, 1986). At least six of these provide the basis for understanding themes frequently expressed by sued doctors in psychotherapy.

Fears of Being Sued Again

This is expressed as anxiety related to specific practice behaviors, specific kinds of patients or diagnostic conditions, or conditions of treatment, such as covering for another doctor. Phobic responses resulting in defensive maneuvers can also create new stresses and retard rather than promote resolution of the doctor's conflicts about litigation.

Shame and Rage Over Vulnerability

Omnipotence as well as active fantasies and universal hope are important psychological factors within the doctor's usual mode of operation. For the sued physician, failure to control the event in question is also a source of shame and rage.

Rage at the Source

Most commonly, sued doctors express rage at the disparity between the ideal and the real expectations in medical practice and at the legal system that regulates that practice. The ideal of medicine is often complicated by intrusions and demands from third parties, and pressures to share authority with the patient within an expanding and unchangeable body of legal rules and responsibilities.

Rage at Those Exempted

Doctors often feel that the demands placed on them by the "system" are more burdensome and that they are held to a higher standard than are other members of society. The attitude of doctors who have never been sued complicates these angry feelings. Non-sued doctors tend to feel, consonant with commonly held perceptions, that litigation is generally warranted by the accused doctor (Charles, 1985). Their need to feel that good practice and good relationships are an effective protective measure makes them "different" from sued doctors, and they often communicate that feeling of superiority to sued colleagues. The perceptions of non-sued physicians change once they themselves are sued, however (Wilbert et al, 1987).

Fear of Loss of Control Over, and Guilt or Shame Resulting From, Aggressive Impulses

This conflict often emerges after a poor outcome or death. The "power" the doctor possesses to do harm as well as good may arise from the same behavior.

Table 3. Selected Coping Responses to Litigation

Source of Stress	Coping Response
The legal system	Become informed about its nature and function. Participate in organized medical efforts to address inequities in the system.
The malpractice complaint	Seek consultation with insurer and legal counsel. Discuss with select peers, spouse, family, and/or staff. If the complaint or some further stage of litigation generates unusual emotional disequilibrium, rearrange office hours, cancel surgery or other procedures for as long as necessary.
Unpredictability in the process	Become acquainted with the legal process and the role of the defendant in the process through consultation with legal counsel and pertinent literature. Participate in mock depositions and trials. Participate in choice of defense experts.
Specific coping mechanisms	Healthy denial and suppression enable the doctor to continue daily work obligations. Engagement in emotion-focused coping expressed as "take one day at a time," "don't let it bother me," "develop an attitude about it," "rationalize it." Engagement in problem-focused coping expressed by implementing control measures as described below, as well as "doing what my lawyer says to do," "try to deal directly with the case."
Control issues in professional life	Review office procedures and make changes which would promote better organization and communication. Review communication processes in place with nurses and staff and change as indicated. Participate in risk management courses. Develop printed procedural forms, such as for informed consent, if indicated. Pay careful attention to record-keeping procedures. Do not practice in situations that tend to compromise personal ethics or standards. Re-evaluate the time related to patient care. This may mean either an increase or decrease of time with each patient depending on the respective needs of patient and doctor. Observe whether any changes have occurred in relating to patients as a result of litigation. Work to neutralize negative feelings. Do not work with patients who create increased anxiety for the defendant during the litigation period.

Table 3. Selected Coping Responses to Litigation (*continued*)

Source of Stress	Coping Response
Control issues in professional life (continued)	Re-evaluate the use of time in medical practice. Is there sufficient time allotted for patient care, record work, continuing education, and time away?
	Work to continue in development of competence. It is a balm to sagging self-esteem?
	Arrange practice to be as manageable and anxiety-free as is possible.
Control issues in personal life	Re-evaluate amount of leisure time and its scheduling.
	Examine the impact of the event on marital and family relationships and take steps to remedy.
	Consult on financial planning and discuss family goals.
	Seek medical consultation if physical symptomatology occurs or persists.
	Seek psychiatric consultation if symptoms or persistence of symptoms warrants it.
	Observe personal use of alcohol and/or self-administered drugs during the period of litigation and seek aid if indicated.
	Schedule "non-working" vacations with spouse/family/ friends.
	Engage in active sports on a regularly scheduled basis.
Control issues related to the process	Become actively involved in the defense of the case.
	Review depositions, especially those of expert testimony.
	Study the literature as it relates to the case at issue.
Social support	Discuss feelings with those with whom you feel most comfortable.
	Understand the concern of legal counsel and the bar to communication about the litigation event. Attorneys counsel their clients not to discuss the case so as not to jeopardize defense. Social support involves discussion of *feelings* about the event.
	If social support is unavailable on an informal basis, seek support from local hospital and medical society organizations.

A given medication may contribute either to a cure or to a disabling side effect. This conflict is exacerbated when a lawsuit follows one of these events.

Sadness Over Losses

The common losses include reputation, referrals, and feelings of self-confidence, as well as those associated with the disruption of personal and professional relationships. The single most common loss is expressed as "medicine isn't fun anymore." This leads to conflicts about changing specialty, early retirement, or to feelings of demoralization.

Psychiatrists as Consultants to Medical Organizations

The emphasis is on developing organized responses to the emotional impact of litigation on the membership. This may include presentations on exploring feelings associated with litigation, stress reduction measures, and effective coping responses to litigation, such as those specifically listed in Table 3. Psychiatrists may also participate in the development of audiovisual aids for educational purposes.

The Development of Support Groups

Model groups have been designed to provide social support for sued doctors within the medical community. These responses may include the development of panels of sued physicians and/or spouses available for informal support, formalized and regularly scheduled educational meetings, and programs designed to explain and provide interventions for the specific stress of litigation. Such efforts by organized medical groups have played a major role in giving tacit permission for doctors to talk about their feelings informally with their peers. In our experience doctors tend not to want involvement in ongoing support groups. This appears related to the increasing willingness of doctors to make themselves available to their sued peers as well as to the intermittent nature of litigation. It also reflects the use of healthy denial so that the sued doctor can continue to work effectively and thereby maintain and increase self-esteem.

CONCLUSION

As the number of physicians sued for malpractice continues to escalate, the role of the psychiatrist in providing support, evaluation, and therapy has also expanded. The goal of the psychiatrist is to provide, against a background of knowledge and understanding, a resource for enabling doctors to effectively work through the stress of litigation so that they can return as rapidly as possible to their work of providing competent and compassionate health care.

REFERENCES

AMA Council on Scientific Affairs: Panel on Physician Mortality, Preliminary Report, May 1985

AMA Council on Scientific Affairs: Results and implication of the AMA/APA Physician Mortality Project: stage II. JAMA 1987; 257:2949–2953

American Psychiatric Association: Diagnostic and Statistical Manual of Mental Disorders, Third Edition, Revised (DSM-III-R). Washington, DC, American Psychiatric Association, 1987

Anwar RA: A longitudinal study of residency-trained emergency physicians. Ann Emerg Med 1983; 12:2024–2055

Bowen OR: Report of the Task Force on Medical Liability and Malpractice. Washington, DC, Department of Health and Human Services, August, 1987

Calabrese JR, Kling MA, Gold PW: Alterations in immunocompetence during stress, bereavement, and depression. Am J Psychiatry 1987; 144:1123–1134

Carlova J: A new and growing malpractice threat. Medical Economics, Oct. 17, 1983

Charles SC, Wilbert JR, Kennedy EC: Physicians' self-reports of reactions to malpractice litigation. Am J Psychiatry 1984; 141:563–565

Charles SC, Wilbert JR, Franke KJ: Sued and non-sued physicians self-reported reactions to malpractice litigation. Am J Psychiatry 1985; 142:437–440

Charles SC, Warnecke RB, Wilbert JR, et al: Sued and non-sued physicians: satisfactions, dissatisfactions, and sources of stress. Psychosomatics 1987; 29:462–468

Charles SC, Pyskoty CE, Nelson A: Physicians on trial: self-reported reactions to malpractice trials with a comparison to previous studies. West J Med 1988; 148:358–360

Charles SC, Warnecke RB, Nelson A, et al: Appraisal of the event: a factor in coping with malpractice litigation. Behav Med (in press)

Clarke TA, Maniscalco WM, Taylor-Brown, et al: Job satisfaction and stress among neonatologists. Pediatrics 1984; 74:52–57

Cohen F. Lazarus RS: Active coping processes, coping dispositions, and recovery from surgery. Psychosom Med 1973; 35:375–389

Danzon PM: The frequency and severity of medical malpractice claims: Rand Study R–2870–ICJ. Santa Monica, CA, Rand Corporation, 1982

Danzon PM: Medical Malpractice. Cambridge, MA, Harvard University Press, 1985

Dohrenwend BS, Dohrenwend BP: Stressful Life Events: Their Nature and Effects. New York, John Wiley & Sons, 1974

Editorial: Quantity versus quality: is stress the link? Fam Pract 1985; 2:125–126

Fairbank DT, Hough RL: Life event classification and event-illness relationship. J Human Stress 1979; 5:41–47

Fox RC: The Human Condition of Health Professionals. Durham, University of New Hampshire, Nov. 19, 1979

Gabbard GO: The role of compulsiveness in the normal physician. JAMA 1985; 254:2926–2929

Gutheil TG, Bursztajn H, Brodsky A: Malpractice prevention through the sharing of uncertainty. N Engl J Med 1984; 311:49–51

Helzer JE, Robins LN, McEvoy L: Post-traumatic stress disorder in the general population: findings of the epidemiologic catchment area survey. N Engl J Med 1987; 317:1630–1633

Horowitz MJ: Stress Response Syndromes. Northvale, NJ, Jason Aronson 1986

Illinois State Medical Inter-Insurance Exchange: Loss Analysis Report, January, 1988

Jones RE: A study of 100 physician psychiatric inpatients. Am J Psychiatry 1977; 134:1119–1123

Katz J: The Silent World of Doctor and Patient. New York, The Free Press, 1984

Keeton W: Prosser and Keeton on the Law of Torts, 5th ed. St. Paul, MN, West Publishing Co., 1984

Krakowski AJ: Stress and the practice of medicine, II: stressors, stresses and strains. Psychother Psychosom 1982; 38:11–23

Lazarus RS, Folkman S: Stress, Appraisal, and Coping. New York, Springer Publishing Co., 1984

Linn LS, Yager J, Cope D, et al: Health status, job satisfaction, job stress, and life satisfaction among academic and clinical faculty. JAMA 1985; 254:2775–2782

Marzuk PM: When the patient is a physician. N Engl J Med 1987; 317:1409–1411

Mawardi BH: Satisfactions, dissatisfactions, and causes of stress in medical practice. JAMA 1979; 24:1483–1486

May ML, DeMarco L: Patients and doctors disputing: patients' complaints and what they do about them. Working paper #7–7, Disputes Processing Research Program. University of Wisconsin at Madison, 1986

McCranie EW, Hornsby JL, Calvert JC: Practice and career satisfaction among residency trained family physicians: a national survey. J Fam Pract 1982; 14:1107–1114

McCue JD: The effects of stress on physicians and their medical practice. N Engl J Med 1982; 306:458–463

Mechanic D: The organization of medical practice and practice orientations among physicians in prepaid and nonprepaid primary care settings. Med Care 1975; 13:189–204

Pearson MM, Strecker EA: Physicians as psychiatric patients: private practice experience. Am J Psychiatry 1960; 116:915–919

Rapp JA, Rapp RT (Eds): Illinois Medical Malpractice: A Guide for the Health Sciences. St. Louis, MO, C.V. Mosby Co., 1988

Rich CL, Pitts FN: Suicide by psychiatrists: a study of medical specialists among 18,730 consecutive physician deaths during a five-year period. J Clin Psychiatry 1980; 41:261–263

Roeske NC: Stress and the physician. Psychiatric Annals 1981; 11:245–258

Schwartz B: The Law in America. New York, McGraw-Hill, 1974

Sonderby M: Relevant ramblings. Cook County Jury Verdict Reporter, May, 1987

U.S. General Accounting Office: Medical Malpractice: A Framework for Action. GAO/HRD–87–73. Washington, DC, U.S. General Accounting Office, May, 1987

Vacarrino JM: Malpractice: the problem in perspective. JAMA 1977; 238:861–863

Vaillant GE, Sobowale NC, McArthur C: Some psychological vulnerabilities of physicians. N Engl J Med 1972; 287:372–375

Valko RJ, Clayton PJ: Depression in the internship. Diseases of the Nervous System 1975; 36:26–29

Welch CE: Medical malpractice. N Engl J Med 1975; 292:1372–1376

Wilbert JR, Charles SC, et al: Coping with the stress of malpractice litigation. Illinois Medical Journal 1987; 171:23–27

Wright MR: Self-perception of the elective surgeon and some patient perception correlates. Archives of Otolaryngology 1980; 460–465

Wright MR: The elective surgeon's reaction to change and conflict. Archives of Otolaryngology 1984; 110:318–322

Chapter 27

Treatment of Violent Patients: Concerns for the Psychiatrist

William H. Reid, M.D., M.P.H.

This chapter is intended to provide practical guidelines for the treatment and management of several kinds of violent patients. It is based on the assumption that the clinician who considers and/or uses these guidelines already understands the diagnostic and basic treatment concepts common to psychiatry, and that he or she will consult additional references (such as those at the end of the chapter) for more detailed information.

An important caveat regarding violence: "Violence" is a generic term which describes a *behavior*, not a diagnosis, disorder, or character style. One cannot treat all violent patients alike any more than one can treat all patients who complain of abdominal pain alike. Nevertheless, many violent people have psychiatric or neuropsychiatric disorders which respond to—and deserve—treatment, and many such persons must be "managed" (as differentiated from "treated") as well.

ETIOLOGY AND PSYCHOPATHOLOGY OF VIOLENCE

It is impossible to describe here the many sources, psychodynamics, and social correlates of violent behavior. We will, however, discuss three etiologic *schemata*: 1) violence due to intolerance of affect; 2) violence as a "best-choice" behavior; and 3) violence due to absence of capacity for alternative nonviolent behavior or communication.

It is important to note that not all violence seen in psychiatric settings is directly related to psychiatric disorders. Simple criminal behavior, for example, and violence used for material gain, should not be diagnosed or treated as emotional illness.

Reactions to staff or milieu in a psychiatric hospital or other institution, even in the presence of psychiatric illness, may not be related to that illness. A patient who is assaulted by staff forcing medication—rare in modern U.S. and Canadian facilities—or a teenager who is confined on a small, locked unit may strike out at others or at objects in the environment. Inpatients or jail inmates may become violent in trying to elope from the institution, or upon being caught. Certain cultures and subcultures expect or condone either outright violence or violent-appearing posturing, which can be mistaken for a psychiatric disorder in the hospital setting.

Intolerance of Affect

One of the most striking functionally based (as contrasted with neurologic dyscontrol) sources of violence is assault to defend oneself against intolerable affect or narcissistic threat. The person may rapidly turn from normal, obsequious behavior to dangerous rage.

HUMILIATION/NARCISSISTIC INJURY.   Many males, in particular, inwardly struggle to maintain an acceptable balance between repugnant (to them) dependent longings or questioned masculinity on the one hand, and feelings of competence and strength on the other. While this is most obvious when it is projected in paranoid defenses, it is present in others as well.

> A 50-year-old Black man was a leader among his peers and had a reputation for sexual prowess. His 27-year-old wife left him and began divorce proceedings. He was despondent over the loss, and begged her several times to return. Each time, she belittled him. On the day that the divorce papers appeared in his mailbox, he sought her out and she bragged that she had cuckolded him.
>
> He was enraged, and had a shotgun nearby. He got the gun, and in view of witnesses pointed it at her. She continued to express her derision, thinking he would not shoot, even daring him to do so. He told her several times to "stop saying that," then shot her repeatedly. He left, drove around for awhile, and returned home to wait for the police. He was completely sober throughout the incident, and had no known psychiatric history.

The absence of any opportunity to "back down" gracefully, or of alternative ways to handle extreme anxiety, coupled with a victim who does not realize the danger of "pushing things too far," can be lethal. The humiliation of such a challenge to a fragile self-image may make destruction of the challenger—and thus symbolic removal of the inner threat as well—more acceptable than physical or emotional retreat.[1]

Other affects that are often difficult to tolerate and that may give rise to violence include severe depression and fear, particularly when either reaches delusional proportions.

"Best-Choice" Behavior

Sometimes violence is an acceptable best choice among several uncomfortable or untenable alternatives. Settings of war or rational defense of one's self or family are common examples in Western culture. Every culture and subgroup seems to have some level of acceptable or expected violence to self or others, sometimes against its own members (as for food or choice of mate) and sometimes against outsiders (as related to cultural preservation or xenophobia). Discussions of these are usually in philosophical or moral contexts, although social scientists may describe them as "psychological" (compare racial or religious conflict).

Limited Capacity for Nonviolent Alternatives

This premise implies that alternatives to violence are almost always better than violence itself. Most anthropologists believe that injury to others of a species, except for culling when survival resources are limited, is wasteful and evolutionarily discouraged. Indeed, many species other than man handle even mating and warlike conflict with show and posturing, stopping short of actual combat.

---

[1]Herbert Thomas, M.D., a New York psychoanalyst, was first to describe this intolerance of narcissistic challenge as a major cause of domestic and "barroom" violence.

At the highest levels of some Eastern martial arts, it is not uncommon for exceedingly capable competitors to face each other, sense who will be the victor, and accept the inevitable outcome without fighting.

Some people appear never to learn behaviors or communication styles that can take the place of violence in threatening or challenging situations. Socially, violence may be a way of life, a way of getting things not otherwise attainable. One's early role models may have been violent, or there may have been a poor repertoire of nonviolent alternatives in the developmental milieu. Conversely, the developmental milieu (that is, parenting environment) may have responded inadequately to the child's attempts at nonviolent defense mechanisms and alternatives during early growth.

Previously existing nonviolent alternatives may be lost, temporarily or permanently, to physical or psychosocial factors. These include toxins of various kinds, intoxicants, disinhibiting drugs, extraordinary stresses in the environment (including the humiliation mentioned above), and brain illness or injury.

Congenital or biogenetic absence of the capacity to develop controls or more adaptive coping mechanisms during early life is a third class of incapacity for nonviolent alternatives. Such persons might be limbically impaired, mentally retarded (although intelligence alone is an incomplete predictor, and retardation should not be considered a precursor to violence), or otherwise predisposed to a neuropsychiatric disorder.

GENERAL TREATMENT AND MANAGEMENT CONSIDERATIONS

Treatment Settings and Resources

For a variety of reasons, many treatment settings for violent patients are in the so-called "public sector." When the treatment is specifically aimed at violence, the patient may have legal entanglements, be in a correctional (or probation) setting, or have sufficient problems with society that he or she cannot afford private care. In addition, private clinics and hospitals often prefer not to treat such patients, and/or merely manage their care until they can be safely discharged or transferred.

Treatment must frequently be carried out in a restrictive setting. The clinician is at once helped and hindered by measures of containment and protection, but in any case must be comfortable treating a patient who may not be able to move about freely. The restrictions may be legal and administrative as well as physical.

Emergency evaluation and intervention, for acute violent behavior or patients known to be potentially violent, usually takes place in an emergency room or detention facility. Occasionally, a patient seen in a mental health clinic or private office becomes violent, or reveals that violence is a problem.

Funding for treatment of violent patients is usually of low political priority, in spite of social attention paid to violence and its effects. It is frustrating to hear on the one hand a great cry for someone to "do something" about violence and know that many forms are amenable to treatment, and on the other hand to realize that the criers do not want to spend tax dollars to search for or implement effective treatment. Some of the reasons for this are discussed later in this chapter.

Although rarely addressed in the literature, outpatient settings can be effective and safe for many patients with histories of violence. In some cases, these are federal, state, or county aftercare centers or special "violence clinics." In others, they are simply offices or clinics where a variety of patients are seen, some of whom have been violent, unexpectedly become violent, or have a potential for violence. In addition, any psychiatric setting is vulnerable to nonpredicted violent or assaultive behavior by patients. Clinician and staff should be reasonably prepared for such a possibility.

Treatment Modalities

Both the public and mental health professionals often see violence simplistically, as determined and shaped by only a few etiologic factors. Social scientists are fond of reducing violence to dichotomies or trichotomies, such as "instrumental versus expressive." Psychiatrists are sometimes asked by courts or journalists to explain violent behavior in a few easy-to-understand words.

Useful understanding of violence may take such descriptive or phenomenologic concepts into account; however, the *biopsychosocial* framework of diagnosis is extremely important. Evaluation of violence, whether as a primary symptom or an accompaniment for any of over two dozen psychiatric disorders, demands medical, psychological, and social understanding of the patient (Reid, 1988; Reid and Balis, 1987).

The treatment of violent patients, with the possible exception of those with characterologic antisocial behavior, is more often successful than not, at least in the short run. The following pages will discuss several treatment approaches, and some of the syndromes for which they are often helpful.

One should note that these are not specific, unitary approaches. Medication, for example, is not given in a therapeutic vacuum; nor is even the strictest behavioral paradigm used in a sterile, laboratory setting. Rather, each is an important part of a biopsychosocial concept. Whenever one omits one or two of "bio-," "psycho-," or "social," treatment response and prognosis suffer.

Unfortunately, some disorders have no effective treatment. Still others have no treatment that is socially or financially acceptable. Many of these are best described as *Diagnostic and Statistical Manual of Mental Disorders, Third Edition, Revised (DSM-III-R)* "v-code" behaviors (American Psychiatric Association, 1987). Nevertheless, this author believes it is very important to focus on what we *can* accomplish, and counter some of the pessimism associated with such patients.

ORGANIC/BIOLOGICAL TREATMENTS. The most common organic treatments are medications. Others include electroconvulsive therapy and neurosurgery.

Acute Violence. Calmatives and sedatives control acute violence with minimal masking of other symptoms or complicating of functional or organic disorders. Short-acting barbiturates are often an excellent choice, provided one understands that the dose should be enough to sedate the patient (lower doses may merely disinhibit him or her [Tupin, 1985]). Sedative benzodiazepines may be equally effective and easier to metabolize; paradoxical rage associated with the benzodiazepines appears to be rare and perhaps overreported.

The sedative and nonsedative neuroleptics (for example, chlorpromazine, haloperidol, thiothixene) should not be used as calmatives unless the violence is known to be related to a neuroleptic-responsive condition such as schizophrenia or mania. These drugs have long half-lives, mask many medical symptoms, and have more side and adverse effects (which may mimic symptoms of schizophrenia or depression) than the barbiturates or benzodiazepines.

Neuroleptics are indicated in violence created by schizophreniform or affective psychosis and, in smaller amounts, may be helpful in organic psychosis as well. The dosage should be commensurate with rapid control; however, one must remember the potential for toxicity (particularly in older or hepatically compromised patients) and adverse effects.

Low-dose regimens are generally as effective as high doses—such as the "rapid neuroleptization" approach (Donlon et al, 1979)—in early control of psychotic symptoms (Reid, 1988). The high-dose proponents recommend the larger amounts (up to 100 mg haloperidol or its equivalent in 5–10 mg increments over 12 hours) for prompt control in emergencies. Caution should be exercised with regard to side and adverse effects and masking of undiagnosed medical illness. Combining a nonsedating neuroleptic with a benzodiazepine such as lorazepam (Salzman et al, 1986) decreased the total amount of neuroleptic needed.

Any medication, but particularly injected ones and those likely to be uncomfortable for the patient, should be given in an atmosphere of humanity and respect. An offer to give it orally (crushed or in liquid form) should be made if feasible, especially if the violence is imminent rather than already under way. One should remember the psychodynamics of misperceived assault or rape that can accompany forced injections.

Electroconvulsive therapy (ECT) is a safe, usually effective treatment for catatonic excitement. A more extensive discussion of pharmacologic and nonpharmacologic emergency treatment may be found in the *American Psychiatric Association Annual Review*, Volume 6 (Soloff, 1987).

Chronic Control and Prevention. One usually does not wish to continue to use barbiturate or benzodiazepine sedation for ongoing control of violent potential. There is no "antiviolence" drug that is specific for severe aggression. Chronic medication is appropriate insofar as it addresses some direct or indirect cause of violent behavior. Thus maintenance neuroleptics are important in thought disorder, antidepressants or ECT in severe or psychotic depression, anticonvulsants (especially carbamazepine) in ictal or quasi-ictal syndromes (Stone et al, 1986), and lithium carbonate (often with other medications) in bipolar disorder and some organic affective disorders.

Neurologic and metabolic sources of violence, particularly ego-dystonic or episodic rage syndromes, are more frequent than commonly assumed, and must be diligently sought during evaluation. Elliott (1988) discusses many of these (such as unusual reactions to alcohol, temporal lobe epilepsy, residual "minimal brain dysfunction," and head injury) in a recent paper. Hypoglycemic episodes are well documented in some cases; blood glucose levels should be assayed as soon as possible after the violent behavior, and specific tests of blood insulin and hypoglycemic response to fasting are recommended (not merely short glucose tolerance tests).

Lithium carbonate has demonstrated effectiveness in decreasing assaults in nonpsychiatric (prison) populations. It is not considered acceptable at this time solely for control of violent behavior, in the absence of other clinical indications (for example, affective disorder, mood swings), however.

Propranolol has been successful in controlling episodic rage and violence syndromes that appear to be associated with organic central nervous system (CNS) trauma or dysfunction (Silver and Yudofsky, 1985). It should be prescribed with attention to medical contraindications and side effects, which may not be familiar to some psychiatrists. Caution should be exercised if propranolol is mixed with neuroleptics, especially thioridazine, as plasma levels of both neuroleptics and anticonvulsants may increase significantly. Cardiac and respiratory side effects of propranolol may also be increased in the presence of neuroleptics (Silver and Yudofsky, 1985).

Carbamazepine may be tried when organic CNS deficit is suspected or confirmed, even in the absence of evidence for epileptiform discharges. Phenytoin is useful less often. L-tryptophan, a serotonin precursor, is safe and sometimes effective in the uncontrollable, primitive assaultive and self-injurious behavior seen in very regressed schizophrenics and the severely mentally retarded. It should be prescribed in doses up to 2–4 grams per day, with attention to possible sedation.

Hormonal approaches may be used for at least two forms of violence. Medroxyprogesterone acetate (MPA) and cyproterone acetate (CPA) are both effective in reduction of sexual violence, including that associated with rape and sexual predation. Neither has become popular in the U.S. (where only MPA is available for general prescription), for reasons that are probably more social and political than clinical. A review published several years ago by Bradford (1983) remains an excellent source of information about the benefits, risks, and special considerations of antiandrogen drug therapy, including issues of informed consent, complex endocrinologic responses, and the unlikely possibility of irreversible effects. "Birth control" drugs may be useful in women with menstrual cycle-related (not just premenstrual) violence.

Methylphenidate, but not other stimulants, has some use in adolescents who have difficulty controlling violent impulses or rage, when it can be shown that the syndrome is related to an attention deficit disorder or similar CNS deficit. It has been tried with so-called "adult hyperactivity," often with disappointing results. Other stimulants, including the amphetamines, have not been prescribed extensively for violent adolescents, although their use in younger children is well established. Pediatric regimens will not be discussed in this chapter.

BEHAVIORAL TREATMENT/MANAGEMENT. Behavioral paradigms in experienced hands are often very successful at shaping human behavior over short periods. The primary issues with regard to practical clinical treatment have to do with 1) recognizing the behaviors (and their antecedents) upon which to focus the treatment; 2) generalizing the usually good results of, for example, conditioning approaches to noninstitutional environments; and 3) preventing the extinguishing of treatment results.

Behavioral analysis, to locate and define behavioral and environmental antecedents and reinforcers, is a complex task which often requires special expertise. The analysis may uncover obvious—or very subtle—precipitants which can be seen and avoided or changed by the patient or those around him. For example:

A muscular 17-year-old Caucasian patient assumes a frightening posture when confronted, yelling, "Get away from me." In examining a behavioral log with his therapist, he accepts the possibility that he does this in order to protect others from his own dyscontrol problem. His ability to hurt others is frightening to him, but he has no good adaptive behaviors in his repertoire for avoiding violence. From time to time his way of *avoiding* violence actually *encourages* it, from adolescents who do not want to give in to his threat, from parents or the police who try to meet challenge with force, and from psychiatric ward staff who are fearful and feel they must control him rather than leave him alone.

Examining a behavioral log helps the patient see the process and consequences of his or her behavior after it has passed. Work with patient and family increases the chance that the patient will use other, less frightening means to avoid hurting others, and that they will be able to back away when he or she assumes an aggressive posture.

Violence, like other behaviors and symptoms, is sometimes rewarding. It may bring capitulation and respect from others, or relief from responsibilities. It becomes part of one's identity, and any change is experienced as a significant loss. Thus return of the symptom, even when it is psychosocial and not neurological, is likely after treatment is over.

Various means have been tried for retaining treatment gains. One of the most successful is psychotherapy that focuses upon showing the patient his gains, helping him see the advantages of his nonviolent life, helping him discover and deal with the rewarding aspects of his former violence, exposing his denial of those rewards or of ways in which the violence was hurting himself and others, and reminding him of the consequences (for example, arrest, divorce, harm to loved ones) of his violence.

Continuing behavioral treatment after the formal clinical work is over is also useful. "Homework" assignments, instructions for "booster" sessions of behavioral therapy at home, or simple reminders such as snapping a rubber band on one's wrist all reinforce the treatment process and may prevent relapse until the new, nonviolent behavior has become a way of life.

A 33-year-old Caucasian pedophile responded well to therapy (described below) for his sexual impulse control disorder. Treated as an outpatient, he finished the strictly behavioral parts of therapy and met with a therapy group weekly. He was surprised when the group expressed disbelief at his statements that he was "completely cured," but listened as patients whose behavior had been similar to his own talked of having to find ways to divert occasional pedophilic fantasies. Forced to consider rationally the possibility and consequences of failure, he and his wife became more open about his earlier "secret" impulses, and he used previously assigned "covert sensitization" techniques at home to gain confidence in his ability to control them.

The most successful behavioral programs try to control all aspects of the patient's stimulus environment and all sources of reinforcement. Since this is quite difficult and expensive, one tends to find such paradigms in inpatient settings, often those specializing in intermediate or long-term care. Attempts to use strict conditioning methods on general psychiatric units, or in acute care hospitals (which may have significant staff turnover or frequent use of "pool" personnel) often fail from lack of the required very consistent environment.

Certain behavioral approaches are a treatment of choice for violence associated with sexual deviance. Abel and colleagues (1984, 1985) have established a combination of structured behavioral, social, and psychotherapeutic modules which include covert sensitization, masturbatory satiation, social skills training, assertiveness training, cognitive restructuring, and sex education.

PSYCHOTHERAPIES. Psychotherapy is useful in two broad ways. It may address the violence directly, or it may augment the effects of other treatments.

If the source of violent behavior is a neurotic or characterologic maladaptation or lack of more emotionally efficient defenses, psychotherapy is indicated, provided the patient is motivated and otherwise qualified for this kind of approach.

> A 31-year-old Caucasian woman was convicted of plotting to kill her husband. History revealed an extraordinarily chaotic and deprived childhood which she had overcome with some success, in part by becoming very active in agencies rescuing children from abusive settings. After a series of particularly gruesome cases, in which the children were severely injured and many of the perpetrators escaped prosecution, she developed a strong suspicion—later shown to be unfounded— that her husband was abusing their young child. She contracted to have him killed.
>
> There was no personal or family history of psychosis. Many primitive narcissistic, borderline, and hysteroid traits were present, which, although psychiatrically obvious, had not interfered markedly in her work or marriage except as sporadic outbursts of unreasonable temper toward her husband. She was verbal, had made several worthwhile attempts to clarify her past (much of which had been suppressed), was able to ponder some psychodynamic material without overwhelming anxiety, and appeared highly motivated for change. Psychoanalytic psychotherapy was recommended as a condition of probation.

In situations of violence or antisocial behavior, the public has a right to expect that some control will be exerted over the patient if he or she is allowed to remain outside an institution. This often is accomplished by means of a probation or parole requirement to attend sessions (and/or take medication and comply with other treatment recommendations).

Most psychotherapists have been taught that the patient must be treated voluntarily. It is now clear, however, that considerable change can often be accomplished in mandated therapy settings. The patient is sometimes unable to tell himself or his peers that he needs treatment, and quietly welcomes an "excuse"—such as a probation requirement—to come to therapy.

For others, the sessions the patient is required to attend can skillfully be used to develop a therapeutic relationship and show the patient that he or she has something to gain by continuing. Some therapists tell their patients in mandated psychotherapy: "You're here; and I'll certify that you've met your requirement. Now that that's out of the way, how can we use the rest of the time we have today?"

Psychotherapy to augment behavioral or organic treatment is important in a wide variety of settings. As already implied, the patient's violence is a part of his life, even if it is ego-dystonic in most respects. It is part of his identity, and it has brought obvious or subtle rewards. In addition, organic treatments, especially, have side effects or adverse effects which mitigate against compliance. Finally, the patient, like all patients with chronic disorders, wants very much to feel "cured," and no longer have any accoutrements of "sickness."

All of these make a consistent, continuing therapeutic relationship with the patient an irreplaceable part of comprehensive psychiatric care. Even if we had some "antiviolence pill," it would not be taken for long without psychotherapeutic support to help the patient adapt to his new lifestyle and make sense of his past.

A word about the qualifications of the therapist: In today's world of cost containment and occasional lowest-common-denominator counseling, the therapist for violent patients must be chosen with care. These patients carry a great risk of countertransference problems (for both patient and therapist), unusually serious consequences for therapeutic misjudgment, and psychodynamic issues that are often different from those usually seen in counseling centers or outpatient practices. If the psychiatrist conducts the therapy, he or she should be experienced and aware of these issues (or should request supervision from a colleague). If he or she refers the patient to someone else, the psychiatrist has an obligation to know something of the second therapist's qualifications.

SOCIAL/ENVIRONMENTAL TREATMENT/MANAGEMENT. The physical and emotional environment plays a large part in precipitating many forms of violence, and can control or prevent it as well. The concept of preventive environments implies avoiding emotional or physical precipitants such as certain kinds of family conflict, alcohol, or drugs which may have a disinhibiting effect, or even idiosyncratic triggers such as specific sights or sounds.

Containing environments are those which prevent the person from acting violently (or at least injuring himself or others). They include secure psychiatric settings, jails, and prisons, and the restraint and seclusion options each may exercise. Chemical restraint is possible in hospitals, and should be differentiated from other roles of medication in the therapeutic environment. Containment may at times also be therapeutic, especially for children and adolescents, but its primary purpose is protection of others through lack of opportunity to act upon the violent impulse, not change of the behavior or its source.

Monitoring environments allow some freedom of movement and other activity while retaining the ability to easily discover and/or prevent inappropriate behavior. Many psychiatric units and correctional settings have this option, the simplest being observation of the potentially violent person. More sophisticated monitoring can be accomplished by such things as electronic transmitters which report, for example, whether one has left home or the probation area.

Monitors may be seen as a form of external conscience or control for people whose internal ones cannot be trusted. Monitoring environments are often therapeutic, as they allow considerable freedom to develop nonviolent alternatives (for example, in psychotherapy or behavioral treatment) in an atmosphere which quickly provides feedback about one's success or failure.

Therapeutic environments are designed primarily for change and growth, although they necessarily include elements of prevention, containment, and monitoring.

Reactions to Violence Important to Treatment

It is impossible to treat violent patients adequately without understanding and dealing with the emotions that violent behavior engenders in the treater and in the society that establishes treatment resources. Anger in ourselves and in the public as a whole, feelings of revulsion for the patient, and fear for the safety of oneself or others all interfere with seeing the violent individual as a patient, or even as a person. Sometimes the violence is such that these feelings are obvious, as in a heinous incident. At other times, however, the problem is much more subtle, and the practitioner is lulled into thinking he is not fettered by prejudice or countertransference.

One of the most insidious of these loosely defined "countertransference" issues is also the most significant for ongoing work with violent patients. Most people guard against unconscious violent wishes and impulses. Our fears of our impulses make us defend ourselves mightily against them with denial, reaction formation, undoing, and other mechanisms which easily get in the way of appropriate clinical work.

A psychiatry resident whose father was severely injured by a drunk driver when she was a child chose an elective rotation in a city jail. Many of her patients had histories of violent behavior or were currently difficult to control. She prided herself on "understanding" them and seeing their emotional pain. Her supervisor one day received a message that the jail personnel were concerned about her placing herself in danger by frequently circumventing safety procedures. When asked about this, she said that the inmates knew she was there to help them, and would not hurt her.

Another therapist asked the author to supervise her psychotherapy of an antisocial patient at a mental health center. She reported consistent success with the treatment, but eventually began to skip supervision sessions. She eventually cancelled supervision and it was assumed that the patient had dropped out of treatment. It was later learned that the patient had threatened and blackmailed the therapist, and stolen from her.

Society's anger at violent patients is expressed in various ways. Psychiatrists are often asked to "do something" about violent people; but our efforts are rarely adequately supported or financed. Those who enter hospitals or outpatient treatment rather than prison are said to be "getting off easy." Clinicians who treat them are held in lowered social regard by their neighbors, and sometimes by their peers.

Society in one way or another blocks even the successful or promising ways of treating and/or managing violent patients. For example, antiandrogenic medications are seen as "chemical castration" or "mind control," rather than as ways in which the physician may help desperately disabled individuals. The combination of societal anger at letting offenders avoid long prison sentences, and unreasonable accusations of "coerced consent" by misguided (in this author's opinion) civil libertarians, shackles many efforts to bring about meaningful change and salvage some otherwise lost lives.

DIFFICULT DECISIONS IN CLINICAL SETTINGS

Notifications/Duties

The duty to warn or protect others from harm by a potentially violent patient is legally defined in many jurisdictions, and has become a part of the ordinary practice of psychiatry. There is no longer very much controversy over whether one should try to minimize danger, but how one goes about it is often confusing. The following discussion briefly touches upon prediction, ways of carrying out one's "duty," and practical conflicts with confidentiality of privilege.

Whether or not psychiatrists or other mental health professionals can predict violence accurately, the fact remains that we are asked to do it every day, and we accept (as we should) this responsibility. We make decisions and recommendations about commitments to institutions, increasing patients' privileges in the hospital, allowing passes or discharge, allowing potentially violent or suicidal outpatients to decide not to come into the hospital, reporting potential child abuse, allowing certain patients to drive or continue to work in sensitive occupations, and the like.

We are rarely, if ever, expected to be perfect in our judgments and decisions. We *are* expected to use the care befitting our profession, and currently accepted clinical criteria, to weigh known pros and cons, potential risks and potential benefits. Any prediction should be limited to a defined setting (for example, supervised, monitored, unsupervised), time frame (the shorter the time predicted, the more accurate), and set of patient characteristics (for example, whether or not the patient is taking prescribed medication). A more detailed discussion of predictors may be found in a recent issue of *Psychiatric Clinics of North America* (Reid, in press).

There are a number of ways to carry out one's obligation to deal in some way with known danger to others. Warning potential victims or notifying a law enforcement agency are the most commonly considered. Talking with the patient about ways to decrease risk and engaging him or her in treatment may be equally (or more) appropriate.

Discussing worry or danger with the patient, including talking about the need to try to prevent harm by notifying others, usually should be considered therapeutic, and not as interfering with the doctor–patient relationship. The clinician should be someone who speaks honestly and frankly, since the same is expected of the patient. One should be very cautious about confronting a potentially violent person alone, however.

It goes without saying that accurate documentation of the decision process is the best way to assure that the clinician's good-faith efforts to help are understood by future reviewers. Courts rarely castigate physicians who make it clear that they considered all reasonable viewpoints and then acted as they saw fit, but it is hard to convey this without a written record. The chart is both record and communication to subsequent health professionals. There is no excuse for omitting complete, legible information.

Confidentiality, or breach of the patient's privilege, is rarely a consideration if the psychiatrist feels that danger to self or others is at issue. Whether or not the patient has been told in advance that suspicion of serious danger will obviate the usual confidentiality, safety must be the first consideration. To do otherwise is foolhardy, especially when threats have been made, violent patients elope from the hospital, children have been abused, or staff are vulnerable to assault.

The clinician's agency, or allegiance to persons other than the patient, often extends even further. He or she may have a legitimate obligation to an employer (especially when working for military, correctional, or law enforcement institutions) or to a hospital's or clinic's risk management procedures. Such an obligation may include reporting of incidents or known risks, or even denial of care for certain patients. Physicians should be certain they understand and accept such policies and procedures from the outset.

Protection of Self and Staff from Assault

Serious assault by psychiatric or mentally retarded patients is unusual, in part because of precautions observed by staff and in part because such patients are not inherently violent. Reid and colleagues (1985) found an average of 2.54 assaults per occupied bed per year in a large, multicenter inpatient study. Most were minor, and severe injury to the victim quite rare. Other authors have found slightly different rates. The assault rate for nonpsychiatric inpatients in the same study was only 0.37 per bed per year. Assaults by outpatients are infrequent (Reid and Kang, 1986), but fatalities have occurred.

The most significant issue in preventing assaults on self and staff has little to do with specific predictors or diagnoses, other than the obvious danger from a currently or recently violent person: *Most assaults occur with little warning.* Thus, it is important to use reasonable precautions (such as care when interviewing alone) at all times. Overconfidence, especially a feeling that one can "feel" or "handle" potential danger, is associated with higher risk of injury.

Staff training for management of violent patients is available readily to hospitals. Psychiatric ward staff and emergency room personnel should be able to recognize escalating potential for violence and contain the patient in appropriate, humane ways. Either routine staff or designated crisis teams (who are immediately available at all times) should have specific training in safe, effective, and pain-free "takedown" procedures, and *practice them regularly*. The physician rarely is trained or called upon to participate in such crisis management, and should generally stay out of the proceedings when violence erupts.

Outpatient clinic and office staff rarely have the sophisticated training suggested for inpatient settings, since there are usually fewer employees available and many are clerical or administrative rather than clinical. Nevertheless, there should be procedures for handling potential or actual violence. Patients come directly from the "street," and thus are less familiar to staff (and may bring in weapons). Training and preparation thus should stress escaping and calling for help, rather than attempting to control a dangerous situation.

The sequelae to violent events in healthcare settings must include attention to the needs of the victim(s), staff, and perpetrator. The victim should receive careful attention and reassurance that his or her safety and feelings are being taken seriously. Administrative action or inquiries that question the victim's motives or judgment should take a back seat to support, especially if serious injury has occurred. The attending physician and/or unit chief should interview the victim to allay untoward feelings.

Unit staff, including those from other shifts, should have a chance to discuss serious incidents in an informal group setting. They are likely to be angry at and fearful of the perpetrator, anger which may be expressed as inappropriate care of the perpetrator in the future, or which may be displaced onto the attending doctor, administration, or victim. If the assailant remains on the ward, the reasons for this should be discussed and feelings aired. The group should not be used as a forum for criticizing staff procedures, although they should be examined whenever a pattern of assaults can be delineated.

Other patients on the unit should be treated as if they were victims themselves. They must live with the assailant (unless he has been transferred), and may be angry or frightened. Wishes to be discharged or transferred; criticisms of the physician, hospital, or themselves; and anger at the perpetrator are all common and must be addressed openly by the counseling staff.

The violent patient should be made aware of the result of his or her actions (such as injury and fear), and should receive whatever consequences are usual. The reason for the consequences should be made clear, as well as ways in which he or she may avoid similar consequences in the future.

Consequences often include brief seclusion or restraint, additional medication, loss of privileges, or transfer to another unit or hospital. It is important to attempt prosecution when the violent act is primarily antisocial or malicious (as contrasted from psychotic), although prosecution from a psychiatric hospital is very difficult.

CONCLUSION

This has not been a complete discussion of the treatment of violent patients. It has, however, highlighted some of the special concerns that are part of the care of such individuals and the protection of others. The physician should see these patients as people in need of psychiatric services, learn to treat them competently, and try to be aware of personal feelings that interfere with clinical judgment.

REFERENCES

Abel GG, Becker JV, Cunningham-Rathner BA, et al: The Treatment of Child Molesters. Atlanta, GA, Behavioral Medicine Laboratory, Emory University, 1984

Abel GG, Becker JC, Skinner LJ, et al: Behavioral approaches to treatment of the violent sex offender, in Clinical Treatment of the Violent Person. Edited by Roth LH. Rockville, MD, NIMH, ADAMHA, US Department of Health and Human Services, 1985

American Psychiatric Association: Diagnostic and Statistical Manual of Mental Disorders, Third Edition, Revised (DSM-III-R). Washington, DC, American Psychiatric Association 1987

Bradford JMW: The hormonal treatment of sexual offenders. Bull Amer Acad Psychiatry Law 1983; 11:159–169

Donlon PT, Hopkin J, Tupin JP: Overview: efficacy and safety of the rapid neuroleptization method with injectable haloperidol. Am J Psychiatry 1979; 136:273–278

Elliott FA: Neurological factors, in Handbook of Family Violence. Edited by Van Hasselt VB, Morrison RL, Bellack, AS, et al. New York, Plenum, 1988

Reid WH: The Treatment of Psychiatric Disorders, Revised for DSM-III-R. New York, Brunner/Mazel, 1988

Reid WH: Clinical evaluation of the violent patient. Psychiatric Clinics of North America (in press)

Reid WH, Balis GU: Evaluation of the violent patient, in American Psychiatric Association Annual Review, Vol. 6. Edited by Hales RE, Frances AJ. Washington, DC, American Psychiatric Press, 1987

Reid WH, Kang J: Serious assaults by outpatients. Am J Psychother 1986; 40:594–600

Reid WH, Edwards G, Bollinger MF: Assaults by inpatients. Psychiatr Med 1985; 2:315–319

Salzman C, Green AI, Rodriguez-Villa F, et al: Benzodiazepines combined with neuroleptics for management of severe disruptive behavior. Psychosomatics 1986; 27(Suppl): 17–26

Silver JM, Yudofsky S: Propranolol for aggression: literature review and clinical guidelines. International Drug Therapy Newsletter 1985; 20:9–12

Soloff PH: Emergency management of violent patients, in American Psychiatric Association Annual Review, Vol. 6. Edited by Hales RE, Frances AJ. Washington, DC, American Psychiatric Press, 1987

Stone JL, McDaniel KD, Hughes JR, et al: Episodic dyscontrol disorder and paroxysmal EEG abnormalities: successful treatment with carbamazepine. Biol Psychiatry 1986; 21: 208–212

Tupin JP: Psychopharmacology and aggression, in Clinical Treatment of the Violent Person. Edited by Roth LH. Rockville, MD, NIMH, ADAMHA, US Department of Health and Human Services, 1985

Chapter 28

When Patients Kill Themselves

by Michael H. Sacks, M.D.

Psychiatrists, like all physicians, must master the stress of patient death and the personal sense of failure and inadequacy at not having prevented it (McCue, 1982). For a psychiatrist, this central and intrinsic stress of medical practice usually means suicide. It need not; patients also die from other causes but the stigma associated with suicide, and the special responsibility that psychiatry assumes for its treatment and prevention, make the suicide of a patient a particularly stressful event.

What is remarkable is that rarely is suicide included in the literature on stress in psychiatry. In a recent article on the impaired psychiatrist, the stresses of psychiatric practice and training are identified; death and suicide were not mentioned (Doyle, 1987). This was omitted despite the fact that there are more than 28,000 deaths from suicide each year in the United States (Taube and Barrett, 1985). Many of these people are in treatment at the time of the suicide. Estimates are that 51 to 81 percent had received professional care for psychiatric problems during the year preceding their suicide, although much of this care may not have been provided by psychiatrists (Robins, 1981; Barraclough, 1974). Dorpat and Ripley (1960) found that 22 percent of patients who completed suicide had some treatment by, or consultations with, psychiatrists in the final year. This would suggest that the number of psychiatrists who have treated a patient who went on to complete suicide is significant. In a recent study, Chemtab and colleagues (1988) found that 51 percent of the respondents in a random survey of psychiatrists listed in the *American Psychiatric Association Biographical Directory* had had a patient commit suicide. The probability of having a second patient commit suicide was about the same. Even if one assumes that those who did not respond did not have the experience of treating a patient who went on to complete suicide—a very unlikely assumption—then 20 percent of psychiatrists have treated at least one patient who committed suicide. It is not an infrequent event.

Also, the stress of a patient suicide may be magnified by the belief that psychiatry is a medical specialty in which death can be avoided. Psychiatrists, in revealing jokes, like to comment on their selecting the specialty in order to avoid physical sickness and death. At least one study suggests that these self-observations are true of third year medical students who wish to become psychiatrists. They have greater anxiety about death than do their classmates who plan to enter specialties (Livingston and Zimet, 1965).

THE PSYCHIATRIST AS A SUICIDE SURVIVOR

This failure to acknowledge patient suicide as a stress for psychiatrists, despite the apparent frequency of successful suicides of patients in psychiatric treatment, is striking but understandable. It parallels a similar lacuna regarding the impact of the suicide on family survivors. This is particularly impressive in suicide studies given the well established clinical insight that the survivor of a suicide is himself at risk for suicide. Resnik (1969) sardonically characterized this omission in a famous editorial entitled "The Neglected Search for the Suicidococcus Contagiosa."

Once the concept of studying suicide survivors took hold, it became readily apparent that it need not only include the widows and orphans of a suicide victim. Friends, employees, students, and colleagues of the person who committed suicide might also be affected (McIntosh, 1985–1986; Henley, 1984). It was then a short but significant step to include the patient's psychiatrist as a survivor. It required an appreciation that "clinical detachment" did not necessarily provide protection against the painful impact of losing a patient, with whom one felt clearly involved, to suicide. Littman (1965) interviewed 200 therapists of patients who had completed suicide and found an intense affective response as the psychiatrists recalled events that had, in many cases, occurred years earlier, leading him to wonder how successfully they had processed the event. Kahne (1968), in a study of a hospital suicide epidemic, found that 22 percent of the therapists had treated a patient who committed suicide. Following the suicide, these psychiatrists were prone to repetitious expressions of guilt, painful awareness of the "silent accusations" of colleagues, implications of the culpability of others, and a marked loss of confidence. Kolodny and colleagues (1979) described the need to work through the personal issues following a suicide and reported the usefulness of group discussions consisting of psychiatrists who have had a patient commit suicide.

Goldstein and Buongiorno (1984) point out that all psychiatrists must face the risk, and possibly the reality, of a patient committing suicide. The small number of their colleagues who had a patient complete suicide and who were willing to participate in their study denied any lasting impact but, interestingly, all said it was necessary to "work it through." The authors believe that this represents an effort to suppress or deny the impact of the event.

PSYCHIATRIC TRAINEES

Estimates of the frequency of patient suicides in psychiatric training programs range from 8 to 30 percent of the trainees at a given time (Sacks et al, 1987; Brown, 1987). During 14 years' experience as an educator, inpatient unit chief, and a leader of second-year resident experiential groups, I have had the opportunity to "debrief" 8 trainees following a suicide, to be present at approximately 15 suicide morbidity conferences, and to conduct 6 year-long experiential groups for second-year residents in which at least 1 of the participants has had a patient commit suicide. I have also interviewed 10 colleagues who have had a patient commit suicide during their careers and who spoke openly with me regarding their reactions. As a result of these experiences, I have come to believe that confronting a patient suicide, either one's own or a colleague's, represents a major, if not central, event in the professional maturation of a psychiatrist. Basic issues of patient responsibility, mastering ambivalence toward patients, and the establishment of professional collegiality seems to crystallize around the resolution of the vulnerability and guilty shame psychiatrists experience in connection with a patient suicide.

THE IMMEDIATE REACTION: DISBELIEF AND DENIAL

The immediate response to a patient suicide is disbelief and denial of the event. One psychiatrist asked for the telephone message to be repeated because he could not understand what he had heard. Another asked what the probability of recovery was after being told that the patient was brain dead. Frequently there is a doubt regarding whether the death was due to suicide and the desperate hope that the death was accidental. If there is definite evidence that it was a suicide, there may be doubts regarding whether or not the patient really intended that the outcome be lethal. This disbelief of the psychiatrist is no different from the denial and repression that occurs in relatives of the person who committed suicide (Resnik, 1972).

The initial denial is followed by a period of depersonalization. Residents will speak of going through the day "on automatic" or feeling "spaced out." An experienced colleague felt "disconnected" for several days, which he later attributed to the intense shame and anger which the suicide evoked in him. One psychiatrist broke into tears when she was told of her patient's suicide and was seized by a panic that she would not be able to function. A year later she described the period afterwards as one of alternating states of "emotional insulation" and "panicky seizures" regarding whether she was crazy or not to be responding as intensely as she was.

SHAME AND GUILT

Shame and guilt are common, and to varying degrees occur in all psychiatrist survivors. They believe they are at fault and everywhere judged. Those who work in institutions feel that the eyes of patients, staff, and colleagues are on them. Those in private practice also worry about what their colleagues might be thinking; how will their referral sources react to it? In the current climate, all worry about the media reporting the death and the possibility of a humiliating malpractice case. In a remarkable first-person account, Herbert Perr, M.D. (1968) described his response to the suicide of a patient after eight years of psychotherapy:

> In those hours following my learning of his death, I blamed myself for the act he had taken. And in the intense guilt that I experienced I felt that there would be certain punishment to come. I anticipated charges of incompetence being leveled against me by his family, and public ridicule, notoriety, and perhaps a lawsuit charging me with malpractice. It reached the point in my fantasy where I was having to leave town, shunned like a leper for the terrible act I had committed. (p. 177)

In a hospital, shame or guilt may also be felt by the doctor on call on the night of the suicide, the doctor who admitted the patient, or the doctor who had treated the patient on an earlier admission. Following a suicide on an inpatient unit, the resident colleagues of the therapist whose patient had committed suicide shared a sense of blame because they had decided not to discuss the secret suicide attempt of another patient at a community meeting the day before because it violated confidentiality. They thought, with guilt feelings, in retrospect, that if they had brought it up, an opportunity might have occurred for the patient (the patient who went on to commit suicide) to express her thoughts and plans.

Guilty self-recriminations can influence the presentation of the case so as to invite blame or punishment. At a suicide review, a psychiatrist gave an incorrectly low dosage for the tricyclic antidepressant that his patient was receiving and did not realize the error even as he listened to a critical discussion of the adequacy of the dose. The guilt associated with a suicide such as this can continue for months and can be expressed indirectly. In another instance, a psychiatric resident acted irresponsibly with a patient. This provocative behavior, uncharacteristic for him, required a disciplinary action. When the situation could be openly discussed several months later, guilty associations to the suicide made it clear that the resident was indirectly seeking punishment for it.

THE FINDING OF OMENS

Frequently the guilt may take the form of a belief that one had a premonition of the suicide and did not act on it. One inpatient physician reported that a patient who completed suicide while on pass looked at her in a strange way as he was leaving the unit, which led her to think he was suicidal. She berated herself for not stopping him. A young schizophrenic patient thanked his therapist for the immense help in recognizing that "things were different" prior to discharge. There was an ambiguity about "things were different" that bothered the psychiatrist, and he felt guilty for not pursuing it further after learning of the patient's suicide one day later.

These "omens" are not uncommon in the aftermath of any disaster. When they occur in the therapist following a suicide they are dismissed by some as the result of a distorted retrospective search for clues which frequently can be found in most patient treatments, but are remembered because in that one situation a suicide actually occurred.

In a study of survivors of death, Maris (1981) found that guilt was three times more frequent (32 percent as opposed to 10 percent) in survivors of those who committed suicide than in survivors of those who died a natural death. He concluded that this relatively high level of guilt supports the interpretation that the survivor was aware of the clues of suicide but was unable or unwilling to prevent it. An alternative and equally likely explanation is that suicide, unlike a natural death, seems more preventable and therefore might be expected to leave a greater burden of guilt, which retrospectively "finds" neglected omens. This is certainly consistent with what many survivors feel.

ANGER AND RELIEF

Anger frequently is present on the part of the surviving therapist. It may be directed toward a staff member in the hospital, a supervisor, an administrator, or the patient's family. In one instance, a therapist blamed the mother of a young schizophrenic for pushing him into suicide because of her refusal to acknowledge that he might never complete college. On the day of the suicide she gave him college course forms for the next semester "in case" he wanted to return. Other sources of anger may be the vacation of a supervisor, absence of senior coverage, inadequate teaching of suicide prevention, lack of aftercare resources, and other limitations or failures of the institution.

Acknowledged anger at the patient is very rare despite the patient's implicit rejection of the psychiatrist's help and because of the latter's unavoidable feeling that the suicide was in some way intended to be vindictive or spiteful. The psychiatrist's guilty rumination, "Why did the patient do it?" often barely conceals the unspoken ". . . to me." The anger towards others, as well as intense self-recriminations, seems to be fueled by the patient's rejection and by the avoidance or repression of anger toward the patient. One psychiatrist trainee was amazed and then relieved during a staff discussion when his inpatient unit chief said he was angry at a patient who had committed suicide. The resident at first thought this was cold, callous, and detached, but felt relief when he realized how angry he was at the patient's family for seeming to cause the suicide, at the patient for doing it, and at his unit chief for not preventing it.

In one instance in which the patient's chronic suicidality was the central focus of the treatment, the therapist acknowledged relief after the patient completed suicide. Another patient committed suicide on the unit shortly after a long suicidal observation had been discontinued. The psychiatrist acknowledged years later in recalling the event that the most difficult thing for him to deal with was the relief at the death . . . and the hatred of the patient which this seemed to him to imply. Often, survivors of a patient who committed suicide attempt to explain a suicide by finding some justification such as pain, sickness, disgrace, and so on. This is thought by Augenbraun and Neuringer (1972) to represent an effort to deny feelings of guilt and responsibility.

SYMPTOMATIC BEHAVIORS

After the suicide the psychiatrist may experience partial identifications with the patient in dreams or fantasies. Frequently reported symptomatic behaviors include imagining seeing the patient in crowds and adopting a patient's gesture. A resident whose patient committed suicide with cyanide hallucinated its odor for a year afterward. A female colleague dreamed that she saw the suicidal patient. His hair was the same color as that of her son, who had experienced a worrisome adolescent depression at the same age as that of the patient. She resumed a personal psychiatric treatment out of a concern that some unresolved ambivalence toward her son may have influenced her professional judgment. Accident-proneness, or suicidal ideation, may occur. One psychiatrist took an incorrect dose of Valium to help him sleep following the suicide of a patient whose death resulted from an overdose of the same drug. Another had thoughts of suicide in which the method was similar to the one used by the patient.

Associated with this initial phase of disbelief, depersonalization, and guilty shame is a panic that another suicide will occur. On inpatient units there is an immediate mobilization of the unit to contain the suicidal act and to prevent another suicide (Sacks and Eth, 1981). Depending on the culture of the unit and hospital, this may result in either community meetings where the suicide is announced and discussed in detail, or in an effort to suppress discussion by pursuing "business as usual." In some instances, opinions for or against either strategy are strongly stated, usually with the not too implicit accusation that the failure to proceed in a particular way will result in further deaths. In either case there is usually an increase in the number of patients on suicide precautions as the fear of another suicide influences the evaluation of status. In the outpatient clinic, the threshold for admitting a patient decreases. These reactions occur not only in the psychiatrist whose patient commits suicide, but in the entire institution. Traditional lore is that after a suicide it takes about a year to regain confidence in one's clinical judgment; several psychiatrists reported that it took about this amount of time to extinguish the startle reaction to late night telephone calls and to the panic at receiving an emergency message.

THE RESPONSE OF PEERS

The psychiatric survivor may be regarded by his or her peers as having erred or having had a lapse in judgment. Discomfort with this thought and a wish by all concerned to avoid talking about a painful topic results in subtle alterations in the interactions between the survivor and his or her peers. Discussion of the patient with the involved physician may be kept to a minimum. This silence only increases the stress further. As a result, the psychiatrist may feel shunned, a partially correct perception that will be amplified by a personal sense of shame.

Alternatively, in some training settings, a resident may receive special attention that is supportive and compassionate following the suicide of his or her patient. Colleagues of the affected resident, seeing the special attention directed toward the trainee, will struggle with the envy this provokes. In the experiential group there will be the fantasy that he has experienced an initiation into the ranks of experienced psychiatrists. This is especially true if there are respected faculty members who acknowledge that the suicide of a patient was an important event in their own professional development. Members of resident groups wonder how they would respond to a patient suicide. To survive it is testimony to one's hardiness, endurance, and being a "real" physician.

Like all survivors, the psychiatrist who has had a patient commit suicide evokes the belief in others that he or she knows something special that can only be acquired as the result of the experience. This "rite of passage" perception of the survivor reflects the special significance attached to the experience. In fact, it can be seen as a response to two disturbing confrontations that a suicide rudely imposes on all psychiatrists: the vulnerability of an individual to an "easeful death" by self-destruction, and the vulnerability of the profession in not being able to prevent it. The doctor who is connected with a suicide may be seen as a hero who has acquired this dangerous knowledge first-hand, or, alternatively, as a fool who has demonstrated ignorance and poor judgment. In either case, he is set apart because he represents a distressing message regarding the possibility of ending human suffering by suicide and the limitations of the profession.

GRIEF: PROFESSIONAL AND PERSONAL

Litman (1965) noted the mixture of professional and personal responses to the patient suicide. The professional grief is facilitated by the series of reports and presentations which the institutional psychiatrists must provide. Private psychiatrists comment on their professional loneliness and on their jealousy of the institutional psychiatrist's apparent support by the peers and procedures of the hospital. The personal grief at the loss of some patients tends to be a private matter. It rarely appears in the professional reports of the suicide; when it occurs at a psychological autopsy of a suicide it is usually in the form of a spontaneous and unplanned remark or an emphasis in the presentation of which the psychiatrist is unaware.

The intensity of the response to the suicide will vary according to a number of factors. Crucial are the intensity of the relationship with the patient, the degree of commitment, the amount of conflict present, the transference–countertransference interaction, the stage of career, and the underlying character structure of the psychiatrist. If the suicide occurs early in training, before one has gained much experience and before professional identity has consolidated, the guilty ruminations will be particularly painful—much more so than if the suicide occurs toward the end of training when one has begun to develop a secure sense of professional competence. An angry or rejecting attitude toward the patient, which, because of inexperience or countertransference was not modified into a useful therapeutic intervention, might be particularly difficult for the therapist. If the patient was liked and the relationship was thought to be one of commitment and trust, the psychiatrist will feel betrayed. The suicide nearly always is felt as an attack or spiteful accusation directed at the therapist, an acting out of some unspoken hatred, or rejection of the therapist and his or her efforts to help. How much this is felt to be deserved will depend on the psychiatrist's characterological patterns of response, as well as on the actual behavior of the psychiatrist that may have contributed to an accurate sense of rejection by the patient.

The long-term outcome of either the personal or professional grieving has not been described in the literature. Goldstein and Buongiorno (1984) noted the affective intensity of psychiatrists in discussing patients who committed suicide years earlier, and concluded that this was evidence of incomplete grieving. The phenomenon they describe does indeed occur. I am unconvinced, however, that this necessarily represents evidence of incomplete grieving—it seems to imply that dispassionate recall is the benchmark of successful grieving. Studies of the impact of suicide on family survivors do emphasize the risk for the mourning process to become stuck or frozen (Lindemann and Greer, 1953). However, some families do succeed in mastering the trauma and gain in increased intimacy and care (Rudestam, 1977). An inability to discuss the loss without becoming emotionally overwhelmed—or an inability to integrate usefully the patient into one's clinical experience—would be evidence of an unsuccessful grieving. It is my impression that all experienced psychiatrists view a suicide as an important lesson about themselves, their patients, and their profession. This might be accompanied by a painful regret that it occurred in the setting of a patient tragedy. I do not agree with Goldstein and Buongiorno (1984) that this affective intensity reflects a denial of the event. It could reflect a successful grieving process in which the dead patient remains an affectively available memory. Two psychoanalysts, both in their mid-50s, remarked on the loss of their "youthful grandiosity" as a result of the impact of a suicide early in their careers. One learned to appreciate that he was more of a limited participant than he thought in the large number of factors impinging on the patient's life; the other began to appreciate the significance of his decisions, and the real elements of uncertainty that entered into them. Both psychiatrists were saddened to recall the event and both continued to work with suicidal patients; but they emphasized their greater respect for the difficulties and risks of the work.

The loss of a youthful professional grandiosity and the acceptance of limitations is easier for mature psychiatrists to acknowledge than it is for trainees still in their professional adolescence. The trainees often describe their response as "traumatic," emphasizing the intensity of the disturbance and the way it affects their personal and professional lives at the time.

Not all grief reactions are successful. At any stage in the professional development of a psychiatrist, experiencing a patient's suicide may result in enduring maladaptations. Some anniversary reactions may be viewed in this perspective. One psychiatrist became apprehensive about a suicide in his patient that seemed without cause, until he realized it was the one-year anniversary of another patient's suicide. Another had lunch with a friend with whom he had discussed the case, which they both recognized as a marking of the one-year anniverary of the patient's death. Other reactions to a suicide are beginning personal psychotherapy, or changing career direction from clinical work to research or from general psychiatry to a selective practice that avoids suicidal patients. One academic psychiatrist who had three patients commit suicide early in his career hospitalized patients quickly if the potential for suicidal behavior became evident and admitted to a reluctance to accepting them back into treatment. "I sort of decided it wasn't worth it . . . I worried too much." Another developed a fatalistic attitude and often publicly addressed the impossibility of preventing, or even of predicting, who would eventually commit suicide.

Another response to the professional grief associated with a suicide is an effort at reparation or repair by writing a clinical report or case study. The suicide is placed in a useful perspective so that others can benefit from the experience. Maltsberger (1986), in the introduction to his book on suicide, notes that it was as a result of "smarting" from the aftereffects of a suicide that he systematically began to study transference—countertransference in suicides.

An interesting example of the use of a clinical report to repair and perhaps memorialize a suicide occurred in a group of residents on an inpatient unit. A patient was admitted on a weekend and shortly thereafter managed to break through a window casement and jump to his death. The residents on the unit were feeling particularly proud of themselves because they were "running" the unit in the absence of a senior resident and attending. Although they had never seen the patient, they were deeply affected by his death and felt it was "their" suicide. They prepared a Grand Rounds presentation on the response of the patients on the unit to the suicide; that is, a study of the patient survivors. They, themselves, of course, were responding as survivors in this situation creatively by investigating the impact of the event and helping others to master it. One of the residents said afterwards that the presentation was like a "funeral." It was seen by her as a way to bury the patient.

Other motives enter into the effort to make something "positive" of the suicide. It can represent an undoing of the guilt and even, as one psychiatrist reports, a wish to enlist "a jury of colleagues to bring back a verdict of 'not guilty'; to agree with me that what had taken place was inevitable and that, in fact, commiseration and praise were due . . ." (Perr, 1968). Finally there can be a "memorialization" wish. One inpatient psychiatrist was "stunned" when he learned that the patients were collecting money to purchase a memorial plaque for the unit following the suicide of a patient until he realized that a clinical report he was preparing for publication may have been motivated by similar dynamics.

THE PSYCHOLOGICAL AUTOPSY

An important event in the processing of a suicide is the "psychological autopsy" or suicide review that occurs in many psychiatric hospitals and training centers. This is a review in which the responsible psychiatrist presents the case and an effort is made to determine how the death occurred, whether issues regarding quality of care need to be considered, and how this particular example relates to our general knowledge of suicide. These are usually experienced as difficult but important tasks for the therapist. The presentation focuses the therapist on the facts of the case and limits speculation and fantasy while encouraging rational thought. These are not always successful. The presenters may find them unproductive, a public shaming, or a masochistic means of "paying one's dues." Goldstein and Boungiorno (1984) found that 12 of 20 psychiatrists at different levels of experience reported that such autopsies "compounded doubt rather than aiding in the process of recovery (from the impact of the suicide)." This may not be an undesirable effect, unpleasant as it seems. The appreciation and acceptance of uncertainty and doubt about a situation that can be as complex as the retrospective reconstruction of a suicide might represent a closer approximation to the truth than a premature closure or finding too easy an explanation. This is not to say that doubt and uncertainty may not have a defensive aspect in the psychological autopsy—the avoidance of responsibility or the denial of a mistake or an error in judgment—but that the pressure at such conferences to find a certain explanation or a scapegoat who can relieve personal and professional guilt or feelings of inadequacy is immense.

One investigator who doubts their scientific value is the sociologist David Light (1980), who describes them as a "tribal ritual intended to bury the case and reaffirm the professional standards that may have been shaken." Light's description of the suicide review as a "tribal ritual" may suggest more than he ironically intended. A suicide does disturb the established order; this certainly includes the profession which is given responsibility for its prevention. But the threat is much larger. We are not far removed from a time when the person who committed suicide was buried at a crossroads and his possessions forfeited to the state. Some religions still refuse them sanctified burial. There is a remnant of taboo and stigma attached to suicide that threatens to disrupt any dispassionate discourse regarding its etiology, evaluation, and treatment. What we expect of the physician at a psychological autopsy of a suicide is that he or she aspire to present the case objectively and that the discussant and colleagues aspire to the same objectivity. That it not infrequently fails, so that the case is "buried," is not the indictment of psychiatry that Light suggests. It is a statement of the difficulty of the task, and a reminder that it is not always easy to attain that goal.

I have no knowledge of how many psychiatrists who have had a patient commit suicide in their private practice seek consultation to review the patient's treatment. Many comment on the loneliness of the experience. Some choose to review the case with a trusted supervisor. Having seen a number of trainees and colleagues who wished to talk about the treatment, I am impressed with their difficulty in thinking about the case in the immediate aftermath. What I frequently do is support their curiosity, draw their attention to whatever acute grieving response is present (especially if there is an indication of excessive guilt), attend to practical matters such as their seeing the family, consider with them the usefulness of attending the funeral, help to provide an initial formulation of the suicide that balances the factors, and share the responsibility in whatever combination of colleague, educator, supervisor, or administrator I am to them. I then make an appointment to meet with them in a few months after they have more time to process the event. I emphasize that they can expect this "processing" to continue for a variable amount of time, to be alert to its impact on the treatment of other patients, and that eventually it is likely to become a valuable reference in one's clinical experience. It is not easy for a psychiatrist to review a suicide. Most welcome the opportunity but some find it an intrusion. Others prefer to keep it in their personal therapy. One young colleague called to cancel an appointment to review a suicide because he felt his reaction was too neurotic. He would leave it for his psychotherapy. Whenever possible I try to discourage this as the exclusive means of reviewing the suicide.

In the remainder of this chapter I shall discuss three other issues that relate to the aftermath of a suicide: ambivalence toward patients, patient responsibility, and collegiality. First, a report of an experiential group that represents some of these broad issues in microcosm.

A REPORT OF A RESIDENT GROUP

In an experiential group of second-year residents in which one of the residents had had a patient commit suicide, the group responded to my cancellation of a session by deciding to meet without me. The meeting was described the following week as one of laughter and silliness. Everyone had brought their own lunch—a "violation" of a "group rule" that I had instituted. This had occurred in the context of my interpreting the large amount of food brought into the group following the patient suicide as a dissatisfaction with me for failing to satisfy their hunger for relief from the painful guilt and fear associated with it. Their behavior at the meeting held in my absence was seen as a manic celebration in which they believed they had overthrown me by meeting in my absence and violating this "sacred" group rule against eating during the meeting time. This was supported by fantasies from some of the group who had felt a vague apprehension underlying the playful fun of the meeting. Many of them had, in fact, bowed in mock deference before the empty chair I usually occupied. The resident whose patient had committed suicide was the first to do this. He recalled thinking at the time, "Wouldn't this really be fun if the suicide hadn't occurred?" I suggested that perhaps they thought of my absence as a suicide (my not being there) and a murder (the rebellion). I added that, similarly, the patient death might be felt as both a suicide and a murder. This was greeted with jokes that only surgeons spoke of their dead patients in that way; but then the doctor whose patient had committed suicide courageously and soberly said that viewing the suicide as a murder made sense to him . . . why else would he feel so much guilt?

This was greeted by an intense effort by the group to convince the resident that he couldn't be feeling that! His efforts to explain himself further were ignored. I compared this group behavior to that of a mob the day after a lynching. They would not "hear" the guilt of the "confessed" individual because it would require an acknowledgement of a group guilt.

In the following sessions, the group divided into two subsections. One was a compliant subgroup which began to acknowledge the symbolic guilt represented in the "totem feast" and saw it as a major event in focusing the events of their second year of psychiatry training. As a subgroup they seemed to compete with each other in bringing material to the group experience which further confirmed the symbolic meaning of their revolt against the group leader. The other subgroup was incredulous. They viewed my interpretations as too fanciful, too analytic, and too Freudian. They competed by becoming defensively biological, steadfastly critical of unconscious motivation, and strongly denied any awareness of guilt for a "group murder." Attempts to focus the attention of both groups on their own competitiveness with each other were not successful. The resident whose patient had committed suicide seemed to belong to neither subgroup and became silent, which was in contrast to his early active and thoughtful leadership in the group. Another resident who had seemed to be having some personal difficulties did not attend for several weeks.

Shortly thereafter, the incredulous subgroup approached the training director with a concern about this absent trainee. When I learned of this, I expressed my belief to the group that there was a scapegoating process that needed to be examined, and cited as evidence the subgroup's failure to discuss their concern with the resident in question or with the entire group. The scapegoated resident rejoined the group after a difficult session and angrily confronted the incredulous group with the destructiveness of their "help" to his career and with the fact that he had, as a result of a private talk with the resident whose patient had committed suicide, recognized his need for professional help, which he had obtained. One member of the incredulous subgroup recognized his own anger and jealousy at the apparent ease with which the scapegoated resident could ask for help, and receive it from another resident. He revealingly related this to his need to be the competent sibling because of a younger brother who suffered from cerebral palsy. The appreciation of becoming a physician, not only out of a desire to help the sick but out of a jealousy toward an ill family member, was not lost on the group. It raised the issue that the object of therapeutic interest and concern might also be the object of a jealous hatred.

There followed a general realization of their ambivalence toward each other, toward their patients, and toward the faculty and me for not providing more help with their painful and frightening feelings of inadequacy. Help in acquiring the skills and knowledge to take care of their demanding psychotic patients did not seem forthcoming either in the group or the training program. They had no choice but to feed themselves. As the full meaning of their "manic feast" was understood they were able to acknowledge their competitiveness with each other. The resident whose patient had committed suicide rejoined the group as the competitiveness that he freely acknowledged was accepted. Part of his guilt was from his failure to seek more supervisory help when he began to appreciate that perhaps there were problems in the treatment.

As the academic year drew to a close, the group playfully decided to have another feast at which they would express their gratitude by having me as a participant. These plans were interrupted by a second suicide. In a remarkable session the group provided a setting for the resident to speak about the patient, the treatment, and the special feelings which the patient had evoked in him. The group members were respectful, perceptive, and empathic. As the hour drew to a close I was asked if I had anything to add. I responded that I had followed their discussion with pride at their working so well with each other and addressing what I thought were the relevant points. The resident whose patient had just committed suicide said he had wanted to thank me for my help but had felt I had just thanked the group, which I in fact had. Someone said, with irony, that I had just been fed.

It is important that during this second postgraduate year of training central questions which the group examined were those of professional responsibility, ambivalence toward patients, and collegiality. These issues were intimately intertwined with the patient suicides, I suppose, because of their extreme impact on the group during this formative period. If there had been no suicide the issues would still be raised because they are core issues in the professionalization of a psychiatrist. Discussion might then focus around a serious suicide attempt. My experience has been that suicide always focuses the issue either by its occurrence or by the threat of its occurrence.

COLLEGIALITY

An immediate impact of a patient suicide is concern regarding the judgment of one's professional competence by peers. Among newly graduated psychiatrists, the judgment of esteemed senior colleagues may be of special importance. The willingness to trust one's professional group and the courage of members of the group to be honest and forthright is at the core of collegiality, and it is in the suicide review that this is most tested. Other untoward patient outcomes are either reversible or do not have the seemingly unnatural finality of a suicide. In the resident group described above, there was an initial reluctance to discuss the group suicide among themselves in the presence of the leader. This was accompanied by the ambivalent perception of the event as an "initiation" into the ranks of "experienced" psychiatrists alongside of the fear that a foolish error had been made.

What is critical to both these fantasies is simply that they reflect the powerful feelings that the suicide provokes in others. It is the psychiatrist's collegial responsibility not only to acknowledge the existence of such feelings but to act in as responsible and rational manner as possible in their presence. It is, in part, the ideals and standards of the profession that enable this to occur. Collegiality, or the critical but supportive evaluation of peers regarding difficult and painful issues, is a reflection of the vitality of the profession's standards and ideals.

When the resident wished to discuss his guilt following the "manic rebellion," his colleagues, out of fear of their own guilt and competitiveness, wanted to bury the issue of culpability by denying it as a possibility. They had become a "mob," subject to the whims of group psychology rather than the rational constraints of professional collegiality. The result was a destructive display of "collegial concern" toward the impaired resident. There is a lesson here for faculty in training institutions and peer reviewers in general. Often the concern for the feelings of a colleague can mask a destructive wish to avoid the mean-

ingful examination of a difficult clinical issue. This destructive collegial interaction may reflect a wish to deny the competitive triumph at a colleague's failure,
the fearful identification with the occurrence of a similar failing in one's self,
and so on. In training institutions the tension between supportive dismissal and
critical blamefinding is often represented in a "split" over the selection of a
discussant for a suicide review. The training director advocates someone who
will attend sensitively to the traumatic response of the trainees, while the medical director seeks someone who will have the courage to address, directly and
forthrightly, the particular clinical issues and judgments that require evaluation.
Of course neither is sufficient without the other. Collegiality involves both.

There are, of course, other professional issues that test the stability and strength
of collegiality. Probably the most significant are autonomy and creativity. The
writing of *Totem and Taboo* (1913), in which the murderous rebellion of the totem
or manic feast is first described, is said to be inspired by Freud's difficulty in
accepting Jung's creative independence. Kohut (1976) addresses the same issue
in his essay on group psychology.

The youth of any group, family or professional, are bound to struggle with
their wishes toward independence and autonomy. The latent murderousness
in these wishes must be mastered during the process of their professionalization.
Winnicott (1971) describes normal adolescence as the murder of parents. It is
also true of professional adolescence. The young colleague must at some time
"seize his independence" . . . an action that inevitably is seen as the unconscious
murder of those who are in authority. Normally this process is contained by
the experience and sympathetic identification of the teacher-leaders until that
point when the adolescent-trainee can acquire sufficient confidence and maturity
to function truly as a colleague. A suicide, or the threat of a suicide, resonates
with this latent murderousness, which, until it is worked through, prevents the
establishment of meaningful collegiality.

That such a process had occurred in the resident group was evident in the
group's response to the second suicide. That it was incomplete was evident in
the request of the resident toward the end of the meeting for the approval of
the leader and the ambivalent comment regarding the leader being "fed" by the
group's behavior. It clearly suggests a further need for approval and anger at
the burden this brings with it.

Within the context of the relationship between the trainee and the professional
group, creative autonomy can only occur in the setting of attaining independence from the group while maintaining a commitment and responsibility for
its standards and ideals. Ultimately, this is seen unconsciously as a murder by
the participants and is subject to confusion with the guilt associated with the
suicide of a patient, or the wish that a patient be dead. It is why older and more
experienced psychiatrists are less traumatized by suicide. Their sense of collegiality and conflict over professional issues is usually more stable and less troubled by these issues.

AMBIVALENCE TOWARD PATIENTS

The ambivalence toward patients is a major aspect of any therapist's confrontation with the reality of a patient killing himself. It is sobering and frightening
to consider the possibility that on some level there is an underlying ambivalence

toward patients that may reflect a frustration or hatred of them, even a wish that they be dead. This may not only reflect a response, which the patient has provoked, but also an earlier anger or jealousy, such as it did for the trainee with the sick brother who had approached the training director to "help" the impaired resident. Only after the group was able to recognize its ambivalence toward the leader and then each other was it possible to begin to acknowledge it as present with patients. The importance of such reaction formations or sublimations regarding a family member in the motivation to become a doctor are widely recognized.

Another example: On the day of the suicide of a young adult patient, a therapist bought a book on dealing with death in young patients. Her conscious thoughts concerned a patient whose son was dying of leukemia. On learning of the suicide she was convinced that the purchase of the book was related to her knowledge or wish concerning the impending suicide in this severely distressed patient. Although this occurrence might be dismissed as coincidental or the retrospective establishment of an "omen" that predicted the event, it nevertheless reflected the therapist's asking herself whether she knew that the patient planned his suicide or perhaps even that she wished for his death. This may be an unanswerable question, but it is sufficient that the therapist asks the question. Maltsberger and Buie (1974) describe how a countertransference aversion or malice toward a suicidal patient is likely to precipitate a suicidal action.

The origins of the literature on the ambivalence of the caretaker is generally attributed to its brilliant beginning in Winnicott's paper "On Hate in the Countertransference." In this paper, Winnicott drew attention to the mother's hatred of her newborn infant and its importance in normal development. Although Winnicott related the natural ambivalence of the caretaker to an infant to the therapist–patient interaction, its relevance to the treatment of suicidal patients is immense. Maltsberger and Buie (1974) systematically outline the ways in which a countertransferential hatred can be denied and destructively expressed in the treatment of a suicidal patient. It represents an important maturational step for a young psychiatrist to fully appreciate that, alongside the wish to help or save, may be wishes to reject, hurt, and even murder the patient.

RESPONSIBILITY

When patients kill themselves, most psychiatrists, perhaps all psychiatrists, question their degree of responsibility. If there was an error in judgment or knowledge, they ask how much this reflects a limitation of the profession, a personal limitation, and most difficult of all, an unconscious countertransference response. Prior to the suicide, in supervision and didactic classes, emphasis is placed on learning how to detect suicidality and how to treat it. The conclusion from most epidemiological or case study follow-ups on suicide is that they occur in the setting of a psychiatric illness and in connection with a recent loss, discharge from the hospital, or the developing of chronicity. The importance of alertness and skill is seen as crucial in attaining a good outcome in the treatment of such patients. Recognition of the inevitability of some suicides is also discussed but not as a source for despair or therapeutic nihilism. The youthful grandiosity of beginning psychiatrists and its unmodified preservation to varying degrees in all psychiatrists often leads to the belief that having a patient commit suicide is true for other psychiatrists . . . never for oneself.

Once the suicide occurs there is a subtle shift or transformation in the discussion. There is now a greater emphasis on its inevitability. Familiar cliches such as "There are two kinds of therapists: those who have experienced suicide and those who will," "You can never prevent a suicidal patient from killing himself," and, finally, "Patients are responsible for their own lives," are repeated. This more fatalistic attitude toward the suicide usually emerges only after the suicide has occurred. It need not. Most investigators have commented on the extreme difficulty in predicting which potentially suicidal patients will actually complete suicide (Pokorny, 1983).

This tension between the inevitability of suicide in some patients versus its representation as a failure in treatment is often seen as a contradiction and rightly experienced as confusing to trainees. It reflects an uncertainty as to what extent suicide is always a treatable medical condition. This is not cause for rejecting, as Light (1983) does, the psychiatrist as an expert in suicide and seeing the profession to be in a collusive struggle to keep its inadequacy hidden. One is impressed, after reviewing a large number of suicides, not at how often they reflect an error of judgment on the part of the therapist, but at how often this seems to be an inadequate explanation for the suicide since in most instances such errors do not have this result. The error of the psychiatrist may be a contributing factor but it rarely is a sufficient condition for suicide. Biological, personal, interpersonal, and social systems factors also play an important role.

It is important that the therapist evaluate these factors. He must distinguish between a *global* assumption of irrational guilt and responsibility that accompanies the initial response to the suicide and a realistic appraisal of the event. This is a critical step in "working through" the suicide. It allows the physician to take more specific responsibility for the suicide and to experience specific guilt for what might *realistically* be his responsibility. Even this assumption of a specific and realistic guilt must ultimately remain ambiguous and uncertain. There is rarely any categorical precision in the assignment of guilt. In the end, it is a responsibility shared by many, including, ultimately, the patient himself.

CONCLUSION

Albert Camus (1959), the philosopher, in the *Myth of Sisyphus*, writes that suicide represents a central problem in philosophy that requires a satisfactory resolution before any other problems can be undertaken. As psychiatrists, most of us would, I suspect, be biased against such a consideration of suicide as a legitimate philosophical solution to life's painful losses and disappointments. We know that more often than not these losses are temporary and that accompanying psychopathological states can be successfully treated by biological and psychosocial treatments, and, if they fail, by time itself. In shifting the discourse of suicide from that of philosophy to psychiatry, in transforming Camus' existentialist hero confronting suicide into a pathologically despairing and medically ill individual, we assume psychiatric responsibility for a subversive behavior that has disturbed man since the moment he realized that, unlike other species, he alone was capable of self-murder. Part of that responsibility is the commitment to diagnosis, treatment, and prevention of suicidal behaviors in our patients.

The impact of a failure to do so successfully has been the subject of this chapter. In dealing with these failures we learn a great deal about ourselves as individuals and professionals. The individual lessons are beyond the scope of this contribution. Professionally, I have argued that there is a grief reaction of varying intensity, occasionally traumatic, especially in the young trainee, that can contribute to a more profound—if somewhat ambivalent—sense of our responsibility to patients; and to the development of our collegial responsibility to evaluate the work of others while simultaneously providing them with the support they may need.

My thanks to the colleagues who shared with me their responses to a patient suicide. Also, thanks to the many colleagues who read early drafts of the manuscript for their encouragement and suggestions; in particular, Jonas Cohler, Allen Frances, William A. Frosch, Howard Kibel, Richard Munich, William Sledge, and Stefan Stein. Finally, the earlier work of Lindemann and Litman (whose influence is acknowledged in the title) was crucial in my thinking.

REFERENCES

Augenbraun B, Neuringer C: Helping survivors with the impact of suicide, in Survivors of Suicide. Edited by Cain C. Springfield, IL, Charles C. Thomas, 1972

Barraclough B, Bunch J, Nelson B, et al: A hundred cases of suicide: clinical aspects. Brit J Psychiatry 1974; 125:355–373

Brown HN: The impact of suicide on therapists in training. Compr Psychiatry 1987; 28:101–112

Calhoun LG, Shelby J, Abernethy CB: Suicidal death: social reactions to bereaved survivors. J Psychol 1984; 116:255–261

Chemtab CM, Hamada RS, Bauer BK, et al: Patients' suicides: frequency and impact on psychiatrists. Am J Psychiatry 1988; 145:224–228

Camus A: Myth of Sisyphus. New York, Random House, 1959

Doyle BB: The impaired psychiatrist. Psychiatric Annals 1987; 17:760–764

Dorpat TL, Ripley HS: A study of suicide in the Seattle area. Compr Psychiatry 1960; 1:349–359

Freud S: Totem and Taboo (1913), in Complete Psychological Works, in Standard Ed. Translated and edited by Strachey J. London, Hogarth Press, 1953

Goldstein LS, Buongiorno PA: Psychotherapists as suicide survivors. Am J Psychotherapy 1984; 38:392–398

Henley SHA: Bereavement following suicide. Current Psychological Research and Reviews 1984; 3:53–61

Kahne MJ: Suicide among patients in mental hospitals: a study of the psychiatrists who conducted their psychotherapy. Psychiatry 1968; 31:32–43

Kohut H: Creativeness charisma and group psychotherapy: reflections on Freud's self analysis, in Freud: The Fusion of Science and Humanism. Edited by Gedo J, Pollock GH. Psychological Issues, Monograph 34–35. New York, International Universities Press, 1976

Kolodny S, Binder RL, Bronstein A, et al: The working through of patients' suicides by four therapists. Suicide Life Threat Behav 1979; 9:33–45

Light D: Becoming Psychiatrists: The Professional Transformation of Self. New York, Norton, 1980

Lindemann E, Greer IM: A study of grief: emotional responses to suicide. Pastoral Psychology 1953; 4:9–13

Litman RE: When patients commit suicide. Journal of Psychotherapy 1965; 19:570–576

Livingston P, Zimet CN: Death anxiety, authoritarianism and choice of specialty in medical students. J Nerv Ment Dis 1965; 140:222–230

Maltsberger JT: Suicide Risk: The Formulation of Clinical Judgment. New York, New York University Press, 1986

Maltsberger JT, Buie DH: Countertransference hate in the treatment of suicidal patients. Arch Gen Psychiatry 1974; 30:625–663

Maris RW: Pathways to Suicide. Baltimore, Johns Hopkins University Press, 1981

McCue JD: The effects of stress on physicians and their medical practice. N Engl J Med 1982; 306:458–463

McIntosh JL: Survivors of suicide: a comprehensive bibliography. Omega 1985–1986; 16:355–370

Perr HM: Suicide and the doctor–patient relationship. Am J Psychoanal 1968; 28:177–188

Pokorny AD: Prediction of suicide in psychiatric patients. Arch Gen Psychiatry 1983; 40:249–257

Resnik HLP: The neglected search for the suicidococcus contagiosa. Arch Environ Health 1969; 19:307–309

Resnik HLP: Psychologial resynthesis: a clinical approach to the survivors of a death by suicide, in Survivors of Suicide. Edited by Cain A. Springfield, IL, Charles C Thomas, 1972

Robins E: The Final Months: A Study of the Lives of 134 Persons Who Committed Suicide. New York, Oxford University Press, 1981

Rudestam KE: Physical and psychological responses to suicide in the family. J Consult Clin Psychol 1977; 45:162–170

Sacks MH, Eth S: Pathological identification as a cause of suicide on an inpatient unit. Hosp Community Psychiatry 1981; 32:36–40

Sacks MH, Kibel HD, Cohen AB, et al: Resident response to patient suicide. Journal of Psychiatric Education 1987; 11:217–226

Taube CA, Barrett SA (Eds): Mental Health, United States. Rockville Md, U.S. Department of Health and Human Services, 1985

Winnicott DW: Hate in the countertransference, in Collected Papers: Through Pediatrics to Psychoanalysis. New York. Basic Books, 1958

Winnicott DW: Contemporary concepts of adolescent development and their implications for higher education, in Playing and Reality. New York, Basic Books, 1971

Chapter 29

The VIP as Patient: Syndrome, Dynamic, and Treatment

by Richard L. Munich, M.D.

From the point of view of the psychiatrist's clinical responsibility, every patient is an important person; but there are certain of our patients who, by virtue of their position, power, and prestige, present unique problems in that their importance alters the treatment situation. Although many are treated quietly and successfully, there is enough collected experience of unfavorable outcome with such patients to suggest a specific name and syndrome and to warrant particular consideration. This chapter will review the literature pertaining to the very important person (VIP) as psychiatric patient and the VIP syndrome, attempt a formulation of the dynamics of the VIP phenomenon—especially splitting and entitlement and their impact on the treater or treatment system—and recommend strategies to minimize the impact of those dynamics on effective treatment.

The VIP syndrome results from a dysfunctional intersection of personality and social system factors in which a patient identified as a VIP is able to convey an exaggerated sense of entitlement onto the social field in which the treatment occurs. Sometimes the exaggerated entitlement exists not in the patient but in their family or its representative. Depending on the vulnerability of the social field to demands for entitlement, the patient gains or at least threatens to gain various priorities from his or her treater or treatment team. A circular and polarizing process is then set into motion in which the social system becomes less responsive and the patient becomes more demanding. The effects include everything from a treatment stalemate in which the patient stays but receives ineffective treatment, to a complete polarization leading to treatment disruption.

LITERATURE REVIEW

Weintraub (1964) collected data from 12 VIP cases treated in a small university psychiatric hospital. Of these cases, only two succeeded in achieving the goals of hospitalization, while the remaining 10 were considered complete therapeutic failures. Weintraub defines a VIP as any patient "who has been able either through personal influence or professional status to exert unusual pressure on the staff" (p. 182). Although systematic and well controlled data do not exist, there are several well-known examples of VIPs whose influential status compromised their treatment. Many of these cases were reported in a GAP report "The VIP with Psychiatric Impairment" (1973). The list in that report goes as far back as George III, King of England from 1760 to 1820, and Ludwig II, King of Bavaria. It includes modern examples such as Paul von Hindenburg, Woodrow Wilson, Franklin D. Roosevelt, Benito Mussolini, and Earl K. Long. In these cases, treatment difficulties had implications well beyond the personal tragedies for each of these men. In the case of James V. Forrestal, the needs of the organization were put above those of the patient. Hotchner (1966) describes how Ernest Hemingway's status contributed to his suicide four days following discharge from a hospital treatment, which included what many would consider an incomplete series of electroconvulsive treatments (Strange, 1980).

Other studies are less general but address the VIP problem in a variety of specific ways: the hateful patient (Groves, 1978); children of the wealthy (Pittman, 1985; Stone, 1972); children or disciples of charismatic individuals (Miller and Roberts, 1967); the famous and the "beautiful people" (Grotjahn, 1975); the physician-patient (Stoudemire and Rhoads, 1983); or the child of a famous mother or father (Stone, 1979). Feuer and Karasu (1978), and Saari and Johnson (1975), along with Weintraub, have written about the special problem of the VIP in the psychiatric hospital.

Patient Factors

The catalogue of contributing features to which these articles allude is extensive and includes from the patient side narcissism, sociopathy, entitlement, incongruence or dissonance between a personal identity and the identity of importance, a denial of illness complicated by legal, financial, social, and professional factors, delay in seeking help, unilateral termination of treatment, and discharges against medical advice. In addition, there may be obstructionism by the family, attempts to control and difficulties in granting respect to the therapist, and special problems concerning the fee and scheduling of sessions. While much of this falls under the rubric of nonacceptance of the patient role, the picture is complicated by specific personality factors and reality-based considerations such as the real need of some VIPs to travel extensively. The problem of confidentiality —as illustrated by the case of Senator Thomas Eagleton, who had to withdraw from a Vice-Presidential candidacy because of the public's response to his prior psychiatric treatment—is a crucial issue for these patients.

Steyn (1980) lists characteristic manic, paranoid, and depressive patterns of behavior that inhibit the VIP as patient from obtaining help in conventional ways. Many of these patterns are deteriorations from behaviors which contribute to the VIPs gaining and sustaining their position. Thus, these patients' aggressiveness, drive, and imagination become assaultiveness, restlessness, and grandiosity; soberness and attention to detail become self-denigration, helplessness, and worthlessness; and vigilance becomes a concern about conspirators. Because of their extremely low self-esteem and covert dependency, which lead to an inability to trust those upon whom they have no claim, Weintraub noted the VIP's difficulty approaching staff members and asking for help directly, a consistent refusal to acknowledge help when the staff members spontaneously offered it, and their insistence that help was received because of their contacts with powerful people. More often than not, being self-made in itself makes asking for help more difficult. Often VIPs fear their treatment will alter the very aspect of their personality that, from their point of view, has accounted for their success.

Therapist Factors

From the side of the therapist or treatment system, contributing features to difficulties with these patients include unacknowledged awe, envy, or contempt, corruptibility, and failure to treat the client as an individual. Unresolved conflicts connected to wealth, social status, and power account for much of the difficulty. These factors are complicated by the fact that treatment is rarely initiated by the VIP himself, or that the psychiatrist is often operating under various constraints imposed upon him, not the least of which is indirect and distorted information about the patient. Many of these factors operate in such a way that the psychiatrist is either restrained from exercising the appropriate amount of control of the situation or exercises too much. If a referring agency is requesting information, the usually reliable boundary around effective treatment is thus threatened from the beginning and made more vulnerable by complicated feelings within the psychiatrist.

The principal focus of the GAP report is on the delicate boundary the psychiatrist must trace between the needs of the VIP and the demands of the family, representative, or organization for which the patient is also important. The situation can be so complex as to compromise the psychiatrist's judgment, especially if he or she is employed by or formally obligated to the agency in which the VIP has authority. Similarly, if restrictions are placed on the psychiatrist's usual functioning—such as requests for secrecy and special meeting places, or efforts to have him misrepresent himself or evaluate the patient surreptitiously— evaluation and treatment may be hampered. At the very least, as the GAP report suggests, data obtained under the above conditions must be evaluated with extreme care.

Treatment System Factors

Much as these problems may beleaguer an individual psychiatrist, they are compounded when the VIP enters a hospital setting. Stanton and Schwartz (1954), Main (1957) and Burnham (1966) have carefully documented the processes of staff splitting which potentially accompany special patients. While these classic papers, like more recent contributions of Gabbard (1986) and Kernberg (1987) do not refer to the VIP per se, they form a theoretical background to understanding the treatment difficulties a VIP can present.

These papers begin with patients whose psychological ailment represents a special appeal to the staff with whom they are involved. This appeal results from an unintegrated aspect of the patient's personality in which intense demands for special help, a special kind of relationship, and exclusive intimacy predominate. Often manifesting itself in multiple dramatic forms of suffering or threats of self-destruction, the appeal strives to locate those individuals in an environment that will provide just the right kind of "all-good mothering" that these patients feel they never had and desperately need. Among other things, they convey a powerful sense of entitlement. Those who respond to the appeal in the desired manner become positively valued and rapidly split off and are differentiated from those who do not and are thus considered all bad. This splitting is often a reflection of an internal split within the patient between an all-good and an all-bad set of self and object representations. These unrealistic polarities are then reinforced within the staff by the arousal of omnipotent feelings in the gratifying members and the attribution to and actual experience of sadistic and malevolent feelings in the ungratifying ones. In both cases, according to Burnham, primitive feelings are mobilized to support the rapidly growing split which tends to exist at first between the psychotherapist and administrative psychiatrist or nursing staff, but may extend to a split between the unit staff and the administrative element of the hospital.

Main reported the split that occurred between the "in-group" and the "out-group." In this configuration, questions by the out-group about the special care given the patient by the in-group led the latter to an increased attentiveness to the patient and a subtle devaluation of the out-group. This resulted in a quiet withdrawal of the out-group where critical feelings about the in-group, the patient, and the treatment were then lost to overall scrutiny. Thus, those closest to the patient became isolated and they, the patient, and the treatment invariably suffered. In the 12 cases of this phenomena which Main reported, open discussion of and personal feelings about the process and the treatment, and especially the treatment's failure, were nearly impossible to discuss during and after hospitalization.

Many of the patients described by Burnham (1966) and Main (1957) arranged to enter hospitals under special circumstances with unusual arrangements in a way that they might already be considered VIPs. Weintraub (1964) suggests that three factors must be present for a VIP problem to develop in a hospital. First, a patient is identified as an important person upon admission. Second, this person has an intense need to be considered special. And third, administrative arrangements must develop within the hospital that promote the "temporary upward transfer of authority within the hospital hierarchy for the purpose of creating special conditions for the politically sensitive patient" (Weintraub, 1964, p. 187).

Perhaps the most important links between the special patient and the VIP, however, are the feelings of omnipotence aroused by these patients in the referring and admitting physicians and the sense of entitlement to special care the patients communicate. Virtually all writers, from Stanton and Schwartz in 1954 to Kernberg in 1987, agree that the splits exacerbated in the treatment staff by interaction with these special patients are usually latent, tolerable, mainly unnoticed, and masked by cooperative feelings and structures used by social systems to defend against disruption. It is our experience that this also holds true for the VIP syndrome.

CLINICAL EXAMPLE

The following clinical example demonstrates many features of the VIP as patient and the ensuing syndrome which may develop:

> After a series of failed outpatient and brief inpatient treatments, the 21-year-old son of a wealthy and socially prominent midwestern family was admitted to a large, private, university teaching hospital in another part of the country. In addition to convincing his parents that his psychiatrists were incompetent, the previous treatment failures resulted from a combination of the patient's resistance to treatment, denial of illness, and grandiose wishes to complete college or work in a high position.
>
> The patient's admission was complicated by several factors. In the months prior to hospitalization, his father arranged a consultation with the hospital's psychiatrist-in-chief who recommended against hospitalization. Several weeks later and without the latter's knowledge, the father arranged for his son to be admitted and brought him to the hospital under the pretext that they would be looking at colleges. The

patient was rapidly transferred from the admission unit to his permanent unit without the usual screening procedure of the permanent unit. In opposition to the parent's wishes, he was assigned an advanced trainee rather than a senior person for the initial workup. Six months later, the patient eloped from his inpatient unit and threw himself in front of an oncoming car on a nearby highway; and although he survived this attempted suicide, his psychiatric course deteriorated until his father arranged for his transfer to another hospital a few months later.

From the time of his admission to the unit, staff members were divided over the issue of the patient's need for treatment. Many staff members shared with the patient his view of himself as "the highest functioning patient on the unit;" these staff members expressed shock and disbelief at his suicide attempt, agreeing that "no one could have predicted" that he would undertake such a violent and desperate act. These attitudes were puzzling, as he had a history of impulsivity and suicidal thoughts. Indeed, the very week of the suicide attempt he twice eloped from the hospital—actions which, under other circumstances, might have been perceived by the staff as clear warning signals to which appropriate measures of restraint could have been applied.

The patient himself was an attractive and superficially charming young man who, from the first days of admission, actively campaigned for his discharge. While he had an essentially unremarkable developmental history with academic, athletic, and social achievement, the history revealed several episodes of anxiety attacks with near-panic states around separations from home in mid- to late adolescence. These episodes were accompanied by insomnia, depression, and obsessional ruminations. Over the next three years, he tried two or three different colleges, psychiatric treatments, jobs, and street drugs. When the patient appeared at home one day after still another flight from college with no thought of the consequences of his repeated failures at school and work, his father initiated the actions just described.

The patient's doctor was only vaguely aware that his objectivity was compromised by his feelings about the parental machinations, extreme family wealth, and the contrast between the appearance of the patient's competence and the reality of the clinical data. He was uncertain about the patient's need for an extended hospitalization. Nevertheless, by the end of the diagnostic period, he was convinced on the basis of the history, the superficiality of the relationship, and the extensive use of denial and projection that the patient suffered from a severe narcissistic personality disorder. This impression was enhanced when the psychiatrist noted that the patient was his charming self so long as the doctor appeared to agree with the patient's own assessment of his capabilities; but if there were the slightest insinuation of psychological problems, then the patient would respond with rageful denunciations of the psychiatrist, belittling his training, credentials, and competence.

The diagnostic impression was consolidated in the patient's case conference. The patient's wish "to do something great with his life" was the central theme of the interview during the conference, which illustrated that there was little, if any, specific content to his wish, and that he had almost no vocational, academic, or interpersonal interests around which he could build an early adult identity. Much to the dismay of the patient, his doctor, and several members of the staff, a long-term hospitalization was recommended and formulated. Many events uncharacteristic of the unit's functioning then ensued: two mainstays of the nursing staff resigned, the head nurse accepted a job on another unit, the patient, already having been elected president of the patient government with unprecedented speed, obtained the highest unit status (unaccompanied), and requested and received permission to enroll in two courses at a local college.

In the meantime, the staff was having difficulty dealing with some important changes in personnel that had occurred by administrative fiat just following the patient's admission to the unit. These changes included the simultaneous arrival of three staff members from another unit in the hospital, a unit which had been in continuous crisis for the previous three years. One was a candidate for the newly vacated assistant head nurse position, but so was a nurse from within the unit. Another, a staff psychiatrist, became the new patient's administrator. And the third, another psychiatrist, was replacing a charismatic educational figure. All three were viewed with quiet hostility and suspicion by the unit staff, who felt betrayed and abandoned by the staff who left. Interestingly, most concern about the patient became localized in these new staff members who were the most articulate advocates of restricting the patient and extending his hospital stay. One of them, for example, was the consultant at the case conference.

The most dysfunctional enactment of the unit's feelings about this cohort who had been imposed upon them occurred in the patient's administrative group where treatment planning took place. The group's administrator, one of the new staff members, was unable to mobilize an effective and cohesive leadership coalition among the staff. Staff members privately complained of his ambivalence about unit philosophy and unclarity in implementing treatment. Patient members saw him as both ineffective and confused: an outsider who did not adequately appreciate the complexities and working structure of the administrative group. In addition, while he was somewhat isolated from the assistant unit chief and unit chief, conflict with the latter was rapidly building.

The patient regarded his administrative group as a tolerable hassle and a joke. More specifically, he communicated to his psychotherapist the feeling that the administrator was defective and beneath him. Even though the psychotherapist was beginning to see the patient in terms of two main conflicting, split off, and unintegrated identity fragments, he agreed with his patient's perception of the administrator. The first fragment, more closely resembling his mother, was that of being the perfect prince who related in an entitled and demanding way and who became enraged, grandiose, and devaluing whenever his wishes were frustrated. The second identity fragment, closely resembling the picture of his father, was one of a deeply damaged self, dependent on others for nurturance and willing to make any sacrifices to maintain the maternal supplies which only a woman could provide. Because of his compromised objectivity, his identification with the imposed-upon staff, and agreement with the patient's view of the new doctor, the therapist felt nowhere near ready to address or interpret these fragments or relate them in any way to the patient's devaluation of the administrator.

Similarly, in the several days before the elopement and suicide attempt, the patient's expressions of ambivalence about hospitalization and treatment, as well as some difficulty in his college courses, were not addressed and, with the exception of a modest change in status, the two elopements were barely responded to. In spite of these loud signals, the otherwise well intentioned and highly perceptive staff continued to accept his devaluation of them, his protestations of competence and promises of compliance, and overlooked his propensity to take flight.

DISCUSSION OF THE CASE

In retrospect, the evolution of this unfortunate concatenation of events might have been predicted and steps taken to prevent the outcome. Some version of it, however, seems to be more the rule than the exception with VIPs as patients. The example also highlights how the interaction with the treatment system and its covert conflicts combine to make the situation problematic. In this example, parallel processes in the patient, his family, the treating physician, and the ward were at work to exacerbate splitting mechanisms, heighten treatment resistance, obfuscate clinical judgment, and block delivery of effective treatment in the form of more attention to the needs of the patient, confrontation of his anger, or limit-setting for his demanding behaviors. What were these processes and how do they relate to aspects of the VIP as patient and syndrome we have outlined so far?

By virtue of his family's extraordinary wealth, important connections, and unusual influence in their community, the patient qualifies for VIP status. This status had already compromised previous treatments from which he was removed prematurely. That the current treatment was in jeopardy from the beginning is indicated by the unusual process of admission and the blocking of the treating staff's access to information from the prior consultation by the hospital's psychiatrist-in-chief: both manifestations of the father's sense of being entitled to manipulate others and control the channels of information. The patient came onto the unit with the sense of having been manipulated into the hospital under false pretenses; and using this betrayal and his own superficial adaptability and borrowing from the parental style, the patient began an active campaign for special treatment with more or less subtle demands to consider him less disturbed than his history indicated. First his therapist and then selected staff members questioned the need for hospitalization. In spite of a case conference which identified his inner impoverishment and need for extended hospitalization, he was allowed to attend college, serve as president of the patient government, and go about the hospital unaccompanied. Thus, a process of isolation of the patient from the staff was in motion.

All of this occurred in the context of a unit quietly and covertly struggling with angry feelings about changes in their staffing which had been imposed upon them. The new staff, representing an out-group, argued for a more restrictive policy; but, fuelled by their own complicated feelings about the patient's importance, the old, intruded-upon-staff became an in-group who identified with the patient and his damaged sense of entitlement, thus helping him and his family ignore the reality of his clinical condition. This process was also enacted in the administrative group's difficulties authorizing their new leader and the covering staff letting the patient leave the unit a third time under their collectively closed eyes.

PERSONALITY CHARACTERISTICS OF THE VIP AS PATIENT

It would be a serious mistake to generalize about the personality characteristics of the VIP as patient. As noted before, there is no systematic or controlled data about the subject. Furthermore, a VIP as patient may have any diagnostic configuration. And finally, it would be a grave disservice to any patient if a preconceived notion of their personality configuration were imposed upon them prematurely. Perhaps the closest generalization that safely can be made involves the dynamics that have been explicated for the special patient in the articles by Burnham and Main. The VIP as patient differs from the so-called special patient, however, in that the former's specialness is reinforced by externally-based social reality. It is also true, of course, that not every VIP as patient generates a full-fledged VIP syndrome.

From this author's experience and the literature cited earlier, the VIP syndrome is marked by splitting and entitlement in the dynamic structure of the VIP as patient or his representatives which, in conjunction with reality-based elements and an inappropriately vulnerable environment, leads to the patient's difficulty accepting the patient role. The situation of illness in an important person represents a kind of split in and of itself, threatening the individual's sense of importance and control. Being a patient is an entitled condition in that others are expected to deliver care; but the potential for humiliation is great in that others examine and minister to the body, extract secrets from the mind, and limit freedom. Intensifying the split intrinsic to an ill VIP, the patient is expected to submit to all of this. Under these conditions, and especially in the inadequately integrated personality, the individual may become acutely sensitive to those aspects of the psychiatrist's personality and elements in the environment which will support their denial of illness and resistance to treatment. If, in addition, a VIP who is a patient or his representatives are actively conveying entitlement by demanding inappropriately special care, then the conditions for the development of a VIP syndrome are in place.

Entitlement is defined by *The Diagnostic and Statistical Manual of Mental Disorders, Third Edition, Revised (DSM-III-R)* (American Psychiatric Association, 1987) as "the expectation of non-obligatory care, respect and affection," and is listed as one of the five categories of signs and symptoms by which one makes the diagnosis of narcissistic personality disorder. Others, however, such as Levin (1970), Kriegman (1983), and Tenzer (1987) believe that, in mild form, disorders of entitlement (and nonentitlement) may be part of the mature personality and, in symptomatic form, cut across diagnostic categories. Linking entitlement with the concept of VIP as patient, Campbell (1981) defines it as "the special privileges that a narcissistic person feels are owed him; for instance, he expects that he will be treated as a VIP" (p. 219).

Freud (1916) alluded to certain patients—"the exceptions"—who, mainly by virtue of their claim that they had suffered enough, were reluctant to submit to the deprivations and lack of immediate gratification of the analytic situation. He believed that attitudes of entitlement related to early, real deprivations in the patient's life. Horney (1950) distinguished between attitudes of entitlement and claims of entitlement: the former, more or less unconscious and unspoken, while the latter are more conscious and interactional. She attributed attitudes of entitlement to an archaically grandiose inner insistence that fulfillment of wishes should come from others. Rothstein (1984) located attitudes of entitlement in the ego where it serves defensive purposes, primarily against the humiliation of being unable to control others, being controlled, or feeling disappointment in a parental object. Blechner (1987) suggested that entitlement defends against feelings of deprivation, especially when experienced in relation to early sibling rivalry. Attributing entitlement behavior to defects in self-esteem, along with an intense rage and a wish to humiliate, destroy, and obliterate others, Grey (1987) listed several elements of exaggerated entitlement which suggest its relationship to the VIP syndrome: It operates like a defense mechanism to enhance status or prestige, and it involves the manipulation and control of others by claiming special privilege beyond the boundaries all would recognize as appropriate to one's role.

Tangential to but different from, antisocial behaviors, entitlement behaviors are common in our culture; for example, the driver who feels that speed limits and stop signs do not apply to him, the caller who has a rapid intolerance of the busy telephone signal, the shopper who cuts into a line, the patient who must be seen immediately, or who parks in a handicapped zone or the hospital's fire lane when a regular space requires extra walking. These behaviors and the attitudes driving them can become subtle features of the commerce between psychiatrist and patient. In setting up appointment times, for example, it is often the case that the psychiatrist finds himself accommodating more to the entitled patient's schedule than to his own. Complications in setting or collecting the fee can often alert the psychiatrist to these same underlying attitudes. Sometimes dismissed as impatience, entitlement may be a thin camouflage for intense dependent longings and a desperate need for special treatment, and exaggerated entitlement is often a precursor to more frankly demanding or grandiose attitudes or behavior. One aspect of passive and dependent behavior (perhaps an earlier way of thinking of entitlement) is the infantile wish that one's needs be met without having to be verbalized.

ACTIVATION OF PATHOGENIC SOCIAL SYSTEM FACTORS

When entitled attitudes and claims are linked with reality-based influence such as wealth, connection, power, and prestige in the treatment situation, the demand takes on a life and power of its own. A wealthy patient or family is entitled in our society to obtain resources which poorer people cannot have, as in the clinical example presented earlier. A patient or family may assume an exaggerated, unrealistic entitlement as in the case of a patient's mother who barely knew, but regularly announced, a close personal relationship with the clinical director. One family instantly assumed VIP status by calling the medical director of a large hospital and influencing him to order an assistant unit chief to write sedative orders for a patient. Another patient's family elevated their sick adolescent to a VIP by enlisting the aid of a state senator to secure admission for her when she had been previously denied admission by the staff.

In these and other situations, entitled demands are backed by implicit threats to the treater or the treatment system. Since considerable resources can be mobilized on behalf of the entitled patient, the reputation of individual practitioners may be at stake; and, in an institution, sanctions may be imposed from above. This can be the case in a corporation, in the military, or in a hospital system. It is especially true when the VIP is a physician, and the confusing and contradictory knowledge base for psychiatric diagnosis and treatment are overtly or covertly shared between client and treater, as may happen in the discussion of medication effect or trials.

A particularly insidious combination between the VIP and the psychiatrist occurs when the latter has unacknowledged entitled, exhibitionistic, voyeuristic, or grandiose trends within his or her own personality. Here a subtle competition between patient and doctor develops, which increases the volatility of the situation. When such countertransference generalizes to the treatment system, strain and dysfunctional processes are activated, even cognitive dissonances. Since the patient's history, diagnosis, symptoms, and course of illness already impinge upon the staff's capacity to see the patient as a person, awe, envy, and the wish to identify oneself with the VIP potentially contribute to this difficulty. These processes can bring particular havoc to psychiatric units that are organized on a therapeutic community model. Where democratic and egalitarian principles are espoused, where roles tend to be diffuse and patients and staff are authorized to feel entitled themselves, resentment and conflict are ignited quickly, splitting ensues, and the VIP is in danger of being scapegoated—usually at first by isolation and then secondarily by an active attack.

This process has been described earlier in the context of the special patient, but it is usually intensified in the case of the VIP patient as hospital administration invariably is called into the fray. When control of the case begins to slip into the hands of professional or administrative staff in the hospital who are external to the VIP's treatment unit, the situation usually has become untenable and treatment failure is virtually inevitable. The VIP's entitlement has, in essence, become communicated or projected into a system which has lost its capacity to respond, manage, or contain it in any useful way for the patient. At this point, the patient is in as much control of his treatment as the professional staff, and his complaints of poor treatment and demands for something better have a substantial reality base.

RECOMMENDATIONS

The clinician undertaking the assessment and treatment of the VIP as a patient is first and foremost advised to be aware of how much energy he or she has available; that is, his or her willingness to embark on such an endeavor. It is work that will probably involve more than the usual pressure on routine policies and practice, and includes a more active taking control of the treatment, setting limits, and protecting the patient's confidentiality. The clinician also is advised that the chances for treatment success are proportional to the awareness of his or her unconscious investment in the patient and the clinician's importance as well as his or her own need for the patient to do well. This includes the psychiatrist's attitudes toward importance, his or her own entitled attitudes, and his or her comfort with multiple negotiations at the many boundaries of the treatment. In the larger sense, this means the awareness and careful monitoring of the psychiatrist's countertransference, especially that involved with awe, envy, and pride. In the more practical sense, it means being available to the patient in the same way he or she is with all of the non-VIPs who are patients.

In a personal communication 25 years after his original contribution to the subject, Weintraub (1987) comments that VIPs as patients are often drawn to VIPs who are physicians. He recommends that this sometimes turns out to be a poor match since both have similar weaknesses and blind spots. Under the circumstances, the therapist's unacknowledged identification with the patient leads to an unwillingness to confront behavior that seems "natural" in the circles in which the patient travels; the therapist's overestimation of the honor of treating someone who can demand and receive the services of any psychiatrist he wants; and, perhaps most important of all, the therapist's inability to resist "playing God" and, in some way, having an influence that goes beyond treating the VIP as patient.

A useful distinction to make in this regard is that between the conditions and content of treatment. The conditions of treatment include all aspects of the treatment contract and the psychiatrist's real relationship with the patient. The content of the treatment is its substance: evaluation, diagnosis, and somatic and psychosocial interventions. Treatment of the VIP often and realistically involves compromises in the conditions of treatment so as to insure and protect its content. For example, a performer who travels cannot be expected to attend sessions on a regular basis. By the same token, a busy surgeon who is on-call cannot be expected to turn off his paging device during sessions, no matter how important the psychotherapeutic moment or material. It is appropriate for the therapist to be flexible about the conditions of treatment as long as he or she acknowledges an exception is being made.

Harry Stack Sullivan was known to have suggested that the only thing a psychiatrist should want from his or her patient was payment of the fee. In this light, the therapist of a VIP as patient should not exploit the financial situation nor enter into any other corrupt agreements about the conditions of treatment that might jeopardize its content in the long run. Similarly, while it is appropriate to accept an irregular appointment schedule as part of the treatment contract, the psychiatrist must be alert to and be prepared to discuss all the implications of sudden cancellations. And, as suggested by the GAP report, the issue of disclosing "public information" about the patient is best left to the VIP and his official family; but as much as possible about the conditions of treatment, including the possibility of disruption of the VIP's usual routines, should be outlined and agreed upon by the VIP and his representatives (when relevant) at the outset of the evaluation and treatment.

The content of treatment should be as close to the accepted standard of care as possible, and some recommendations in this regard appeared earlier in this chapter. Specifically, the psychiatrist and treatment team need to be protected from retaliation and intrusion by both the patient, his official family, and the hospital hierarchy if reasonable and objective treatment is to take place. Also, the psychiatrist is advised to evaluate with extreme care data about the patient that have been obtained when the conditions of treatment have been compromised.

Just as it is in the conditions of treatment where the psychiatrist implements his or her recognition that treatment of the VIP is not the usual, as Weintraub advised, the hospital must be prepared to show the VIP special consideration.

For example, a unit was inappropriately unable to adjust its usual admission policy, which required the presence of parents, when the actively suicidal son of a hospital board member presented for admission when his father was on a business trip in Europe. Ideally, the VIP can be hospitalized in a facility where his influence is not so great. A clear and open line of communication must exist between the head of the treatment team, the clinical director, hospital administration, and those people in the community who are in the official family. While some special considerations around admission, room, and therapist assignment may appropriately be made, at the same time, the boundary around the content of the staff's treatment must be protected.

A great deal has been made in this review about the intersection between attitudes of entitlement and their enactment into overt claims through staff countertransferences in the genesis of the VIP syndrome. It is, therefore, recommended that a staff about to launch into the treatment of a VIP meet before the patient arrives, and regularly thereafter, for the purpose of bringing into awareness, exploring, and working through complex feelings about the patient's importance and how he is being treated. Special privileges that have been granted to the patient must be explained to the staff in detail. When a VIP is on a psychiatric unit, staff process must be attended to even more scrupulously than usual, especially those that indicate processes of splitting and an isolation of the patient. Naturally, scapegoating and its deceptive opposite, making the patient into a "pet," needs immediate attention. Pedantic though it may seem, reminders to the staff about confidentiality must be made while requests to the patient for seemingly innocuous favors are forbidden, even when the latter has completed treatment.

A critical variable in the prevention of the VIP syndrome is the role of the unit chief. Jointly identified with the unit and its endeavors and the hospital administration and its needs, it is his or her primary role to identify the warning signals inherent in these dysfunctional processes and manage this precarious boundary (Munich, 1986). The VIP syndrome is the maximum test of this capacity. Similarly, the patient's hospital psychiatrist sits on the boundary between the patient and the unit and experiences much the same kind of inner strain. Both of these individuals are at great risk for contributing to the divisiveness and the splitting we have described and must feel authorized in their roles and at some inner ease with the dilemma. This authorization is as much an administrative issue as a clinical and personal one.

CONCLUSION

The predominantly negative experience of treating the VIP as psychiatric patient that appears in the literature probably does an injustice to the number of favorable outcomes that go unrecorded. When attitudes of entitlement and reality-based importance do not interfere with the assumption by the VIP of the patient role, and when the psychiatrist and his or her team are in touch with the potential difficulties that attend VIP treatments, then treatment has a good chance for success. When any of these factors does not apply, then the potential for an untoward outcome is enhanced. This chapter has outlined the many processes by which a VIP syndrome may develop. It has especially defined and emphasized the reciprocal and dysfunctional mobilization of attitudes of entitlement between the VIP and treaters, and the split which develops between the former's heightened pressure and the latter's quiet withdrawal. Acknowledgement of the VIP as special, attention to warning signals, monitoring personal countertransferences, and addressing latent staff conflict can protect against the troubles outlined in this review and lead to treatment success and treater gratification.

REFERENCES

American Psychiatric Association: Diagnostic and Statistical Manual of Mental Disorders, Third Edition, Revised (DSM-III-R). Washington, DC, American Psychiatric Association, 1987

Blechner MJ: Entitlement and narcissism: paradise sought. Contemporary Psychoanalysis 1987; 23:244–255

Campbell RJ (Ed): Psychiatric Dictionary, 5th edition. New York, Oxford University Press, 1981

Burnham DL: The special problem patient: victim or agent of splitting? Psychiatry 1966; 29:105–122

Feuer EH, Karasu SR: A star-struck service: impact of the admission of a celebrity to an inpatient unit. J Clin Psychiatry 1978; 39:743–746

Freud S: Some character types met with in psychoanalytic work (1916), in Complete Psychological Works, Standard Edition, vol. 14. Translated and edited by Strachey J. London, Hogarth Press, 1961

Gabbard G: The treatment of the 'special' patient in a psychoanalytic hospital. International Review of Psychoanalysis 1986; 13:333–347

Grey A: Entitlement: an interactional defense of self esteem. Contemporary Psychoanalysis 1987; 23:255–263

Grotjahn M: The treatment of the famous and the "beautiful people" in groups, in Group Therapy 1975: An Overview. Edited by Wolberg LR, Aronson ML. New York, Stratton Intercontinental, 1975

Group for the Advancement of Psychiatry: The VIP with Psychiatric Impairment. Vol. VIII, Report No. 83, January 1973

Groves JE: Taking care of the hateful patient. New Engl J Med 1978; 298:883–887

Horney K: Neurosis and Human Growth: The Struggle Toward Self-Realization. New York, Norton & Co., 1950

Hotchner AE: Papa Hemingway. New York, Random House, 1966

Kernberg O: Projective identification, countertransference, and hospital treatment. Psychiatr Clin North Am 1987; 10:257–272

Kriegman G: Entitlement attitudes: psychosocial and therapeutic implications. J Am Acad Psychoanal 1983; 11:265–281

Levin S: On psychoanalysis of attitudes of entitlement. Bulletin of the Philadelphia Association for Psychoanalysis 1970; 20:1–10

Main TF: The ailment. Br J Med Psychol 1957; 30:129–145

Miller MH, Roberts LM: Psychotherapy with the children or disciples of charismatic individuals. Am J Psychiatry 1967; 123:1049–1057

Munich RL: The role of the unit chief: an integrated perspective. Psychiatry 1986; 49:325–336

Pittman FS: Children of the rich. Fam Process 1985; 24:461–472

Rothstein A: The Narcissistic Pursuit of Perfection. New York, International Universities Press, 1984

Saari C, Johnson SR: Problems in the treatment of VIP clients. Social Casework Dec. 1975; 599–604

Stanton AH, Schwartz MS: The Mental Hospital. New York, Basic Books, 1954

Steyn RW: Psychiatric problems of the VIP. Milit Med 1980; 145:482–483

Stone MH: Treating the wealthy and their children. International Journal of Child Psychotherapy 1972; 1:15–46

Stone MH: The child of a famous father or mother, in Basic Handbook of Child Psychiatry. Edited by Noshpitz JD. New York, Basic Books, 1979

Stoudemire A, Rhoads JM: When the doctor needs a doctor: special considerations for the physician-patient. Ann Intern Med 1983; 98:654–659

Strange RE: The VIP with illness. Milit Med 1980; 145:473–475

Tenzer A: Grandiosity and its discontent. Contemporary Psychoanalysis 1987; 23:263–271

Weintraub W: The VIP syndrome: a clinical study in hospital psychiatry. J Nerv Ment Dis 1964; 138:181–193

Chapter 30

The Psychotherapeutic Stalemate

Dianna E. Hartley, Ph.D.

Since the beginning of the practice of psychotherapy, treatment impasses or stalemates, premature terminations, and negative outcomes have been important clinical and theoretical problems, approached from many different angles. The phenomenon has been called by many names, including negative therapeutic reaction, resistance, and transference–countertransference bind. For the purposes of this review, a stalemate or impasse is defined as a relatively long-lasting period in the course of treatment in which the patient's presenting problems and overall level of coping do not improve or significantly worsen, in ways that are not merely transient effects or random fluctuations due to life stresses. Paolino (1981) identified two basic reasons for such therapeutic failure: 1) the patient was not suitable for the type of therapy offered for any of a variety of reasons; and 2) the therapeutic techniques were incorrectly applied by the therapist.

A recent survey of leading clinicians across the country revealed that certain patients are considered inherently more difficult to treat than others. These therapists included in the category of difficult patients those with paranoid, borderline, narcissistic, and antisocial personality disorders. They also believed that it was not only the patient, but a severely pathological family system, that made treatment difficult (Wong, 1983).

A number of other therapists, however, disagree with the idea that the problem lies within the patient. Stolorow and colleagues (1983) argue that there is no such person as a difficult patient, and contend that stalemates arise from the interaction between patient and therapist; that therapeutic impasses and disasters cannot be understood apart from the intersubjective context in which they develop. They usually are the product of prolonged transference–countertransference disjunctions, in which the therapist assimilates the material expressed by the patient into configurations that distort its actual subjective meaning for the patient, resulting in chronic misunderstandings and countertherapeutic spirals that intensify, rather than relieve, the patient's suffering and fail to correct the underlying psychopathology.

In this view, stalemates may also result from intersubjective conjunctions in which the patient's experiences are assimilated into similar central configurations in the mind of the therapist. If the conjunction reflects a mutual defensive posture, resistance and counterresistance in the treatment may be strengthened. They recommend that therapists be sufficiently aware of themselves that they are able to decenter, in the Piagetian sense, from their own subjective worlds in order to grasp the meaning of their patients' experience of difficulties in treatment.

HISTORY OF THE CONCEPT

Both definitions and attributions of causes of stalemates have changed over the course of history of psychoanalysis and psychotherapy. Freud (1918) first used the term "negative reaction" in his discussion of the case of the Wolf Man. It seemed to him that every time something was cleared up, the patient contradicted the new insight by an aggravation of his symptoms, like a child violating a prohibition one last time before giving up the forbidden behavior. Later, he wrote about "negative therapeutic reactions," saying that "something in these people" opposes recovery and dreads its approach (Freud, 1937). Freud viewed this phenomenon as the result, in part, of defiant attitudes toward the analyst, secondary gain of the symptoms, or narcissistic inaccessibility to a relationship with the analyst; but he attributed it primarily to a "moral factor," in that the illness seemed to be a way to atone for unconscious guilt.

Abraham (1918/1948) attributed some treatment failures to the inability of some narcissistic patients to tolerate the humiliation and diminished self-love involved in facing ego-dystonic facts. Writing from a Kleinian perspective about negative reactions in analysis, Riviere (1936) said that some patients used hypomanic denial and infantile omnipotence to defend against depression, with its accompanying sense of dependent vulnerability and helplessness. Gero (1936) also saw negative therapeutic reactions as characteristic of depressed patients. Sullivan (1953), working in a different conceptual framework, wrote of negative reactions in sadomasochistic patients who, when they are stressed and most in need of tenderness, act in defensive, malevolent ways that bring malevolence back into themselves.

Thus, most traditional psychoanalytic theorists tended to attribute treatment stalemates and failures to something inside the patient, generally to some form of internalized sadomasochistic tendencies. Wilhelm Reich (1933), however, was among the first to take a more interactive perspective, and to see that existing technique was often inadequate for dealing with latent negative transferences and treatment impasses.

Recent conceptualizations of both stalemates and treatment failures in the clinical and psychotherapy research literatures emphasize gains made in understanding regressive transference manifestations (Blanck and Blanck, 1986; Gedo, 1979, 1986), and in adopting more dynamic family-systemic (Lerner and Lerner, 1983) and interactional (Langs, 1982; Gorney, 1979) perspectives. A recent issue of *Psychoanalytic Inquiry* (1987, vol. 7, no. 2), in which analysts representing different theoretical positions commented on the same case material, gives some idea of the vast differences of opinion on the subject of impasses that exist even among a relatively homogeneous group of therapists.

If we consider stalemates from an interactional perspective, we must raise questions about 1) the patient's contribution; 2) the therapist's contribution; 3) the treatment situation or framework; and 4) the social context of the treatment.

Some early ideas about the patient's contribution have been outlined above and will be further explicated later. Here we will consider the therapist's contribution in terms of personal and technical factors, apart from countertransference (which is detailed in Chapter 25). In his work on therapeutic alliance, Bordin (1979) pointed out that different forms of therapy make different demands on both the therapist and the patient in terms of their personal qualities and their working contract. Langs (1982) has been particularly active in explicating the effects of violations of the basic framework, or implicit working contract, inherent in the psychotherapy relationship on the therapeutic process and on the patient's level of functioning. Lerner and Lerner (1983) emphasized the importance of the patient's family system with regard to the dynamic stresses and reactions that are set off by change in the individual. The explicit and implicit messages the patient gets from family members could potentially undermine strides toward autonomy or higher levels of functioning.

THE DIFFICULT PATIENT

Early in the history of psychoanalysis and psychotherapy, negative therapeutic outcomes and stalemates were attributed almost exclusively to intrapsychic characteristics of patients, such as unconscious guilt, sadomasochistic tendencies, intolerable envy of the therapist, or defenses against depression. More recent object-relational and interactional perspectives focus more on the patient's perception of the therapist and the therapeutic relationship, and his or her ability to make constructive use of the person and the expertise of the therapist. While our formulations have changed, the fact remains that many cases of therapeutic impasse involve patients who are legitimately described as "difficult to treat," because of such characteristics as masochism (Parkin, 1980), unconscious preoedipal or oedipal guilt (Kernberg, 1986; Modell, 1971), narcissistic envy (Rosenfeld, 1975), or an imbalance of libidinal and aggressive impulses (Loewald, 1972).

Only a few authors have focused on the adaptive and reparative meanings of these characteristics (Colson, 1982). Some patients, usually on the basis of early family dynamics, seem to feel deeply that they do not have a right to a better life, and that any gains they make result in suffering for others. Thus, they are "good" and either sacrifice their own development or punish themselves whenever they do something to enhance their lives.

For whatever reasons, many patients do become hostile, disorganized, or dependent in the therapy relationship to an extent that their treatment progress is halted or compromised. While it is clear that competent therapists disagree about the characteristics of this population and the etiology of the problem, it is a major concern in the field.

In a major study in which experts were asked about negative effects in psychotherapy, several participants stressed that a thorough diagnostic assessment in the initial phase of therapy was the best safeguard against antitherapeutic processes and the negative outcomes which usually result (Strupp et al, 1977). Such an assessment should include a full description of the symptom picture, as well as a comprehensive understanding of the patient's strengths and weaknesses, general level of ego functioning or personality organization, and the role the symptoms might play in maintaining a personal and a family-systems equilibrium. In the absence of a comprehensive understanding, the therapist may probe too deeply too soon, and provoke negative reactions, or may not challenge the patient to change for the better to the fullest extent possible.

The present consensus seems to be that patients with borderline personality disorder are more prone than the patient population in general to negative experiences in psychotherapy. For example, Colson and colleagues (1985) reexamined 11 cases from the Menninger Foundation Psychotherapy Research Project who were rated as treatment failures, and compared them with the 10 most successful cases. Paradoxically, they found that the patients with poorer outcomes had higher levels of educational and occupational achievement, and concluded from a careful reading of the clinical write-ups that misdiagnoses in the direction of overestimating ego strength had consistently been made. The negative outcome group included primarily patients with borderline personality organization, particularly those marked by a desperate, angry search for satisfaction or chronically thwarted needs for nurturance. They had enormous difficulty establishing mature relationships, and most resorted to substance abuse. Because they had achieved relatively high social status despite significant psychopathology, they "tended to receive treatments which, at least at the outset, were mismatched in terms of the amount of support, containment, and structure required for a successful outcome" (Colson et al, 1985, p. 67).

Mays and Franks (1985), in a major review of negative effects in psychotherapy, concluded that borderline patients seem to do worse than other patients, especially in psychoanalysis or insight oriented psychotherapy. Their conclusion may be biased because of the fact that psychoanalytically oriented clinicians and researchers tend to look at their data in terms of such personality variables, which often are ignored by adherents of other types of therapy. The extremely maladaptive interpersonal patterns of these patients are likely to be equally disruptive in all approaches to therapy. Since patients with borderline personality organizations constitute approximately 10 percent of the total patient population, it is especially important to find ways to help them use therapy. Mays and Franks listed five characteristics of high risk patients: 1) impaired or conflicted social support; 2) disturbances in the ability to communicate with others; 3) disturbances in mood or affect regulation; 4) disturbances in identity and sense of self; and 5) disturbances in impulse control.

Psychological testing and structured clinical interviews increase diagnostic accuracy among these high risk patients. Testing has been shown to be more accurate than any other single source, or combined sources, of information in the diagnosis of borderline disorders (Appelbaum, 1977; Maltas, 1978). Specific interviews for diagnosing borderline disorders have been developed by Gunderson (1977) and by Kernberg (1986).

THE DIFFICULT THERAPIST

While theoretical formulations of the problem of therapeutic impasses focus on the patient's contribution, many clinicians and researchers cite primarily therapist factors, such as poor clinical judgment; deficiencies in training and skills; inappropriate personality traits, such as exploitativeness, sadistic or masochistic trends, narcissism, or obsessionalism; or lack of authenticity (Strupp et al, 1977). While there is disagreement about the relative importance of therapist and patient factors in producing stalemates, a consistent finding is that the more disturbed the patient, the more therapist skill and personal qualities appear to be critical to the avoidance of negative events. Therapist characteristics which increase the likelihood of stalemates and negative reactions can be separated into two categories: those which are perceived as excessively stimulating or threatening to the patient (for example, high levels of confrontation, unacceptable interpretations); and those which are perceived as providing too low levels of support (such as excessive interpersonal distance, lack of warmth, passivity).

Weiner (1982) believes that different factors are involved for relatively inexperienced and more experienced therapists. For neophyte therapists, errors in diagnosis and technical errors are the most common contributors to impasses.

The most common diagnostic error is the overestimation of ego strength, while the most common technical error is the attempted application of inappropriate techniques, based either on bias or naivete. For more experienced therapists, Weiner thinks that patient factors account for a greater number of stalemates. Unfortunately, an all too common practice in institutional settings, especially those with training programs, is to assign the most difficult, undesirable cases to the least experienced or least well trained therapists. With anxious and naive therapists, particularly those whose time commitment to the treatment is limited, failures are almost inevitable.

Once an impasse is developing, therapists may perpetuate or exacerbate it either by neglecting to deal with the feelings involved, for fear of losing control of the process, or by responding defensively to justify their own behavior, rather than helping patients examine the realistic and unrealistic sources of their perceptions and feelings (Mays and Franks, 1985). Therapists usually feel angry, guilty, and impotent at times of impasse. These feelings may be enacted by being late for or cancelling sessions, being sarcastic or cold, allowing dependency, or giving up on attainable goals, all of which exacerbate the situation and may lead to premature termination or poor outcome of the therapy.

Colson and colleagues (1985) found that therapists in their negative-outcome group were often slow to recognize the lack of progress in treatment and to shift to more appropriate therapeutic strategies. Particularly in psychoanalysis or psychoanalytic psychotherapies which are intended to be long term, inertia may be seen as less undesirable than impatience; but their evidence suggests that inactivity can be just as harmful to the treatment.

It is easy to say that high-risk patients should be treated only by therapists who are able to offer high levels of empathy, warmth, and genuineness and who have the greatest knowledge of personality dynamics, interpersonal style, and potential pitfalls of treatment. However, the results of studies of therapists' contribution to the psychotherapy process and common lore among therapy researchers suggest that such consistently "high functioning" therapists are rare (Mitchell et al, 1977; Strupp, 1980a, 1980b, 1980c).

MISALLIANCES

Many therapeutic stalemates are precipitated by failure to deal with issues of the contract (Weiner, 1982), the framework (Langs, 1982), or the therapeutic alliance (Greenson, 1967; Hartley, 1985). A major component of the therapeutic alliance is the explicit or implicit understanding between the therapist and the patient about the goals they will work toward and the means they will use in their pursuit. The process of establishing and maintaining an alliance may go awry at many points and in many ways. Bordin (1979) specified three components of the therapeutic alliance that need to be considered: 1) the bond between the therapist and patient as two adults who, to a reasonable degree, like and trust each other; 2) agreement on the ultimate goals of the therapy; and 3) division of responsibility for accomplishing the work of the therapy. The therapist and the patient must be both willing and able to engage genuinely in the relationship and to accomplish the tasks required of them for the particular kind of therapy they undertake.

Colson and colleagues (1985) found that the therapy process for patients with negative outcomes in the Menninger study was notable for the absence of cooperative and collaborative activity by the patient, based in part on the attitude that the therapist should cause the patient to feel better without the patient's active work. Therapy proceeded as though the patient had to extract solutions from a harsh, ungiving therapist. They also noted that the therapists were remarkably inconsistent in addressing blatant violations of basic aspects of the therapeutic contract, unwittingly tolerating behavior that undermined the therapies' chances of success:

> Frequently the treatments were marked by inconsistent attendance, lateness, delinquent payment of the bill, interminable contacts with the therapists at odd hours outside the treatment sessions, persistent verbal assaults on the treater, inconsistent use of medication, and a variety of other forms of "acting out" within and outside the treatment hours. In far too many instances the therapists patiently tolerated the continuation of such behavior, perhaps expecting that such behavior would yield to the "right" interpretations. In not one case did the treater insist that continuation of treatment would depend on an alteration in such behaviors. From our current perspective it would have been quite appropriate, and in some instances necessary, for the therapist to support treatment structures by putting the treatment itself on the line (Colson et al, 1985, pp. 72–73).

When a therapist fails to insist that basic treatment structures be adhered to, he or she has indeed violated the therapist's part of the framework, and may have conveyed to the patient that such violations are acceptable or tolerable.

The results of the Menninger study, the treatments of which were conducted 20–30 years ago did, in fact, teach us much that we now take for granted about the importance of the therapeutic alliance (Horwitz, 1974) and firm insistence on the patient adhering to the basic treatment structure (Kernberg, 1986). In the recent review of the cases, it is clear that the therapists' tolerance of maladaptive behavior in the context of the therapy perpetuated their patients' problems, while insisting that they follow the more mature adult aspects of the contract might have led to further development in other relationships as well. Such neglect of the basic framework of the treatment often feeds into the patient's poor sense of personal responsibility, poor reality testing, and poor impulse control, and ultimately creates a chronic impasse in the treatment that is exceedingly difficult for the patient and therapist to resolve or dilute.

THE SOCIAL ENVIRONMENT OF THE TREATMENT

Considering the fact that therapy rarely occupies more than a few hours a week, it is suprising how little attention has been paid to events occurring outside the consulting room. For example, impasses often have a significant impact on patients' family members. Their reactions may at times undermine the patient's self-confidence as well as his or her confidence in the therapist, or may reinforce the idea that the patient is bad or uncooperative.

When there is no detectable family reaction to an impasse, we may wonder about the importance of the patient's symptoms or weaknesses in maintaining some particular balance in family dynamics. Colson and colleagues (1985) concluded that among negative outcome cases, "significant people in the patient's life colluded to an extraordinary degree, either to sabotage treatment or to undermine opportunities for health" (p. 67). The usual pattern was one of overindulgence and encouragement of self-destructive behavior and hostile dependence on family members, alternating with periods of harsh control and rejection.

Voth and Orth (1973), in their book about these cases, were struck by the parallel between the impasses in the therapies of these patients and the impasses of development in the separation–individuation phases that are, in theory, associated with borderline pathology. Gurman and Kniskern (1978) suggested that the development of alliances with key family members may reduce both deliberate and unwitting sabotage of therapy.

Lerner and Lerner (1983) emphasize that failures to change often can be understood by considering the adaptive functions served by the patient's symptoms or developmental failures in the context of the family system. They see the patient as caught between the competing pulls of change, represented by the treatment contract and the therapeutic relationship, and homeostasis, represented by loyalty to the family's overt or covert injunctions to remain the same or "change back." Behavior toward the therapist that appears to be oppositional or devaluing may take on different meanings when the systemic vantage point is adopted. Once these meanings are formulated by the therapist, they are interpreted to the patient in a neutral way, thus freeing the therapist from a position of urging the patient to change and allowing the patient to decide whether or not to change. The systemic approach can be used not only for addressing current family activity, but also with patients who are geographically distant or emotionally disengaged from family or whose key family members are deceased. The essential aspects are a conceptual framework and techniques that allow gathering information about how the family system works and how the patient's symptoms and resistance are embedded in it.

RESOLVING STALEMATES

Obviously, it is better to anticipate and deal with an impending stalemate than with a fully developed one. Several clues may point to potential difficulties. For example, if the therapist makes a therapeutic contract that differs dramatically from the usual, such as setting an extremely low fee or allowing extensive outside contact, problems often ensue. Recognition of early stages of an impasse requires that the therapist have in mind a goal for treatment and the means by which to reach the goal; that is, the beginnings of a sound therapeutic alliance. During extended periods when no change occurs or when interactions are consistently empty or negative, a reexamination of the contract may reveal that neither therapist nor patient is working toward the original goal.

At a point of suspected impasse of uncertain etiology, the therapist needs, first, to observe the therapeutic process closely, then perhaps to obtain consultation, to transfer the patient to another therapist, or to suggest a vacation from therapy (Weiner, 1982). The patient should also be involved in the process of observation and reflection on the process of the therapy in order to diagnose and decide what to do about the problem. By asking the patient to participate in the process, the therapist indicates that both are responsible for the outcome of the therapy.

Obtaining Consultations from Other Clinicians

Consultation may take such forms as scheduling independent interviews with another therapist, having another person (a supervisor or colleague) observe a video or audiotape, or referring the patient for psychological testing. Cognitive and intellectual testing can be useful in detecting patients whose capacity for abstract thinking is impaired, or for whom other deficits make it difficult or impossible to attain the conceptual integration necessary for verbal therapies. Projective testing can identify problems with impulse control, impaired reality testing, or other aspects of personality organization which may alert the therapist to the need for more ego-building approaches to the treatment (Blanck and Blanck, 1986). In addition to these more formal or structural aspects of cognitive style and personality organization, testing may alert the therapist to psychological themes that have been missed because of inexperience, countertransference problems, or other sources of empathic failure.

The process of deciding whether to obtain a consultation can itself give clues about the nature of the difficulty. A patient's hesitation to see a consultant when the therapist suggests it may indicate unwillingness to engage significantly with the therapist, a lack of motivation for the therapy, a conscious or unconscious sense that the consultation threatens the pathological gratification inherent in the impasse, or a fear that this is the first step toward abandonment by the therapist.

When it is the patient who requests a consultation, the therapist may either suggest consultants or allow the patient to select one. While a therapist has an obligation to state clearly his or her own professional advice, therapists who feel strongly about whom the patient sees or even whether the patient should ask for another opinion, must examine their own wish to control their patients, or other potentially antitherapeutic attitudes.

For nonmedical therapists or physicians who prefer not to use medications with their own psychotherapy patients, multiple treatment is an alternative to transferring patients who require biological interventions. A separate physician manages medications while the psychotherapist continues psychological treatment. This practice is most feasible within an institutional setting or in a situation where frequent communication between treaters is possible.

Transferring the Patient

When it becomes clear through exploration and observation or through consultation that the therapist does not offer the kind of treatment the patient needs or that something in the patient–therapist interaction blocks effective collaborative work together, transfer of the patient should be considered. When this occurs, both the transferring and the receiving therapists share the responsibility to help in working through the loss, resolving the problematic dynamics as much as possible, and making the attachment to the new therapist.

Termination or Vacation from Therapy

Raising the question of stopping treatment has long been used to deal with impasses (Freud, 1937). When temporary or permanent termination of treatment is a realistic alternative, and not a manipulation, the therapist's mentioning it may motivate the patient to examine all the possibilities for resolving the impasse.

Some patients may find that the therapist's nondefensive willingness to discuss stopping the treatment makes them feel freer to air their own feelings and ideas about the problems in the relationship. The dangers of raising this possibility are the same as those of raising the more general issue of the impasse itself: The patient may act impulsively, or may feel demoralized or abandoned.

POSITIVE ASPECTS OF STALEMATES

Since both patients and therapists have strong emotional reactions to stalemates, it is important to work with these feelings as a problem in the therapist–patient relationship, not just as an intrapsychic phenomenon. Clear discussion of the stalemate itself can be a valuable experience for a patient whose previous relationships have been based on mutual blame instead of mutual responsibility. Anger, guilt, helplessness, frustration, and other negative feelings often can be turned to therapeutic advantage by direct expression. Weiner (1982) stresses that mutual exploration must take place in the context of an adequate therapeutic alliance, and not be used to seduce patients into remaining in therapy or to substitute for the patient's self-examination.

In addition to the positive effects that open discussion of stalemates can have in individual cases, it often has been the case that treatment impasses have provided the impetus for major revisions of theory and technique, and are thus beneficial to the profession as a whole when they are productively examined. To take an early example, an impasse and premature termination in the case of Dora led Freud to his conceptualization of transference. More recently, Kohut's (1979) paper about his reanalysis of Mr. Z, which indicates his willingness to examine his mistakes and his thinking processes about them, provides a valuable model for questioning "received wisdom," for listening carefully to patient's associations with an open mind, and for reformulating ideas about the etiology and treatment of relatively common forms of psychopathology. Gedo (1986), in a scholarly review of the history of ideas in psychoanalysis and current controversies in the field, clearly illustrated how many significant advances in both theory and practice developed from failures to deal adequately with certain types of psychopathology.

RELEVANT RESEARCH FINDINGS

No research has addressed directly the problem of therapeutic stalemates and their resolution. However, it is possible to find relevant information in existing research on negative outcomes and on psychotherapy process with measures that allowed the examination of negative events during sessions. Orlinsky and Howard (1986) point out that the "macro-outcome" of a psychotherapy is the net result of an extended series of incremental "micro-outcomes" seen in the sessions and between sessions in the daily life of the patient during therapy.

The first step toward empirical examination of impasses is the development of reliable and valid process measurements for the relevant variables. The Psychotherapy Research Group at Vanderbilt University, under the direction of Hans Strupp, has made substantial progress in this area in the past two decades. They recently developed the Vanderbilt Negative Indicators Scale, which specifically identifies a number of in-session occurrences which have been shown to be associated ultimately with poor outcomes (Sachs, 1983; Suh et al, 1986). They have also included in other process scales the possibility of assessing negative, as well as positive, signs of therapeutic interaction and therapeutic alliance (Gomes-Schwartz, 1978; Hartley and Strupp, 1983).

For example, the Vanderbilt Psychotherapy Process Scale (VPPS) comprises eight subscales: Patient Participation, Patient Hostility, Patient Psychic Distress, Patient Exploration, Patient Dependency, Therapist Exploration, Therapist Warmth and Friendliness, and Negative Therapist Attitude. The 80 items on the scale are rated by observers who watch or listen to the therapy sessions. Unfortunately, in most of the process-outcome studies using the VPPS, these subscales have been collapsed in ways that make it impossible to examine the impact of the identified negative patient or therapist qualities on outcome.

An interesting exception is a study of therapist characteristics associated with differential outcome by Suh and O'Malley (1982). They divided their sample into four groups by crossing prognosis and outcome (for example, high prognosis–low outcome, low prognosis–low outcome, and so on). They found that it was not the absolute level of the therapist quality, but the *pattern of change* over the early sessions that discriminated among these groups. Patients who were categorized as high prognosis–low outcome had therapists "characterized by initially high levels of Negative Therapist Attitude which increased across sessions with a concomitant decrease in Therapist Warmth and Therapist Exploration. . . . Therapists for low prognosis–low outcome cases not only exhibited high initial levels of Negative Therapist Attitude but there was a decrease in Therapist Warmth over sessions" (Suh et al, 1986, p. 301). These results indicate that there was a sample of patients who, according to other indicators, including their own willingness and ability to participate in psychotherapeutic exploration, would have been expected to have good outcomes. However, for some reason, the stance of the therapist toward them was somewhat negative from the beginning of the therapy, and the therapist progressively withdrew both in terms of warmth of interaction and in terms of his engagement in the process of exploration of the patient's difficulties. There was also a sample of patients who could be identified early as having significant problems with the interpersonal and/or the intrapsychic aspects of therapy. While their prognosis was thus poor from the beginning, their therapists' negative attitude and lack of warmth did not help overcome the obstacles to their treatment.

Another measure developed by this group, The Vanderbilt Negative Indicators Scale (VNIS), is the best existing measure for examining the kind of events in therapy sessions that generally are associated with impasses and eventual poor outcome. Growing out of the work of Strupp, Hadley, and Gomes-Schwartz (1977), this scale includes 42 patient, therapist, and interaction items. The subscales include: Patient Qualities, Therapist Personal Qualities, Errors in Technique, Patient–Therapist Interaction, and Global Factors. Sachs (1983) found that the subscale Errors in Technique showed the strongest and most consistent relationship to outcome, while Therapist Personal Qualities were not significantly associated with outcome. This subscale, however, has consistently been the most difficult to achieve adequate interrate reliability, suggesting that judges have different opinions about this important facet of the therapy process. The authors recommended using as raters for the VNIS only well-trained therapists familiar with a broad range of therapeutic practices. This solution may reduce some of the variance; but because the VNIS calls for value judgments, there is considerable room for legitimate disagreement as to what constitutes poor practice. This scale is anchored in psychodynamic concepts, and may therefore be less applicable to other types of therapy.

In a study using the Vanderbilt Therapeutic Alliance Scale, Hartley and Strupp (1983) found that the alliance ratings for patient contribution, therapist contribution, and interaction factors increased over the first few sessions for cases with positive outcomes, and decreased during the early sessions for the poorer outcome cases.

The correlations between process and outcome measures found in these and other studies give us reason to be hopeful about the possibility of empirically examining therapeutic stalemates. However, the kind of microscopic analysis that could tell us more about how they evolve, how they either do or do not become resolved, and how they affect the eventual outcome of the therapy has not been done. A promising direction was taken by Foreman and Marmar (1985) in a study of patients who showed low scores on a measure of therapeutic alliance early in therapy and higher scores later in the treatment. In each case in which the alliance had become better, the therapist had explicitly addressed the issue of the poor working relationship and explored with the patient what changes were necessary.

CONCLUSIONS AND RECOMMENDATIONS

Selection and Training of Therapists

Graduate programs in clinical psychology and psychiatric residencies rely heavily on academic rather than personal qualifications for admission. As the contribution of the therapist's personality to the process and outcome of psychotherapy becomes clearer, these programs must find ways to assess variables relevant to clinical practice. The best chance for decreasing therapist-induced difficulties lies in eliminating those applicants who are likely to be unsuitable practitioners. Even now, enough is known about potentially noxious personality characteristics to institute screening procedures for such traits as sadism, exploitativeness, and pathological narcissism.

In addition to screening applicants, training directors can make sure that their curricula include both didactic and experiential components that teach students to assess areas of vulnerability, such as fragile ego organization in their patients, and to intervene appropriately. The importance of determining the patient's status prior to beginning treatment cannot be overemphasized.

Implications for Clinical Practice

Therapists should be willing and able to recognize impending and actual impasses in their practices and to assess the relative contributions of the patient's dynamics, their own possible errors or lack of adequate training, the need of the patient for a different therapeutic approach, and the interaction of the patient with family or significant other people in the environment. The occurrence of persistent dissatisfaction must be regarded as a signal that something is seriously amiss in the patient–therapist relationship.

Therapists can also act to *prevent* impasses through awareness of their personalities, their interpersonal impact, and the influence these factors have on their approach to therapy. A therapist who expresses chronic anger through aggressive interpretations or attacks on defenses, or who fosters dependency to gratify his/her own needs, or who enjoys a sense of omnipotent power by manipulating patients is likely to produce many negative results.

In addition to such self-awareness, therapists can minimize stalemates by assessing not only the patient's personality resources for the therapy undertaken, but also by assessing how realistic and achievable the patient's goals are. Impasses associated with mismatches could be reduced, and the therapist could correct any misapprehensions or misperceptions about therapy the patient might have.

In addition to increased use of such diagnostic techniques as psychological testing and structured interviews, the use of more experienced and skilled therapists in the initial assessment process seems warranted. Unfortunately, the therapists who are least capable of handling high-risk cases are also those most likely to underestimate the severity of patient psychopathology and the degree of immediate psychological distress (Beutler, 1983). Using more expert diagnosticians initially might also help avoid the formidable problems associated with transferring patients with borderline disorders, or other high-risk patients, after a relationship is established.

Therapists who treat difficult patients successfully are not superhuman, and do respond in natural human ways to the stresses of consistently being in emotional struggles with other people and of dealing with professional frustrations. Ongoing consultation, supervision, or discussion with peers is the best antidote to therapist burnout. Antitherapeutic behaviors and attitudes are relatively easy to identify, even by relatively inexperienced clinicians, such as clinical psychology graduate students (Sachs, 1983). Therapists are often reluctant to admit angry, sexual, or dependent feelings to colleagues for fear of being seen as unprofessional; but consultation can be invaluable in sorting out the sources of such feelings and putting them in perspective.

Recommendations for Patients

It is hard for a patient to evaluate whether feelings of frustration and hostility or a sense of neediness and dependency toward a therapist are based in their past experience with other people or arise from therapeutic mismanagement. Even the most positive therapy experience is likely to include periods when the emotional intensity is subjectively experienced as nearly unbearable. Patients are well advised to have realistic expectations for the work and stress inherent in most psychotherapies, to select a therapist whose approach is compatible with their goals and values, to clarify the working contract with the therapist, to explore fully any strong negative feelings they have about their therapy or therapist, and to seek a consultation if talking with the therapist does not seem to help. Some relatively knowledgeable or naturally assertive patients may come to therapy already capable of accomplishing all the tasks on this list; but most patients, particularly in public or institutional settings, will need to be specifically advised and encouraged to act on their own behalf and to pursue actively the best possible treatment for themselves.

Research Directions

The study of therapeutic impasses is an integral part of the study of the process and outcome of psychotherapy more generally. Much has been written about the concept of negative outcome in psychotherapy. Little has been done to allow adequate examination of negative outcomes, and even less to explore the process by which these negative outcomes were produced. While some patients are worse at termination or follow-up points because of external life circumstances, it seems far more likely that seeds of such an outcome could be detected in the form of poorly handled impasses during the therapy. Kiesler (1973) stressed that any meaningful therapeutic changes must be evident within the therapy sessions themselves. This statement is as true of negative events as it is of positive changes. Even with recent advances in process research, we still lack systems of measures and data analysis procedures that would allow us to track whether or not the patient–therapist interactions occurring as difficult times in the therapy are mastered.

It is unethical to design studies in which impasses are experimentally induced, and it is unlikely that impasses induced by irresponsible clinicians will become available for scientific scrutiny. However, one excellent source of information already exists in the form of the recorded psychotherapy sessions from several major process-and-outcome studies. Patient–therapist dyads that are known to have resulted in poor outcomes should be subjected to close scrutiny in order to learn more about factors that might have led to the outcome. Cases in which there were clear struggles and temporary impasses could also be examined to tell us more about the process of overcoming such strains and successfully completing treatment.

REFERENCES

Abraham K: A particular form of neurotic resistance against the psychoanalytic method (1918), in Selected Papers. London, Hogarth Press, 1948

Appelbaum S: The Anatomy of Change: A Menninger Foundation Report Testing the Effects of Psychotherapy. New York, Plenum, 1977

Beutler L: Eclectic Psychotherapy: A Systematic Approach. Elmsford, NY, Pergamon, 1983

Blanck G, Blanck R: Beyond Ego Psychology. New York, Columbia University Press, 1986

Bordin ES: The generalizability of the psychoanalytic concept of the working alliance. Psychotherapy Theory, Research and Practice 1979; 16:252–260

Colson D: Protectiveness in borderline states: a neglected object relations paradigm. Bull Menninger Clin 1982; 46:305–320

Colson D, Lewis L, Horwitz L: Negative outcome in psychotherapy and psychoanalysis, in Negative Outcome in Psychotherapy and What To Do About It. Edited by Mays DT, Franks CM. New York, Springer, 1985

Foreman S, Marmar C: Therapist actions that address initially poor therapeutic alliances in psychotherapy. Am J Psychiatry 1985; 142:922–926

Freud S: From the history of an infantile neurosis (1918), in Complete Psychological Works, Standard Edition, Vol. 17. London, Hogarth Press, 1955

Freud S: Analysis terminable and interminable (1937), in Complete Psychological Works, Standard Edition, Vol. 23. London, Hogarth Press, 1964

Gedo J: Beyond Interpretation: Toward a Revised Theory for Psychoanalysis. New York, International Universities Press, 1979

Gedo J: Conceptual Issues in Psychoanalysis. Hillsdale, NJ, The Analytic Press, 1986

Gero G: Construction of depression. Int J Psychoanal 1936; 17:423–461

Gomes-Schwartz BA: Effective ingredients in psychotherapy: prediction of outcomes from process variables. J Consult Clin Psychol 1978; 46:1023–1035

Gorney J: The negative therapeutic interaction. Contemporary Psychoanalysis 1979; 15:288–337

Greenson R: The Technique and Practice of Psychoanalysis. New York, International Universities Press, 1967

Gunderson JG: Characteristics of borderlines, in Borderline Personality Disorders: The Concept, the Syndrome, the Patient. Edited by Hartocolis P. New York, International Universities Press, 1977

Gurman AS, Kniskern DP: Deterioration in marital and family therapy: empirical, clinical and conceptual issues. Fam Process 1978; 17:3–20

Hartley D: The therapeutic alliance in psychotherapy research, in American Psychiatric Association Annual Review, vol 4. Edited by Hales RE, Frances AJ. Washington, DC, American Psychiatric Press, Inc., 1985

Hartley D, Strupp HH: The therapeutic alliance: its relationship to outcome in brief psychotherapy, in Empirical Studies of Psychoanalytical Theories, vol I. Edited by Masling J. Hillsdale, NJ, Analytic Press, 1983

Horwitz L: Clinical Prediction in Psychotherapy. New York, Jason Aronson, 1974

Kernberg O: Severe Personality Disorders. New Haven, Yale University Press, 1986

Kiesler D: The Process of Psychotherapy. New York, Plenum, 1973

Kohut H: The two analyses of Mr. Z. Int J Psychoanal 1979; 60:3–27

Langs R: Psychotherapy: A Basic Text. New York, Jason Aronson, 1982

Lerner S, Lerner SE: A systemic approach to resistance: theoretical and technical considerations. Am J Psychotherapy 1983; 37:387–399

Loewald HW: Freud's conception of the negative therapeutic reaction with comments on instinct theory. J Am Psychoanal Assoc 1972; 20:235–245

Maltas CP: Therapeutic uses of psychological testing of borderline adolescents. J Adolesc 1978; 1:259–272

Mays DT, Franks CM: Negative Outcome in Psychotherapy and What To Do About It. New York, Springer, 1985

Mitchell KM, Bozarth JD, Krauft CC: A reappraisal of the therapeutic effectiveness of accurate empathy, nonpossessive warmth and genuineness, in Effective Psychotherapy: A Handbook of Research. Edited by Gurman AS, Rasdin AM. New York, Pergamon, 1977

Modell A: The origin of certain forms of pre-oedipal guilt and the implications for a psychoanalytic theory of affects. Int J Psychoanal 1971; 52:337–346

Orlinsky DE, Howard KI: Process and outcome in psychotherapy, in Handbook of Psychotherapy and Behavior Change, 3rd Ed. Edited by Garfield SL, Bergin AE. New York, Wiley, 1986

Paolino TJ: Psychoanalytic Psychotherapy: Theory, Technique, Therapeutic Relationship and Treatability. New York, Brunner/Mazel, 1981

Parkin A: On masochistic enthrallment: a contribution to the study of moral masochism. Int J Psychoanal 1980; 61:307–314

Reich W: Character Analysis. New York, Orgone Institute Press, 1933

Riviere J: A contribution to the analysis of the negative therapeutic reaction. Int J Psychoanal 1936; 17:304–320

Rosenfeld H: Negative therapeutic reaction, in Tactics and Techniques in Psychoanalytic Theory, vol. II: Countertransference. Edited by Giovacchini P. New York, Jason Aronson, 1975

Sachs J: Negative factors in brief psychotherapy: an empirical assessment. J Consult Clin Psychol 1983; 51:557–564

Stolorow RD, Brandchaft B, Atwood GE: Intersubjectivity in psychoanalytic treatment: with special reference to archaic states. Bull Menninger Clin 1983; 47:117–128

Strupp HH: Success and failure in time-limited psychotherapy: a systematic comparison of two cases (comparison 1). Arch Gen Psychiatry 1980a; 37:595–603

Strupp HH: Success and failure in time-limited psychotherapy: a systematic comparison of two cases (comparison 2). Arch Gen Psychiatry 1980b; 37:831–841

Strupp HH: Success and failure in time-limited psychotherapy: further evidence (comparison 4). Arch Gen Psychiatry 1980; 37:947–954

Strupp HH, Hadley SW, Gomes-Schwartz B: Psychotherapy for Better or Worse: The Problem of Negative Effects. New York, Jason Aronson, 1977

Suh CS, O'Malley SS: The identification of facilitative therapist factors: methodological considerations and research findings of a study. Paper presented at the Society for Psychotherapy Research, Smugglers Notch, VT, 1982

Suh CS, Strupp HH, O'Malley SS: The Vanderbilt process measures: the psychotherapy process scale (VPPS) and the negative indicators scale (VNIS), in The Psychotherapeutic Process. Edited by Greenberg L, Pinsof W. New York, Guilford, 1986

Sullivan HS: The Interpersonal Theory of Psychiatry. New York, Norton, 1953

Voth HM, Orth MH: Psychotherapy and the Role of the Environment. New York, Behavioral Press, 1973

Weiner MF: The Psychotherapeutic Impasse. New York, The Free Press, 1982

Wong N: Perspectives on the difficult patient. Bull Menninger Clin 1983; 47:99–106

Afterword to Section V

by William H. Sledge, M.D.

There are several general themes that are repeated in these chapters on difficult situations in clinical practice. These are the roles of technical knowledge, self-awareness, clarity concerning accountability and responsibility, and the role of professional peer relations.

TECHNICAL KNOWLEDGE

There are many gaps in our knowledge about psychiatric practice; furthermore, the means–ends relationships among technical knowledge, skill, and effort and outcome are ambiguous. Nevertheless, the continuing acquisition of new knowledge and the development and reassessment of skills is essential in avoiding serious problematic consequences that may arise from the inevitable difficulties of psychiatric practice. In addition to the acquisition of technical knowledge, the continued study of developments in the field has a salutary effect on reducing the isolation that can become associated with solo psychiatric practice.

SELF-KNOWLEDGE

A clear and enduring idea of oneself as a practitioner, including awareness of the personal motivations for pursuing the work, are essential guides through the difficulties of psychiatric practice. Furthermore, self-knowledge reduces the potential for inappropriate feelings of guilt by helping the clinician establish clear, realistic expectations. An ability to perceive accurately social reality is essential to personal success in the conduct of psychiatric practice. While it is no longer fashionable to require intensive psychotherapy or psychoanalysis for all psychiatrists, a "didactic" psychoanalysis or psychotherapy for practitioners of intensive clinical work still is an important adjunct to professional development. If character is destiny, character need not be vulnerability as a practitioner.

RESPONSIBILITY AND ACCOUNTABILITY

There are forces within modern medical practice that are shifting the focus of responsibility and accountability from the interaction between doctor and patient toward an institutional definition of responsibility. Under such conditions it is inevitable that regulatory and other bureaucratic entities will become involved in the commerce between doctors and patients. The rules of accountability are changing as institutions become more involved. In most instances these changes do not alter the fundamental nature of the doctor–patient relationship for the provision of most psychiatric services; however, when there are influences on the doctor–patient relationship (such as the peer review of a prolonged treatment by a third party) the practitioner needs to be fully aware of the social realities of accountability and responsibility.

THE ROLE OF PEERS

In these complex times, relationships with peers are all the more important, especially in the practice of psychiatry. Peers assist in reducing the potential for professional isolation and can provide an alternative view of difficult situations.

One aspect of the perception of social reality is the pitfall of coming to see oneself as indispensable in the patient's care and well-being. Working intimately and closely with others can lead to a feeling of the specialness of the relationship (as indeed it is) with a related feeling of its uniqueness (which, probably, it is not). The practitioner may come to overvalue his or her role along grandiose lines. Regular, candid discussion with peers about these matters can reduce tendencies in this direction and assist the practitioner in avoiding hubris.

Peers help one to know oneself. The gentle confrontation that comes naturally with familiarity and respect in the context of a collegial work group serves the purpose of increasing self-knowledge.

CONCLUSION

While psychiatric practice clearly is filled with many potential difficulties, there are strategies available to master and prevail over them. Self-knowledge, honest professional peer relationships, and continued efforts to inform and to remain informed are the cornerstones to coping effectively with whatever problems may come with time.

Afterword

Afterword

by Allan Tasman, M.D., Robert E. Hales, M.D., and
Allen J. Frances, M.D.

We hope that you have found the time spent with this lengthy and challenging volume rewarding. While the amount of material precludes being able to absorb it all in one reading, we feel confident that there is much here which can be directly applied to daily practice. The tremendous advances in the knowledge base of psychiatry and its applications to clinical practice are reflected in the wealth of information included here, and the persistent reader will be rewarded by frequent returns to these pages. We hope that our efforts have been of assistance to you in the difficult task of keeping up to date.

Volume 9 of the *Review of Psychiatry* is already in the initial stages of preparation. A new editorial leadership consisting of Allan Tasman, M.D., Stephen M. Goldfinger, M.D., and Charles Kaufmann, M.D., will be working to uphold the high standards of the series. Robert M. Post, M.D., will be editing a section on treatment of refractory mood disorders; Stephen M. Goldfinger, M.D., and Carolyn B. Robinowitz, M.D., will be coediting a section on AIDS and its applications to psychiatry; Charles A. Shamoian, M.D., Ph.D., will edit a section on geriatric psychiatry; Robert E. Hales, M.D., returns in a new role as a section editor with Troy L. Thompson II, M.D., for an update on psychiatric consultation to special populations; and Jerald Kay, M.D., will be editing a section on the applications of psychoanalytic work in self psychology to psychotherapy practice. We are confident that we have an outstanding volume planned and look forward to being with you in these pages again next year.

Index

AA, *see* Alcoholics Anonymous
AAPAA, *see* American Academy of
   Psychiatrists in Alcoholism and
   Addictions
Abandonment
   BPD issues with, 50, 54-60
   depression, 52
   fears, chronic, 12, 26, 50, 54-60
Abstinence, from alcohol, 273, 275, 276,
   278-280, 294, 326
   complete, need for, 306, 346, 347, 350
   early, levels of impairment, 335
   inability to abstain, 296, 304
   rates, 343
   riboflavin for, 368, 374
   syndrome, 277, 279, 368, 374
   violation effect, 281
Abstractions, alcohol-related impairment,
   284
Abuses, psychiatric, 385
   See also Alcohol abuse; Child abuse;
      Countertransference; Sexual abuse;
      Substance abuse
Acceptance, of BPD patient, 91
Accountability, therapist's, 515-517
   clarity concerning, 609-610
Acetaldehyde syndrome, 367
ACoAs, *see* Children, of alcoholics
Acquired immunodeficiency syndrome
   (AIDS) and alcoholism, 342, 344, 355
   exposure of children to, 471
Acting-out behaviors, 12, 17, 62, 305
   blocking, 50
   of primitive conflicts, 51
   in retarded adolescents, 231
   self-destructive, 11-13, 17, 18, 50, 55,
      59-62, 96-97
Action
   disorders, 37, 39, 44
   and feeling, connections between, 50,
      55
Activated countertransference, 523-528
Active-passivity, versus apparently
   competent person, 88-89
Actus reus, 451-452
Adaptation
   brain system processes for response to
      stimulation, 303, 316
   to unexpected external stimuli, LC
      system, 316
Addiction
   cocaine, 280
   opioid, 280, 319, 344, 347
   power theory of, 285
   psychodynamic theories of, 283
   relationship to other psychopathology,
      281-282
   self-help approaches to, 341-343,
      347-350, 353-354

societally created, 285
   therapists, researchers, and the AA
      community, 270, 342, 344, 354, 355
   withdrawal from, 319
   See also Alcoholism
Addiction Severity Index (ASI), 334
ADHD, *see* Attention-deficit hyperactivity
   disorder
Adler, G., 26, 44, 53, 55, 58, 59
Adolescents, psychiatry with, 132-262
   ADHD outcome, 145
   alcohol abuse and criminality, onset,
      301
   anxiety disorders in, 132, 162-176
   BPD in, 28, 61, 71-72, 104
   in combat, PTSD, 169-170
   conduct disorders in, 132-133, 180-192
   family intervention techniques, 256
   independence and autonomy, 575
   lithium resistance in, 212
   mood disorders in, 133, 197-213
   overanxious disorder in, 163-164
   pedophilic, 475
   personality deviance in mentally
      retarded, 231
   recurrence of separation/individuation
      dilemma, 26
   schizophrenic disorders in, 133, 242-257
   waiver to adult courts, 390, 478, 485
   See also Age; Children
Adoptability, 469
Adoption, and BPD life course, 117-118
Advocacy, mental health, needs-oriented
   rather than rights-oriented, 387
Affect
   blunting of, 252
   instability, 11
   intense, accompanying schema
      triggering, 87
   intolerance of, 549-550
   and mood, relationship between, 197
   negative family climate, 256
Affection, parental, consistent, 186
Affective contact, biologic, inability to
   form, 243
Affective disorders
   biogenetic overlap with BPD, 123
   and conduct disorders, 188
   genetic link to BPD, 33, 36
Affective dyscontrol, 19
Affective dysregulation, 44, 96, 98, 109,
   284, 350
   alcohol for self-medication of, 286
   and BPD, 19, 20, 27, 88
Age
   aggression by, 191
   behaviors normal for, 219
   BPD prevalence by, 9
   of onset, 164-165, 242, 243, 246, 294-296,
      305-306

Art
  talent in, effect on BPD outcome, 112,
    118, 119
  therapy, 256
ASI, see Addiction Severity Index
Assault, preventing, 558-561
Assessment, behavioral, 89
Assessment instruments
  ADHD, 146-149
  for alcoholic comorbidity, 333-334
  for BPD, 14-16
  for conduct disorders, 180, 186
  IQ and adaptive functioning, 226
  nonverbal techniques, for mentally
    retarded persons, 231-234
  standardized to cultural background,
    221, 226
  and therapeutic impasse, 596, 603, 605
Assumptions, cognitive, underlying, 86,
  93
Attention
  control, difficulties in, 88
  disordered, 246, 249-250
  getting BPD patient's, 92
  to suicidal behaviors, 96-97
Attention deficit disorder, 134-138, 141
  BPD as effect of, 71, 77
Attention-deficit hyperactivity disorder
    (ADHD), 132, 134-154
  cognitive deficits in girls, 139, 141
  core features of the disorder, 135,
    137-138
  epidemiology, 141-145
  family genetic factors, 142
  gender effects, 139, 141
  history of classification, 134-139
  and maternal smoking during
    pregnancy, 144
  and mental retardation, 141
  methylphenidate for, 149-151
  natural history and outcome, 145-146
  neurophysiology and -chemistry,
    143-144
  related disorders, 132, 139-141, 187-188,
    198, 297
  soft signs, 139
  stimulant medication, and tics or
    Tourette's syndrome, 140
  treatment, 149-154
  under- and overarousal, 143
Attention Span Task (AST), 249, 250
Attractiveness, in females, effect on BPD
    outcome, 112, 118, 119
Attributions
  internal, stable, and global, 205
  retraining, 212
Australia, conduct disorder rate, 183
Authority
  defiance of, 180, 181

lack of trust in, 346
provocative opposition to, 188
Autism, 245-246, 251, 252
  and fragile-X syndrome, 228
  infantile, 234, 242, 243, 246
  outcome, 253
  residual, 234
Autonomic nervous system, high
    reactivity, disposition to, 88-89,
    248, 362
Autonomy
  creative, 575
  schemas about, 86
Autopsy, psychological, 569, 571-572
Avoidance behaviors, 91

Baby Doe case, 479
Baby M case, 479
Badness, inner, feelings of, 20, 25, 44,
  53-55, 60
Bayley Scales of Infant Development, 226
Beck Depression Inventory, 333, 334
Behavior therapy
  assessment, 89
  for BPD, 84-99
  for childhood anxiety, 174
  for childhood schizophrenia, 256-257
  for conduct disorder, 189-190
  dialectical, 84-85, 90-98
  with and without pharmacotherapy,
    98, 99
Behaviors
  acting-out, 12, 17, 50, 51, 55, 62,
    231, 305
  alcohol-seeking, 303-304
  antisocial, 180, 182, 189
  avoidance and escape, 91
  coping, 87, 96, 544-545
  destructive, 59
  exploratory appetitive, 304
  grooming, and OCD, 172
  inhibition, activation, and maintenance
    of, 303
  noncompliant, 94-95
  normal for age, 219
  parasuicidal, 84, 85, 92, 93
  parenting, 256
  pharmacological dissection, 66
  responses to stimulation, 303, 316
  self-destructive, 11-13, 17, 18, 50, 55,
    59-61, 96-97, 231, 233
  self-stimulatory, 217, 228, 231, 234, 374
  suicidal, 18, 19, 71, 77, 91, 105
  therapy-interfering, 94-95
Benzodiazepines
  for children, 174-175
  and ethanol, 311, 317-319, 362, 371-372
  paradoxical rage response, 552
  in treatment of alcohol withdrawal, 270,
    362, 364, 374

Confidentiality, of treatment, 388, 402, 403, 426, 516, 558-560
and child psychiatry, 477
Conflict
versus deficit, in etiology of BPD, 49, 51, 54
family, 32
See also Anger; Rage; Violence
Confrontation, with BPD patients, 49-54, 56, 63
of pathological splitting, 57-58
Connectedness, schemas about, 86
Consent
children's, 476-477
coerced, 413-414, 558
informed, 78, 388, 409-428, 479
Consolidation, of recovery, 55
Consultant strategy, in DBT BPD therapy, 91, 98
Consultation, with other physicians and specialists, 405, 564, 572-575, 610
Contact
affective, biologically provided, 243
erotic, 389, 404, 473, 525-526
eye, 225, 230
See also Communication; Countertransference; Sexual abuse
Containment
for difficult patients, 49, 51-54, 56
modalities, 62, 63, 557
of self-destructive acts, 61
Continuous Performance Test (CPT), 249, 250
Contraindications, in psychotherapy for BPD, 62-63, 80-81, 98
Control
cognitive and behavioral, 460
degree of, and litigation stress, 538
over drinking, loss of, 268, 273, 278, 279, 293, 296, 324, 325, 327
of emotions, 285
future outcomes, ability to, 205
loss of, meaning of, 11
physicians' difficulty in conceding, 413, 537
and sanity, 456-457
Coping, 87
with malpractice litigation, 544-545
nonsuicidal, 96
Core
deficits, in schizophrenic individuals, 246, 247, 257
features, of ADHD, 135, 137-138
issues, in professionalization of a psychiatrist, 572-577
Costs
of alcoholism treatment, 344, 347
conduct disorder treatments, 191-192
medical, 536

of programs for mentally ill, 387-388
for treatment of violent patients, 551, 557, 558
Countertransference, 389, 404, 516, 518-530
activated, 523-528
with BPD patients, 50, 51, 56-57
in custody cases, 472
defined, 518-520
eroticized, 389, 404, 525-526
hatred, 59, 60, 567, 576
managing, 529-530
negative, 514
normative, 519
versus personal limitations, 59
with physician-patients, 542
prevention, through training, 526, 529-530
and suicide, 569, 570, 576
therapist's need to believe therapeutic alliance exists, 58
during trial period, 60
turning-away, 520-523, 525
unconscious enactment, 528
with violent patients, 557-558
with VIP patient, 589-591
withdrawal-from-reality type, 56-57
Court, psychiatrist in, 461, 485-501
Craving, alcohol, 268, 273, 275, 285, 293
after priming drink, 268, 326
learning to live with, 351
and relapse, 279
self-regulatory and self-reflective abilities, 280
Crime
defined, 451-452
and type 2 alcoholism, 305
violent, aggressive, 180
See also Violence
Crises, unremitting, 80
versus inhibited grieving, 88, 89
Cruelty
to animals, 117, 181, 248
parental, 28, 31, 112, 117, 185, 390, 467-468
physical, 181
Cultural effects
on alcoholism, 267-268, 284, 285, 298-299, 328
on BPD, 9-10
See also Gender; Socioeconomic factors
Cutoff points, *DSM-III-R* BPD diagnosis, 13, 15
Cytomegalovirus, prenatal infection, 224, 226, 229

Danger, stages of response to, 209
See also Stress

on alcohol dependence, 267, 269-270, 323-324
attention deficit disorder, 134-138, 141
on BPD, 5, 8, 14, 20
on childhood depression, 198-201, 210
comorbid Axes I and II disorders in alcoholics, 282
inclusion of autism, 242, 251
Diagnostic and Statistical Manual of Mental Disorders, Third Edition, Revised (DSM-III-R)
attention-deficit hyperactivity disorder, 135-138
on conduct disorder, 181-182
cutoff point for BPD diagnosis, 13, 15
dependence syndrome construct, 278
on depression, 198-201, 210
diagnosis of alcoholism, 267, 323-329
diagnostic criteria for anxiety disorders, 162-163
diagnostic criteria for BPD, 20-21
diagnostic criteria for mental retardation, 219
diagnostic criteria for schizophrenic disorders of childhood and adolescence, 242-245
early forms of childhood psychoses, 246
SPD definition, 65
Diagnostic and Statistical Manual of Mental Disorders, Fourth Edition (DSM-IV), optimal criteria for BPD, 20-21
Dialectical behavior therapy (DBT), 84-85, 90-98
collaborative focus, 94-95
consultant strategy in, 91, 98
problem-solving strategies, 91, 95
Dialectical processes, in BPD therapy, 90-91, 94, 98
Dichotomization
in BPD, 86, 90
and collegiality, 575
and premature closure, 518
about violence, 552
Difficult patients, spectrum of, 49, 594
Disbelief, in response to suicide, 565
Discipline
parental, 28, 31, 32, 112, 117, 185, 186, 390, 467-468
therapist's, 515
Disclosure, for informed consent, 412-413
Discouragement, therapist's, 528
Disease concept, of alcoholism, 274-277
Disillusionment, with everyday imperfections of therapist, 54, 55
Distractibility, in children of schizophrenics, 249
Distress-tolerance skills, 89-90, 96, 98, 350
Disulfiram
adverse effects, 349, 350, 353, 367-369, 373

depot pellets, 369
systematic clinical trial, 270, 367-369
Divorce, and child custody, 469-470
See also Marriage
Do-not-resuscitate (DNR) orders, 413
Documentation, of significant information and decisions, 405-406, 559
Dopamine
in BPD, 42, 43
variation in rate of turnover, 304
Down's syndrome, 224, 225, 228, 234
Alzheimer's-like changes, 229, 234
congenital and acquired associated conditions, 229
and hypothyroidism, 229, 232, 234
Dreams, of death and violence, 248
Driving
while drinking, 295, 296, 328
injuries to third parties while on psychotropics, 402
reckless, 18
Drug Abuse Screening Test, 333
Drugs
abuse in BPD, 71, 77, 79
for ADHD, 149-151
adverse effects, 389, 400-402
for alcoholism, 270, 349, 350, 353, 359-375
antiandrogen, 554, 558
for child and adolescent schizophrenics, 251, 254-257
for childhood anxiety, 174-175
for childhood depression, 211
heterogeneity of BPD response to, 6, 65-66, 81
informed consent for, 424-425
involuntary treatment, 424-425, 437-442
physician abuse of, 541
precipitating decompensation in adolescents, 251
psychiatric malpractice issues, 400-402, 424-425
psychotropics, and mental retardation, 235
right to refuse, 424-425, 437-442
side effects, failure to warn of, 389, 401
social context, 80
suicide risk, 79, 92, 97, 211
DSM, DSM-II, DSM-III, DSM-III-R, DSM-IV, see Diagnostic and Statistical Manual of Mental Disorders entries
DST, *see* Dexamethasone suppression test
Durable powers of attorney, 421
Duress, offenders under, 451
Durham v. United States, 455
Durham Rule, D.C., 457
Duties
to maintain confidentiality of treatment, 388, 402, 403, 426, 477, 516, 558-560

P300, in children of alcoholics, 297-298, 304, 318
Excited countertransference, 523-528
Exercise, in treatment of alcoholics, 351
Expert witness, 390, 488, 495-497
  amicus, 488
  constraints on, 488-490
  as educator, 497
  standards for, 397
  ultimate question, 461
Explanatory models
  of alcoholism, 268, 273-289, 294-295, 324, 332
  of BPD, 50-56, 72-77, 86-92
  of childhood mood disorders, 199-207
Exploitativeness, 17, 597
Expressive psychotherapy, 49, 51-52
Extratherapeutic contacts, demands for, 59
Eye contact, disturbances in, 225, 230
Eye movements
  rapid (REM), latencies, 19, 27, 41-42, 202
  smooth pursuit (SPEM), deviant, 250

Failure
  and formation of the cognitive triad, 204
  therapeutic, 594-606
Family
  adaptability and tolerance, 145
  alcoholic, 298-303, 352-353
  with antisocial children, 190
  of childhood schizophrenic, 256
  conflict, 32
  early dynamics, and patient's right to a better life, 596
  history, and genetic tree, 225, 253, 342
  invalidating, 88
  in maintenance of depression, 206-207, 212-213
  studies, of BPD, 6, 18, 28-39, 61-62, 114-116
  systems, 206-207, 212-213, 282, 594, 599-600
  therapy, 256, 352-353
  traumatic, 61-62, 114-116, 596
Fantasies
  of death and violence, 248
  differentiating from delusions and hallucinations, 232, 242
  masochistic, 54
Fathers
  alcoholic, 286-288, 294-295, 298, 301
  of BPD patients, 28, 29, 32, 185
  child custody, 470-472
  homosexual, 471-472
  irritable, punitive, or criminal, 185
  loss, by death or divorce, 28, 185

Fatigue
  avoiding, in ADHD, 152
  and depression, in children, 198
Fears
  of abandonment, chronic, 12, 26, 50, 54-60
  of change, 87, 95, 96, 169, 243, 245, 252
  of dependence, 98
  of invasiveness (intrusiveness), in BPD, 50, 54-60
  of merger, 53, 54, 58
  of termination, 87
  of uncertainty, 294
  of violent patients, 557-558
Feelings
  and actions, connections between, 50, 55
  with BPD patient, 50, 51, 56-58, 60, 94
  likeability, of BPD patient, 60, 94, 112, 118, 119
  of others, sensitivity to, 252, 257, 262, 515, 520, 521
  therapist's, 50, 51, 56-58, 60, 94, 598, 605
  See also Countertransference; Emotions; Transference
Fetal alcohol syndrome, 229, 344
Fetal forensics, 468
Fighting, 18
  when drinking, 295, 296
  See also Anger; Conflict; Violence
Finlay v. Finlay, 467
Fire setting, 112, 117, 180, 181
Forensic psychiatric services, 389, 451-464, 485-501
  child, 390, 467-469
  clinical evaluation for court use, 459-461, 490-495
  terms of involvement, 488
Forgetfulness, 149, 169, 284, 335-336, 346
  therapist's, 520
Foster care, 390, 467-469
Fragile-X syndrome, 224, 228, 231
Friedman, Lawrence, 505
Friends
  of the court, 488
  imaginary, 232
  stability of friendships, as measure of ego strength, 61, 62
Frustration
  optimal, 54
  and self-destructive behavior, 60-61
Functional family therapy, for conduct disorders, 190
Funding, for treatment of difficult patients, 191-192, 344, 347, 387-388, 536, 551, 557, 558
Future, negative view of, 204

GABA, *see* Gamma amino-butyric acid receptor complex
Gambling, pathological, and criminal violence, 390
Gamma amino-butyric acid (GABA) receptor complex, effects of ethanol on, 269, 270, 317-318
GAP, *see* Group for the Advancement of Psychiatry
Gender
  and ADHD, 139, 141
  and alcoholism, 286, 295-299, 302-303, 305-306, 335-336
  and anxiety disorders, 164, 165, 170
  and BPD, 9, 29, 36, 112, 115, 117, 119
  and childhood schizophrenia, 247
  in conduct disorder, 183
  and depression, 208, 335-336
  divorce research, 470, 471
  –linked stereotypes, clinician's, 9-10, 513, 528
  in OCD, 171
  in separation anxiety, 170
  suicide, 117, 119
General Social Survey, 296
Generalized anxiety disorder, childhood equivalents, 162, 163, 170
Genes, brain-related, 310
  See also Family; Hereditary factors
Goals, treatment, BPD, 96
Good-faith efforts
  to discharge confidentiality duty, 403
  to treat patient appropriately, 405, 559
"Good mother" countertransference paradigm, 56-57
Gravely disabled criteria, for commitment, 435
Grief
  inhibited, versus unremitting crises, 88, 89
  professional and personal, in suicide survivor, 568-571
Groups for the Advancement of Psychiatry (GAP), "The VIP with Psychiatric Impairment," 580, 582, 590
Groups, therapy or support
  for adolescent child abuse victims, 474-475
  for alcoholics, 118-119, 341-343, 347-354
  for psychiatrists losing patients to suicide, 564
Growth, deleterious effects of stimulants on, 149
Guilt, 17, 20
  in connection to patient suicide, 564-566
  about drinking, 296
  and sickness, 455, 463-464

unconscious oedipal or preoedipal, 53, 596
Guilty but mentally ill
  alternative to insanity defense, 463-464
  legal and mental health criticisms, 464
Gunderson, J.G., 54-55, 59, 61-62
  definition of BPD, 103

Halfway house programs, 341, 347
Hallucinations
  in children, 232, 242, 252
  religious, common, 252
Haloperidol, development of school phobia on, 174
Handicaps
  multiple, 219, 223, 226, 234
  organic, in preschizophrenics, 247
  See also Mental retardation
Hangover, 328
Harm avoidance, 303
  high, 294, 304, 305
  low, 286, 295, 304
Hatred, countertransference, 59, 60, 567, 576
Hazelden Treatment Center, Minnesota, 343
Head, trauma to, 27
  and violence, 553
Helplessness deficits, 205
Hereditary factors
  in ADHD, 142
  in alcoholism, 268, 277-279, 286, 293-306
  in BPD, 5, 27-28, 33-39, 43
  in childhood depression, 202-203
  in childhood schizophrenia, 246-247
  in conduct disorder, 183-184
  in mental retardation, 224, 228
  in personality, 303
Herpes, prenatal infection, 224, 226, 229
Hinckley, John, debate over trial, 389, 457, 463, 485
Hippocampus
  ethanol effects, 316-317
  P300 ERPs, 297-298
Hispanics, sex-bias hypothesis, BPD, 9-10
History taking, family and genetic, 253
  when diagnosing alcoholism, 342
  establishing mental retardation, 225
Holding environment, for difficult patients, 49, 51-54, 56, 59
Holding introjects, 53, 54, 56, 59
Homeless, mentally ill, 386, 434, 442
Homework, DBT, 94-95
Homosexuality
  and alcoholism, 342
  and BPD, 112, 117
  and child custody, 471-473
Hope, despite slow progress, 98
Hormonal treatment, for sexual violence, 554

Hospitalization
  of BPD patients, 61-62
  conjoint marital, for alcoholism, 352
  involuntary, 386, 433-437
  as response to suicide risk, 97
  security or forensic, 461-462
Hostility, 44, 115
Husbands, motherly, 107
Hybrid model, of alcoholism, 286-288
Hyperactive child syndrome, 134, 141, 297
Hyperactivity, See Attention-deficit
    hyperactivity disorder
Hypnosis, 493
Hypochondriasis, in BPD, 14
Hypoglycemia, and violence, 553
Hypothyroidism, and Down's syndrome,
    229, 232, 234
Hypotonia, in young childhood
    schizophrenics, 252, 253
Hysteria
  dysphoric, 27
  in parents of hyperactive child, 142
  primitive oral, 65

Iatrogenic injury, see Malpractice
ICD-9-CM, see International Classification of
    Diseases, Ninth Revision, Clinical
    Modification
Identification
  with the aggressor, 59
  with patients, 515
  projective, 56, 58, 520
Identity
  in the alcoholic, 350
  in BPD, 10-12, 19, 71, 85
  defined, 86
  development of, 88
  disturbance, 10-12, 19, 71, 85, 105,
    251-350
  as tied to relationships, 90
  weak or unstable sense of, 86
Immune system
  regulation by neuronal events, 311
  stressful life events, 277, 535, 538
Impasse, therapeutic, 594-606
  positive aspects, 602
Impulse disorders, 37, 39, 44, 45
Impulsivity, 88, 135
  and anxiety or mood disorders in
    children, 140
  and BPD, 11-12, 18, 71
  control of, 96
  as dimension cutting across diagnostic
    categories, 17
  medication strategies against, 77
Inattentiveness, and anxiety or mood
    disorders in children, 140
  See also Attention

Incest victims, 390, 462-468, 473-475
  BPD, 112-113, 117, 119
Incompleteness, issues of, 53
Inconsistency, comfort with, 91
Indications, for psychotherapy in BPD,
    62-63, 80-81, 98
Individuation, problems in, 350
Indolamine, cortical, disturbance in
    metabolism, 27
Infantile autism, 234, 242, 243, 246
Infants
  legal, 451
  low birth weight, 223, 229
  over- or understimulation, 230
  temperament in, 184
  See also Age; Children
Infertility, increases, 469
Information processing, 249
  central executive control lack, 257
  cortical, and alcohol, 316
  impairments, 250
  neuron circuits or ensembles, 310, 311
  reception, and storage, 303, 316
Informed consent, 388, 409-428
  children's, 476-477
  coerced, 413-414, 558
  components, 412-419
  exceptions to, 419-420
  for pharmacotherapy in BPD, 78
  surrogacy, 479
Inhibited grieving syndrome, 88, 89
Injury litigation, 392-393
Inner badness, feelings of, 20, 25, 44,
    53-55, 60
  projection, 55
Insanity defense, 455-461
  disposition of acquittees, 461-463
  guilty but mentally ill alternative,
    463-464
  legal definition of insanity, 389
  psychiatric evaluation for, 459-461
  standards for determining, 456-459
Insanity Defense Reform Act of 1984, 458
Insemination, artificial, 480
Instability, affective, 11
  as dimension cutting across diagnostic
    categories, 17
Institutionalization, in the mid-1950s, 433
Insurance, 531-532
  medical malpractice, 392
Integration
  of addiction treatment approaches, 270,
    342, 344, 346-351, 353-355
  biopsychosocial framework for
    understanding violence, 552
  biopsychosocial models of alcoholism,
    268, 276-279, 285-288, 342
  developmentally oriented
    biopsychosocial model of childhood
    disorders, 199, 262

of libidinal and aggressive self and
  object representations, 51
neuroscientific data avalanche, 268-269,
  310-311
of patterning, within CNS functioning,
  243
pharmacotherapy with BPD, 81
of research explosion with clinical work,
  5, 268-269, 310-311
of responses to stimulation, 303, 316
unifying hypothesis of ethanol actions,
  319
Intelligence quota (IQ), 217-221, 226, 231
  and BPD, 112, 118, 119
  and perinatal stress, 144
  prognostic significance, 253
  verbal, 250, 257
Interdependence, versus independence,
  98
International Classification of Diseases,
  Ninth Revision, Clinical Modification
  (ICD-9-CM), 278
  alcohol dependence syndrome, 267
International Pilot Study of Schizophrenia
  (IPSS), 104, 106
Interpersonal skills, 89, 190
  See also Relationships, interpersonal
Interpretation, with difficult patients,
  49-54, 56
Intimacy
  capacity for, 62
  renunciation, for stability, by BPDs, 119
Intoxication, alcohol, 269, 310
  drinking to, frontier style, 285
  GABAergic mechanisms, 317-318
  sequence of cellular events, 312, 318
  subjective feelings of, 297
  treatment of, 359-361
Introjects, holding and soothing, 53,
  54, 56, 59
  introjective failure in BPD, 26
Intrusiveness/invasiveness, BPD fears
  of, 50, 54-60
Invalidation, versus emotional
  vulnerability, 88
IPSS, *see* International Pilot Study of
  Schizophrenia
Irreverent-communication strategies, 91
Irritability, parental, 185

Jealousy, pathological, in paranoid
  borderline, 115
Jellinek, E.M., 268, 274, 281, 284, 286
Juvenile rights, 477-478

Kaimowitz v. Michigan Department of Mental
  Health, 413
Kernberg, Dr. Otto F., 5, 8, 14-15, 25-26,
  44, 50-53, 56-57, 59, 62

Lability, affective, in BPD, 11, 87, 88
Labor, difficult, 225, 229
Lake v. Cameron, 432
Language
  deficits, in girls, 139, 141
  disorders, severe, 243
  therapy, 256
Lanterman–Petris–Short Act, 385, 433
Latent schizophrenia, 65
Law, psychiatry and, 385-505
  child-related, 467-480
LC, *see* Locus coeruleus
Lead
  and ADHD, 140, 144
  toxicity, 229, 230
Learned-helplessness theory, of
  depression, 205-206, 212
Learning
  deleterious effects of stimulants on, 149
  disabilities, 27, 71, 77, 134, 229, 553
Least-restrictive alternative doctrine,
  386, 432
Liability, 531
  limitations on, 396
Life events, stressful, 277, 311, 535, 538
Life style, and alcoholism, 342, 351
Likeability, of BPD patient, 60, 94, 112,
  118, 119
Limbic system
  abnormal regulation, 39-40
  reactivity, 27-28, 88
Limitation, statutes of, 396
  for sexual abuse, 468
Limits
  for ADHD child, 152
  for BPD patient, 50, 54-60, 62-63,
  80-81, 98
  flexible and compassionate, 97
  setting, 50, 54-60
  therapist's, 59, 95
  to treatment continuation, after
  alcoholic relapses, 350
Lipid-focused hypothesis, of physical
  dependence on alcohol, 269, 309, 312
Literacy, and nonverbal techniques for
  psychiatric assessment, 231-234, 422
Lithium carbonate, for BPD, 71-72
Litigation, 392-406, 531-546
  malpractice, coping with, 538-539,
  544-545
  process, 540
Liver
  disorder, 296
  end-stage pathology, from alcohol, 274
Living with Children, 153
Living wills, 421
Locus coeruleus (LC)
  activity in alcohol withdrawal, 270

adaptation to unexpected external
stimuli, 303, 316
alcohol effects, 315-316, 319
Loneliness, in BPD, 53-54, 57, 71
chronic, with impulsivity and/or
unstable relationships, 12
Loss
of control, see Control
depressive reactions to, 305
parental, 28-29
repetitive, 89
stages of response to, 209
See also Grief; Suicide
Love object, ambivalence toward, 203
L-tryptophan, for very regressed
schizophrenic and severely mentally
retarded, 554
Luck, and BPD, 118-119
Lying, by children or adolescents, 180,
181

Magical thinking, 225, 253, 516
in BPD, 115
Magnesium, binding, and ethanol, 313
Mahler, M., 26, 52-53
Mainstreaming, retarded children, 218,
231
Major depressive disorder
comorbidity with BPD, 18
in sued physicians, 534
Maldevelopment, in BPD, 43
Male-limited alcoholism, 286-288, 294-295
Malice, 453, 561
countertransference, toward suicidal
patient, 576
true, and rebelliousness, spectrum
between, 115-116
Malnutrition, fetal, 229
Malory Weiss syndrome, 349
Malpractice, defined, 394
Malpractice, medical
associated stress, 531-546
coping strategies, 538-539, 544-545
countertransference, 542
emotional and physical reactions,
534-535
Malpractice, psychiatric, 388-389, 392-406
frequency and severity of claims,
392-395
in prescribing medication, 400-402
prevention, 405-406
proof, 394-396
suicide and parasuicide issues, 398-400
Management, of countertransference
difficulties, 529-530
See also Treatment
Mania, and schizophrenia, differentiating,
251
Manipulation, 17, 44, 597

Markers
alcoholism, 268, 279, 296-297
BPD, 6
depressive state, 202
neurodevelopmental pathology, 71, 77
of vulnerability to schizophrenia,
246-247, 249, 250
Marriage
alcoholic, 343, 352
child custody questions, 390, 467,
469-472
conflict in, 29, 32, 207
demeaning attitudes, rejection, 32
therapist's, 525, 527-528
tightly bonded, excluding attention,
support, or protection of children, 29
Masochism, 25, 54, 595, 596
Masterson, J., 26, 52-53, 55, 57-58
MCMI-II, see Millon Clinical Multiaxial
Inventory-II
Melancholia, triggered by carbamazepine,
71
Membranes, fluidity of, and ethanol, 269,
309, 312, 360-361
Memory
deleterious effects of stimulants on, 149
evocative, 26, 44, 53, 59
problems, alcoholic, 284, 335-336, 346
verbal and behavioral, relation to age,
169
Mens rea, 451-452, 455, 457
Menstrual cycle, violence related to, 554
Mental disorders, in retarded children,
218, 231-235
Mental health law reform, 385-390
first wave, 385, 386
right to treatment, 386-387
Mental retardation, in children and
adolescents, 133, 217-236
acquired childhood diseases, 224, 229
and ADHD, 141
associated handicaps, 219, 223, 226
as CNS dysfunction, 221-224
concept and definition, 219-221
concerns about sexuality, 231
early alterations of embryonic
development, 224, 226, 229
environmental and behavioral
diagnostic group, 224, 230
etiologic diagnosis, 223-226
hereditary disorders, 224, 226-228
management of mental disorders in,
234-235
mood disorders in, 233-234
normalization of, 218, 231
perinatal factors, 221-226, 229
personality development in, 230-231
pervasive developmental disorders
in, 234
psychiatric diagnosis, 232

Proteins, within neuronal membranes, alcohol effects, 312-313
Protracted abstinence syndrome, in detoxified alcoholics, 277, 279
Pseudomemories, 493
Pseudoneurotic schizophrenia, 65, 104
Pseudoreality, and pseudoidentity, in BPD, 56
Psychiatrists
    in court, 389, 461, 485-501
    ethical responsibilities as physicians, 389
    as patients, 542
    stressful situations, 513-610
    suicide rates, 541-542
    See also Therapists
Psychiatry, forensic, 389, 390, 451-464, 467-469, 479-480, 485-501
Psychodynamic therapy, indications for, 350
Psychological autopsy, 569, 571-572
Psychopharmacology, pediatric, rating scales and assessment instruments, 148
Psychosocial principal, of alcoholism, 284-285
Psychosomatic illness, 311, 535, 538
Psychotherapy
    for childhood schizophrenia, 255-257
    for conduct disorder, 189-190
    emotional environment of, 56
    supportive/suppressive versus exploratory/expressive, 6, 49, 51-54, 59-60, 62, 255-256
    trial, with BPD, 59-60, 96
Psychotic disorders, in mentally retarded, 233
Public Law 94-142, 219, 230
Public Law 99-457 of 1987, 219

Queen Victoria, influence on evolution of insanity defense, 457, 463

Race
    and alcoholism, by subtype, 297
    BPD prevalence by, 9-10
Rage, 50
    in BPD, 71
    paradoxical, in response to benzodiazepines, 552
    patient's, therapist and patient surviving, 53
    See also Anger; Hatred; Violence
Rape
    BPD outcome in victims, 112
    coercive paraphilic, 390
Rapid eye movement (REM) latency
    in BPD, 19, 27, 41-42
    in children, 202

Rapprochement, separation/individuation subphase, 26, 43, 52-53
Reading, deficits, 182
Reality testing, by BPD patient, 50, 51, 55-56
Rebelliousness, and true malice, spectrum between, 115-116
Receptors, ethanol, 269
Record keeping
    of decision to warn, 559
    psychiatric, inadequate, 405-406
Recovery
    from addiction, long-lasting, 348
    consolidation of, in BPD, 55
    from impact of suicide, 568, 571
    See also Remission
Reenactment, post-traumatic, 163, 169, 473
Rehabilitation, alcoholic, 341, 346-347, 365-374
Relapse, alcoholic, 327, 344, 350
    precipitants, 332
    prevention, 351, 375
    processes leading to, 276, 279-281
    maintaining progress after, 351
Relationship strategies, in DBT, 91, 94, 97-98
Relationships, interpersonal and intrafamilial, 284
    cognitive problem-solving deficits, 257
    gross impairment in, 243, 245
    identity as tied to, 90
    maladaptive behaviors, 190
    pathological, in BPD, 61-62, 80, 97-98
    patient–therapist, 49, 59, 405, 597-598, 605
    skills, 96, 97, 98, 190
    social disinhibition, in children, 138
    stable friendships, 88
    therapist's, with peers, 564, 572-575, 610
    unstable–intense, 11-13
    unusual demandingness, 14
Relief, at suicide, 567
Relocation syndrome, in mentally retarded, 233
Remission, from alcoholism, 275, 278, 324, 329, 348
Reparenting, BPD, 61, 97
Rescue, pathological countertransference, 56
Resistance, 594
Responsibility
    criminal, 389, 452-464, 485
    exaggerated sense of, 536
    for patients with severe and dangerous conditions, 515-517
    professional, development of, 572-574, 576-577
    therapist's, clarity concerning, 609-610

Revictimization, 473
Reward dependence, 303
  high, 294, 304, 305
  low, 286, 304
Riboflavin, and alcoholic abstinence,
    368, 374
Rights
  concerning pregnancy, 478-480
  to die, 432
  Fifth Amendment, 460-461
  juvenile, 477-478
  to life, 479
  to psychiatric assistance on criminal
    justice issues, 485
  to refuse treatment, 387, 388, 419-421,
    423, 437-442
  retarded patient's, 217-219, 230-232,
    234-235
  Sixth Amendment, 460-461, 476, 485
  to treatment, 386-387
  women's, 478
Rinsley, D., 26, 52-53, 62
Risk
  and consequences, anticipating, 284
  factors, for developing alcoholism,
    282-283, 296-305
  taking, 295
Rite of passage, suicide survival as,
    564, 568
Roe v. Wade, 479
Rogers Criminal Responsibility
    Assessment Scales, 460
Rubella, prenatal infection, 224, 226, 229
Running away, 18
Rush, Dr. Benjamin, 268, 273, 409

Sadism, 595
  identification with the aggressor, 59
Safety, protecting self, staff, and third
    parties from violent patients, 558-561
Sameness, desire for, 243, 245, 252
Scapegoating, 573, 589, 591
Schedule, treatment, compliance with,
    57-59, 94-97
Schemas, cognitive
  dysfunctional, in BPD, 86, 87
  states of mind, 90
Schizophrenia
  activity level and muscle tone, 252, 253
  adolescent-onset, 251-253
  adult-onset, 242
  age of onset, 242, 243, 246, 250, 252,
    253
  childhood, 133, 242-257
  core symptoms, 246, 247, 252, 253, 257
  follow-back studies, 247
  inherited predisposition, 246-247
  lack of central executive control
    functions, 257

and mania, differentiating, 251
  parental, 248-250
  vulnerability markers, 246-247, 249, 250
Schizotypal borderline, 65
Schizotypal personality disorder (SPD),
    42, 248
  and BPD, 12, 16, 17, 38, 44, 115
  DSM-III-R definition, 65
  long-term outcome, Chestnut Lodge
    patients, 110
School
  phobia, 164, 166, 174
  problems, serious, 145-146
  refusal, 163, 170, 174
Searles, H.F., 55-56
Seduction, vulnerability to, 525-526
Seizure disorders, BPD as effect of, 71, 77
Self, sense of
  failure to internalize, 26
  false, 58
  shifting, 105
Self-absorption, 17
Self-awareness, therapist's, and difficult
    situations, 609
Self-care
  in alcoholics, 350
  individual, 98
Self-control model, of depression, 206, 212
Self-destructive behaviors, 11-13, 17, 18,
    55, 59
  in BPD, managing, 60-61, 96-97
  clarification and confrontation, 50
  intrapsychic mechanisms related to, 60
Self-discipline, effect on BPD life course,
    118, 119
Self-esteem
  clinician's professional, 514
  lowered, in children, 197
Self-help programs, 341, 346-348,
    351-354, 375
  partnership between therapist and, 270,
    342, 344, 346-347, 353-354
Self-injurious behaviors, 11-13, 18,
    231, 233
Self-punishment, 50, 53
Self-report inventories, BPD, 15-16, 20
  See also Assessment instruments
Self-stimulation, 217, 228, 231, 234
  intracranial, 374
Sensory motor integrative therapy, 256
Sensory processing, 297
Sentimentality, 294
Separation
  alcoholic problems with, 350
  anxiety, 12, 170
  BPD issues with, 59-60
  child's reaction to, 253
  severe depressive responses to, 295, 305

psychiatric trainees, and suicide, 564
questioning stance, 58
refusal to see certain patient types, 535
selection and training, 99, 564, 598, 604
special challenges of the work, 390, 468,
    513-517
supervision/support, 99, 564, 572-575,
    604, 610
for violent patients, 557
See also Countertransference
Thiamine, for alcoholic withdrawal, 362,
    364, 365, 374
Thoughts, automatic, 86, 93
Threat
    actual/fantasied, 514
    destructive or self-destructive, 59
    to property, 403
    stages of response to, 209
    See also Violence
TIQs, *see* Tetrahydroisoquinoline
    hypothesis
Tolerance, deemphasis in *DSM-III-R*, 324,
    327-328
TORCH, prenatal infection, 224, 226, 229
Tort law, 394-397, 531
Total Justice, 505
Totem and Taboo, 575
Tourette's syndrome
    and ADHD, 140
    development of school phobia with
        haloperidol or pimozide use for, 174
    OCD in families, 171
Toxoplasmosis, prenatal infection, 224,
    226, 229
Training, therapist's, 99, 564, 598, 604
    in child forensic psychiatry, 468
Tranquilizers, for BPD, 70-71
Transference, 515
    acting out, 51
    in BPD psychotherapy, 6, 50, 51
    in the here and now, 50, 55
    selfobject, 54, 58
    and suicide, 570
    See also Countertransference
Transference–countertransference
    bind, 594
Transitional object, BPD reliance on, 26
Transmuting internalization, 54
Trauma
    childhood, 169-170, 253
    head, 27
    psychic, damages related to, 468
    severe, and BPD, 27, 114-116
    See also Child abuse; Post-traumatic
        stress disorder
Treatment
    of ADHD, 149-154
    of alcoholic comorbidity, 331-333

of alcoholism, 270, 305-306, 323,
    331-333, 341-355
of BPD, 49-63, 65-81, 84-99
of childhood schizophrenia, 254-257
clinicians' preferences for modes of, 343
conditions, and content of, 590
of conduct disorder, 180, 189-191
costs, and funding, 191-192, 344, 347,
    387-388, 536, 551, 557, 558
early phases, 596, 600
engagement in, 57-60, 77-78, 82-93
failed, sources of, 514
goals, BPD, 90-91, 96
impasses, 594-606
indications, contraindications,
    limitations, 62-63, 80-81, 98
of insanity acquittees, 462-463
involuntary, 432-447, 461-464
management of mental disorders in the
    retarded, 234-235
managing countertransference
    difficulties, 529-530
for mood disorders in children, 211-213
outpatient, 442-446, 552, 556
for patients with history of violence,
    461-464, 549-561
of prisoners, 461-464
refusal, right to, 387, 388, 479
right to, 386-387
schedule and boundaries, compliance
    with, 57-59, 94-97
of self-destructive actions, 60-61
social/family support, 61-62
of sued physicians, 539-546
of VIP patient, 582-583, 589-591
Trial by Jury, 527
Trial period, for BPD psychotherapy,
    59-60, 96
Truancy, 180, 181
    See also School
Tuberous sclerosis, 228
Turning-away countertransference,
    520-523, 525
12-Step programs, 118-119, 341-343,
    347-350, 353-354

Unconscious countertransference
    enactment, 528
Underinvolvement, parental, 29, 30, 32
Understanding, legal sense, 416-417
Uninvolvement, therapist's, 515
United States v. Byers, 461
Unrelenting-crises syndrome, 88, 89

Vacation, from therapy, 601-602
Validation, in BPD, 55
    patient's need for therapist's, 54
    strategy, DBT, 91, 93-97